CARDIOLOGY SCIENCE AND TECHNOLOGY

CARDIOLOGY SCIENCE AND TECHNOLOGY

DHANJOO N. GHISTA

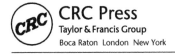

CRC Press
Taylor & Francis Group
Boca Raton London New York

CRC Press is an imprint of the
Taylor & Francis Group, an **informa** business

CRC Press
Taylor & Francis Group
6000 Broken Sound Parkway NW, Suite 300
Boca Raton, FL 33487-2742

First issued in paperback 2019

© 2016 by Taylor & Francis Group, LLC
CRC Press is an imprint of Taylor & Francis Group, an Informa business

No claim to original U.S. Government works

ISBN-13: 978-1-4200-8806-9 (hbk)
ISBN-13: 978-0-367-86424-8 (pbk)

Visit the Taylor & Francis Web site at
http://www.taylorandfrancis.com

and the CRC Press Web site at
http://www.crcpress.com

With deep gratitude, I dedicate this book to James M. Gere,
Alfred L. Erickson, and Harold Sandler.

James M. Gere, PhD, Professor Emeritus, Civil Engineering Department, Stanford University, Stanford, California, was my doctoral advisor. He was a terrific professor and a dedicated adviser. From 1960 to 1970, he was Associate Dean of the School of Engineering, and from 1967 to 1972, he served as Chairman of the Department of Civil Engineering. He cofounded the John A. Blume Earthquake Engineering Center and retired from Stanford University in 1988.

He authored outstanding textbooks, which are used in engineering courses around the world, among them being: *Theory of Elastic Stability* (with S.P. Timoshenko, McGraw-Hill 1961); *Matrix Analysis of Framed Structures* and *Matrix Algebra for Engineers* (with W. Weaver, Van Nostrand 1980); *Mechanics of Materials* (Thomson Learning 2004); *Moment Distribution* (Van Nostrand-Reinhold 1963); *Earthquake Tables* (John A. Blume Earthquake Engineering Center, 1983); *Structural and Construction Design Manual* (with H. Krawinkler); *Terra Non Firma: Understanding and Preparing for Earthquakes* (with H.C. Shah, Freeman 1984). I remember him most for his warm personality and his inspirational mentorship for my doctoral studies.

Alfred L. Erickson, Chief of Structural Dynamics Branch, NASA Ames Research Center, Mountain View, California, gave me my first appointment after I finished my PhD at Stanford University. He was a great mentor with a very endearing personality. He was the sort of research leader to whom NASA entrusted its most complicated problems. During World War II, as Lockheed encountered the problems of flutter on aircraft, Al Erickson devised techniques in the Ames 16-foot wind tunnel to measure flutter and design a solution. That led to his lifelong involvement in unsteady aerodynamics, instrumentation design, and computational methods.

In 1960, director Harvey Allen (who I also remember warmly) tasked Al Ericksen to form the structural dynamics branch to solve the structural dynamic problems in NASA's launch vehicles; Al's Structural Dynamics branch became famous for the breadth of its engineering acumen. It was indeed a pleasure to work in his branch. Every morning, he made it a point to go around and speak with every member of his team. Under his guidance, I worked on aerospace engineering problems, culminating in biomedical engineering studies of physiological problems encountered by astronauts in weightlessness. Al was indeed a wonderful leader and guide.

Harold Sandler, MD, a renowned cardiologist, pioneered aerospace medicine and its biomedical engineering in the space age at NASA Ames Research Center. From 1965 to 1987, he directed aerospace medical research on the study of physiological adaptation to varying gravity environments at NASA Ames Research Center (Mountain View, California), NASA's lead center in Space life sciences. As Chief of the Biomedical Research Branch,

Hal studied the impact of space flight on the human body, for which he devised the bedrest method for simulating the impact of weightlessness, and invented many novel biomedical instruments. Through his research on circulation in hyper- and micro-gravity, he became a world-renowned expert in aerospace cardiology.

Now, let me talk about our relationship. After I had been at Ames Research Center for a year or so, I attended his seminar in which he invited colleagues to work with him in aerospace cardiology. That started my lifelong research collaboration and partnership with him. We published our first paper "An analytic elastic-viscoelastic model for the shape and forces of the left ventricle" in the *Journal of Biomechanics* in 1969. We also coauthored (with Israel Mirsky, Harvard University) *Cardiac Mechanics*, the first book on the subject (Wiley, 1974). He gave me deep insight into the biomedical engineering of heart function, which has eventually led to this book. I wish him lots of happiness.

Contents

Section I   Left Ventricular Wall Stress, Cardiac Elastances, Cardiac Contractility Measures, Cardiomyopathic Ventricular Remodeling and its Surgical Restoration, Active Wall Stress and Systolic Pressure Generation, Vector Cardiogram Characteristics, and Their Implications in Clinical Cardiology

Section II   ECG Signal Analysis, Left Ventricular Pumping (Intra-Ventricular, Aortic and Coronary Flow) Characteristics, Coronary Bypass Surgery Design, and Their Implications in Clinical Cardiology and Cardiac Surgery

Preface

Cardiology Science and Technology comprehensively deals with the science and biomedical engineering formulations of cardiology. As a textbook, it addresses the teaching, research, and clinical aspects of cardiovascular medical engineering and computational cardiology.

The book consists of two sections. The first section deals with left ventricular (LV) wall stress, cardiac contractility, ventricular remodeling, active wall stress and systolic pressure generation, and vector cardiogram characteristics, with applications in cardiology. The second section covers ECG signal analysis for arrhythmias detection, LV pumping (intra-LV, aortic and coronary flow) characteristics, and coronary bypass surgery design, with applications in cardiology and cardiac surgery.

This book is like an exciting train ride through the heart and into blood flows within its chamber, the coronary tree, the aorta, and finally into the coronary bypass grafting.

The train starts from the central station of the heart, and we are treated to the fascinating scenery as it journeys to the stations of heart wall stresses, cardiac contractility measures to characterize heart failure, and the noninvasive contractility index formulated as the maximum value of pressure-normalized wall stress. We take a break at this novel cardiac contractility station. The train then takes us to exciting places of active stress generation and the setting up the systolic heart pressure for cardiac output. Then we are shown how the cardiomyopathic and infarcted heart undergoes remodeling with decreased contractility and its surgical ventricular restoration. Next, we get into the theory of ECG and vector cardiogram (VCG) derivation and medical applications. Finally, we reach the junction of the heart and blood flows.

At this junction, we get down and take another train. We first arrive at the ECG waveform station and study how heart rate variability signal processing is carried out to detect cardiac arrhythmias. We then travel into the heart chamber to witness the amazing intricate flow patterns that constitute the outcome of heart contractility. Then we see how pressure pulse wave propagates into the aorta and into its branches, and learn how to measure pulse wave velocity and the arterial elastic property. We then climb into the mountainous coronary tree and look at the fascinating scenery of coronary flows and myocardial perfusion that governs cardiac contractility. We then learn how to analyze intra-cardiac flow patterns from Doppler echo flow mapping. Finally, we arrive at coronary bypass grafting and can see how it has been modernized by the new sequential anastomosis (SQA) design. This is indeed a fascinating journey, and we can appreciate how it will transform cardiology and take it into the era of science, technology, engineering, mathematics (STEM).

Section I. Left Ventricular Wall Stress, Cardiac Elastances, Cardiac Contractility Measures, Cardiomyopathic Ventricular Remodeling and its Surgical Restoration, Active Wall Stress and Systolic Pressure Generation, Vector Cardiogram Characteristics, and Their Implications in Clinical Cardiology

Chapter 1. Left Ventricular Wall Stress Compendium to Analyze Heart Function

In understanding heart function and dysfunction, left ventricular wall stress is the first lesson. Wall stress develops passively in the left ventricle (LV) due to LV filling pressure in the diastolic phase. Then, LV wall stress develops actively due to LV contraction and results in intra-LV pressure development in LV systolic phase, which leads to ejection of blood into the aorta (as shown in Chapter 6). Cardiologists and physiologists have long been interested in the quantification of LV wall stress. This is because (1) wall stress is viewed as an important stimulus for the remodeling of the failing heart, (2) systolic wall stress represents a primary determinant of myocardial oxygen consumption ($M\dot{V}O_2$) in LV pressure and volume overload demands on the LV, and (3) systolic wall stress normalized with respect to LV pressure can also be employed as a noninvasive index of LV contractility (as is shown in Chapter 3), and hence as a measure of LV failure. Therefore, the level and distribution of wall stress and its cyclic variation provide a quantitative evaluation of the response and adjustment of the LV to heart disease.

This chapter deals with biomechanics analyses, analytical and computational models used to characterize LV wall stress, and clinical methods available for monitoring in vivo data to determine LV wall stress. We have provided a compendium of the major types of wall stress models: pioneering thin-wall Sandler–Dodge models based on LaPlace law, thick-wall shell models, our elasticity theory based dynamic shape models, thick-wall large deformation models, and finite element models. We have compared the mean stress values of these models and the variation of stress across the wall. All of the thin-wall and thick-wall shell models are based on idealized ellipsoidal and spherically shaped geometries. However, the elasticity model's shape throughout the cardiac cycle is adjusted to correspond to the monitored shape of the LV and approximates an ellipsoidal shape. Finite element models have more representative geometries but are more time consuming for medical application. Therefore, thick-wall shell models and the Ghista–Sandler elasticity model are better for medical applications. This chapter will enable our readers to clinically employ these LV wall stress models and to gain the understanding of how the LV copes with after-load demands and other disorders such as cardiomyopathy.

Chapter 2. Cardiac Function Assessment in Filling and Systolic Phases: Passive and Active Elastances of the Left Ventricle

In a bioengineering sense, the heart can be described as a blood pump, and its physiological behavior can be understood in terms of time-varying relationship between ventricular blood pressure and volume. In order to study LV pump function, we have developed expressions for LV passive elastance and active elastance, and have employed them to study LV pressure–volume relationship during a cardiac cycle. The passive elastance E_p governs LV stiffness variation due to volume increase during the filling phase and due to volume decrease during the ejection phase, and active elastance E_a governs LV pressure increase due to LV myocardial contraction.

In our clinical study, we have shown how (1) E_a increase (due to force development in the myocardial sarcomere) and constant E_p, during isovolumic contraction, contribute to LV pressure increase, (2) E_a increase during systolic ejection (due to sarcomere force development) and E_p decrease (due to blood volume decrease) contribute to LV pressure dynamics during ejection phase, and (3) E_a decrease and E_p increase (due to blood volume increase) contribute to pressure dynamics during filling phase. We have also shown a high degree of correlation of $E_{a,max}$ with dP/dt_{max}, which justifies the use of $E_{a,max}$ as a contractility index.

Chapter 3. Novel Cardiac Contractility Index and Ventricular-Arterial Matching Index to Serve as Markers of Heart Failure

Cardiac contractility constitutes the prime mechanism by which intra-LV pressure is increased and made available for the ejection of blood into the aorta. It is affected by myocardial perfusion from the coronary circulatory system. Traditionally, cardiac contractility has been assessed in terms of dP/dt_{max}. However, this measure of contractility is based on the outcome of contractility in generating LV pressure for blood ejection. In a way, it is an afterthought, in addition to its requiring invasive measurement of LV pressure. The LV pressure increase is caused by the generation of active wall stress due to contractile stress developed in the myocardial structural unit between the myocardial sarcomere's myosin and actin filaments. Hence, it is more appropriate to develop a measure of cardiac contractility in terms of LV systolic wall stress. We have therefore developed the formula of this new LV contractility index as the maximum rate of change of LV systolic wall stress normalized to intra-LV pressure, $d(\sigma/P)/dt_{max}$ or $d\sigma^*/dt_{max}$, where $\sigma^* = \sigma/P$. This contractility index can be determined noninvasively in terms of myocardium volume and maximum outflow rate.

In this chapter, we have provided its derivation and demonstrated (1) its good correlation with the traditional contractility index dP/dt_{max}, in patients with varying ejection fractions (EFs), and (2) its capacity to diagnose heart failure (HF) with normal EF (HFNEF, or diastolic HF) and with reduced EF (HFREF, or systolic HF). We have then studied the interaction of LV with the arterial system. For this purpose, we have formulated a ventricular-arterial matching (VAM) index, as the ratio of the contractility index and the arterial elastance. We have then employed this VAM index in patients with elevated N-terminal pro B-type natriuretic peptide (NT-proBNP), as a marker of HF. The NT-proBNP is secreted by the heart ventricles in response to excessive stretching of cardiomyocytes, and is a strong predictor of mortality among patients with acute coronary syndromes and a strong prognostic marker in patients with chronic coronary heart disease. We have been able to see a strong correlation between the VAM index and NT-proBNP. In patients with elevated NT-proBNP levels, the value of this VAM index is shown to decrease, due to impaired LV contractility (as caused by LV myocardial infarction) as well as due to elevated arterial elastance. Hence, in patients with HF (HFREF) and arteriosclerosis, requiring more contractile effort by the LV with impaired contractility, this VAM index can be employed as an effective marker of HF.

Chapter 4. Cardiomyopathy Effect on Left Ventricle Function (Shape and Contractility) and Improvement after Surgical Ventricular Restoration

Cardiomyopathy literally means heart muscle disease, involving measurable deterioration of the ability of the myocardium to contract. In cardiomyopathy, the heart muscle becomes enlarged, thick, or rigid. In rare cases, the muscle tissue in the heart is replaced with scar tissue. As cardiomyopathy worsens, the heart becomes weaker. It is less able to pump blood throughout the body and maintain a normal electrical rhythm. This can lead to arrhythmia and HF. Ischemic dilated cardiomyopathy (IDCM) is caused by coronary artery disease, i.e., myocardial infarction (MI) and heart attack. In IDCM, the heart's ability to pump blood is decreased, because the LV is enlarged, dilated, and weak.

In this chapter, we have quantified heart dysfunction caused by IDCM, by studying ten IDCM patients and ten normal subjects, using magnetic resonance imaging (MRI) and gadolinium-enhancement imaging to determine the extent of myocardial infarct. The LV shape in IDCM patients differed from those in normal subjects in several ways. First, the IDCM LVs had a more spherical shape (greater sphericity index), reduced curvedness at end-diastole and end-systole, increased peak systolic wall stress (implying increased oxygen demand) and decreased cardiac contractility (as measured by our $d\sigma^*/dt_{max}$ index). We then present our study of 40 patients who underwent surgical ventricular restoration (SVR) for restoring LV function. Following SVR, it is noted that (1) the LV end-diastolic and end-systolic volume indices were significantly reduced from 156 ± 39 to 110 ± 33 and from 117 ± 39 to 77 ± 31 mL/m^2, respectively; (2) the end-systolic stresses in all the three zones (infarcted zone, border zone, remote zone) were reduced; and (3) the global systolic function was improved, in terms of EF increase from 26 ± 7 to 31 ± 10, and the contractility index $d\sigma^*/dt_{max}$ value increase from 2.69 ± 0.74 to 3.23 ± 0.73 s^{-1}.

Chapter 5. Cardiac Contractility Measures for Left Ventricular Systolic Functional Assessment in Normal and Diseased Hearts

The heart is an electrically activated muscle pump, and LV contraction is the basis of LV pumping function. The determination and quantification of LV contractility can provide diagnostic indication of HF and prognostic indication of the success or failure of a given therapy. In the patient care setting, the evaluation of cardiac contractility (with data obtained with echo or MRI or even catheterization procedure) constitutes an essential component of clinical cardiology. In this chapter, we have shown the modeling and formulation of relevant contractility indices at different LV physiological levels in terms LV elastance, LV wall elastic modulus, pressure-normalised wall stress, myocardial sarcomere contractile dynamics, and Intra-LV blood flow profile. We have also shown how these indices can be employed to assess patients with different types of cardiac disorders.

The LV active elastance index enables us to reconstruct the variation of LV pressure from LV volume data during filling and ejection phases; it also provides an explanation of LV suction phenomenon as a mechanism of LV filling during the early diastolic phase. Then, from our pioneering LV elasticity model of wall stress, strain, and elastic modulus, the maximum value of the effective elastic modulus is shown to determine how well LVs with valvular diseases have compensated for hypertrophy by the restoration of their systolic modulus value to the normal range so that there is adequate reserve contractile capacity. Our contractility index of maximum rate of increase of normalized LV wall stress $d\sigma^*/dt_{max}$ is shown to have decreased value in cardiomyopathy, and following surgical ventricular restoration. We then develop a novel mechatronic thick shell model of the LV, with myocardial fibers oriented helically in the wall. Its myocardial structural unit's contractile force versus shortening velocity and power index are employed as contractility indices. The area of the loop of contractile force versus shortening velocity and the value of power index decreases in patients with MI. Finally, we arrive at the outcome of the LV contraction process in terms of setting up favorable intraventricular maps of blood flow velocity and pressure gradients that are conducive to effective ejection of adequate blood volume. In patients with myocardial infarcts, there is inadequate intra-LV pressure gradient toward the aortic valve, which is shown to improve following the administration of coronary vasculature's vasodilating agents. This can enable the cardiologist to assess the viability of this LV for improved performance following coronary bypass surgery. This chapter promotes the employment of these contractility indices into routine cardiology practice by clinical applications of these indices in a large pool of patients with varied etiology of cardiac disorders. In this way, we can develop a range of values of these contractility indices for normal patients and for cardiac disease states so that they can be effectively employed in differential diagnosis.

Chapter 6. Analysis for Left Ventricular Pressure Increase during Isovolumic Contraction Phase due to Active Stress Development in Myocardial Fibers

During diastolic filling, LV wall stress builds due to the LV chamber pressure passively acting on the LV wall. When the LV starts contracting as the myocardium gets electrically activated, the force development in the myocardial fibers causes development of what might be termed as "active stress" in the myocardium, which in turn deforms the LV (including causing its twisting) and thereby decreases its chamber volume. Then, because of the high value of the bulk modulus of blood, there is a substantial rise in LV pressure from the start of isovolumic contraction. Therefore, in this chapter, we analyze that the LV pressure generated during isovolumic contraction and the LV twist angle are caused by the active stress state in the LV wall (equivalent to LV twisting and compression), due to contractile stress in the helically wound myocardial fibers. The LV is modeled as a thick-walled, fluid-filled cylindrical elastic shell (of hyperelastic material) closed at both ends and attached to the aorta at its top base. We simulate the phenomenon of LV isovolumic contraction (which causes the intra-LV pressure to rise very quickly during 0.04–0.06 s of isovolumic contraction) by means of a finite-elasticity analysis of this thick-walled LV cylindrical shell under incremental pressure increase.

In this LV model, we employ the monitored instantaneous LV pressure and dimensions (expressed in terms of the monitored LV volume and myocardial volume) as inputs. The deformation of this LV cylindrical model due to the monitored rise in its chamber pressure (Δp) is represented by a decrease in its chamber volume (ΔV) in terms of blood bulk modulus (K). The resulting changes in the length and radius of the LV cylindrical model are expressed in terms of this chamber volume decrease (ΔV). These changes in the LV cylindrical length and radius along with the LV twist angle (whose reasonable values are assumed in this analysis) constitute the LV deformations. By employing finite elasticity and large-deformation analysis, we express (1) the stretches and strains within the LV cylinder wall in terms of these deformations and (2) LV wall stresses in terms of these stretches and strains, by means of the strain energy density function and its material parameters. We then carry out the equilibrium analysis of wall stress in terms of the monitored chamber pressure. By solving these equilibrium equations, we determine the values of (1) the myocardial material parameters of the strain energy density function, (2) stretches and strains, and (3) stresses. We then go back and determine the principal stresses and principal angle. We associate the principal compressive stress with that of the contractile stress in the myocardial fibers and the principal angle with the myocardial fiber angle. Thus, by means of this inverse analysis, we determine the stresses and the orientation of the activated and contracted myocardial fibers, which cause LV deformation (shortening and twisting) and rapid chamber pressure rise during the isovolumic contraction phase. Finally, we determine and compute the torque and the axial compressive force induced in the LV due to its contraction and the activation of the helically wound myocardial fibers. This induced torque, causing the twisting of the LV and the resulting chamber pressure increase, is an important aspect of LV contraction process and pressure increase during isovolumic contraction.

Chapter 7. Left Ventricular Remodeling due to Myocardial Infarction and its Surgical Ventricular Restoration

Myocardial infarct (MI) reduces the contractile capacity of the LV, and hence the LV is unable to attain its tight contracted curved shape in systole. In other words, an infarcted LV undergoes remodeling, with decreased systolic shape curvedness and decreased contractility, and progresses to HF. This LV remodeling can be quantified and characterized in terms of local curvedness index and diastole-to-systole change in curvedness (%ΔC). In this chapter, we present the (1) course of LV cardiomyopathy (with myocardial infarcts) progressing to HF through cardiac remodeling and decreased contractility and (2) recovery of LV through surgical ventricular restoration (SVR), by the restoration of myocardial ischemic segments, reversal of remodeling, and improvement in contractility.

For this purpose, we first provide a methodology for the detection of myocardial infarcts. We then present a clinical study involving normal subjects and patients after MI. It is seen that the diastole-to-systole change in curvedness (%ΔC) is significantly lower in MI patients compared to the normal group, which characterizes or quantifies LV remodeling following MI. Then, we present a study showing how SVR combined with coronary arterial bypass grafting (CABG) is able to increase (1) the diastolic-systolic change in sphericity index SI (i.e., SIED–SIES) and (2) the value of the contractility index $d\sigma^*/dt_{max}$. So we see that as MI progresses into HF, the LV size increases, LV function deteriorates, and symptoms of HF become evident. Thus, cardiac remodeling (expressed in terms of the regional curvedness of the LV) constitutes a measure of the progression of HF after MI. It is then seen that an intervention by SVR combined with CABG causes some reversal of this LV remodeling process and improves mortality in patients with HF. Hence, in this chapter, we demonstrate how the curvedness index, sphericity index, and contractility index enable us to track and assess LV progression to HF, and its recovery following CABG and SVR intervention.

Chapter 8. Vector Cardiogram Theory and Clinical Application

It is common to have ECG analysis carried out for cardiac diagnosis. The ECG lead system is based on Einthoven's triangle (EIT), whose vertices (A, B, C) are three bipolar leads, and the equivalent-dipole heart electrical-activity vector (HAV) is located at its centroid. The three-lead ECG voltages are derived from the projection of the equivalent-dipole HAV on the sides of the EIT. It is useful to know the bioelectricity basis and derivation of this EIT, which we have provided in this chapter by developing expressions for potential differences between the vertices of the EIT, as scalar components of the HAV along the sides of the EIT. The three bipolar lead voltages can be expressed as the projections of the heart vector onto each side of the EIT. Conversely, since the three-lead voltages can be monitored, they can be employed to reconstruct the HAV, from which we can then generate the VCG.

In this chapter, we present the theory, development, and clinical application of VCG. We have demonstrated VCG development by illustrating the progression of the equivalent-dipole HAV during the QRS complex from the onset of the QRS until the end of the depolarization stage. We have constructed VCGs for a normal subject, and three patients with ventricular hypertrophy, bundle branch block, and inferior MI. Then in order to distinguish the VCG shapes of diseased and normal subjects, we have introduced two VCG diagnostic parameters—VCG loop area and loop sling length. We have constructed a VCG parametric space with loop area and loop sling length as coordinates for 35 subjects representing healthy control and abnormal electrocardiological states. It can be seen that each diagnostic class has its own zone in the parametric space. Subtle changes in the ECG are distinctly reflected in the VCG loop and in the VCG parametric space. Hence, VCG can even help to diagnose cardiac disease at an early stage.

Section II. ECG Signal Analysis, Left Ventricular Pumping (Intra-Ventricular, Aortic, and Coronary Flow) Characteristics, Coronary Bypass Surgery Design, and Their Implications in Clinical Cardiology and Cardiac Surgery

Chapter 9. ECG Waveform and Heart Rate Variability Signal Analysis to Detect Cardiac Arrhythmias

The electrocardiogram is currently the most commonly used noninvasive technology to monitor the heart's electrical activity, to evaluate the heart condition of patients with cardiac complaints, cardiac arrhythmias, ischemic heart disease, and myocardial infarct (MI). The origin of the electrocardiogram dates back to 1811, when Dr. Augustus Waller, a British physiologist at St. Mary's Medical School in London, published the first human electrocardiogram, using a capillary electrometer with electrodes placed on the chest and back of a human; he demonstrated that electrical activity preceded ventricular contraction. Many years later, Dr. Willem Einthoven, a Dutch physiologist, further refined the capillary electrometer and was able to demonstrate five deflections, which he called ABCDE. To adjust for inertia in the capillary system, Einthoven implemented a mathematical correction, which resulted in the curves that we are familiar with today; he called these deflections PQRST. Einthoven coined the term *electrocardiogram* to describe the cardiac electrical activity wave forms at the Dutch Medical Meeting of 1893. He went on to develop (in 1901) a new string galvanometer, which he used in his electrocardiograph device. As the string galvanometer electrocardiograph became available for clinical use, improvements were made to make it more practical. The earlier electrocardiograms used five electrodes, one on each of the four extremities and the mouth, with 10 leads derived from different combinations. Einthoven reduced the number of electrodes to the three-lead system used to construct the Einthoven's triangle (EIT), which is an important concept to this day and is referred to in this chapter. In 1924, Einthoven was awarded the Nobel Prize in physiology and medicine for the invention of electrocardiogram. By 1930, the importance of electrocardiogram in diagnosing the cause of cardiac chest pain had become universally recognized and adopted.

So with this historical background, we embark, in this chapter, on ECG waveform analysis to detect cardiac arrhythmias, and thereafter conduct heart rate variability (HRV) signal processing and analysis to detect cardiac arrhythmias. We first study the electrical activity of the heart and the different phases of the action potential. We then discuss the EIT, the relationship between the Einthoven vector and each of the three frontal limb leads (leads I, II, and III), and the method of measuring ECG by using electrodes attached to the body surface and connected to an instrumentation amplifier. We then present (1) how the

ECG waveform evolves and develops the PQRST complex, (2) detection of P, QRS, and ST segments of the ECG waveform, and (3) ECG waveform abnormalities in terms of P-wave amplitude, PR interval, and QRS width. Since visual analysis of ECG waveform is highly subjective, there is a need for more objective digital signal analysis strategies. The HRV signals, obtained from the measurements of the time interval between two consecutive R waves, are reliable, accurate, reproducible, yet very simple to measure and process. In this chapter, we review how the HRV signal can be analyzed using methods based on time domain, frequency domain, time-frequency domain, and also geometric and nonlinear methods for detection of cardiac arrhythmias. We also present a predictive analytics framework of a HRV analysis technique for arrhythmia detection that involves the following steps: (1) continuous wavelet transform (CWT) application, resulting in a series of wavelet coefficients in the form of a scalogram signal, and (2) principal component analysis (PCA) of the wavelet coefficients, resulting in eigenvalues that provide information about the patterns in the HRV signal. We have studied the distribution of these eigenvalues over the normal sinus rhythm (NSR) and the four arrhythmias and have found considerable overlap for some arrhythmias. Hence, we have developed a single physiological index number called the HRVID Index by combining these eigenvalues, and observed that this index can effectively separate out the different classes of arrhythmia from NSR. We therefore make a case for the adoption of this HRVID Index for arrhythmia detection.

Chapter 10. Left Ventricular Blood Pump Analysis: Intra-LV Flow Velocity and Pressure for Coronary Bypass Surgery Candidacy

Cardiac contractility manifests in the form of intra-LV blood flow patterns. Regional variations in LV wall distensibility and contractility caused by diseased myocardial segments or intramyocardial conduction abnormalities influence wall motion kinematics during the filling and systolic phases of the cardiac cycle, and thereby set up variations in characteristic intra-LV flow and pressure gradient distributions. In order to address this problem, we have developed a method of computing intra-LV blood flow velocity and pressure-differentials at different instants of the cardiac cycle derived from sequentially digitized cine-ventriculograms, to assess left ventricular pumping efficiency. By employing finite element modeling, we can determine intra-LV flow velocity and pressure gradient distribution from sequential analog images of contrast ventriculograms. The intra-LV flow velocity distribution can identify the presence of stagnant or recirculating flow zones and can help delineate the sites of mural thrombus formation. The intra-LV pressure gradients during ejection constitute a signature of regional myocardial function. We present herein the requisite analysis, technology, and methodology for the computation of flow velocity distribution in the LV and the results of clinical applications in three of patients suspected of having coronary artery disease.

In this chapter, a 2D inviscid fluid flow finite element analysis is carried out in the anteroposterior projection plane of the LV, by assuming a quasi-steady flow in the time intervals between successive frames. The blood flow is governed by the potential equation $\nabla^2\phi = 0$, where ∇^2 is the Laplacian operator, ϕ is the velocity potential, and $\nabla\phi$ is the velocity vector. In order to solve this equation for the velocity potential (ϕ), the requisite boundary conditions are (i) specification of ϕ over a part of the boundary, and (ii) specification of the normal derivative of the velocity potential, $\partial\phi/\partial n$ ($=V_n$, the normal velocity of the boundary or the normal velocity of blood in contact with the boundary), over the remaining part of the boundary. Now, from the LV endocardial outlines of the sequential instants, we obtain the value of LV wall motion velocities, which equal the blood velocities at the endocardial boundary; therefrom, the values of $\partial\phi/\partial n = V_n$ can be determined. We then compute the values of instantaneous ϕ in the interior of the LV chamber by solving the potential equation by using the finite element method, for the designated instantaneous V_n at the wall boundary. From the computed values of ϕ at each internal point, we obtain the instantaneous maps of blood flow velocity patterns inside the LV chamber. The intra-LV pressure-differential distribution at points within the LV chamber is then obtained from the Bernoulli equation for unsteady potential flow. The clinical application of the finite element methodology is carried out for three subjects with coronary artery disease. For these patients, we have obtained and displayed the superimposed sequential diastolic and systolic endocardial frames. Then from the instantaneous wall displacements and the endocardial wall velocities during the diastolic and systolic time intervals, the intra-LV blood flow velocities are computed by finite element analysis; the intra-LV pressure-differential distribution is then obtained from the Bernoulli equation. We then compare their computed intra-LV flow velocity and pressure distributions before and after the administration of nitroglycerin (a vasodilating agent). Following the administration of nitroglycerin, the intra-LV velocity distributions have demonstrated improved filling-flow and ejection-phase flow velocity patterns. For one patient, when the diastole pressure-differential distributions before and after nitroglycerin administration were compared, we noted substantially deleterious pressure gradient characterizing resistance-to-LV filling before nitroglycerin administration, and reduction of this pressure gradient after nitroglycerin administration. Likewise, we observed improvement in the systolic pressure gradient conducive to more effective ejection, following administration of nitroglycerin. This patient was thereby deemed to be a candidate for coronary bypass surgery.

Chapter 11. Cardiac Perfusion Analysis and Computation of Intra-Myocardial Blood Flow Velocity and Pressure Patterns

Myocardial perfusion is an important designation and determinant of cardiac function, as it affects cardiac contractility, ejection fraction (EF) and blood supply to all the organs and to the coronary tree. Hence mapping and quantification of myocardial perfusion is very important. This chapter is composed of two main parts: (1) the quantification of cardiac myocardial perfusion and function by single photon emission computed tomography (SPECT) imaging in terms of intramyocardial radionuclide tracer maps and (2) substantiation of myocardial perfusion by computing intramyocardial pressure and velocity distribution patterns. In Section 11.2, we start out with myocardial ischemia physiology, ischemia cause and diagnosis, and coronary autoregulation. With exercise stress, tissue accumulation of metabolites occurs, which relaxes the arteriolar wall smooth muscle cell contraction. The coronary blood flow (CBF) in nonstenosed arteries expands more than in stenosed arteries, because arterioles supplied by the stenosed arteries are semi-dilated even before exercise begins. Hence, the coronary flow reserve (CFR), defined as the ratio of stress to rest CBF, is lower in stenosed arteries compared to normal arteries. To assess CBF and CFR, we carry out radionuclide myocardial perfusion imaging (MPI) by SPECT acquisition technique. The MPI is performed with intravenously injected technetium-99 m-based agents. These tracers are trapped in the myocardium in proportion to the regional CBF. SPECT enables 3D image reconstruction and good separation of the different heart chambers in space. The acquisition, computer processing, and display of scintigraphic (radionuclide imaging) data by high-speed computing constitute fundamental steps in the process of nuclear imaging. SPECT allows the evaluation of perfusion patterns in reconstructed thin slices of the myocardium. The comparison of stress and rest images helps in differentiating ischemia from infarct scar. A perfusion abnormality present in the stress study that is resolved in the rest study represents ischemia, whereas a perfusion abnormality on both the stress and rest studies represents a scar. We present the studies of myocardial perfusion SPECT imaging of patients with myocardial infarcts. The regional tracer uptake is normalized with respect to the maximum tracer activity detected count in the myocardium and then displayed according to the deciles of percentage maximal counts by using a stepped color scale. We then present automated SPECT quantization of myocardial perfusion (and the software algorithms for it), quantified as polar maps wherein the count activities are displayed as successive annular rings of increasing radii as the slices progress toward the base of the LV. Finally, we present left ventricular ejection fraction (LVEF) assessment from gated perfusion SPECT measurements (of technetium-99m tracer). We display a patient study of quantitative wall motion assessment of gated perfusion SPECT. From transmural radionuclide count profiles, the endocardial and epicardial surfaces are determined, from which LV cavity and myocardial volumes are estimated and the EF is calculated. Also, regional wall motion (endocardial surface displacement) and wall thickening are evaluated. Post-stress-gated SPECT in this patient shows normal wall motion in all segments. We can conclude that gated SPECT LVEF measurements are generally accurate and reliable, even in the presence of large defects.

Section 11.3 primarily deals with the perfusion analysis of the myocardium. In order to gain further quantitative insight into LV intramyocardial flow, we have developed a biomechanics model of intramyocardial blood flow through a porous myocardium medium, using a modified form of Darcy's law in which the blood velocity is dependent on intramyocardial pressure-gradient (Δp), myocardial permeability (k), and myocardial-stress-dependent hydrostatic-pressure (H). The governing equations required to compute intramyocardial pressure and velocity distributions include equations for the incompressible and viscous fluid (blood), incompressible and elastic solid (myocardium), and fluid–solid interaction. Specifically, these equations are (1) continuity equation for the fluid, (2) momentum equations for both the fluid and solid mediums, (3) constitutive equations for both solid and fluid mediums, and (4) Darcy's law. We express the blood velocity in terms of the pressure head gradient, myocardial tissue permeability, and blood viscosity and density. The pressure head ϕ is a function of the fluid pressure and potential gradient. Darcy's law is expressed in terms of the hydraulic conductivity C, as a function of myocardial permeability and blood viscosity. Finally, we can express the blood velocity V in terms of C and the spatial derivative of pressure. We provide a flow chart of this poroelastic fluid structure analysis for computing the streamlines, pressure, and velocity distributions. We then display the computed results of intramyocardial pressure and velocity distributions in annular myocardial segments, based on specified inlet and outlet pressures. This chapter therefore provides the methods for (1) determining myocardial perfusion by SPECT imaging and detecting ischemia regions, based on myocardial radionuclide tracer maps, and (2) quantifying myocardial perfusion in terms of pressure and velocity distributions in the myocardial segments.

Chapter 12. Arterial Pulse Wave Propagation Analysis: Determination of Pulse Wave Velocity and Arterial Properties

In the circulatory system, the pulse wave travels along with the exchange of energy between the flowing blood and elastic vessel walls. In the aorta, the pressure increases with left ventricular ejection, and blood flows through it as it dilates and relaxes (or contracts). Arterial pulse wave velocity (PWV) describes how fast a blood pressure pulse travels from one point to another in an artery. PWV, by definition, is the distance traveled (Δx) by the wave divided by the time (Δt) for the wave to travel that distance: PWV = $\Delta x/\Delta t$. PWV can be measured between two sites a known distance apart, using the pressure "foot" of the waveform to calculate the transit time. In the aorta, PWV is typically measured between the carotid and femoral arteries. Typically, the pulse wave is detected by pressure transducers or arterial tonometry. We can also measure PWV noninvasively by Doppler ultrasound. Based on its formula, $(Eh/2a\rho)^{1/2}$, PWV is a measure of arterial stiffness and an indicator for arteriosclerosis. Hence, PWV is a well-established technique for measuring the arterial stiffness parameters in the aorta. Arterial stiffness is now recognized as a major driver of cardiovascular disease; an increase in arterial stiffness elevates central systolic and pulse pressure and left ventricular afterload and decreases coronary artery perfusion pressure.

In this chapter, we derive the expression for PWV. We then analyze and determine arterial stiffness properties in terms of (1) the arterial wall stress–strain relationship or the elastic modulus (E) as a function of arterial wall stress (σ) and (2) arterial impedance z, the ratio of the amplitudes of the pressure and flow-rate pulses, representing the incremental pressure pulse response to the incremental flow-rate pulse. We then analyze pulse wave reflection at aortic bifurcation. In the aorta, the forward pressure and flow waveform comes from the heart, and the reflected wave comes from various locations in the arterial system (such as from bifurcations). The pulsatile pressure and flow can thus be viewed as the sum of forward and reflected pulse wave fronts. Based on arterial impedance and the pressure wave reflection coefficient, we have shown that the reflected wave can be either in phase or out of phase with the incident wave, and hence can either increase or decrease the afterload on the LV. Finally, we present noninvasive methods of measurement of PWV.

Chapter 13. Simulation of Blood Flow in Idealized and Patient-Specific Coronary Arteries with Curvatures, Stenoses, Dilatations, and Side-Branches

Atherosclerosis is the main disease affecting coronary arteries, and it tends to be localized in regions of curvature and branching in the coronary arteries. Atherosclerotic coronary arteries cause myocardial ischemia and infarcts, resulting in diminished cardiac contractility and output. Using computational blood flow simulation, researchers have shown that there are complex hemodynamic changes in S-shaped arteries in terms of the large changes of pressure and wall shear stress (WSS). It has been found that atherosclerotic plaques and wall thickening in left and right coronary arteries (RCAs) are localized almost exclusively on (1) the outer wall of one or both daughter vessels at major bifurcations and T-junctions and (2) along the inner wall of curved segments, where WSS is low. It has also been discovered that high WSS induces plaque growth at bifurcations by producing endothelial injury and disruption. Large WSS gradients can also induce morphological and functional changes in the endothelium in regions of disturbed flow and promote the occurrence of plaque. In this chapter, we present simulations of blood flow in idealized and patient-specific coronary arteries with curvatures, stenoses, dilatations, and side-branches. In all these coronary arterial models, the blood flow is governed by the incompressible Navier–Stokes equation and continuity equation. For the solid segment of the artery, the elastic mechanics equation of motion is employed. The coupling of fluid and solid domains is carried out by means of the compatibility equations of stress and displacement. The two-way fluid-structure interaction (FSI) analysis between the blood vessel wall (and its constitutive properties) and the blood has thus been carried out. The flow simulation is based on the physiologically realistic boundary conditions of pulsatile blood flow velocity and pressure boundary conditions at the inlet and outlet of the artery, acquired with an electrocardiography-gated intravascular Doppler ultrasound and pressure probe.

Four types of coronary arterial models are analyzed in this chapter. We start with an analysis of transient blood flow in a curved coronary artery with progressive amounts of stenosis and determine the variation of WSS and wall pressure gradients (WPGs) with the degree of stenosis. A two-way FSI analysis is carried out between the blood vessel wall and the blood in elastic arteries with eccentric stenotic plaques, and the boundary conditions of time-varying velocity and pressure waves are applied at the inlet and outlet of the artery. Next, we present an analysis of blood flow in coronary arteries with varying degrees of curvature and stenosis, and determine the WSS and WPG profiles in idealized artery models and realistic arteries. Our results show that the increasing values of WSS and WPG are associated with the increasing narrowing of the lumen and degree of curvature. The WSS and WPG are then determined in patient-specific RCAs, and it is likewise seen that WSS is maximum in the stenotic region and the wall pressure gradient is maximum in the most curved artery. We then conduct analysis of pulsatile blood flow in straight coronary arteries with varying degrees of stenosis and dilatations. The results indicate that both WSS and WPG properties are shown to demonstrate significant increments at segments where the artery is more stenosed. Finally, we study blood flow in RCAs with varying degrees of curvature and side-branch bifurcation angles. Therein, we employ computational fluid dynamics (CFD) to computationally analyze the WSS and WPG variations in idealized and realistic RCA models. Our study results show low WSS regions located at the inner wall of the arterial curve and opposite to the flow divider, and increased values of WSS and WPG with higher values of curvature angle and branch bifurcation angle. In summary, we have provided quite a comprehensive study of the effect of coronary arterial bending, curvature and atherosclerotic plaques on (1) average wall shear stress, and (2) the pressure drop ΔP between the inlet and outlet of the blood vessels (representing the flow resistance). This chapter can provide the basis for analysis of patient-specific coronary arteries, to study their pathologies and thereafter determine how to carry out remedial measures by means of coronary stents or coronary bypass surgery.

Chapter 14. Intra-Left Ventricular Flow Velocity Distributions, Based on Color Doppler Echo Vector Flow Mapping of Normal Subjects and Heart Failure Patients

Intracardiac flow is useful for evaluating cardiac function, as it is the end result of cardiac myocardial abnormalities. The vortex flow pattern during left ventricular filling is a critical determinant of directed blood flow during ejection and can offer a novel index of cardiac dysfunction. The vector flow mapping (VFM) technique has been developed recently to generate flow velocity vector fields by post-processing color Doppler echo images. In this technique, axial velocity is measured from color Doppler images, while radial velocity is computed by deconstructing the flow into basic nonvortical laminar flow component and a vortical flow component. In normal subjects, after flow ejection into LV, the direction of flow is reversed toward the apex, with a brief appearance of vortex at the early stage of isovolumic relaxation time. The major diastolic anterior vortex develops immediately after the onset of the early diastolic phase. This vortex continues during diastasis, persists into late LV filling phase and throughout isovolumic contraction phase, and dissipates with the opening of the aortic valve and LV ejection. Color-Doppler-derived VFM helps to (1) determine the intraventricular vortex flow for the detection of pathologically altered flow characteristics and (2) identify new pathophysiologic mechanisms in the development of cardiac disease.

We have carried out clinical studies to determine intra-LV flow patterns for HF patients (both HFNEF and HFREF) and normal subjects. Color Doppler flow images were captured in the three-chamber view for the visualization of both inflow through the mitral valve and outflow into the aorta. Intra-LV flow was determined by using the VFM analysis package. In this technique, color Doppler velocity (axial velocity, $\mathbf{u}$) profile was analyzed across an arc at each echo depth. The measured Doppler velocity $\mathbf{u}$ is composed of basic nonvortical laminar flow ($\mathbf{u}_b$) and vortex flow ($\mathbf{u}_v$) components. The vortex flow velocity components $\mathbf{u}_v$ (along the Doppler beam) and $\mathbf{v}_v$ (perpendicular to the Doppler beam) are obtained in terms of the stream function $\psi(r, \theta)$. The flow velocity $U(r, \theta)$ is then calculated in terms of (1) $\mathbf{u}_b$ and $\mathbf{u}_v$ in the axial Doppler beam direction and (2) $\mathbf{v}_b$ and $\mathbf{v}_v$ in the radial direction perpendicular to the Doppler beam. The contractility index $d\sigma^*/dt_{max}$ is also evaluated by measuring the maximal flow rate into the aorta (using VFM) and the myocardial volume. In diastolic flow patterns, in the rapid filling phase, a straight flow is seen to rush into the LV from the LA; circulating flow patterns are seen at the anterior and posterior walls of the LV in all subjects. In systolic flow patterns, it is seen that LV contraction produced recirculating flow patterns and directed flow toward the aortic valve. The flow is ejected into the aorta rapidly at mid systole and is gradually reduced at the end of systole. The results show (1) substantially reduced values of contractility index for HFREF patients and (2) marked reduction of peak systolic outflow rate in HFREF patients. We have been able to demonstrate the use of the VFM technique to visualize blood flow patterns in HF patients and normal subjects, abnormal circulating flow patterns in filling, and irregularly directed flow patterns toward the aortic valve for HFREF patients.

Chapter 15. Coronary Blood Flow Analysis and Coronary Bypass Graft Design

Coronary artery disease (CAD) remains one of the primary causes of morbidity and mortality worldwide, because the coronary arteries are most vulnerable to lesions restricting blood flow. Coronary circulation is complex due to its bifurcations and branches, which cause considerable spatial and temporal variations in the hemodynamic parameters (HPs) of WSS and wall pressure. Hence, coronary circulation is highly prone to atherosclerosis and consequently to myocardial ischemia, which causes decreased cardiac contractility and decreased EF, leading to risk of HF. Hence, understanding the mechanism and mechanics of atherosclerosis and its initiation and association with the complex features of CBF dynamics is very important. The spatial complexities of blood flow in the cardiovascular system cannot be visualized with current imaging methods; hence, analytical modeling combined with computational solution methodology is a necessity. CFD methods utilized in conjunction with monitored or experimental data (as boundary conditions) are employed to simulate blood flow behavior and disturbances (such as flow separation, secondary flow, flow stagnation, reversed flow, and turbulence), and subsequently estimate the HPs. Restoration of coronary flow perfusion to the myocardium is required to sustain cardiac output and prevent HF. In this regard, coronary bypass grafting (CABG) surgical procedure constitutes an effective remedy for high-risk CAD patients. However, its complications and patency are known to be intertwined with the hemodynamics and vascular mechanics of bypass-grafted arterial vessels at the anastomotic sites. In particular, hemodynamic analysis of CABG blood flow at distal anastomotic sites (which are prone to disturbed flow patterns and HPs) is important, in order to develop anastomoses designs that can enhance the CABG patency. Computational modeling is employed to study how the distal anastomotic geometry affects the blood flow patterns and the HPs influencing CABG patency.

In this chapter, we provide insights into (1) the current methods of blood flow studies in coronary arteries and CABGs by means of computational fluid–solid mechanics and (2) innovative designs of CABG distal anastomotic configuration for the enhancement of patency and the prevention of restenosis. Myocardial ischemia, a major cause of morbidity and mortality in the United States and worldwide, is transmurally heterogeneous, and the subendocardium is at a higher risk than the mid-wall or epicardium. This requires looking into the CBF determinant of subendocardial vulnerability by studying the dynamics of the CBF system as an integrated system, involving the complex coronary vasculature embedded in the myocardium and of the associated biomechanical interactions. In Section 15.2 of this chapter, computational methodologies of blood flow analysis are employed to formulate and illustrate three types of coronary circulatory flows (in porcine models): pulsatile flow in the epicardial coronary tree, steady-state flow in the entire coronary arterial tree, and wave propagation in the coronary arterial tree. For the epicardial coronary tree pulsatile flow analysis, we have developed a finite element model for pulsatile flow analysis based on CT scans and physiological measurements in porcine models. The HPs indicate that the sites at the flow divider are prone to atherosclerosis due to the presence of low WSS; the branch sites with high values of WSS are susceptible to increased permeability of LDL. In the future, the model can be made patient specific through medical imaging to guide diagnosis, intervention, and therapy. For the steady-state laminar flow model in the entire coronary arterial tree of porcine model, we have determined the pressure distribution in the entire coronary arterial tree model down to the first capillary segments. It is seen that the pressure distribution is fairly uniform in larger vessels and changes significantly in smaller vessels (<100 μm), which shows that the myocardial resistance mainly resides in the arteriolar bed. Finally, we have carried out a hybrid Womersley-type 1D wave propagation model in the entire coronary arterial tree of a Porcine model, using the inlet pulsatile pressure boundary condition obtained from experimental measurements. Our 1D wave propagation model can determine the transient blood flow waves sequentially at different spatial positions along the main trunk, starting from the inlet of LAD artery into the various primary branches. There is decrease of flow amplitude along the main trunk, and the flow waves at the inlet of primary branches show different amplitudes. This wave propagation model can be made patient specific by interface with patient-specific anatomy of large epicardial vessels obtained from CT, MRI, or other imaging techniques. In Section 15.3, we have provided an overview analysis of CABG, the preferred treatment for high-risk CAD patients. The importance and role of HPs in restenosis of CABG is analyzed. We have presented various attempts to design an optimal distal anastomotic configuration, in terms of the anastomotic angle, graft caliber (i.e., graft-to-host diameter ratio), and influence of out-of-plane graft curvature. A smaller distal ETS anastomotic angle (≤30°) seems to bring about a less disturbed and more uniform, smooth flow from the graft into the coronary artery. Smaller grafts typically present an increased risk of early graft failure due to thrombosis. Further results of computational studies indicate that the graft caliber should always be maximized in order to minimize the spatial and temporal gradients of WSS. As regards the influence of out-of-plane graft curvature, investigations have revealed reductions in the magnitudes of the peak time-averaged WSS and mean oscillatory shear in the nonplanar models as compared to the planar configurations, which imply a corresponding reduction in the spatial extent of wall regions exposed to physiologically unfavorable flow conditions. This chapter provides the knowledge base for how coronary circulation and obstruction (stenosis) occurs, how

CABG can address the stenosis problem, and how a smoother hemodynamics-based design of the distal anastomosis geometry can enhance CABG patency.

Chapter 16. Coupled Sequential Anastomotic Bypass Graft Design

In CABG, the design of anastomosis is very important for enhancing its patency. In this context, the sequential bypass grafting is a technique in which two or more coronary artery anastomoses are made with a single graft, usually the saphenous vein (SV). Intraoperative studies demonstrate a higher blood flow and a higher velocity in the proximal (pre-anastomotic) segment of a sequential graft than in a single coronary graft with an end-to-side (ETS) anastomosis. Higher patency rates have also been observed through post angiograms in the side-to-side (STS) anastomoses than in the ETS anastomoses. It is well established that in the conventional ETS distal anastomotic region, the impingement of blood flow on the artery floor and the flow recirculation at the heel play a critical role in the restenosis of the CABG distal anastomosis. We have conducted several studies, both numerically and experimentally, in order to investigate the effects of geometrical parameters, including anastomotic angle, out-of-plane graft, and complete CABG modeling. Optimization of these parameters in a conventional ETS anastomosis can improve the flow field and distributions of HPs to some extent. However, in order to further improve the hemodynamics and alleviate the drawbacks of the available CABG anastomosis designs, we have developed a novel coupled sequential anastomotic (SQA) configuration design. The investigation of the flow field in this SQA design (by means of numerical simulation of pulsatile Newtonian blood flow) and its comparison with a conventional CABG ETS anastomosis is presented in this chapter.

We have developed an innovative distal SQA geometrical configuration for enhancing the patency of CABG. Computational and in vitro simulations of blood flow through this novel design have shown improvements of the hemodynamic parameters that can contribute to its enhanced patency, namely, (1) an increase in the time-averaged WSS on the artery bed of the ETS anastomosis of the SQA (as compared to the conventional ETS anastomosis), (2) reduction of the time-averaged WSS gradient at the heel and bed of the ETS component and at the toe and suture line of the STS component of the novel SQA (as compared to conventional ETS and typical parallel STS anastomoses, respectively), and (3) reduction of the oscillatory shear index (OSI) at the ETS anastomosis of the SQA at the heel region and on the artery wall and bed opposite to the heel (in comparison with the conventional ETS anastomosis). In addition, this design provides a spare route for blood flow to the coronary artery, in order to avoid reoperation in case of restenosis in either of the anastomoses. This design can also be employed by using autologous grafts without the need for any additional training.

Acknowledgments

Over the years, Prof. Ru San Tan, Dr. Liang Zhong and I have had numerous research collaborations and coauthored publications. Together, we have contributed significantly to biomedical engineering formulation of heart function and cardiovascular medicine. One of our innovations has been our noninvasive cardiac contractility index, based on LV wall stress normalized with respect to LV intracavitary pressure (P), as given by $d(\sigma/P)/dt_{max}$ or $d\sigma^*/dt_{max}$, where $\sigma^* = \sigma/P$. As shown in Chapter 3, this cardiac contractility index can be expressed as

$$d\sigma^*/dt_{max} = \left. \frac{d(\sigma_\theta/P)}{dt} \right|_{max} = \frac{3}{2V_m} \left. \frac{dV}{dt} \right|_{max}$$

where V denotes LV volume and V_m denotes LV myocardial volume. It can be noted that this cardiac contractility index can be determined solely from a noninvasive assessment of LV myocardial volume and its maximum outflow rate. Normalizing LV wall stress to LV pressure obviates the need for invasive LV pressure measurement for the traditional contractility index dP/dt_{max}. This concept originated from our reckoning that while in diastole the LV wall developed passive stress in response to LV filling pressure, in LV systole, the myocardium contracts and develops stress; it is this active LV wall stress that develops LV pressure, which ultimately results in blood ejection through the aortic valve. So we need to base our contractility index on this active wall stress that causes LV pressure development. The chapters in this book present the details of our collaborative works.

I am deeply grateful for the help of Prof. Ghassan Kassab in getting this book ready for publication. He has contributed significantly to Chapters 3, 4, and 7. Chapter 15 reflects his insights into the intricacies of CBF, which results in benefitting myocardial perfusion and cardiac contractility as represented by the above defined cardiac contractility index. He has been a great friend and asset to me. I wish him success with his high-profile California Medical Innovations Institute, a prime innovator of bioengineering mechanisms of organ pathologies bioengineering technologies in medicine and surgery.

I am also grateful to Dr. Foad Kabinejadian for his immense help in preparing the manuscript ready for production. In addition to his contribution to Chapters 6, 10, 12, 15, and 16, he helped me with small details in the formatting of other chapters. He has contributed greatly to the enhancement of patency of coronary bypass grafting through the SQA technique, presented in Chapter 16. He has a great career ahead of him in biomedical engineering.

Author

Professor Dhanjoo N. Ghista is a pioneer and world authority on biomedical engineering. He has developed biomedical engineering programs and departments and has had senior academic and administrative appointments at universities in the United States, Canada, India, United Arab Emirates, and Singapore. He has published several books on many aspects of biomedical engineering, including physiological mechanics, human body dynamics, cardiovascular engineering and physics, orthopedic mechanics, osteoarthro mechanics, spinal injury medical engineering, biomechanics of medical devices, cardiac perfusion and pumping engineering, biomedical and life physics.

In his previous book, *Applied Biomedical Engineering Mechanics* (CRC Press, Boca Raton, FL, 2008), he demonstrated the use of a problem-based approach to quantify physiological processes, formulate diagnostic and interventional procedures, develop orthopedic surgical procedures and guidelines for prostheses design, and apply the results in tertiary care. This book also contains an analysis of sports fitness and explains how to optimize performance in sports such as soccer, baseball, and gymnastics.

Professor Ghista has an international standing in education and research, in making university institutional developments, and planning and modeling universities. He has had senior academic and administrative appointments at universities (in the United States, Canada, India, United Arab Emirates, and Singapore). He is committed to promoting the concept of Global Education for Global Harmony.

Professor Ghista's academic involvements span engineering, medicine, hospital management, and social sciences in which he has authored a definitive book, *Socio-economic Democracy and the World Government*, World Scientific, 2004, to provide the basis of a new norm of civilian participatory democracy, economically sustainable communities and global peace.

In an academic career spanning over 45 years, he has taught many courses, including biomechanics, physiological engineering, clinical engineering, cardiovascular engineering, sports science, and organ systems to medical students. He has published more than 480 papers in peer-reviewed journals and conference proceedings. His 28 books have been in biomedical engineering and physics, physiological mechanics, cardiac engineering and physics, orthopedic and spinal biomechanics, life science, and social sciences. He has guided several PhD students and postdoctoral fellows, many of whom have gone on to hold responsible positions in universities and research institutes.

Among his many innovations is his new concept of nondimensional physiological index (NDPI) in medical assessment, for quantifying physiological and organ systems and analyzing medical test data. In physiological medicine, the use of NDPIs can provide a generalized approach by which a number of physiological and medical parameters (such as the parameters of a second-order differential equation representing a physiological system function or a medical test data) can be integrated into one nondimensional physiological index (or physiological number) to characterize normal or abnormal physiological or organ system function. In this way, NDPI can be employed as a medical diagnostic index.

Dr. Ghista has been editor of *Automedica and Renaissance Universal*, and has served on the editorial boards of *Journal of Mechanics in Medicine and Biology* and *Biomedical Engineering Online*. He has been reviewer of grant proposals for several national agencies, including the International Spinal Trust, the Medical Research Council (Canada), the Ontario Research Foundation, and the Agency for Science and Technology (Singapore).

Of significance is his novel formulation of a new field of STEM translational medicine. This book conveys this theme of how to translate engineering science formulations of anatomical and physiological systems into medical and surgical procedures and systems. Thereby, *Cardiology Science and Technology* addresses the teaching, research, and clinical needs of biomedical engineering in cardiovascular medicine.

This book can be termed to belong to the field of what can be termed *computational medicine*. Professor Ghista is at the forefront of this field, which will contribute to the evolution of STEM precision medicine.

Contributors

U. Rajendra Acharya
Department of Electronics and Computer
    Engineering
Ngee Ann Polytechnic
Singapore

Leok Poh Chua
Department of Mechanical and Aerospace
    Engineering
Nanyang Technological University
Singapore

Ernie Fallen
Department of Medicine
McMaster University
Hamilton, Ontario, Canada

Yunlong Huo
Department of Mechanics and Engineering
    Science
College of Engineering
Peking University
Beijing, China

Sridhar Idapalapati
School of Mechanical and Aerospace
    Engineering
Nanyang Technological University
Singapore

Reginald Jegathese
Department of Mechanical Engineering
PET Engineering College
Tamil Nadu, India

Foad Kabinejadian
Department of Biomedical Engineering
University of Michigan
Ann Arbor, Michigan

Ghassan S. Kassab
California Medical Innovations Institute
San Diego, California

Li Liu
Bumi Armada
Singapore

Thu-Thao Le
National Heart Centre Singapore
Singapore

Guiying Liu
Guangdong Provincial Key Laboratory of
    Medical Biomechanics
Department of Anatomy
School of Basic Medicine Science
Southern Medical University
Guangdong, People's Republic of China

Israel Mirsky
Harvard Medical School and Peter Bent
    Brigham Hospital
Boston, Massachusetts

Thurairaj Nagenthiran
School of Mechanical and Aerospace
    Engineering
Nanyang Technological University
Singapore

Eddie Y.K. Ng
School of Mechanical and Aerospace
    Engineering
Nanyang Technological University
Singapore

Harold Sandler
Biomedical Research Branch
Ames Research Center
National Aeronautics and Space
    Administration
Moffett Field, California

Jian-Jun Shu
School of Mechanical and Aerospace
 Engineering
Nanyang Technological University
Singapore

Vinitha Sree Subbhuraam
Cyrcadia Health
Reno, Nevada

K. Subbaraj
Department of Biophysics
College of Medicine and Health Sciences
United Arab Emirates University
Al Ain, UAE

Yi Su
Institute of High Performance Computing
Agency for Science, Technology and Research
Singapore

G. Swapna
Department of Applied Electronics and
 Instrumentation
Government Engineering College
Kerala, India

Ru San Tan
National Heart Centre Singapore
and
Duke-NUS Graduate Medical School
Singapore

Kelvin K.L. Wong
School of Medicine
Western Sydney University
New South Wales, Sydney, Australia

Jianhuang Wu
Shenzhen Institutes of Advanced
 Technology
Chinese Academy of Sciences
Shenzhen, People's Republic of China

Liang Zhong
National Heart Centre Singapore
and
Duke-NUS Graduate Medical School
Singapore

Section I

Left Ventricular Wall Stress, Cardiac Elastances, Cardiac Contractility Measures, Cardiomyopathic Ventricular Remodeling and its Surgical Restoration, Active Wall Stress and Systolic Pressure Generation, Vector Cardiogram Characteristics, and Their Implications in Clinical Cardiology

1

Left Ventricular Wall Stress Compendium to Analyze Heart Function

Dhanjoo N. Ghista, Harold Sandler, and Israel Mirsky

CONTENTS

1.1 Introduction

In 1963, two eminent cardiologists, Hal Sandler and Harold Dodge, published their pioneering paper on left ventricular (LV) tension and stress in man (Sandler and Dodge). This phenomenal paper stirred a huge amount of activity and inquiry into LV wall stress, its importance and implications. As a result, by 1969, three more pioneering works were published by Wong and Rautarharju (1968) at Dalhousie University,

Ghista and Sandler (1969) at NASA Ames Research Center, and Mirsky (1969) at Harvard University. Since, this activity has kept burgeoning until today. So, let us recognize and pay tribute to the pioneers Dr. Sandler and Dr. Dodge, as we embark on the exotic trail of LV wall stress.

Cardiologists and physiologists have long been interested in the quantification of LV wall stress. This is because (1) wall stress has been viewed as an important stimulus for the remodeling of the failing heart (Mann, 2004; Zhong et al., 2009a,b); (2) systolic wall stress, generated by LV contraction, is responsible for the development of intraventricular pressure; (3) wall stress is one of the determinants of myocardial oxygen consumption (MVO$_2$) and plays an important role in the mechanical behavior of the coronary circulation (Jan, 1985); (4) wall stress contributes to adverse consequences for energy metabolism, gene expression, and arrhythmia risk (Schwitter et al., 1992; Di Napoli et al., 2003; Alter et al., 2010); (5) systolic wall stress represents a primary determinant of MVO$_2$ in LV pressure and volume overload, and MVO$_2$ increases in diseases when myocardial hypertrophy becomes inadequate in coping with pressure and volume demands imposed on the left ventricle (Grossman, 1980); (6) systolic wall stress normalized with respect to LV pressure can also be employed as a noninvasive index of LV contractility (as is shown in Chapter 4), and hence as a measure of LV failure. Hence, the level and distribution of wall stress and its cyclic variation provide a quantitative evaluation of the response and adjustment of the LV to heart disease.

The joint use of imaging and modeling of the heart has opened up possibilities for a better thorough understanding and evaluation of the LV wall stress (see, for instance, the Physiome Project [Smith et al., 2002; Hunter et al., 2003; Crampin et al., 2004]). However, still due to the limitations of medical imaging and modeling capabilities, the application of heart models to employ human in vivo data for their use in clinical applications still remains a challenge, which this chapter attempts to address.

Traditionally, most works on LV wall stress have been based on 2D and 3D models that are represented by simplified idealized geometry analyses (e.g., a sphere, spheroid, or ellipsoid is used to approximate the shape of the ventricle) (Wong and Rautarharju, 1968; Ghista and Sandler, 1969; Mirsky 1969; Moriarty, 1980). The accuracy of these simplified geometry models is compromised because of the complex geometrical shapes and deformations of the left ventricle (Gould et al., 1972; Solomon et al., 1998). Finite element analysis (FEA), an engineering technique utilized to study complex structures, can overcome some of these limitations (Ghista and Hamid, 1977; Janz, 1982; Guccione et al., 1995; Bovendeerd et al., 1996; Costa et al., 1996a,b). Research in the past two decades has elucidated characteristics of LV wall stress, and clarified how they should be properly analyzed so that these concepts can be applied in translational research (Guccione et al., 2003; Dang et al., 2005a,b; Walker et al., 2005, 2008; Wall et al., 2006).

From the clinical applications consideration, the assessment and relevance of LV wall stress in heart failure (HF) has been studied by using angiography (Sandler and Dodge, 1963; Ghista and Hamid, 1977; Pouleur et al., 1984; Hayashida et al., 1990), echocardiography (Douglas et al., 1987; Feiring and Rumberger, 1992; Turcani and Rupp, 1997; Rohde et al., 1999; De Simone and Devereux, 2002), and cardiac magnetic resonance imaging (MRI) (Fujita et al., 1993; Balzer et al., 1999; Delepine et al., 2003; Prunier et al., 2008; Zhong et al., 2009b). In this regard, due to the different imaging modalities, some differences may occur in the data on LV geometry. However, most importantly, in order to properly bring to bear the clinical application of LV wall stress, we also need a clear understanding of the theories and analyses of LV wall stress (Mirsky, 1974).

Direct measurement of wall force in the intact heart using various types of strain gauge transducers coupled directed to the myocardium has also been attempted over the years (Hefner et al., 1962; Huisman et al., 1980). Some of the limitations (e.g., insertion of transducer damages the tissue) and problems associated with these direct measurement techniques have been extensively discussed by Huisman et al. (1980). They have demonstrated that much of the uncertainty in the measured values of wall stress was related to the degree of coupling between the transducer and the muscle wall.

This chapter deals with the biomechanical analyses, analytical and computational models used to characterize LV wall stress as well as clinical methods available for monitoring in vivo data to determine LV wall stress. We present the available methods for calculating ventricular wall stress and provide the reader with enough information to allow evaluation of the trade-off in accuracy between simplified models and more representative models for the purpose of clinical evaluation and applications of LV wall stress. We have provided herein a compendium of major type of wall stress models: thin-wall models based on Laplace's law, thick-wall shell models, elasticity theory dynamic shape model, thick-wall large deformation models, and finite element models (FEMs). We have compared the mean stress values of these models as well as the variation of stress across the wall. All of the thin-wall and thick-wall shell models are based on idealized ellipsoidal and spherical-shaped geometries. However, the elasticity model's shape varies throughout the cardiac cycle, to match the monitored LV shape and size. The FEMs have more representative geometries and are still shown to yield stress distribution (for radial, meridonial, and hoop stresses) across the wall that very closely match those obtained analytically in the elasticity model. We have prepared this chapter to enable our readers to obtain a comprehensive perspective of LV wall stress models, and of how to employ them to determine wall stresses, and employ them in medical applications to determine how LV copes with the after load demand and disease states like cardiomyopathy, as well as to noninvasively determine LV contractility to characterize LV failure.*

1.2 Left Ventricular Wall Stress

Stress is defined as the force acting on a surface divided by the cross-sectional area over which the force acts. Usually stress has many components, some of which act perpendicular to a surface (normal stresses) and others parallel to the surface (shear stress). An example of the stress components in a spherical coordinate system is shown in Figure 1.1. The unit of stress is Pascal.

In order to accurately assess LV wall stress, an appropriate characterization of the myocardial structure and properties is required. In the 1970s, in LV models the myocardium was assumed to be homogeneous and isotropic (Wong and Rautarharju, 1968;

---

* This chapter is based on Zhong L, Ghista DN, Tan RS, Left ventricular wall stress: A compendium, *Computer Methods in Biomechanics and Biomedical Engineering*, 15(10), 2012. With permission of Taylor & Francis.

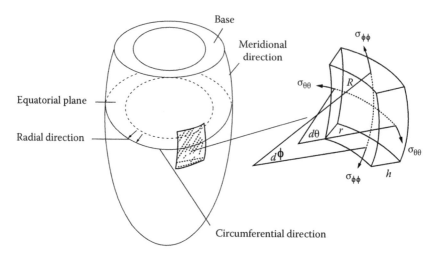

FIGURE 1.1
Stress concept, illustrating the principal directions and corresponding normal wall stress components in the spherical coordinates system. For the wall element, R is the meridional radius of curvature and r is the circumferential radius of curvature. (Adapted from Yin, F.C., *Circ. Res.*, 49, 829, 1981.)

Mirsky, 1969). However, studies made by some researchers (Streeter and Hanna, 1973a,b; Nielsen et al., 1991a,b) have shown that the architecture and orientation of myocardial fibers have significant effects on the mechanical properties of myocardium and on wall stress. Also, in a few studies, existing analytical models were modified to simulate anisotropic behavior of the wall tissue in the wall by introducing transmural variations in axial and circumferential stiffness of the material (Misra and Singh, 1985).

Myocardial properties include passive and active components. One of the simplest approaches for deriving the passive material properties of the myocardium is the uniaxial tension test. However, due to the 3D constitutive behavior of the myocardium, uniaxial stress–strain data are insufficient for the purpose (Costa et al., 2001). Triaxial testing is considered as the ideal approach, but it remains a challenging and difficult practice. It is thus the common practice for researchers (Yin et al., 1987; Huyghe et al., 1991; Nielsen et al., 1991a,b) to characterize myocardial material properties by biaxial tissue testing. In general, for its constitutive behavior, the myocardium is assumed to be hyperelastic with the strain energy density function formulated from biaxial experimental data. Based on this consideration, researchers have come up with different constitutive laws to describe the passive myocardial behavior (Humphrey et al., 1990; Guccoine et al., 1991; Hunter, 1997; Vetter and McCulloch, 2000).

Active muscle constitutive law is a relation between stress and strain rate, and is based on the sarcomere model of series elastic element, parallel elastic element, and contractile element, which is based on interaction between the actin and myosin filaments. Many constitutive laws have been proposed, including Hill's three-component model (Hill, 1950), Huxley's sliding-filament model (Huxley, 1957), Ghista's 3D rheological model (Ghista et al., 1973), Hunter's fading memory model (Hunter et al., 2003), Bestel–Clement–Sorine (BCS) model (Arts et al., 2001; Bestel et al., 2001; Costa et al.,2001; Hunter et al., 2003), and mechatronic sarcomere contractile model (Ghista et al., 2005). However, until now, there is still somewhat lack of reliable constitutive laws to describe the active properties of the myocardium during the systolic phase.

1.3 Left Ventricular Wall Stress Based on Laplace's Law: Sandler–Dodge Model

Despite its simplicity, the Laplace's law has been widely accepted by many investigators. With the simultaneous measurement of LV pressure and geometry, it is possible to quantify LV wall stress. Laplace derived the relationship relating the pressure inside a membrane to the radii of curvature and wall stress, way back in 1805 (Laplace, 1805). The generalized form of Laplace's law for a thin-walled prolate spheroid can be written as (Sandler and Dodge et al., 1963)

$$\frac{\sigma_\xi}{R_\xi} + \frac{\sigma_\theta}{R_\theta} = \frac{P}{h}, \quad \text{with } h \le R_\xi \text{ and } R_\theta \tag{1.1}$$

where
   σ_ξ and σ_θ are the circumferential and meridional stresses
   R_ξ and R_θ are the respective radii of curvature of the endocardial surface
   h is the wall thickness

Using this equation, Sandler and Dodge derived two formulas for the meridional and circumferential wall stresses at the equator, based on the following assumptions (Sandler and Dodge, 1963): (1) that the ventricle is isotropic and homogeneous and (2) that the stress across the wall is constant (a constant stress across the wall implies that there are no shear forces and bending moments). Their formulas for the stresses at the equator are

$$\sigma_\xi = \frac{P R_\theta^2}{(2R_\theta + h)h}, \quad \sigma_\theta = \left(\frac{Pb}{h}\right)\left(1 - \frac{b(b/a)^2}{(2b+h)}\right) \tag{1.2}$$

where
   a and b are the semimajor and semiminor axes of the internal elliptical cross section, respectively
   $R_\theta = b$
   $R_\xi = a^2/b$

If we assume that $h \ll b$, then the resulting expressions (for midwall geometry) are

$$\sigma_\xi = \frac{Pb}{2h}, \quad \sigma_\theta = \left(\frac{Pb}{h}\right)\left(1 - \frac{b^2}{2a^2}\right) \tag{1.3}$$

where a and b are, respectively, the semimajor and semiminor axes of the midwall elliptical cross section.

For the sphere, $a = b$, and so, from Equation 1.2, we have

$$\sigma_\theta = \sigma_\xi = \frac{Pa^2}{(2a+h)h} \tag{1.4}$$

where a is the internal radius, and

$$\sigma_\theta = \sigma_\xi = \frac{Pa}{2h}, \quad \text{for } h \ll a \tag{1.5}$$

Mirsky (1969) developed expressions for LV stress for a thick prolate spheroid (which we will present in the subsequent section), using thick shell theory (Mirsky, 1969). He then compared the meridional and circumferential average stresses in a prolate spheroid obtained from thick shell theory (for $h/b = 0.5$) expressions (1.8) and (1.9) (presented later), with those evaluated on the basis of Equation 1.2, as shown in Figure 1.2. It is seen, from this figure that the Laplace's law given by formula (1.2) yields stresses in reasonably close agreement (within 15%) with the thick wall theory.

This Laplace's law can provide a useful and reasonably accurate formula for calculating average ventricular stresses, which can be employed for determining LV contractility index ($= \sigma/P_{max}$), as developed and clinically applied by us (Zhong et al., 2007, 2009).

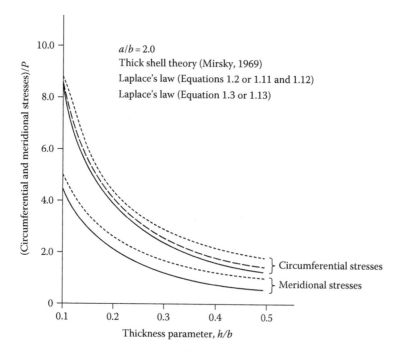

FIGURE 1.2
Comparison of stress distributions obtained by Laplace's law with thick-wall shell theory as shown in expressions (1.9) and (1.10). (Adapted from Mirsky, I., *Biophys. J.*, 9, 189, 1969.)

The major problem with Laplace's law and thin shell theory is that there is no variation of stress through the wall. The thick shell theory (and elasticity theory) provides this variation, which depicts the stress at the endocardial wall boundary to be maximum. This aspect has a bearing on the reason why myocardial infarcts are seen to generally occur at the inner wall of the left ventricle.

1.4 Left Ventricular Wall Stress Based on Thick-Shell Theory

In the late 1960s, there was a tremendous surge in research work on LV stresses, inspired by Sandler and Dodge pioneering paper on LV stress in *Circulation Research* in 1963. These works were on the development of LV stress based on thick shell theory, elasticity theory, and large elastic deformation theory. The thick-wall shell theory enables determination of stress variation across the LV wall from endocardium to epicardium. It can also include the effects of transverse normal stress (radial stress) and transverse shear deformation that accompanies bending stresses. These effects, which are physiologically significant for the left ventricle, are neglected in the development of Laplace's law. In this section, we will highlight the two principal works of Wong and Rautharju (1968) and Mirsky (1969).

1.4.1 Wong and Rautharju Thick Ellipsoidal Shell Model

The Wong and Rautharju model analysis (for LV approximated as a thick ellipsoidal shell) was employed by Hood et al. (1969) to determine stress distribution in the LV wall. Wong and Rautaharju (1968) developed equations which yielded nonlinear stress distribution across a thick-walled ellipsoidal shell. This made it possible, for the first time, to compare the mean stresses from thin- and thick-walled ellipsoidal models. In the Wong and Rautaharju model (1968), the ventricular wall is subjected to three types of stresses: radial stress (acting perpendicular to the endocardial surface), longitudinal stress, and circumferential stress (acting within the wall at right angles to each other).

The circumferential stress has been shown to be related to MVO$_2$ (Graham et al., 1971). Peak systolic circumferential stress has been adopted as the force factor in the application of the Hill force–velocity concept in intact man (Gault et al., 1968). Additionally, peak systolic circumferential stress has been shown to have a bearing on compensatory wall hypertrophy in chronic heart disease (Hood et al., 1969). All these studies employed thin-walled models for quantifying mean circumferential stress. The validity of thin-wall models could only be resolved after the availability of nonlinear distribution of stress across an ellipsoidal shell model of LV by Wong and Rautaharju (1968). Although this model is more sophisticated than that of Sandler and Dodge, it should be emphasized that some common basic assumptions have been made in both models, namely, that wall stress is considered in its passive sense (to be incurred passively form LV pressure), and the heart myocardial material is an isotropic and homogeneous. Consequently, the factor of fiber orientation and contraction is disregarded. In both models, other wall forces such as wall shear and bending moments are neglected.

Wong and Rautaharju developed a general equation for stress at any level from apex to base, whereas Sandler and Dodge solved for stress only at the equator of the ellipsoidal LV model. Consequently, for the purpose of comparison, circumferential stress calculations were made only at the equator. Application of thick-wall theory at the equator permits simplification of the general Wong and Rautaharju (W&R) equation into an expression using the same terms as that of Equation 1.2. If μ is taken to be 0.5, the circumferential stress, at any thickness depth (T) within the wall in the plane of the equator, is given by (Hood et al., 1969):

$$\sigma = \frac{PR_o^{(n+R)/2}R^{(n-R)/2}}{(R_o+h)^n - R_o^n}\left[1+\left(1-\frac{3b^4}{2(a^4+a^2b^2+b^4)}\right)\left(\frac{R_o+h}{R}\right)^n\right] \tag{1.6}$$

where

    a is the major semiaxis (cm)
    b is the minor semiaxis (cm)
    P is the pressure (dynes/cm²)
    h is the wall thickness (cm)
    R_o is the longitudinal radius of curvature at the endocardium = a^2/b
    $R = R_o + T$
    $n = (2a^2 + b^2)/b^2$

Hood et al. (1969) then employed this W&R equation (1.6) to calculate the stress at the endocardium, at the epicardium, and at nine evenly spaced points between the endocardium and epicardium. The mean circumferential stress was then calculated from the following expression:

$$\bar{\sigma}_{W\&R} = \frac{1}{h}\int_0^h \sigma(T)dT \tag{1.7}$$

which, at the equator becomes

$$\bar{\sigma}_{W\&R} = \frac{2PR_o^{(n-R)/2}}{h\left[(R_o+h)^n - R_o^n\right]}\left[\frac{(R_o+h)^{(n-1)/2}-R_o^{(n-1)/2}}{n-1}+\frac{(R_o+h)^n\left((R_o)^{-(n+1)/2}-(R_o+h)^{-(n+1)/2}\right)}{n+1}\left(\frac{2a^4-b^4}{2(a^4+a^2b^2+b^4)}\right)\right] \tag{1.8}$$

where all the model parameters are defined in Equation 1.6.

    For calculating stress based on this expression, biplane angiograms (obtained at a filming speed of 8 s⁻¹ for 5 s) were employed to derive chamber dimensions and wall thickness of the left ventricle throughout the cardiac cycle (Hood et al., 1969). The major semiaxis (a) of the chamber was taken to be one-half the longest length measurable within the cavity silhouette on either the antero-posterior or lateral film. The planimetry silhouette area and measured longest length from each x-ray film were substituted into the equation for the area of an ellipse, in order to derive the minor axis. Then the minor axes from each antero-posterior and lateral film pair were averaged (geometric mean) and divided by 2, to give the minor semiaxis (b) of an idealized prolate ellipsoid. The wall thickness (h) was derived as the average width of a 4 cm segment of free wall immediately below the equator on each antero-posterior film. The mean stress based on Sandler and Dodge model and Wong and Rautaharju model are then compared in terms of the percent error, with the thick-wall stress being taken as the standard of reference: percent error = $(\sigma_{S\&D} - \sigma_{W\&R})/\sigma_{W\&R} \times 100\%$.

Selected mean circumferential stress and dimensional data from all subjects have been summarized in Table 1.1 (Hood et al., 1969). It can be seen that the degree of overestimation in terms of percent error usually varies between 5% and 15% in individual patients and overall averaged about 10%.

Comparison of calculated stress at end-diastole shows that the thin-wall equation overestimates mean thick-wall stress by more than 15%. Furthermore, even at end-systole when h/b has its maximum value, the percent error between the two formulae is also around 10%. The Sandler and Dodge formula is simpler and more convenient to use in clinical application compared to Wong and Rautajarju formula. However, the Sandler and Dodge formula permits calculation only of mean stress and only at the equation, whereas, the Wong and Rautaharju analysis permits calculation of stress at any depth within the wall. It also theoretically allows quantification of stress at any point on the ventricle, although difficulties in measuring wall thickness from angiocardiograms in human subjects can limit stress determination to the wall regions at the equator.

1.4.2 Mirsky Thick-Walled Ellipsoidal Shell Model

The Mirsky thick-walled ellipsoidal model, illustrated in Figure 1.3, includes the effects of transverse normal stress (radial stress) and transverse shear deformation. The model presents a system of differential equations for the stress equilibrium in the wall of the thick-walled prolate spheroid. These equations were derived from the 3D equations of elasticity, by employing the method of the calculus of variations. The analysis for the LV stress involves the solution of these differential equations by numerical integration and asymptotic expansion of displacement and stress formations. The geometrical data employed in the evaluation of the stresses were obtained from biplane angiocardiography. The results indicate that maximum stresses occur in the circumferential direction on the endocardial surface at the equator of the ellipsoid, which we all know now. Also, during a cardiac cycle, this stress is found to be maximum either prior to, or at the time of peak left ventricular pressure (LVP).

For the analysis, the following assumptions were made: (1) the myocardium is composed of an isotropic and homogeneous elastic material, having Poisson's ratio = 0.5'; (2) throughout the cardiac cycle, the geometry of the ventricle is approximated by a prolate spheroid of uniform wall thickness; (3) instantaneous measurements of geometry and LVP were employed in a static analysis for the evaluation of instantaneous stresses throughout the cardiac cycle; (4) ventricular wall stress and deformations are independent of the circumferential coordinate and are due to the LVP only; (5) the effects of transverse normal stress (radial stress) and transverse shear are included; (6) the quasi-static analysis is performed over short intervals of time for which the deformations are small.

The model coordinate system, the shell element (in deformed and undeformed states), and the stress and moment resultants are illustrated in Figure 1.3.

Simplified expressions for the equatorial stresses were obtained as follows:

$$\sigma_{\xi\xi} = \frac{\left[\sigma_{\xi ME} + (2\xi/h)\sigma_{\xi BE}\right]}{(1 + \xi/b)}$$

TABLE 1.1

Thin-Wall Versus Thick-Wall Stress Analysis

Group	No.	End-diastole					Peak systole					End-systole				
		h/b	a/b	σ_{SsD}	σ_{WsR}	% error	h/b	a/b	σ_{SsD}	σ_{WsR}	% error	h/b	a/b	σ_{SsD}	σ_{WsR}	% error
Normal left ventricle (EDV = 140 ± 11)	6	0.35 ± 0.03	2.1 ± 0.1	32 ± 6	29 ± 5	7.2 ± 0.8	0.44 ± 0.03	2.1 ± 0.1	326 ± 24	304 ± 24	7.0 ± 0.8	1.05 ± 0.09	2.6 ± 0.1	123 ± 0.22	115 ± 21	7.8 ± 0.9
Mitral stenosis (EDV = 121 ± 8)	9	0.30 ± 0.02	1.0 ± 0.1	42 ± 7	39 ± 6	7.4 ± 0.4	0.38 ± 0.03	2.0 ± 0.1	359 ± 29	333 ± 28	8.0 ± 0.9	0.6 ± 0.04	2.3 ± 0.1	195 ± 34	180 ± 32	8.0 ± 0.7
Volume overload (EDV = 239 ± 22)	19	0.31 ± 0.01	1.8 ± 0.03	53 ± 6	48 ± 5	9.3 ± 0.5	0.43 ± 0.03	2.0 ± 1.0	354 ± 19	328 ± 18	8.2 ± 0.5	0.77 ± 0.09	2.2 ± 0.03	147 ± 20	130 ± 18	9.0 ± 0.6
Pressure overload compensated (EDV = 123 ± 20)	5	0.43 ± 0.07	2.0 ± 0.1	33 ± 3	31 ± 3	8.0 ± 1.0	0.53 ± 0.05	2.2 ± 1.0	393 ± 43	385 ± 41	7.6 ± 0.7	1.29 ± 0.28	2.6 ± 0.1	122 ± 38	113 ± 36	8.8 ± 0.7
Pressure or volume overload, decompensated, and primary myocardial disease (EDV = 314 ± 51)	9	0.35 ± 0.03	1.7 ± 0.04	1.7 ± 0.04	67 ± 14	11.2 ± 0.7	0.38 ± 0.03	1.7 ± 0.04	386 ± 15	347 ± 15	11.6 ± 0.05	0.52 ± 0.05	1.8 ± 0.1	198 ± 36	176 ± 32	12.3 ± 0.8
Idiopathic myocardial hypertrophy (EDV = 101 ± 41)	2	0.82 ± 0.24	2.0 ± 0.2	2.0 ± 0.2	39 ± 17	14 ± 7	1.05 ± 0.06	2.5 ± 0.6	171 ± 26	155 ± 7	11.5 ± 7.0	2.38 ± 0.39	2.5 ± 0.6	68 ± 16	59 ± 18	18.5 ± 10.5

Source: Adapted from Hood, W.P. et al., *Circ. Res.*, XXIV, 575, 1969.

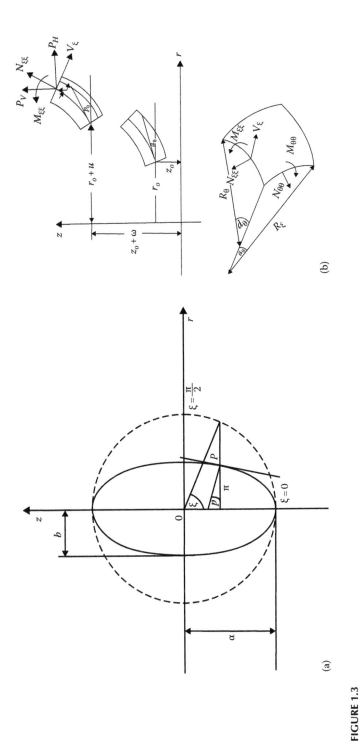

FIGURE 1.3

Ellipsoidal thick-shell model: (a) With reference to the cylindrical coordinate system (r, θ, z), the middle surface of a closed ellipsoidal shell of revolution is represented as: $r = b\sin\xi$, $z = -a\cos\xi$, $0 \leq \xi \leq \pi$, where a and b are, respectively, the semimajor and semiminor axes of the elliptical cross section of the middle surface; the coordinate ξ represents the eccentric angle of ellipse. (b) Elements of the shell in deformed and undeformed states, and stress and moment resultants acting on the shell element. (Adapted from Mirsky, I., *Biophys. J.*, 9, 189, 1969.)

$$\sigma_{\theta\theta} = \frac{\left[\sigma_{\theta ME} + (2\xi/h)\sigma_{\theta BE}\right]}{(1 + \xi b/a^2)} \tag{1.9}$$

$$N_{\theta\theta} = \sigma_{\theta\theta} h$$

where the membrane stresses $\sigma_{\xi ME}$, $\sigma_{\theta ME}$, and the bending stresses $\sigma_{\xi BE}$, $\sigma_{\theta BE}$ are given by

$$\sigma_{\xi ME} = \left(\frac{pb}{2h}\right)\left(1 - \frac{h}{2b}\right)^2$$

$$\sigma_{\theta ME} = \left(\frac{pb}{h}\right)\left(1 - \frac{h}{2b}\right)\left(1 - \frac{hb}{2a^2}\right) - \left(\frac{pb^2}{2a^2h}\right)$$

$$\left[1 - \left(\frac{h}{b}\right) + \left(\frac{h^2}{9b^2}\right)\right]\left\{4.5 + 3\left(\frac{b}{a}\right)^2 + 2.25\left(\frac{b}{a}\right)^4 + 2.5\left(\frac{b}{a}\right)^6 - 10\left(\frac{b}{a}\right)^8\right\}\right]$$

$$\sigma_{\xi BE} = \frac{6M_{\xi\xi}}{h^2} = \left(\frac{p}{4}\right)\begin{bmatrix} 1 + 3\left(\dfrac{b}{a}\right)^2 - \left(\dfrac{8}{3}\right)\left(\dfrac{b}{a}\right)^4 - \left(\dfrac{4}{3}\right)\left(\dfrac{b}{a}\right)^6 \\ -\left(\dfrac{h}{b}\right) + 0.25\left(\dfrac{h}{b}\right)^2 + 0.55\left(\dfrac{h}{a}\right)^2 + 0.9\left(\dfrac{hb}{a^2}\right)^2 \end{bmatrix}$$

$$\sigma_{\theta BE} = \frac{6M_{\theta\theta}}{h^2} = -\left(\frac{p}{2}\right)\begin{bmatrix} 1 - 2.5\left(\dfrac{b}{a}\right)^2 + 1.167\left(\dfrac{b}{a}\right)^4 + 0.333\left(\dfrac{b}{a}\right)^6 \\ -0.323\left(\dfrac{h}{b}\right)^2 + 0.23\left(\dfrac{h}{a}\right)^2 + 0.5\left(\dfrac{hb}{a^2}\right)^2 - 1.42\left(\dfrac{b^2h^2}{a^4}\right) \end{bmatrix} \tag{1.10}$$

For the purpose of comparison of the stress values obtained by expressions (1.9) and (1.10) with those obtained by Laplace's law, we will (for the sake of convenience) again provide the Laplace's law thin shell expressions. For a prolate spheroid, the meridional mean stress $\sigma_{\xi\xi}$ at the equator (obtained by equilibrating the forces to the pressure loading) is given by

$$\sigma_{\xi 1} = \frac{pb_i^2}{(2b_i + h)h} \tag{1.11}$$

and the circumferential mean stress $\sigma_{\theta\theta}$ is given by

$$\sigma_{\theta 1} = \left(\frac{pb_i}{h}\right)\left[1 - \frac{b_i(b_i/a_i)^2}{(2b_i + h)}\right] \tag{1.12}$$

where a_i and b_i are, respectively, the semimajor and semiminor axes of the internal elliptical cross section.

If we assume midwall geometry for the radii of curvature, the resulting expressions are

$$\sigma_{\xi 2} = \frac{pb}{2h}$$

$$\sigma_{\theta 2} = \left(\frac{pb}{h} \right) \left[1 - \left(\frac{b^2}{2a^2} \right) \right] \tag{1.13}$$

where a and b correspond to the midwall cross section.

For a spherical-shaped model, the meridional and circumferential stresses are equal and independent of the angular coordinates and are given by

$$\sigma_{\theta 3} = \sigma_{\xi 3} = \frac{pb_i^2}{h(2b_i + h)} \tag{1.14}$$

For $h \ll b_i$, the stresses at internal wall and midwall are given by

$$\sigma_{\theta 4} = \sigma_{\xi 4} = \frac{pb_i}{2h} \tag{1.15}$$

$$\sigma_{\theta 5} = \sigma_{\xi 5} = \frac{pb}{2h} \tag{1.16}$$

where
b_i is the internal radius of the sphere
b is the midwall (or mean) radius

The exact result for the mean stress is

$$\sigma_{\theta 6} = \frac{pb_i(4b_i^2 + b_o^2 + b_i b_o)}{4(b_o^3 - b_i^3)} \tag{1.17}$$

where b_o is the outer radius of the sphere.

For two patients (HW and WER), the stresses in Equations 1.9 and 1.10 were computed from LV biplane angiocardiogram-derived geometry and intraventricular pressure measurements. In Figure 1.4, the time histories of these two patients HW and WER are depicted for the maximum (endocardial equatorial) circumferential stress ($\sigma_{\theta\theta}$), along with the circumferential force/unit length ($N_{\theta\theta}$), in relation to the LVP. It is seen that the maximum stress occurs either prior to, or at the time of peak intraventricular pressure. This result demonstrates the relationship of stress on LV systolic geometry and pressure.

The stress distributions through the wall thickness are depicted in Figure 1.5 for three values of ξ (= 0°, 50°, and 90°) at the time of maximum stress, for patient WER. It can be noted that the stress gradients through the wall increase as we proceed from the equator to the apex, where the bending stresses become more significant. As expected, the

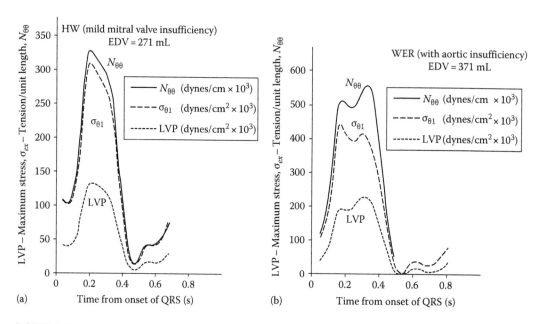

FIGURE 1.4

Left ventricular pressure, circumferential stress ($\sigma_{\theta\theta}$) and tension/unit length ($N_{\theta\theta}$) versus time for (a) a patient with mild mitral valve insufficiency, (b) a patient with aortic insufficiently. *Note*: dynes/cm^2 = 0.1 Pa. (Adapted from Mirsky, I., *Biophys. J.*, 9, 189, 1969.)

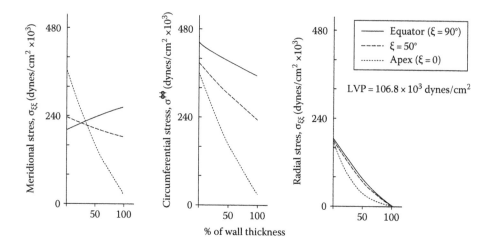

FIGURE 1.5

Thick-wall stress distributions through the wall at three values of ξ for patient WER. *Note*: 1 dynes/cm^2 = 0.1 Pa. (Adapted from Mirsky, I., *Biophys. J.*, 9, 189, 1969.)

stresses decrease from a maximum value on the endocardial surface to a minimum on the epicardial surface. Also, as expected, the circumferential and meridional stresses are tensile, where the radial stress is always compressive. It can be noted that the maximum (endocardial) circumferential stress is 2.5 times the LV pressure (or the maximum radial stress on the endocardial surface). This validates the use of thick shell analysis. In the

TABLE 1.2

Comparison of Thick Shell Theory and Laplace's Law with Exact Solution for a Sphere

	Maximum Stress		Average Stresses				
	$\sigma_{\theta 1}/P$					Laplace	
h/b	Exact	Present	Exact	Present	$\sigma_{\theta 3}/P$	$\sigma_{\theta 4}/P$	$\sigma_{\theta 5}/P$
0.1	4.78	4.77	4.51	4.51	4.51	4.75	5.25
0.2	2.35	2.30	2.07	2.03	2.03	2.25	2.75
0.3	1.52	1.49	1.22	1.21	1.20	1.42	1.92
0.4	1.13	1.09	0.81	0.82	0.80	1.00	1.50
0.5	0.91	0.86	0.59	0.58	0.56	0.75	1.25

Source: Adapted from Mirsky, I., *Biophys. J.*, 9, 189, 1969.
Note: The stresses $\sigma_{\theta 1}/P$, $\sigma_{\theta 3}/P$, $\sigma_{\theta 4}/P$, and $\sigma_{\theta 5}/P$ are given by Equations 1.12, 1.14, 1.15, and 1.16, respectively; the exact stress is given by Equation 1.17.

development of Laplace's law, this stress is neglected entirely. These equatorial stresses agree with the results obtained by Wong and Rautaharju (1968) and this is because the effects of bending stresses, which were neglected in Wong and Rautaharju analysis, are insignificant at the equator. It is interesting that for the thick-walled spherical elasticity solution of wall stress expression (Equation 1.2), the maximum endocardial stress is 1.6 times of the LV pressure.

In Table 1.2, the stresses based on this thick-shell analysis are compared with the stresses based on (1) the exact solution (Equation 1.17) based on the classical theory of elasticity for a thick spherical shell (Timoshenko and Goodier, 1951) and (2) Laplace's law, for the special case of the sphere. In this table, it is relevant to observe the results for the realistic case of $h/b = 0.3$. We find that the thick-shell analysis value is almost equal to the exact solution for both maximum and average stresses. However, for the average stress, only the Laplace analysis for $\sigma_{\theta 3}$ gives results corresponding to the exact solution and is hence valid to employ.

In the earlier Figure 1.2, we can observe the comparison of the meridional and circumferential average stresses in a prolate spheroid obtained from this thick shell theory ($\sigma_{\zeta\zeta}$ and $\sigma_{\theta\theta}$ in Equations 1.9 and 1.10) with those evaluated on the basis of the two versions of Laplace's law ($\sigma_{\zeta 1}$ and $\sigma_{\theta 1}$, and $\sigma_{\zeta 2}$ and $\sigma_{\theta 2}$, in Equations 1.11 through 1.13). It is noted that the modified form of Laplace's law based on internal geometry and given by formulae (1.11) and (1.12) are in closer agreement with the thick-wall analysis result. The meridional stresses are actually identical, and the circumferential mean stresses differ by no more than 15% from the thick-wall theory for relatively thick shells ($h/b = 0.5$). Thus Laplace's law formulae, as given by Equations 1.11 and 1.12, are useful and reasonably accurate for calculating average (or mean) ventricular wall stress.

The important significance of this thick-shell theory is the variation of circumferential wall stress through the wall. As seen in Figure 1.5, the high stress in the endocardial wall implies that in systole the myocardial oxygen demand is very high in the endocardial region. Further the high stress in this region has the effect of squeezing the coronary vessels in the inner wall region of the LV, which increases the resistance to coronary flow. This decreases myocardial perfusion in the inner wall region. Thus, there can arise a situation of oxygen perfusion versus demand mismatch, resulting in the formation of a myocardial infarct. This is why there is a preponderance of myocardial infarcts in the inner wall of the LV.

1.5 Ghista–Sandler 3D Elasticity Model of the LV

We have gone over the 3D LV models based on thick shell theory of ellipsoidal shell (Wong and Rautarharju, 1968; Mirsky, 1969), which have certain assumptions compared to the use of elasticity theory. So, we will now study the Ghista and Sandler 3D elasticity model of the LV. The model simulates the instantaneous 3D geometry of the LV by a quasi-ellipsoidal shaped geometry, as depicted in Figure 1.6 (Ghista and Sandler, 1969, Ghista et al., 1971, 1973). The noteworthy feature of this model is that its shape is adjustable with the varying shape of the LV, as it becomes more ellipsoidal and thicker during systole.

This model comprises of superposed: (1) Line Dilatation system, over a length "*a*" along the longitudinal axis of LV, of amplitude parameter A (Figure 1.6a), (2) and a hydrostatic stress system, of amplitude parameter B. Incorporating LV catheterization and cineangiography monitored LV pressure and geometry data in patients, this model yields (1) the expression for LV wall stresses (whose variations across the wall are depicted in Figure 1.6c), (2) the principle stress-trajectory surfaces (shown in Figure 1.6a), having approximately ellipsoidal LV geometry, and (3) the expressions for the displacements at these stress-trajectory surfaces. Based on elasticity theory, the model provides for (1) shear in the ventricular wall, (2) normal stress in the ventricular wall, and (3) variation of stresses across the wall.

For employment of the Ghista–Sandler model, we have first to determine the shape parameters so that the model's instantaneous major dimensions (maximum length L, maximum width W, and thickness H) match the corresponding dimensions of the LV, recorded as shown in Figure 1.6d.

1.5.1 Shape Parameters of the Model

The analytical model is derived (in cylindrical coordinates) by superposing a line dilatation force system (obtained by distributing point dilatations along a portion of length $2a$ of the y-axis of revolution) of intensity A, and uniform hydrostatic stress system of intensity B. Stress trajectories of the combined system are drawn in a plane containing the axis of revolution, with coordinates $\bar{r} = r/a$, $\bar{y} = y/a$. The two trajectories, whose intercepts' ratios $R_1 (= \bar{y}_1/\bar{r}_1)$, $R_2 (= \bar{y}_2/\bar{r}_2)$ on the axes $\bar{r}$, $\bar{y}$ equal the ratios of length-to-width of the inner and outer surfaces of the LV, namely, L/W and $(L + 2H)/(W + 2H)$, are selected to represent the inner and outer boundaries of the geometrically similar model (see Figure 1.6). These intercepts' ratios R_1 and R_2 are referred to as the shape parameters of the model.

Now, to make the geometrically similar model match the actual model in size, we select the values of the factor "*a*" (the size parameter of the model) equal to the ratio of half-the-width ($W/2$) of the inner surface LV chamber and the "*r*" intercept $\bar{r}_1$ of the inner boundary of the geometrically similar model. At this stage, the stresses due to the constituent stress systems of the model are functions of the stress intensity parameters A and B.

The parameters A and B of the two stress systems are obtained by satisfying the boundary conditions that (1) the instantaneous change in stress on the inner surface of the model must equal the instantaneous change in chamber pressure ΔP, and (2) the stress on the outer surface of the model must be zero. Once the intensity of parameter A and B are obtained in terms of the data quantities of the LV chamber pressure and dimensions, the stresses in the model are also expressed completely in terms of these data quantities.

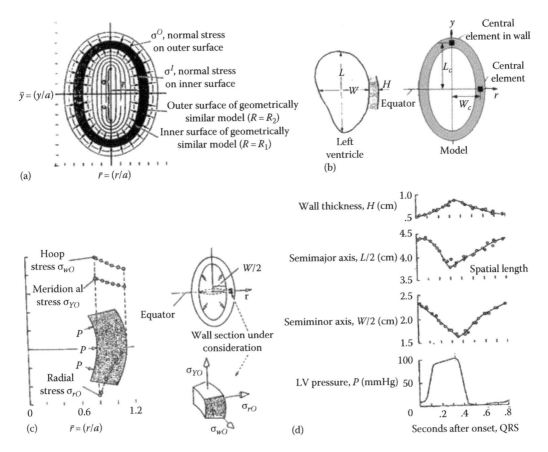

FIGURE 1.6
(a) Stress trajectories for the analytical LV model: the radial stress at the inner surface of the LV equals the LV pressure and that at the outer surface of LV is zero, for evaluating the stress intensity parameters A and B; (b) Comparison of actual left ventricle geometry with corresponding model geometry: The LV model expressions for incremental circumferential and meridional strains at the central equatorial element (in terms of the instantaneous modulus E) are made to match the computed incremental strains (based on LV geometry data), to evaluate E of the LV; (c) 3D stress distribution across the left ventricular wall, depicting the maximum endocardial hoop stress value to be equal to twice the value of chamber pressure; (d) LV pressure and dimensions during a cardiac cycle, constituting the data for the model application. These figures are based on the Ghista–Sandler model. (Adapted from Ghista, D.N. and Sandler, H., *Med. Biol. Eng.*, 13(2), 151, 1975.)

1.5.2 The Stress in the Model

The instantaneous stresses in the instantaneous model of the LV (the instantaneous model simulates the LV at an instant during the cardiac cycle) are given in dimensionless $(\bar{r}, \bar{y})$ as follows:

$$
\sigma_{rr} = \frac{A}{a^2}\left[
\begin{array}{l}
-\dfrac{2}{\bar{r}^2}\left\{ \dfrac{(\bar{y}+1)}{\left[(\bar{y}+1)^2+\bar{r}^2\right]^{1/2}} - \dfrac{(\bar{y}-1)}{\left[(\bar{y}+1)^2+\bar{r}^2\right]^{1/2}} \right\} \\[4ex]
+2\left\{ \dfrac{(\bar{y}-1)}{\left[(\bar{y}+1)^2+\bar{y}^2\right]^{3/2}} - \dfrac{(\bar{y}+1)}{\left[(\bar{y}-1)^2+\bar{y}^2\right]^{3/2}} \right\}
\end{array}
\right] + B
$$

$$\sigma_{ry} = \sigma_{yr} = \frac{A}{a^2}\left[2\bar{r}\left\{\frac{1}{\left[(\bar{y}+1)^2+(\bar{r})^2\right]^{3/2}} - \frac{1}{\left[(\bar{y}-1)^2+(\bar{r})^2\right]^{3/2}}\right\}\right]$$

$$\sigma_{yy} = \frac{A}{a^2}\left[2\left\{\frac{\bar{y}+1}{\left[(\bar{y}+1)^2+(\bar{r})^2\right]^{3/2}} - \frac{\bar{y}-1}{\left[(\bar{y}-1)^2+(\bar{r})^2\right]^{3/2}}\right\}\right] + B$$

$$\sigma_{ww} = \frac{A}{a^2}\left[\frac{2}{\bar{r}}\left\{\frac{\bar{y}+1}{\left[(\bar{y}+1)^2+(\bar{r})^2\right]^{1/2}} - \frac{\bar{y}-1}{\left[(\bar{y}-1)^2+(\bar{r})^2\right]^{1/2}}\right\}\right] + B \qquad (1.18)$$

where
$$\bar{r} = r/a$$
$$\bar{y} = y/a$$

In Equation 1.18, the parameters A and B are given in terms of the instantaneous values of chamber pressure and dimensions as follows:

$$A = \frac{-\Delta P}{\frac{4}{a^2}\mu\left\{\frac{1+2(d_1/a)^2}{(d_1/a)^2\left[(d_2/a)^2+1\right]^{3/2}} - \frac{1+2(d_1/a)^2}{(d_1/a)^2\left[(d_2/a)^2+1\right]^{3/2}}\right\}} = \frac{(\Delta P)a^2}{\mu k_1}$$

$$B = \frac{-(\Delta P)(d_1/a)^2\left[(d_1/a)^2+1\right]^{3/2}\left[1+2(d_1/a)^2\right]}{\left\{(d_1/a)^2\left[1+2(d_2/a)^2\right]\left[(d_1/a)^2+1\right]^{3/2} - (d_1/a)^2\left[1+2(d_1/a)^2\right]\left[(d_2/a)^2+1\right]^{3/2}\right\}} \qquad (1.19)$$

where
d_1 and d_2 are given in terms of the instantaneous width (W)
H, wall thickness, as follows: $d_1 = W/2$, $d_2 = (W/2) + H$

We need to note that the stresses given by Equations 1.18 and 1.19 are due to the instantaneous changes (ΔP) in pressure P and hence provide instantaneous changes ($\Delta\sigma$) in the stresses (Equation 1.18). In order to obtain stress at an instant, we can sum up the instantaneous stresses ($\Delta\sigma$) or even put the term P instead of ΔP in Equation 1.19.

Now, for the central equatorial element shown in Figure 1.6, the stresses are given by

$$\sigma_{rr} = -\frac{4A}{a^2}\frac{(2d_c^2+1)}{d_c^2(d_c^2+1)^{3/2}} + B$$

$$\sigma_{ry} = 0 = \sigma_{yr}$$

$$\sigma_{yy} = -\frac{4A}{a^2} \frac{1}{(d_c^2 + 1)^{3/2}} + B$$

$$\sigma_{ww} = -\frac{4A}{a^2} \frac{1}{d_c^2 (d_c^2 + 1)^{1/2}} + B \qquad (1.20)$$

where $d_c = \dfrac{W + H}{2a}$.

The Ghista and Sandler (1969) model has added intrinsic features that the shell models do not have; this is because it is an elasticity model. As can be seen from Figure 1.6a, the model resembles a thick-walled ellipsoid of revolution but allows for a variation in shape during a cycle as well as for simulation of enlarged LVs of persons (say, due to regurgitant aortic valve). It can be seen (from the shape of the stress trajectories) that the model becomes less oval-shaped as the internal cavity gets bigger as diastolic filling proceeds and becomes more oval-shaped as it becomes smaller as during systolic ejection phase. It can also be seen that simulation of enlarged LV chambers will yield model geometries that are less oval-shaped. This corresponds to the clinical situation, wherein enlarged LV chambers become less oval-shaped and more spherically shaped.

This model is hence more representative of the cyclic LV geometry compared to shell models. This model also then yields a more representative stress distribution in the LV wall. Further, it being an elasticity model, there is flexibility to make the model shape even more representative of the LV geometry during the diastole and systolic phases. For instance, we can shorten the length of the line dilation along the *y*-axis to make the model more conical in shape. We can also make the model more innovative by superposing additional stress systems corresponding to a series of pressurized sphere along the wall, to simulate the pressure of coronary artery vessels in the wall. We can then study the variation of the size of these coronary artery vessels across the wall thickness, so as to get an idea of how the LV wall stress affects the wall perfusion.

1.6 Left Ventricular Wall Stress Based on Large Deformation Theory

Thick-wall elasticity and shell models have been developed by Ghista and Sandler (1969), Wong and Rautaharju (1968), and Mirsky (1969). For thick-wall structures, the model should include the effects of transverse normal stress (radial stress) and transverse shear deformation, which always accompanies bending stresses. The analysis then yields a nonlinear stress distribution through the wall thickness, a result that cannot be predicted by Laplace's law.

This far, in the models presented, linear elasticity has been assumed, that is, deformations of the order 5%–10% are assumed to take place. However, during the contractile and ejection phases, substantial changes in the ventricular dimensions can occur. For such large deformation, it is more appropriate to apply the large elastic deformation theory in order to obtain a more accurate description of the stress distribution.

Mirsky (1973) investigated the specific effect of large deformations on stresses in the LV, which was approximated by a thick-walled sphere composed of isotropic, homogeneous,

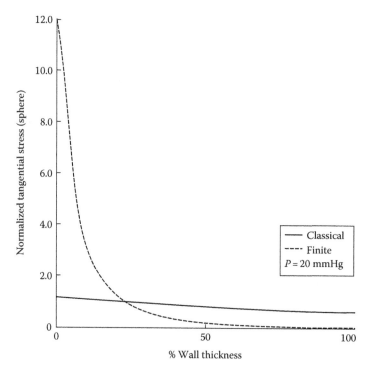

FIGURE 1.7
The circumferential stress (normalized to the Laplace stress $\sigma = Pa/2h$, based on the classical theory and large deformation theory) is shown plotted as a function of wall thickness. There is a marked difference in the stresses, particularly in the endocardial layer. (Adapted from Mirsky, I., Review of various theories for the evaluation of left ventricular wall stress, in *Cardiac Mechanics*, Mirsky, I., Ghista, D.N., and Sandler, D. eds. Wiley, New York, 1973, pp. 381–409.)

and incompressible material. The stresses at a given pressure level were calculated from a strain energy density function. Using data from dog studies (Spontnitz et al., 1966), he evaluated this function at the midwall, based on strains and cavity and wall volumes at that particular cavity pressure. The nonlinear relation between stress and strain was assumed to be of exponential form. The major finding of this study is that inclusion of nonlinear stress–strain properties predicts a very high stress concentration at the endo-cardium, which is almost 10 times higher than predicted by linear elasticity theory, as depicted in Figure 1.7. This stress concentration is noted to increase markedly as the LV cavity pressure is increased, such as during systole it may well be that such an analysis could provide some insight into the mechanisms causing ischemia in the endocardial lay-ers of the LV, based on strain energy values, evaluated in this region.

Another noteworthy contribution to the application of large deformation shell theory LV is by Chaudhry et al. (1996, 1997), who employed a more realistic circular-conical shell model (closed at the apical end). Both Mirsky (1973) and Chaudhry et al. used dog studies data of Spontnitz et al. (1966) to demonstrate how LV stresses can be determined.

For the Mirsky LV model, let the spherical coordinate system (R, θ, ψ) refer to the strained state of the model (with its origin at the center of the shell), and (r, θ, ϕ) coordinate system refer to the unstained state. Denoting the internal and external radii of the LV shell in the unstrained and strained states by r_1, r_2 and R_1, R_2, respectively, we have the following relations based on the incompressibility condition:

$$r^3 - R^3 = r_1^3 - R_1^3 = r_2^3 - R_2^3 \tag{1.21}$$

$$Q(R) = \frac{r}{R} = \left(1 + \frac{r_1^3 - R_1^3}{R^3}\right)^{1/3} \tag{1.22}$$

The strain energy density function W (the amount of mechanical energy required to deform a given volume of material) is generally a function of the strain components r_{ij}, namely γ_{11}, γ_{22}, γ_{33}, the radial, circumferential, and meridional strains. However, for the special case of spherical symmetry with an incompressible material, the strain energy density function W was taken to be a function of the strain invariant I, given by:

$$I = Q^4 + \frac{2}{Q^2} \tag{1.23}$$

so that W is expressed as $W = W(I)$.
The radial and circumferential stresses are given by

$$\tau^{11} = 2Q^4 \frac{\partial W}{\partial I} + P_H \tag{1.24}$$

$$R^2 \tau^{22} = (2/Q^2) \frac{\partial W}{\partial I} + P_H \tag{1.25}$$

where P_H, the hydrostatic pressure, is determined from the equilibrium equation as:

$$P_H = -Q^4 \phi + 2 \int^{Q} (Q^3 + 1) \phi \, dQ + C \tag{1.26}$$

where $\phi = 2\partial W/\partial I$ and C is a constant of integration to be determined from the boundary conditions:

$$\tau^{11} = -P \text{ on } R = R_1; \quad \tau^{11} = 0 \text{ on } R = R_2 \tag{1.27}$$

Equations 1.24 through 1.27 yield the following relations:

$$\tau^{11}(R = R_1) = -P = 2 \int^{Q_1} (Q^3 + 1) \phi \, dQ + C \left(Q_1 = \frac{r_1}{R_1}\right)$$

$$P_H = -Q^4 \phi + K(R) - P = -2Q^4 \left(\frac{\partial W}{\partial I}\right) + K(R) - P \tag{1.28}$$

where

$$K(R) = 2\int_{Q_1}^{Q} (Q^3 + 1)\phi \, dQ$$

$$\tau^{11} = K(R) - P$$

$$R^2\tau^{22} = \left(\frac{1}{Q^2 - Q^4}\right)\phi + K(R) - P$$

$$K(R_2) = P \tag{1.29}$$

The equilibrium condition $K(Q_2) = P$, given by

$$P = K(R_2) = \int_{Q_1}^{Q_2} 4(Q^3 + 1)\left(\frac{\partial W}{\partial I}\right)dQ = \left(\frac{\partial W}{\partial I}\right)_m \left[\left(Q_2^4 - Q_1^4\right) + 4(Q_2 - Q_1)\right] \tag{1.30}$$

serves to determine the deformed radius R_1 if the pressure P and the strain energy density W are known, since R_2 can be expressed in terms of R_1 via the incompressibility condition (Equation 1.21).

From the stress expressions (1.24) and (1.25), $\partial W/\partial I$ is evaluated by employing midwall values for the stress components $(\tau^{11}, R^2\tau^{22})$, as obtained from the classical theory of elasticity for a thick spherical shell (Timoshenko and Goodier, 1951). These classical theory stresses are given by

$$R_m{}^2 r_m{}^{22} = P\left(\frac{V}{V_w}\right)\left[1 + 0.5\left(\frac{R_2}{R_m}\right)^3\right]$$

$$\tau_m{}^{11} = P\left(\frac{V}{V_m}\right)\left[1 - \left(\frac{R_2}{R_m}\right)^3\right] \tag{1.31}$$

where
  V is the LV volume
  V_w is the LV wall volume
  the subscript m denotes the midwall value

Thus, $(\partial W/\partial I)_m$ is given by

$$\left(\frac{\partial W}{\partial I}\right)_m = \frac{Q_m{}^2\left(R_m{}^2 r_m{}^{22} - \tau_m{}^{11}\right)}{2\left(1 - Q_m{}^6\right)} = 0.75P\left(\frac{V}{V_w}\right)\left(\frac{R_2}{R_m{}^2}\right)^2 \frac{Q_m{}^2}{\left(1 - Q_m{}^6\right)} \tag{1.32}$$

TABLE 1.3

Pressure–Volume Data and Strain Energy Density for the Left Ventricle

P (mmHg)	V (mL)	R_1	R_m (cm)	R_2	$(\partial W/\partial I)_m$ (mmHg)	I_M
5	31.5	1.96	2.56	3.15	3.73	3.56
10	40.0	2.12	2.67	3.22	6.82	3.86
15	46.7	2.23	2.74	3.27	9.9	4.1
20	52.0	2.31	2.80	3.31	13.0	4.28
25	56.5	2.38	2.85	3.34	16.1	4.44
30	60	2.43	2.90	3.37	19.3	4.56

Source: Adapted from Mirsky, I., *Biophys. J.*, 13, 1141, 1973.
Wall volume $V_w = 100$ mL. At zero pressure, $V = 12$ mL, $R_1 = 1.42$ cm, $R_2 = 2.99$ cm.

which can be evaluated for each pressure level P if the pressure–volume and pressure–radii data are known. Now, in order to determine the stress distribution through the wall of the left ventricle, we require $\partial W/\partial I$ to be expressed as a function of I (which, as can be seen from Equation 1.22, is a function of the deformed radius R).

For this purpose, for each pressure level, P, the function $\partial W/\partial I$ was evaluated at the midwall by employing relation (1.32), and this midwall value for $\partial W/\partial I$ was then plotted against I_m, the average of the values for I at the endocardial and epicardial surface, that is, $I_m = (I_1 + I_2)/2$. These data were fitted by an exponential curve: $\partial W/\partial I = A + Be^{CI}$, where A, B, and C are constants determined from a nonlinear regression analysis. These constants were then adjusted until the equilibrium condition (Equation 1.30), $P = K(R_2)$, agreed to within 5% of the experimental dog pressure–radius (P versus R_1) data.

Mirsky used pressure–volume data (Table 1.3) obtained from dog studies by Spontnitz et al. (1966) to obtain

$$\frac{\partial W}{\partial I} = -6.1 + 0.4e^{0.93I} \tag{1.33}$$

With this expression for $\partial W/\partial I$, the expression (1.30) for $K(R_2)$ was computed at 5 mmHg pressure increments over the range 5–30 mmHg, as shown in Table 1.3. The calculated $K(R_2)$ versus R_1 pressure–radius curves matched with the experimental P versus R_1 curves.

Using this $\partial W/\partial I$ expression, in Equations 1.24 and 1.25, we can determine the stress distribution through the wall of the LV. Mirsky computed the circumferential and meridional stresses from Equations 1.24 and 1.25. The earlier Figure 1.7 depicts LV circumferential stress (τ^{11}) based on both the classical theory (Equation 1.31) and large deformation theory (Equations 1.24 and 1.25), plotted as a percentage of the wall thickness for a ventricular pressure $P = 20$ mmHg. The circumferential stresses are normalized to $(PR_1/2h)$, which is the mean stress as given by the Laplace's law for a sphere (Mirsky, 1969). This figure depicts a marked difference in the stress distributions, showing a 10-fold increase in the stress at the endocardial surface over that predicted by the classical theory.

As we have stated earlier, Mirsky (1973) as well as more recently Chaudhry et al. (1996, 1997) used experimental dog studies data to demonstrate how LV stresses can be determined by using large deformation theory for thick shells. However, they did not indicate how this large deformation theory can be applied to human data, which we will now indicate in the following.

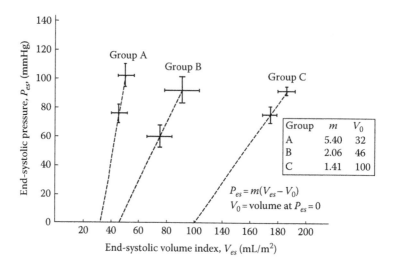

FIGURE 1.8
Average values for left ventricular end-systolic volume and pressure at two levels of systolic load are plotted for subjects with normal contractile function (group A, ejection fraction $\geq 0.6\%$), intermediate function (group B, ejection fraction = 0.41–0.59), and poor contractile function (group C, ejection fraction <0.40). (Adapted from Grossman, W. et al., *Circulation*, 56, 845, 1977.)

It can be seen that for the computation of LV stresses from Equations 1.24 and 1.25, we need to know the LV undeformed state dimensions r_1 and r_2 (the inner and outer dimensions) of the LV at zero internal pressure. It is possible to determine these dimensions from dog studies for zero internal pressure. However, this cannot be done in human clinical applications. So in human application, in order to determine r_1 and r_2, we need to first determine the value of LV volume V_0 at zero pressure, from LV geometry and pressure for at least two cardiac cycles. Then from the cyclic pressure–volume plots, we can determine the volume (V_0) at zero pressure by the method employed by Grossman et al. (1977), as illustrated in Figure 1.8. Herein, it is seen that V_0 can be obtained from two successive values of end-systolic pressure (P_{es}) and end-systolic volume (V_{es}).

As can be seen, the slope of the LV end-systolic pressure–volume relation was relative steep in subjects with normal contractile function (Group A), but became progressively less steep with greater degrees of impairment in contractile function. The extrapolated V_0 value is small (32 mL/m²) for the group with normal contractile function, and larger (46 mL/m² and 100 mL/m²) for the groups with intermediate and poor contractile function, respectively. From the value of V_0, we can determine r_1 (the inner radius of the LV model) at zero pressure. The value of r_2 (outer radius of the model) can be thereby obtained from the incompressibility condition of Equation 1.21.

So in this way, the Mirsky large-deformation model can be applied to human data. There is an added application of Figure 1.8. The parameter m in the equation $P_{es} = m(V_{es} - V_0)$ represents the LV systolic elastance E_{es}, which has an important bearing on how well an LV matches with the aorta. The ratio of E_{es} to E_a (aortic elastance) represents the degree of matching. This LV–aorta matching ratio value is significantly disturbed for cardiomyopathy LVs. Surgical ventricular restoration (SVR) is supposed to improve the value of E_{es}, and the degree to which SVR improves LV systolic function is based on the improved value of E_{es}/E_a following SVR. So in the clinical application, we will see how to noninvasively determine and clinically apply this LV–aorta matching index (E_{es}/E_a).

Aside from Mirsky and Chaudhry not applying their work into large-deformation models to assess in vivo stress in humans, these models also did not incorporate twisting moments. In fact, the reason why LV is able to generate such a high increase of pressure (of the order of 50–100 mmHg) during ventricular contraction and able to eject such a high volume of blood into the aorta (of the order of 70–140 mL) is because of its twisting. This reason for LV twisting when it contracts is because of the spirally wound myocardial fibers. It is easy to comprehend how contraction of these spirally wound myocardial fibers can cause the LV to twist. Now the LV model to demonstrate these effects of LV twisting, due to contraction of the spirally wound myocardial fibers, is that of Ghista et al. (2009). Chapter 3 presents this LV model, of how LV contraction develops contractile forces in the helically wound myocardial fibers, which causes the LV to twist and to suddenly develop the high intra-LV pressure during the isovolumic contraction phase.

1.7 Left Ventricular Wall Stress Based on Precise In Vivo Geometry and Using Finite Element Modeling

1.7.1 The Finite Element Model Trail

A more accurate description of the geometry of the heart requires the use of the finite element model (FEM) for calculation. The FEMs have been developed to incorporate non-linear and anisotropic material properties, fiber architecture, and nonlinear strains from animal data. These models were pressurized to simulate the mechanics of the LV. These LV FEMs provide us useful insights into LV physiology, wall stress distributions, and deformations during diastole and systole.

It is noteworthy that LV models have also been developed to account for the influence of intramyocardial coronary blood volume upon the stress distribution in the myocardial tissue (Smith et al., 2000). This is an area that needs extensive work, because it can provide insights into how wall stress influences intramyocardial blood flow and myocardial perfusion, and hence into the formation of myocardial infarcts in the LV wall.

One of the earliest FEMs of LV was formulated by Gould et al. (1972), who incorporated a realistic longitudinal cross section of the LV wall into an axisymmetric FE representation. The effects of the geometric complexity were examined using rings of isotropic, homogeneous shell elements. The additional geometric flexibility of this model permitted the wall curvature changes (from concave to convex inwards) and hence a shift in the location of the peak wall stress from the endocardium to the epicardium, which idealized geometrical models could not predict.

Janz and Grimm (1972) proposed FE models by incorporating material anisotropy and heterogeneity, along with more realistic LV geometry. The main results of this work were that deformations were significantly affected by the degree of heterogeneity and anisotropy of the myocardium. The isotropic model underestimated the deformed lumen radius by approximately 8%, and the stress predicted by the isotropic model differed by factors of two or three from those predicted by the heterogeneous model. While providing some qualitative insights into predicted myocardial stress distributions, the quantitative accuracy of predicted stresses was limited by the use of small-strain elasticity theory. Then, Janz et al. (1974) extended their earlier FEM to include large deformation theory.

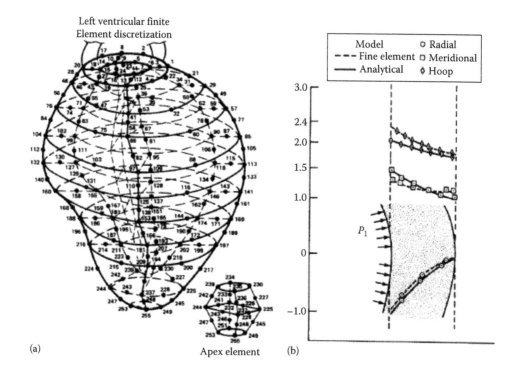

FIGURE 1.9

(a) Ghista and Hamid left ventricular finite element model (made up of 20-node, 3D isoparametric elements), whose irregular shape is developed from single plane cineangiocardiogram; (b) Comparison of the wall stress distributions of this finite element model with that obtained from the Ghista and Sandler elasticity model, indicates close matching of stresses both in magnitude and distribution across the wall. (Adapted from Ghista, D.N. and Hamid, S., *Comp. Prog. Biomed.*, 7, 219, 1977.)

The earliest 3D FE model applied to human data was by Ghista and Hamid (1977). Figure 1.9 illustrates this model, made up of 20-node, 3D isoparametric elements, which precisely simulates the LV geometry. This figure also displays the stress distributions across the LV wall by both this FE model and that obtained by Ghista and Sandler elasticity model (Figure 1.6). It can be seen that the Ghista and Hamid finite element model yields stress distribution (for radial, meridional, and hoop stresses) across the wall that very closely match those obtained analytically by Ghista and Sandler (1969). This gives a measure of confidence into both the Ghista and Sandler elasticity model and the Ghista and Hamid FE model for realistic portrayal of the stress distributions in the LV wall.

The first non-axisymmetric large deformation FEM of the LV was proposed by Hunter (1975). This model represented the ventricular myocardium as an incompressible, transversely isotropic material and incorporated the transmural distribution of fiber orientations measured by Streeter and Hanna (1973a,b). In this study, ventricular geometry was measured by mounting silicone-filled canine hearts onto a rig and using a probe to record the radial coordinates of the endocardial and epicardial surfaces at several predefined angular and axial locations. Hunter (1975) used this rig to also measure fiber orientations throughout the ventricular walls, and this work was subsequently completed by Nielsen et al. (1991).

More recent anatomical studies have revealed that the ventricular myocardium should not be viewed as a uniformly continuous structure, but as a composite of discrete layers of myocardial muscle fibers bound by endomysial collagen (Le Grice et al., 1995). It was

Nash (1998) who first formulated the anatomically accurate FE model of ventricular geometry and fibrous structure based on the earlier work of Nielsen et al. (1991). This model incorporated the orthotropic constitutive law, based on the 3D architecture of myocardium, to account for the nonlinear material response of the myocardium. The strain results showed good overall agreement with reported observations from experimental studies of isolated and in vivo canine hearts from Nielsen et al. (1991), which offered credibility to the derived stress. The computed tensile fiber stress was greatest near the endocardial region of the apex, while small tensile stresses were obtained for epicardial fibers at the apical and equatorial regions. Also, smaller fiber stresses were obtained for epicardial regions near the base.

Later, other animal FE models from rat (Omens et al., 1993) and rabbit (Lin and Yin, 1998; Vetter and McCulloch, 2000) were also developed. Figure 1.10 shows the equibiaxial fiber and cross-fiber stress–strain relations in rabbit, dog, and rat. It shows that rat myocardium is less stiff than the canine myocardium, and that both materials are stiffer in the fiber direction than in cross-fiber direction, which is to be expected.

With the development of modern imaging modalities, some more sophisticated LV models were developed, which incorporated realistic 3D geometry and fiber architecture, constitutive law for nonlinear anisotropic elastic properties of myocardium, and boundary conditions of physiologically realistic constrains under normal or diseased conditions (Guccione et al., 2003; Dang et al., 2005a,b; Walker et al., 2008). Cupps et al. (2003) used end-systolic stress, as determined by MRI and FEA, as a noninvasive clinically applicable index of regional LV function for early identification of LV decompensation. Generally, this kind of finite element heart modeling includes (1) in vivo heart geometry from MRI, (2) detailed helical fiber angles from diffusion tension MRI (Walker et al., 2005), and (3) myocardial material properties (Moonly, 2003). Material properties were generally iteratively determined by comparing the FE models with experimentally tagged MRI strain measurements.

In fact, in order to develop advanced realistic FE model, connective tissue (Hooks et al., 2002), conduction system (Tranum-Jensen et al., 1991), and ventricular and coronary fluid mechanics (Smith et al., 2000) should also be incorporated. These physiological processes are interlinked. The electrical activation of the heart initiates mechanical contraction through intracellular calcium release and is also influenced by cell stretching in terms of mechano-electric feedback. The supply of oxygen and metabolic substrates via coronary flow is finely tuned to ATP consumption by cross-bridges, membrane ion pumps, and other cellular processes. Ventricular fluid inflow is driven by myocardial diastolic recoil and atrial contraction, and coronary flow is driven by systolic contraction. The coupling of these processes has been initiated in the Physiome Project (Hunter et al., 2003; Crampin et al., 2004). A more detailed account of Physiome Project can be obtained from a recent review by Hunter et al. (2003).

1.7.2 Features of Constructed Finite Element Models

Here, we briefly introduce the framework for the development of advanced FE models, involving FE geometry determination and computation of stress and strain.

1.7.2.1 Finite Element Geometry

To achieve the simulation of cardiac mechanics, the myocardium geometry and the myocardial fiber orientations are needed as anatomical inputs into LV models. Figure 1.11a through d illustrates the preparation of the 3D finite element model by Vetter and

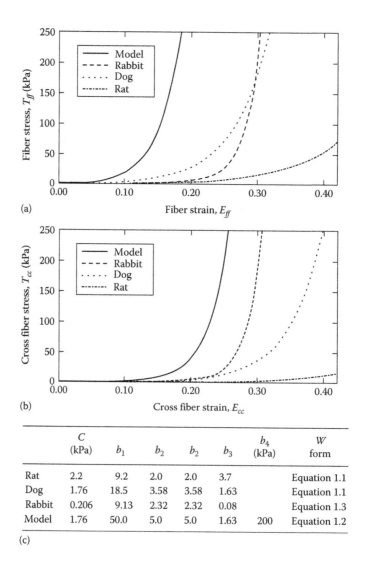

FIGURE 1.10

Equibiaxial fiber (a) and cross-fiber (b) stress–strain relations from models of the dog (Omens et al., 1993), rat (Omens et al., 1993), rabbit (Lin and Yin, 1998), and model by Vetter and McCulloch (2000). The material parameters used to model the stress–strain relation in the rat (Omens et al., 1993), dog (Omens et al., 1993), and rabbit (Lin and Yin, 1998) myocardium and the parameters in Vetter model (2000) are tabulated in (c). The constitutive law, function of the principal strain invariants, is given by

$$W = \frac{1}{2}C(e^Q - 1) - b_4\left(\det[C] - 2\sqrt{\det[C]} + 1\right)$$

$$Q = b_1(I_1 - 3)^2 + b_2(I_1 - 3)(I_4 - 1) + b_3(I_4 - 1)^2$$

The material parameters C, b_1, b_2, and b_3 are determined from the myocardial deformation under different loading conditions. (Adapted from Vetter et al., *Ann. Biomed. Eng.*, 28, 781, 2000.)

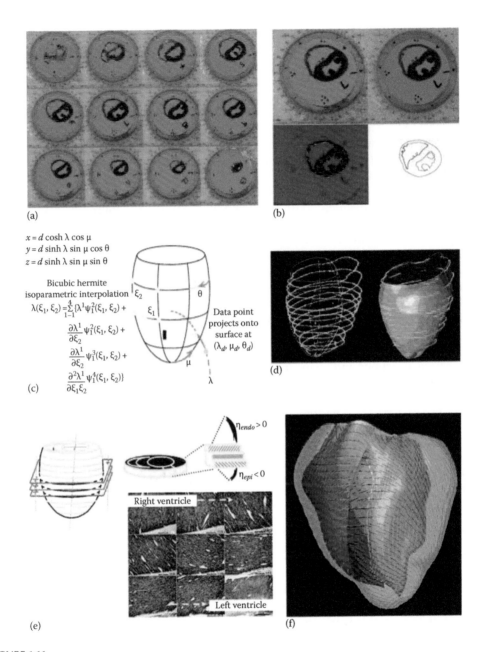

The equations shown in panel (c):

$$x = d \cosh \lambda \cos \mu$$
$$y = d \sinh \lambda \sin \mu \cos \theta$$
$$z = d \sinh \lambda \sin \mu \sin \theta$$

Bicubic hermite isoparametric interpolation

$$\lambda(\xi_1, \xi_2) = \sum_{1-1}^{4} \{ \lambda^1 \psi_1^2(\xi_1, \xi_2) + \frac{\partial \lambda^1}{\partial \xi_2} \psi_1^2(\xi_1, \xi_2) + \frac{\partial \lambda^1}{\partial \xi_2} \psi_1^3(\xi_1, \xi_2) + \frac{\partial^2 \lambda^1}{\partial \xi_1 \xi_2} \psi_1^4(\xi_1, \xi_2) \}$$

Data point projects onto surface at $(\lambda_d, \mu_d, \theta_d)$

$\eta_{endo} > 0$

$\eta_{epi} < 0$

Right ventricle

Left ventricle

FIGURE 1.11
(a) Successive series images of the short-axis slices of myocardium cast in dental rubber. After each image was captured, 2–3 mm of the tissue/rubber plug were pressed out of the tube and sliced off exposing the myocardium and rubber of the next image. Successive images are shown in rows stating at the base (upper left) and ending at the apex (lower right). (b) Segmentation of the ventricular myocardium. (c) The rectangular Cartesian "model" coordinate system is convenient for modeling cardiac geometry. The curvilinear parameter coordinates (ξ_1, ξ_2, ξ_3) used in fitting and subsequent analysis are the local finite element coordinates. (d) Fitted 3D LV geometry with fiber orientation. (e) Schematic of a block cut from a tissue slice, showing the transmural variation in fiber angle η and typical images of series cross sections of unstained tissue from the inferior septum with averaging measured fiber angle in the first section is −104° and in the last section is +43°. (f) Anterior (left) and posterior lateral (right) views of the fitted 3D finite element model showing interpolated fiber angles superposed on the epicardial and endocardial surfaces. (Adapted from Vetter, F.J. and McCulloch, A.D., *Prog. Biophys. Mol. Biol.*, 69, 157, 1998.)

McCulloch (1998, 2000). The excised LV was fixed by filing its cavity with quick-setting dental rubber, and then its short-axis digital images were acquired. From these images, the geometrical contours of the rubber tissue were segmented (Figure 1.11a, b) and the geometrical coordinates of the fiducial markers were recorded by image-processing software (Figure 1.11c). The LV geometry was then constructed by fitting a surface through the myocardial contours on tagged MRI slices, using a prolate spheroidal coordinate system aligned to the central axis of the LV (Vetter and McCulloch, 1998) (Figure 1.11d).

The transmural variations of the myocardial fibers were measured from the blocks of tissue cut from the slices (Figure 1.11e). Most diffusion tensor imaging and dissection analysis have depicted an elevation angle (angle between the fiber and the short-axis plane) varying from around +70° on the endocardium to around −70° on the epicardium (Guccione et al., 1991; Hsu and Henriquez, 2001), and being horizontal in the short-axis plane at midwall. Herein, due to the smoothing in the discretization and averaging per tetrahedron, the imaged fiber orientations are seen to follow a linear variation between +90° and −90° (Figure 1.11e) (Vetter and McCulloch, 1998).

The FE model was then created by placing nodes at equal angular intervals in the circumferential and longitudinal directions, and by fitting radial coordinates to the inner and the outer surfaces. The models were subsequently converted into a rectangular Cartesian coordinate system, with the long axis of the ventricle oriented along the x-axis and the y-axis directed toward the centre of the right ventricle. The resulting model consisted of a number finite elements with their geometry interpolated (1) in radial direction using Lagrange basis functions and (2) in circumferential and longitudinal direction using cubic Hermite basis functions. The elements were solid blocks or thin surfaces shells.

The fitted 3D ventricular geometry and fiber angles by Vetter and McCulloch (1998) are shown in Figure 1.11f. Over 22,500 measurements are represented by 736 degrees of freedom, with a RMSE of ±0.55 mm in the geometric surface and ±19 in the fiber angles. A comparison of the measured fiber angles and the fitted transmural distribution is shown in Figure 1.12. The fitted fiber distributions (by assigning the coordinates) are seen to be in close agreement with the measured angles and the fitted distribution in the dog (Nielsen et al., 1991).

1.7.2.2 Computing Stress and Strain Using FEA

We have presented the description of LV FEM construction, based on the work of Vetter and McCullogh (1998). Once the geometrical construction is done (as per Figure 1.11), the material properties, boundary, and initial conditions are assigned, and LV pressure simulation can be carried out. We will now move on to the work of Vetter and McCulogh published in 2000. In this work, the earlier model (Figure 1.11) was modified to serve as a computational model for passive LV inflation simulating the control group experiments of Gallagher et al. (1997).

1.7.2.3 Material Law and Determination of Material Parameters

The myocardium was modeled (by Vetter and McCulloch, 2000) as a transversely isotropic, hyperelastic material with an exponential strain energy function (Guccione et al., 1991; Omens et al., 1993)

$$W = \frac{1}{2}C(e^{Q} - 1)$$

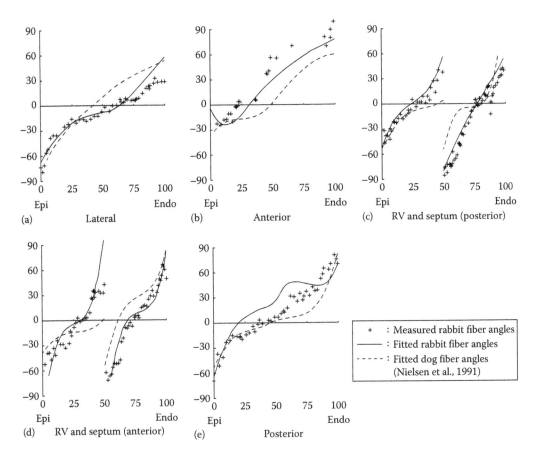

FIGURE 1.12
Measured and fitted fiber angles for the rabbit (crosses and solid lines) and fitted fiber angles for the dog. Horizontal axes are normalized wall depth (%); vertical axes are fiber angle (degrees). (Adapted from Vetter, F.J. and McCulloch, A.D., *Prog. Biophys. Mol. Biol.*, 69, 157, 1998.)

$$Q = b_1 E_{ff}^2 + b_2 \left(E_{rr}^2 + E_{cc}^2 + E_{rc}^2 \right) + 2b_3 \left(E_{fr}^2 + E_{fc}^2 \right) \tag{1.34}$$

where the Lagrangian Green's strains E_{ij} are referred to the local fiber coordinate system consisting of fiber (f), cross-fiber (c), and radial (r) coordinate directions. The material parameters C, b_1, b_2, and b_3 have been described in detail by Guccione et al. (1991); briefly, the material constant C scales the stress; b_1 and b_2 scale the material stiffness in the fiber or cross-fiber direction, respectively, and b_3 scales the material rigidity under shear in the fiber–radial and fiber–cross-fiber planes.

The LV passive inflation was simulated. The model strains were compared with experimental measurements, and the material parameters were adjusted to improve the agreement: b_1 and b_2 were modified to minimize discrepancies in fiber and cross-fiber strains and b_3 was modified according to differences in shear strain. Vetter and McCulloch computed the root mean squared error (RMSE) of the objective function $\hat{E}_{ij} - E_{ij}$, where $\hat{E}_{ij}$ are the model strains and E_{ij} are the epicardial strains measured by Gallagher et al. (1997) at LV pressures of 5, 10, 15, 20, and 25 mmHg. The parameters that minimized the RMSE were accepted as the best estimates of myocardial material parameters.

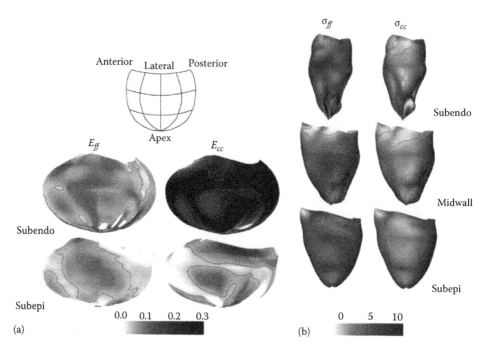

FIGURE 1.13

(a) Hammer projection maps of fiber strain (E_{ff}) and cross-fiber strain (E_{cc}) in the LV free wall at 25 mmHg pressure. Contours are drawn at 0.05, 0.10, 0.20, and 0.25 strain levels. (b) Cauchy stresses (kPa) resolved in fiber (σ_{ff}) and cross-fiber (σ_{cc}) directions in the LV free wall and apex at 10 mmHg pressure. Contours are drawn at 0, 2, 4, 6, and 8 kPa stress levels. (Adapted from Vetter, F.J. and McCulloch, A.D., *Ann. Biomed. Eng.*, 28, 781, 2000.)

1.7.2.4 Boundary Conditions and Computational Approach

The boundary conditions were specified by constraining the model displacement degrees of freedom. The model coordinates and their circumferential and transmural derivatives were constrained at the base on the LV epicardium and RV endocardium. The LV was passively inflated. The fiber strains and cross-fiber strains distributions are depicted in Figure 1.13a.

The resulting Cauchy stress distribution is depicted in Figure 1.13b. Over the lateral wall and apex, the Cauchy stress resolved in the fiber direction is seen to be on an average higher than that in the cross-fiber direction, which can be expected. For the region shown in Figure 1.13, the mean fiber stress was 2.91 ± 3.93 kPa and the mean cross-fiber stress was 1.47 ± 3.51 kPa. At the midventricle, the fiber stress tended to be larger than cross-fiber stress transmurally. At the epicardium and midwall, the cross-fiber stress is seen to be more uniform than the fiber stress, while the fiber stress was greater. The apex and papillary insertions at the subendocardium show the greatest magnitude and regional variability in both directions, while the negative stresses are seen to occur predominately at the regions of negative curvature.

1.7.3 Anatomically Accurate Bio-Elasticity Passive–Active LV Finite Element Model

A representative FE model needs to include the heart's macroscopic (left and right ventricular) components and microstructure architecture (of myocardial fibers and sheets), so as to incorporate the contractile properties of the ventricular myofibers (by means of the intracellular Ca concentration–fiber tension relationship). This enables the LV model to simulate (the effect of contractile wave propagation along the myocardial fibrous network, in terms of) the ventricular apex-to-base twist, which is the prime factor behind the LV pressure rise during isovolumic contraction to initiate ejection of blood into the aorta. This is the feature of the Nash model, which was built up from silicone-filled canine hearts (Nash, 1998).

The model consists of 60 high-order finite elements and 99 nodes, defined with respect to a prolate spheroidal coordinate system. The ventricular mechanics model incorporates the orthotropic pole-zero constitutive law. The nonlinear elastic properties of passive myocardium were modeled by using 3D orthotropic relationships between the components of the second Piola–Kirchhoff stress tensor and Green's strain tensor, to simulate the diastolic phase of the cardiac cycle.

In the model, the contractile forces are generated along the axes of cardiac fibers and are related to the strain in the fiber. The contractile properties of ventricular myofibers are approximately by means of a relationship between the fiber extension ratio, intracellular calcium concentration, and active fiber stress. In this way, the LV model framework incorporated a somewhat realistic model of active myocardial mechanics.

The ventricular mechanics was analyzed for three of the four main phases of the heart cycle. The diastolic filling phase inflated the unloaded and residually stressed ventricles to physiological end-diastolic LV and RV cavity pressure of 1 kPa (75 mmHg) and 0.2 kPa (15 mmHg), respectively. During diastolic filling, the LV volume increased from 32 to 52 mL, while the RV volume decreased from 28 to 22 mL. This was accompanied by an increase in the LV long-axis dimension from 73 to 76 mm. The average end-diastolic long-axis rotation (or apex-to-base untwist angle) was about 5°.

Following end-diastole, the level of activation was increased consistently throughout the myocardium (in terms of Ca concentration) to simulate myofiber contraction, while the ventricular cavities were held at their end-diastolic volumes. By the end of this isovolumic contraction phase, the LV and RV cavity pressures increased to 92 kPa (69 mmHg) and 39 kPa (29 mmHg), respectively, and the LV long-axis dimension decreased to 75 mm.

Ventricular ejection was simulated by decreasing the afterload impedances imposed on each of the cavities. End-systole occurred when the LV ejection fraction had reached 44%. At this stage, the LV and RV cavity volumes had decreased to 29 and 20 mL, respectively, and the LV and RV cavity pressures had decreased to 55 kPa (41 mmHg) and 16 kPa (12 mmHg), respectively. During ejection, the LV long-axis dimension decreased to 69 mm. Ventricular twist was calculated in terms of the circumferential rotation (relative to the end-diastolic state) with respect to the long-axis coordinate. The rotations were clockwise, when viewed from the apex toward the base; the mean systolic twist was about 5°.

Figure 1.14a illustrates anterior and posterior views of the computed epicardial and endocardial end-diastolic fiber stress distributions superimposed on the inflated ventricles. At end-diastole, due to LV filing pressure, the tensile fiber stress was greatest near the endocardial region of the apex, while small tensile stresses were obtained for epicardial fibers at apical and equatorial region. Small compressive fiber stresses were obtained for the epicardial regions near the base, because of the stiff constraining effects of the basal ring on the mechanics of the ventricles.

Figure 1.14b and c illustrates anterior and posterior views of the predicted epicardial and endocardial fiber stress distributions, superimposed on the deformed ventricles at the end of isovolumic contraction and ejection phases of systole, respectively. At the end of isovolumic contraction, small compressive stresses were obtained for the most of the LV

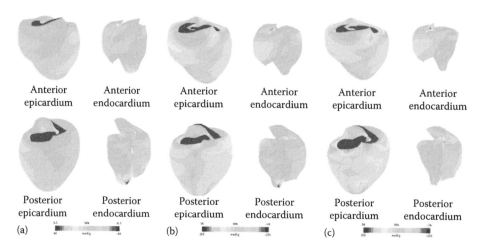

FIGURE 1.14

(a) End-diastolic fiber stress distribution superimposed on the inflated ventricles. Fiber stress distributions superimposed on the deformed ventricles at the end of isovolumic contraction (b) and end-ejection. (c) Stresses are referred to the unloaded residually stressed state. Lines represent element boundaries of the FE mesh. (Adapted from Nash, M., Mechanics and material properties of the heart using an anatomically accurate mathematical model, PhD thesis, The University of Auckland, New Zealand, 1998.)

endocardium, associated with contraction of the fibers. At end-systole, small comprehensive stresses were obtained in most of the LV endocardium.

The ventricular mechanics model's results of (1) cavity pressure versus volume relationship, (2) longitudinal dimension changes, (3) torsional wall deformations, and (4) regional distributions of myocardial strain, during diastolic filling as well as isovolumic contraction and ejection phases of the cardiac cycle, showed good overall agreements with observations derived from experimental studies of isolated and in vivo canine hearts.

In spite of the physiological useful results of this LV FE model, it can still be kept in mind that this model has not been applied to human data. Hence, there still remains the need to demonstrate (1) how the model can be developed from human data for the important phases of the cardiac cycle (namely, start of diastole, end-diastole, end-isovolumic contraction, and end-systole), (2) how the model deformation can be monitored (especially LV twist), and (3) how the LV pressure measurements can be synchronized with LV geometry and structural measurement. Then only we can clinically utilize all the features of this model to (1) develop indices for cardiac contractility, (2) obtain insight into stress variation across the wall, and (3) relate LV fiber structure to LV twist and pressure rise during isovolumic contraction.

1.8 Comparison of Left Ventricular Wall Stress Based on LV Models

Several geometric models of the LV have been used to estimate cavity volume and wall volume (V_w) (De Simone et al., 1996; Devereux et al., 1996), the most common being ellipsoidal and spherical-shaped models. With regard to stress calculations, many formulas have also been proposed.

We will first compare the wall stress distribution values obtained from the popular thick-wall models of LV. Huisman et al. (1980) compared the stresses predicted from several of the previously presented thick wall models, by using the same angiographic data obtained in a number of disease states as input to each model (Wong and Rautarharju, 1968; Ghista and Sandler, 1969; Mirsky, 1969). In each case, the material was assumed to be isotropic, homogeneous, and incompressible. The absolute magnitude of the calculated wall stress differed, depending on the model used. The difference in mean stress predicted by a thin sphere compared to a thick-wall sphere was about 12% at end-diastole and 20% at end-systole.

The stress distributions across the wall for the various models are also compared (Figure 1.15). These thick-walled models yield both quantitatively and qualitatively different results. The circumferential stress gradients predicted by all models decreased from endocardium to epicardium, but by different amounts. Without experimental verification, the discrepancy between the thick-walled models makes it somewhat difficult to compare their accuracy. The longitudinal stress decreased by 26% from endocardium to epicardium for the Ghista and Sandler model (1969), but increased by 36% for the Mirsky (1969) model. At the midwall, all the models' stresses vary by about 16%.

Mirsky and Pasipoularides (1990) proposed a simplified analysis for LV stress, based on a thick spherical shell model, which requires measures or estimates of the cavity volume V and wall volume V_w. By assuming a spherical geometry for the left ventricle,

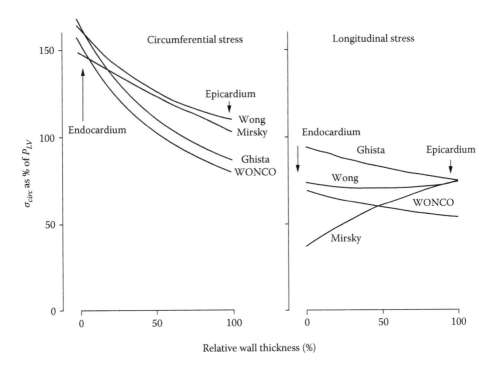

FIGURE 1.15
Comparison of the stress distribution across the wall for the thick-walled ellipsoid models demonstrating marked quantitative and qualitative differences between the models. The WONCO model is a modification of the model of Wong and Rautaharju (1968) with transverse shear taken into account. (Adapted from Huisman, R.M. et al., *Med. Biol. Eng. Comput.*, 18, 133, 1980.)

the chamber inner radius (R_i), outer radius (R_o), and midwall radius (R_m) are obtained from relationships.

$$R_i = \left[\left(\frac{3}{4\pi}\right)V\right]^{1/3}, \quad R_o = \left[\left(\frac{3}{4\pi}\right)(V+V_m)\right]^{1/3}, \quad R_m = \frac{(R_i+R_o)}{2} \tag{1.35}$$

Then, midwall circumferential stress can be estimated from measured pressure, cavity volume, wall volume, and R_m according to the following (Mirsky and Pasipoularides, 1990):

$$\sigma = \left(\frac{3}{2}\right)P \times \left(\frac{V}{V_m}\right) \times \left(\frac{R_o}{R_m}\right)^3 \tag{1.36}$$

Thus, for each value of pressure and volume obtained during the measurement, a value for σ and R_m can be obtained from Equations 1.35 and 1.36.

We now provide some comparison of stresses obtained from some popular analytical stress expressions used in cardiology and echocardiography with the stresses obtained from FE models for (1) spherical, (2) ellipsoidal, (3) anatomic axisymmetric, and (4) anatomic non-axisymmetric chambers developed by Ingrassia et al. (2008).

The Laplace's law for a sphere expresses circumferential stress as a function of pressure, radius of curvature, and thickness, in a simple way as:

$$\sigma = \frac{P(r_{long})}{2h} \tag{1.37}$$

where
r_{long} is the longitudinal radius of the curvature
h is the wall thickness

Mirsky and Pasipoularides (1990) provided the following expression for circumferential stress at the equator of an ellipsoid (based on Laplace's law):

$$\sigma = \left(\frac{Pb}{h}\right)\left(\frac{1-b^2}{(2a^2)} - h(2b) + \frac{h^2}{(8a^2)}\right) \tag{1.38}$$

where a and b are the midwall semimajor and semiminor axes, respectively. This formula is a slight modification of the expression given by Equation 1.12.

Janz (1982) proposed a circumferential stress expression, applied to general axisymmetric geometries, as follows:

$$\sigma = \frac{Pr_{circ}r_{long}\left(2 - r_{circ}/r_{long}(\sin\varphi)\right)}{2h\sin\varphi(r_{long} + h/2)} \tag{1.39}$$

where
r_{circ} is the circumferential radius of curvature
r_{long} is the longitudinal radius of curvature
φ is the angle between r_{long} and the axis of symmetry

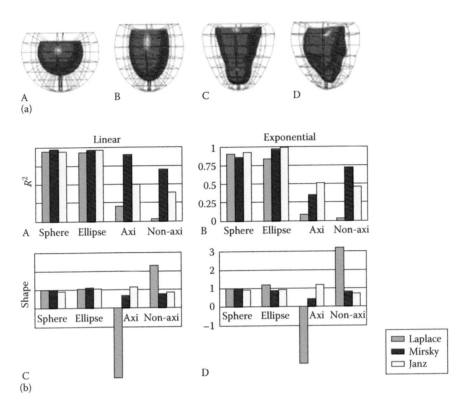

FIGURE 1.16
(a) Illustration of finite element models for spherical, elliptical, anatomic axisymmetric, and anatomic non-axisymmetric chambers. Solid surface and wire mesh represent inner and outer surfaces, respectively. (b) Regression results of R^2 values from corrections between stresses obtained from each analytic equation and the finite element method using (A) linear and (B) exponential material properties; their corresponding slopes are shown in (C) and (D). (Adapted from Ingrassia, C.M. et al., Evaluation of analytic estimates of ventricular wall stress using the finite element method, in *Proceedings of the ASME 2008 Summer Bioengineering Conference*, SBC2008-193262, Marco Island, FL, 2008.)

For validation of these expressions, Ingrassia et al. (2008) developed a series of LV FE model chambers (Figure 1.16a), to compute and compare the circumferential stress with the analytical expressions (Equations 1.37 through 1.39).

The FEMs developed consisted of 64 incompressible elements defined in prolate spheroidal coordinates, with hybrid cubic–Hermite linear–Lagrange tensor product basis functions to yield smooth geometric surfaces and ensure convergence of regional wall stress. Figure 1.16a shows examples of the four levels of geometric complexity: spherical, elliptical, anatomic axisymmetric, and anatomic non-axisymmetric chambers. The anatomic non-axisymmetric shape was developed from magnetic resonance image slices of an isolated canine LV (Costa et al., 1996). From this model, the LV anatomic axisymmetric shape was constructed as a solid of revolution about the long axis, using longitudinal slices through the anterior papillary muscle. Each LV model shape was scaled to achieve a variety of chamber sizes and radius-to-thickness ratios, yielding a wider range of stress values for the analysis. Chamber inflation was simulated by incrementally loading it to cavity pressure ranging from 1.5 to 3 kPa. Two constitutive laws were used in the model to encompass a range of material complexity. The first law concerns the strain energy potential (W).

$$W = k(I_c - 3) \tag{1.40}$$

expressed as a linear function of the first strain invariant, I_c, with the stiffness parameter k set to 3 kPa. This represents a hyperelastic, isotropic neo-Hookena material with a linear stress–strain relationship (Costa et al., 1996). Then, in order to model a more realistic complex nonlinear anisotropic relationship, W was expressed as a Fung-type exponential function of Cauthy–Green strain tensor components, E_{ij}, referred to fiber coordinates (Guccione et al., 1991):

$$W = k(e^{Q(E_{ij})} - 1) \tag{1.41}$$

where

$$Q(E_{ij}) = b_1 E_{FF}^2 + b_2 \left(E_{RR}^2 + E_{CC}^2 + E_{RC}^2 \right) + 2b_3 \left(E_{RF}^2 + E_{FC}^2 \right)$$

wherein subscripts R, F, and C denote radial, fiber, and cross-fiber directions, respectively. The local muscle fiber angle varied linearly from 83° at the endocardium to −37° at the epicardium. The material parameter values ($k = 0.44$ kPa, $b_1 = 18.5$, $b_2 = 3.58$, and $b_3 = 1.63$) were adopted from Guccione et al.'s work (1991).

The stress values estimated by each of the analytical formulae (Equations 1.37 through 1.39) were compared with the finite element results using linear regression. The resulting values of R^2 and slope were grouped by model geometry and material type, to determine the range of applicability of each equation. Figure 1.16b(B) summarizes the results of the regression analysis. All the three analytical expressions for stress yielded (correlation coefficient) R^2 values and slopes (between FEM and analytical Equations 1.37 through 1.39) near 1 for the spherical and elliptical geometries (A and B), independent of material type. However, Laplace's law did not work when it was applied to the anatomically shaped axisymmetric geometry (C), for which the Janz's equation was originally derived. In terms of slope, Janz's expression (Equation 1.39) was superior to that of Mirsky's expression (Equation 1.38), for the anatomic axisymmetric geometry.

However, for the anatomic non-axisymmetric geometry, both Mirsky and Janz expressions compared favorably in terms of slope, indicating that they give reasonable approximations of the overall average stress in the FE models. Overall, the results suggest that the reliability of each of the expressions (Equations 1.37 through 1.39) of circumferential wall stress depends more strongly on the geometry of the chamber than on the complexity of the material.

1.9 Discussion

In this LV wall stress compendium, we have presented (1) LV thin-wall models for stress based on Laplace's law, (2) LV thick-shell ellipsoidal small-strain models, (3) LV thick-wall elasticity dynamic-shape model, (4) LV thick-shell large-deformation model, and (5) LV FE models. Let us compare the stresses obtained by these models.

Table 1.1 provides comparison of circumferential wall stress values of subjects computed by Sandler and Dodge expression (Equation 1.2) for a thin-walled ellipsoidal shell LV model with the mean stress values computed by Wong and Rautahraju model expression (Equation 1.8) for a thick-wall ellipsoidal shell. It is seen that the Sandler and Dodge (1963) expression overestimates the stress by only 10%–15% at different values of h/b at end-diastole, peak systole, and end-systole. These stress calculations utilized LV catheterization and biplane angiogram data.

Table 1.2 presents comparison of maximum and average stress values computed by Mirsky thick-shell spherical model expressions (1.9) and (1.10) (for $b = a$) with (1) the stresses computed from expression (1.17) based on elasticity theory (in Timoshenko and Goodier, 1951), and (2) the stresses computed by Laplace's law expressions (Equations 1.14 through 1.16) for various values of h/b. The stresses were computed from monitored biplane angiography and intraventricular pressure data. It is seen that the discrepancy between the maximum stress values of thick-shell model and elasticity theory is less than 6%. There is also close agreement of stresses computed by Laplace's law expression (Equation 1.14) and that computed by the exact solution (Equation 1.17) based on elasticity theory.

Figure 1.4 provides the cyclic variation of $\sigma_{\theta\theta}$ based on Mirsky model (1969), circumferential with respect to the cyclic variation of LV pressure. In view of $\sigma_{\theta\theta}$ being a somewhat complex function of LV pressure and ellipsoidal geometry parameters, it is interesting to note that $\sigma_{\theta\theta}$ becomes maximum at the start of the ejection phase. Mind you, this relationship is still based on the passive stress model. Figure 1.5 shows the variations across the wall of maximum meridional, circumferential, and radial stresses obtained from Mirsky thick-shell ellipsoidal model. As expected, the circumferential stresses are maximum on the endocardial surface, and equal to 2.5 times the radial stress on the endocardial surface.

Now, in comparison with the use of fixed-shaped thick-shell models of Wong and Rantaharju (1968) and Mirsky (1969), Ghista and Sandler (1969) employed elasticity theory to obtain instantaneous geometries of the LV model corresponding to monitored angiographic data of LV geometry and stress distributions for monitored LV chamber pressures. The noteworthy feature of Ghista and Sandler (1969) elasticity model is that the model shape is more akin to actual LV shape, as the stress trajectories become less oval-shaped for increasing values of r and y. This means that it is possible to appropriately simulate both more oval-shaped systolic LV geometries and dilated less oval-shaped LVs as well as dilated LVs due to regurgitant aortic valve.

Figure 1.15 provides comparison of the three thick-wall models of Wong and Rantaharju, Mistry and Ghista and Sandler circumferential and longitudinal stress variations across the wall. All the models depict this trend of maximum value of circumferential stress at the endocardial surface decreasing to about 50% of this value at the epicardial surface. However, because the Ghista and Sandler model has no restrictive assumptions of shell theory, it can be deemed to be the most representative of LV shape and stress distribution compared to the other models.

To note the effect of using large-deformation theory, Figure 1.7 provides comparison of across-wall variation of LV circumferential stress based on Mirsky (1973) large-deformation spherical thick-shell model Equations 1.24 and 1.25 and the classical thick-shell elasticity theory Equation 1.31 from Timoshenko and Goodier (1951), normalized with respect to Laplace stress for a sphere ($\sigma = PR/2h$). It is seen that the large-deformation model stress value at the endocardium is over 10 times greater than the stress based on classical theory. These stress computations were based on dog heart data. For using large deformation theory, it is necessary to know the undeformed radii (r_1 and r_2) of the LV at conceptual zero internal pressure. Now, since Mirsky employed dog pressure–volume data (as depicted in Table 1.3), it was possible to obtain these unde-formed radii. So to enable application of this large-deformation model to human data, we have indicated (in Figure 1.8) how we can make use of two successive values of LV end-systolic pressure–volume values (from two successive cycles) to extrapolate the values of V_0 and thereby obtain the values of r_1 and r_2 by utilizing the incompressibility condition.

1.10 Conclusion and Future Perspectives

In this chapter, we have comprehensively surveyed LV wall stress models based on Laplace's law, thick-shell (small-strain) theory, elasticity theory, thick-shell large deforma-tion theory, and the advanced finite element method (FEM). We have presented an in-depth analysis of all these models' theories, derivations, and results. We have compared the LV wall stress results based on analytical expressions with those obtained from FEMs. This enables the reader to assess the representativeness of the models, the simplicity ver-sus complexity of the stress computations, and which model is appropriate for them to use physiologically or clinically.

There are two comments that we want to make. First, the FE models need to be based on human data, in order to be assessed to be employable. Then also, the complexity of their computations needs to be weighed against the relative ease of employing analytical mod-els. Second, these models are all based on simulating LV as passive chamber under pres-sure, resulting in stresses in the wall. In other words, the stresses are assumed to result from the pressure in the LV chamber.

Now it is somewhat recognized that LV wall stress can have some association with cardiac pathophysiology, but that needs unraveling. The pathophysiology is based on what hap-pens at the sarcomere level. In an infarcted LV, the bioelectrical wave will skirt the infarcted segments, and also not properly excite the ischemic segments. As a result, certain sets and segments of myocardial fibers will not be contracted, and this will reflect on the wall stress distribution. However, all this requires that we first determine the infarcted segments' loca-tions, incorporate them in the LV FEMs, make the sarcomeres in the infarcted segments not contractile, and determine the associated wall stress distribution. Then only we will be able to figure out how wall stresses can reflect pathology based on non-perfused damaged myo-cardial segments. This then remains as our future avenue to embark upon.

References

Alter P, Rupp H, Rominger MB, Czerny F, Vollrath A, Klose KJ, Maisch B. 2010. A new method to assess ventricular wall stress in patients with heart failure and its relation to heart rate vari-ability. *Int J Cardiol.* 139(3):301–303.

Arts T, Bovendeerd P, van der Toorn A, Geerts L, Kerckhoffs R, Prinzen F. 2001. Modules in cardiac modeling: Mechanics, circulation, and depolarization wave. In: *Functional Imaging and Modeling of the Heart* (FIMH'01), Lecture Notes in Computer Science (LNCS), Springer, Vol. 2230, pp. 83–90.

Balzer P, Furber A, Delepine S, Rouleau F, Lethimonnier F, Morel O, Tadei A, Jallet P, Geslin P, Le Jeune JJ. 1999. Regional assessment of wall curvature and wall stress in left ventricle with magnetic resonance imaging. *Am J Physiol Heart Physiol.* 277:H901–H910.

Bestel J, Clement F, Sorine M. 2001. A biomechanical model of muscle contraction. In: *Medical Image Computing and Computer-Assisted Intervention (MICCAU'01)*, Lecture Notes in Computer Science (LNCS), Niessen W and Viergever M (eds.), Berlin, Germany: Springer, Vol. 2208, pp. 1159–1161.

Bovendeerd PH et al. 1996. Regional wall mechanics in the ischemic left ventricle: Numerical modeling and dog experiments. *Am J Physiol.* 270:H398–H410.

Chaudhry HR, Bukiet B, Davis AM. 1996. Stresses and strains in the left ventricular wall approximated as a thick conical shell using large deformation theory. *J Biol Syst.* 4(3):353–372.

Chaudhry HR, Bukiet B, Regan T. 1997. Dynamic stresses and strains in the left ventricular wall based on large deformation theory. *Int J Nonlinear Mech.* 32:621–631.

Costa KD et al. 1996a. Three-dimensional FEM for large elastic deformations of ventricular myocardium I: Cylindrical and spherical polar coordinates. *J Biomech Eng.* 118(4):452–463.

Costa KD et al. 1996b. Three-dimensional FEM for large elastic deformations of ventricular myocardium II: Prolate spheroidal coordinates. *J Biomech Eng.* 118(4):464–472.

Costa KD, Holmes JW, McCulloch AD. 2001. Modeling cardiac mechanical properties in three dimensions. *Philos Trans R Soc Lond A.* 359:1233–1250.

Crampin EJ, Smith NP, Hunter PJ. 2004. Multi-scale modeling and the IUPS physiome project. *J Mol Histol.* 35:707–714.

Cupps BP, Moustakidis P, Pomerantz BJ. 2003. Severe aortic insufficiency and normal systolic function: Determining regional left ventricular wall stress by finite element analysis. *Ann Thorac Surg.* 76(3):668–675.

Dang AB, Guccione JM, Mishell JM. 2005a. Akinetic myocardial infarcts must contain contracting myocytes: Finite-element model study. *Am J Physiol Heart Circ Physiol.* 288(4):H1844–H1850.

Dang AB, Guccione JM, Zhang P. 2005b. Effect of ventricular size and patch stiffness in surgical anterior ventricular restoration: A finite element model study. *Ann Thorac Surg.* 79(1):185–193.

De Simone G, Devereux RB. 2002. Rationale of echocardiographic assessment of left ventricular wall stress and midwall mechanics in hypertensive heart disease. *Eur J Echocardiogr.* 3:192–198.

De Simone G, Devereux RB, Ganau A, Hahn RT, Saba PS, Mureddu GF, Roman MJ, Howard BV. 1996. Estimation of left ventricular chamber and stroke volume by limited M-mode echocardiography and validation by two-dimensional Doppler echocardiography. *Am J Cardiol.* 78:801–807.

Delepine S, Furber AP, Beygui F, Prunier F, Balzer P, Le Jeune JJ, Gesline P. 2003. 3-D MRI assessment of regional left ventricular systolic wall stress in patients with reperfused MI. *Am J Physiol Heart Circ Physiol.* 284:H1190–H1197.

Devereux RB, Alonso DR, Lutas EM, Gottlieb GJ, Campo E, Saches I, Reichek N. 1996. Echocardiographic assessment of left ventricular hypertrophy: Comparison to necropsy findings. *Am J Cardiol.* 57:450–458.

Di Napoli P, Taccardi AA, Grilli A, Felaco M, Balbone A, Angelucci D. 2003. Left ventricular wall stress as a direct correlate of cardiomyocyte apoptosis in patients with severe dilated cardiomyopathy. *Am Heart J.* 146:1105–1111.

Douglas P, Reichek N, Plappert P, Muhammad A, Sutton M. 1987. Comparison of echocardiographic methods for assessment of left ventricular shortening and wall stress. *J Am Coll Cardiol.* 9:945–951.

Feiring A, Rumberger J. 1992. Ultrafast computed tomography analysis regional radius to wall thickness ratio in normal and volume overloaded human left ventricle. *Circulation.* 85:1423–1432.

Fujita N, Duerinckx A, Higgins C. 1993. Variation in left ventricular regional wall stress with cine magnetic resonance imaging: Normal subjects versus dilated cardiomyopathy. *Am Heart J.* 125:1337–1345.

Gallagher AM, Omens JH, Chu LL, Covell JW. 1997. Alterations in collagen fibrillar structure and mechanical properties of the healing scar following myocardial infarction. *Cardiovasc Pathobiol.* 2(1):25–36.

Gault JH, Ross J Jr, Braunwald E. 1968. Contractile state of the left ventricle in man: Instantaneous tension-velocity-length relations in patients with and without disease of the left ventricular myocardium. *Circ Res.* 22:451–463.

Ghista DN, Advani SH, Gaonkar GH, Balachandran K, Brady AJ. 1971. Analysis and physiological monitoring of human left ventricle. *J Basic Eng.* 93:147–161.

Ghista DN, Brady AJ, Ranmakrishnan S. 1973. A three-dimensional analytical (rheological) model of the human left ventricle in passive-active states. *Biophys J.* 13:32–54.

Ghista DN, Hamid S. 1977. Finite element stress analysis of the human left ventricle whose irregular shape is developed from single plane cineangiocardiogram. *Comput Programs Biomed.* 7(3):219–231.

Ghista DN, Liu L, Chua LP, Zhong L, Tan RS, Tan YS. 2009. Mechanism of left ventricular pressure increase during isovolumic contraction, and determination of its equivalent myocardial fibers orientation. *J Mech Med Biol.* 9(2):177–198.

Ghista DN, Sandler H. 1969. An analytic elastic-viscoelastic model for the shape and the forces of the left ventricle. *J Biomech.* 2(1):35–47.

Ghista DN, Sandler H, Vavo WH. 1975. Elastic modulus of the human intact left ventricle determination and physiological interpretation. *Med Biol Eng.* 13(2):151–160.

Ghista DN, Zhong L, Chua LP, Ng EYK, Lim ST, Chua T. 2005. Systolic modelling of the left ventricle as a mechatronic system: Determination of myocardial fiber's sarcomere contractile characteristics and new performance indices. *Mol Cell Biomech.* 2:217–233.

Gould P, Ghista DN, Brombolich L, Mirsky I. 1972. In vivo stresses in the human left ventricular wall: Analysis accounting for the irregular 3-dimensional geometry and comparison with idealized geometry analysis. *J Biomech.* 5(5):521–539.

Graham TP Jr, Jarmakani JM, Canent RV Jr, Anderson PAW. 1971. Evaluation of left ventricular contractile state in children; normal values and observations with a pressure overload. *Circulation.* 44:1043–1052.

Grossman W. 1980. Cardiac hypertrophy: Useful adaptation or pathologic process? *Am J Med.* 69:576–584.

Grossman W, Braunwald E, Mann T, McLaurin L, Green L. 1977. Contractile state of the left ventricle in man as evaluated from end-systolic pressure-volume relations. *Circulation.* 56:845–852.

Guccione JM, Costa KD, McCulloch AD. 1995. Finite element stress analysis of left ventricular mechanics in the beating dog heart. *J Biomech.* 28:1167–1177.

Guccoine JM, McCulloch AD, Waldman LK. 1991. Passive material properties of the intact ventricular myocardium determined from a cylindrical model. *ASME J Biomech Eng.* 113:42–55.

Guccione JM, Salahieh A, Moonly SM. 2003. Myosplint decrease wall stress without depressing function in the failing heart: A finite element model study. *Ann Thorac Surg.* 76(4):1171–1180.

Hayashida WT, Kumada R, Nohara H, Tanio M, Kambayashi N, Ishikawa Y, Nakamura Y, Himura Y, Kawai C. 1990. Left ventricular wall stress in dilated cardiomyopathy. *Circulation.* 82:2075–2083.

Hefner LL, Sheffield LT, Cobbs GC, Klip W. 1962. Relation between mural force and pressure in the left ventricle of the dog. *Circ Res.* 11:654–663.

Hill AV. 1950. Mechanics of the contractile element of muscle. *Nature.* 165:415.

Hood WP, Thomson WJ, Rachley CE, Rolett EL. 1969. Comparison of calculation of left ventricular wall stress in man from thin-walled and thick-walled ellipsoidal models. *Circ Res.* 24:575–585.

Hooks DA, Tomlinson KA, Marsden SG, LeGrice IJ, Smaill BH. 2002. Cardiac microstructure: Implication for electrical propagation and defibrillation in the heart. *Circ Res.* 91:331–338.

Hsu E, Henriquez C. 2001. Myocardial fiber orientation mapping using reduced encoding diffusion tensor imaging. *J Cardiovasc Magn Reson.* 3:325–333.

Huisman RM, Elzinga G, Westerhof N, Sipkema P. 1980. Measurement of left ventricular wall stress. *Cardiovasc Res.* 14:142–153.

Humphrey JD, Strumpf RK, Yin FCP. 1990. Determination of a constitutive relation for passive myocardium: I Parameter estimation. *J Biomech Eng.* 112:340–346.

Hunter PJ. 1975. Finite element analysis of cardiac muscle mechanics. PhD thesis, University of Oxford, Oxford, UK.

Hunter P. 1997. Myocardial constitutive laws for continuum mechanics models of the heart. In: *Molecular and Subcellular Cardiology: Effect of Structure and Function*, Sideman S and Beyar R (eds.), Plenum Press, New York, pp. 303–318.

Hunter P, Pullan A, Smail B. 2003. Modeling total heart function. *Ann Rev Biomed Eng.* 5:147–177.

Huxley AF. 1957. Muscle structure and theories of contraction. *Prog Biophys Chem.* 7:255.

Huyghe JM, van Campen DH, Arts T, Heethaar RM. 1991. The constitutive behavior of passive heart muscle tissue: A quasi-linear visco-elastic formulation. *J Biomech.* 24:841–849.

Ingrassia CM, Jani SY, Costa KD. 2008. Evaluation of analytic estimates of ventricular wall stress using the finite element method. In: *Proceedings of the ASME 2008 Summer Bioengineering Conference*, SBC2008-193262, Marco Island, FL.

Jan KM. 1985. Distribution of myocardial stress and its influence on coronary blood flow. *J Biomech.* 18:815–820.

Janz RF. 1982. Estimation of local myocardial stress. *Am J Physiol Heart Circ Physiol.* 242:H875–H881.

Janz RF, Grimm AF. 1972. Finite-element model for the mechanical behaviour of the left ventricle: Prediction of deformation in the potassium-arrested rat heart. *Circ Res.* 30:244–252.

Janz RF, Kubert BR, Moriarty TF, Grimm AF. 1974. Deformation of the diastolic left ventricle-II. Nonlinear geometric effects. *Journal of Biomechanics*, 7(6):509–516.

Laplace PS. 1805. Theorie de l'Action Capillarie. In: *Traité de Mecanique Celeste, Supplement au livre X.*, Coarcien, Paris, France.

Le Grice IJ, Smaill BH, Chai LZ, Edgar SG, Gavin JB, Hunter PJ. 1995. Laminar structure of the heart: Ventricular myocyte arrangement and connective tissue architecture in the dog. *Am J Physiol.* 269(38):H571–H582.

Lin DHS, Yin YCP. 1998. A multiaxial constitutive law for mammalian left ventricular myocardium steady-state barium contracture or tetanus. *J Biomech Eng.* 120(4):504–517.

Mann DL. 2004. Basic mechanisms of left ventricular remodeling: The contribution of wall stress. *J Cardiac Fail.* 10(6):S202–S206.

Mirsky I. 1969. Left ventricular stresses in the intact human heart. *Biophys J.* 9:189–208.

Mirsky I. 1973. Ventricular and arterial wall stresses based on large deformations analyses. *Biophys J.* 13:1141–1159.

Mirsky I. 1974. Review of various theories for the evaluation of left ventricular wall stress. In: *Cardiac Mechanics*, Mirsky I, Ghista DN, Sandler H (eds.), Wiley, New York, pp. 381–409.

Mirsky I, Pasipoularides A. 1990. Clinical assessment of diastolic function. *Prog Cardiovasc Dis.* 32:291–318.

Misra JC, Singh SI. 1985. Distribution of stresses in the left ventricular wall of the intact heart. *Bull Math Biol.* 47:53–70.

Moonly S. 2003. Experimental and computational analysis of left ventricular aneurysm mechanics. University of California, San Francisco, CA.

Moriarty TF. 1980. The law of Laplace, its limitations as a relation for diastolic pressure, volume or wall stress of the left ventricle. *Circ Res.* 46:321–331.

Nash M. 1998. Mechanics and material properties of the heart using an anatomically accurate mathematical model. PhD thesis, The University of Auckland, Auckland, New Zealand.

Nielsen PM, Hunter PJ, Smail BH. 1991a. Biaxial testing of membrane biomaterials: Testing equipment and procedures. *J Biomech Eng.* 113:295–300.

Nielsen PMF, LeGrice IJ, Smail BH, Hunter PJ. 1991b. A mathematical model of the geometry and fibrous structure of the heart. *Am J Physiol.* 260:H1365–H1378.

Omens JH, MacKenna DA, McCulloch AD. 1993. Measurement of strain and analysis of stress in resting rat left ventricular myocardium. *J Biomech.* 26(6):665–676.

Pouleur H, Rousseau M, Van Eyll C, Charlier A. 1984. Assessment of regional left ventricular relaxation in patients with coronary artery disease: Importance of geometric factors and changes in wall thickness. *Circulation.* 69:696–702.

Prunier F, Brette S, Delepine S, Geslin P, Le Jeune JJ, Furber AP. 2008. Three-dimensional MRI assessment of regional wall stress after acute myocardial infarction predicts postdischarge cardiac events. *J Magn Reson Imaging.* 27(3):516–521.

Rohde LE, Aikawa M, Cheng GC, Sukhova G, Solomon SD, Libby P, Pfeffer J, Pfeffer MA, Lee RT. 1999. Echocardiography-derived left ventricular end-systolic regional wall stress and matrix remodeling after experimental myocardial infarction. *J Am Coll Cardiol.* 33:835–842.

Sandler H, Dodge HT. 1963. Left ventricular tension and stress in man. *Circulation*. 13:91–101.

Schwitter J, Eberli FR, Ritter M, Turina M, Krayenbuehl HP. 1992. Myocardial oxygen consumption in aortic valve disease with and without left ventricular dysfunction. *Br Heart J*. 18:815–820.

Smith NP, Mulquiney PJ, Nash MP, Bradley CP, Nickerson DP, Hunter PJ. 2002. Mathematical modeling of the heart: Cell to organ. *Chaos Solitons Fractals*. 13:1613–1621.

Smith NP, Pullan AJ, Hunter PJ. 2000. Generation of an anatomically based geometric coronary model. *Ann Biomed Eng*. 28:14–25.

Solomon SD, Martini M, Rosario L. 1998. Regional wall stress following myocardial infarction estimated by echocardiography-based structural analysis. *J Am Soc Echocardiogr*. 32:1819–1824.

Spontnitz HM, Sonnenclick EH, Spiro D. 1966. Relation of ultrastructure to function in intact heart: Sarcomere structure relative to pressure-volume curves of intact left ventricles of dog and cat. *Circ Res*. 18:49–59.

Streeter DD, Hanna WT. 1973a. Engineering mechanics for successive states in canine left ventricular myocardium: I Cavity and wall geometry. *Circ Res*. 33:639–655.

Streeter DD, Hanna WT. 1973b. Engineering mechanics for successive states in canine left ventricular myocardium: II Fibre angle and sarcomere length. *Circ Res*. 33:656–664.

Timoshenko S, Goodier JN. 1951. *Theory of Elasticity*. McGraw-Hill, New York.

Tranum-Jensen J, Wilde AAM, Vermeulen JT, Janse MJ. 1991. Morphology of electrophysiologically identified junctions between Purkinje fibres and ventricular muscle in rabbit and pig hearts. *Circ Res*. 69:429–437.

Turcani M, Rupp H. 1997. Etomoxir improves left ventricular performance of pressure-overloaded rat heart. *Circulation*. 96:3681–3686.

Vetter FJ, McCulloch AD. 1998. Three-dimensional analysis of regional cardiac anatomy. *Prog Biophys Mol Biol*. 69:157–184.

Vetter FJ, McCulloch AD. 2000. Three-dimensional stress and strain in passive rabbit left ventricle: A model study. *Ann Biomed Eng*. 28(7):781–792.

Wall ST, Walker JC, Healy KE, Ratcliffe MB, Guccione JM. 2006. Theoretical impact of the injection of material into the myocardium. *Circulation*. 114:2627–2635.

Walker JC, Ratcliffer MB, Zhang P, Wallace AW, Fata B, Hsu EW, Saloner D, Guccione JM. 2005. MRI-based finite-element analysis of left ventricular aneurysm. *Am J Physiol Heart Circ Physiol*. 289(2):H692–H700.

Walker JC, Ratcliffe MB, Zhang P, Wallace AW, Hsu EW, Saloner DA, Guccione JM. 2008. Magnetic resonance imaging-based finite element stress analysis after linear repair of left ventricular aneurysm. *J Thorac Cardiovasc Surg*. 135(5):1094–1102.

Wong AYK, Rautarharju PM. 1968. Stress distribution within the left ventricular wall approximated as a thick ellipsoidal shell. *Am Heart J*. 75:649–662.

Yin FC. 1981. Ventricular wall stress. *Circ Res*. 49:829–842.

Yin FCP, Strumpf RK, Chew PH, Zeger SL. 1987. Quantification of the mechanical properties of noncontracting canine myocardium under simultaneous biaxial loading. *J Biomech*. 20:577–589.

Zhong L, Sola S, Tan RS, Le TT, Ghista DN, Kurra V, Navia JL, Kassab G. 2009a. Effects of surgical ventricular restoration on LV contractility assessed by a novel contractility index in patients with ischemic cardiomyopathy. *Am J Cardiol*. 103(5):674–679.

Zhong L, Su Y, Yeo SY, Tan RS, Ghista DN, Kassab G. 2009b. Left ventricular regional wall curvedness and wall stress in patients with ischemic dilated cardiomyopathy. *Am J Physiol Heart Circ Physiol*. 296:H573–H584.

Zhong L, Tan RS, Ghista DN, Ng EYK, Chua LP, Kassab GS. 2007. Validation of a novel noninvasive cardiac index of left ventricular contractility in patients. *Am J Physiol Heart Circ Physiol*. 292(6):H2764–H2772.

2

Cardiac Function Assessment in Filling and Systolic Phases: Passive and Active Elastances of the Left Ventricle

Dhanjoo N. Ghista, Liang Zhong, and Eddie Y.K. Ng

CONTENTS

2.1 Introduction

Heart failure is a leading cause of death in developed countries. This clinical syndrome may be a manifestation of left ventricular (LV) filling abnormalities and/or inadequate LV myocardial contraction (due to myocardial ischemia or infarct and/or electrical contraction abnormality). Cardiologists have been using simple clinical measurements such as heart rate, ECG patterns, blood pressure, and ejection fraction to diagnose cardiac pathologies. However, these measurements do not provide adequate scientific insight into the heart's complex electromechanical machinery involved in its functional performance and clinical syndromes. This chapter constitutes study of biomechanical mechanisms and phenomena of the heart function, leading to the development of new indices of assessment of heart function and impairment.

In a bioengineering sense, the heart can be described as a blood pump and its physiological behavior can be understood in terms of the time-varying relationship between ventricular blood pressure and volume. For many years, clinicians have used this relationship as a measure of cardiac function [1–14]. Concomitant with this approach, we have developed the concept of LV myocardial stress and modulus [15–17] to characterize both diastolic and systolic performance.

An understanding of LV function mechanisms in terms of its myocardial properties is important to characterize the underlying ventricular pump function. Pressure and volume are the fundamental measurable physical variables, from which to derive and express the biomechanical properties of the LV. Some of the earlier works of Ghista et al., on this intrinsic characterization of LV function [15,17], have in fact been adopted clinically.

Characterizing the LV as a pump is not simple, as the LV function is a complex phenomenon. It depends both on its myocardial properties and chamber geometry, as well as on the preload (i.e., end-diastolic pressure) and afterload (i.e., aortic pressure). Therefore, it is necessary to know the bioengineering characteristics of LV shape dynamics and LV muscle contraction during physiological and pathological conditions. Hence, we need to develop appropriate LV bioengineering models, to characterize the LV in vivo anatomy and physiology as well as its sarcomere properties, and link them to LV clinical performance.

Analytical modeling is necessary for such a quantitative understanding of the cardiac function and dysfunction during diastolic-filling and ejection phases. In this regard, the primary objectives of this chapter are to (1) develop LV pressure–volume-based model to determine LV passive elastance and active elastance, and propose the maximum value of the LV active elastance as a cardiac contractility index, (2) present another noninvasively determinable cardiac LV contractility index based on LV normalized wall stress with respect to LV intracavitary pressure, and (3) provide clinical validation for these two contractility indices.*

---

* This work was first reported in [12], and then incorporated in Chapter 2 of *Applied Biomedical Engineering*, D.N. Ghista, CRC Press. It is also based on Chapter 11: Assessment of cardiac function in filling and systolic ejection phases: A mathematical and clinical evaluation, L. Zhong, D.N. Ghista, E.Y.K. Ng, R.S. Tan, S.T. Lim, *Advances in Cardiac Signal Processing*, R. Acharya U, J. Suri, J.A.E. Spaan, S.M. Krishnan (eds.), Springer Verlag GmbH, Berlin, Germany (with permission from Springer Verlag).

2.2 History of Research: LV Diastolic and Systolic Dysfunction

2.2.1 Ventricular Diastolic Dysfunction Characterization

From a physiological point of view, the LV is an integrated muscle-pump system. LV diastole starts when active relaxation has been completed and includes the diastasis and the left atrial (LA) contraction phase. Diastole is interpreted as "the dilatation or period of dilatation of the LV, coinciding with the interval between the second and first heart sounds" [18]. In this interpretation, it is the part of the cardiac cycle, which starts with the isovolumic relaxation phase and ends with cessation of mitral flow; the passive biomechanical properties of the LV are associated with this phase [19,20].

The functional properties of the LV during diastole have mostly been described in terms of either the rate at which it relaxes in early diastole or its stiffness when it is fully relaxed in the later part of diastole. Hence, diastolic dysfunction can be divided into relaxation abnormalities (due to ischemia and cardiomyopathy), decreased compliance (i.e., LV stiffness due to hypertrophy and myocardial fibrosis) and abnormal high heart rate [21,22]. Common conditions associated with diastolic dysfunction are shown in Figure 2.1.

However, the filling pattern of the LV depends on a complex and continuous interaction of multiple factors, of which only some relate directly to the diastolic properties of the LV itself. Other factors relate to the hemodynamic conditions imposed on the LV, including venous return, LV suction, resistance-to-filling and LA contraction. Therefore, diastolic dysfunction can be regarded as the result of a diversity of physiological abnormalities of myocardial relaxation or decreased ventricular compliance.

2.2.2 Left Ventricular Systolic Dysfunction Assessment

LV systolic function can be defined in terms of the myocardial cells generating appropriate coordinated contractile force to develop adequate LV pressure to open the aortic valve, and then contracting and shortening the LV wall to pump an appropriate stroke volume. This means systole is a process of converting biochemical energy into biomechanical energy in the myocardial sarcomere cross-bridges for contraction. The functional properties of the LV during systole have mostly been described in terms of its contractility property at different levels. Hence, systolic dysfunction can be defined in terms of the LV not being able to contract and eject an adequate stroke volume into the circulation.

How to intrinsically assess the systolic function of the LV has long been a major problem in physiology and cardiology. This is addressed in this chapter and in Chapter 3 of this book.

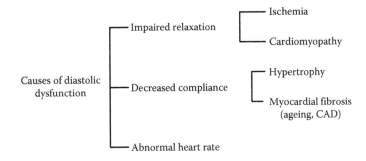

FIGURE 2.1
Causes of diastolic dysfunction.

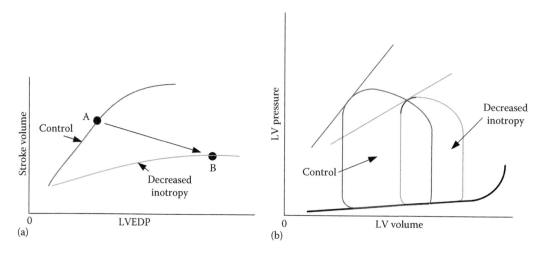

FIGURE 2.2
(a) The Frank–Starling relationship showing the effects of systolic dysfunction on stroke volume and left ventricular end-diastolic pressure (LVEDP). (b) Effects of left ventricular systolic dysfunction on left ventricular pressure–volume loop.

The systolic function of the LV has been viewed at different levels [23]. In 1895, Frank characterized ventricular function in terms of the pressure–volume diagram. In 1918, Starling first viewed the LV as a pump to generate cardiac output (proportional to its filling) against an afterload. The loss of cardiac inotropy (i.e., decreased contractility), associated with LV systolic dysfunction, causes a downward shift in the Frank–Starling curve (Figure 2.2). This results in a decrease in stroke volume and a compensatory rise in preload (i.e., end-diastolic pressure). The rise in preload is considered compensatory, because it activates the Frank–Starling mechanism to help maintain stroke volume despite decreased inotropy. The effects of decreased inotropy on stroke volume, left ventricular end-diastolic pressure (LVEDP), and LV pressure–volume loop are depicted in Figure 2.2. Hill [24] and Huxley [25,26] investigated muscle contraction by means of muscle force–velocity relationship at the micro-structural level (cross-bridge theory). Then, more recently, Suga [27] proposed that the systolic function of the LV is a process of converting the cross-bridge biochemical energy into the biomechanical energy during contraction.

2.3 Clinical Indices of Cardiac Function

The use of LV biomechanical properties or indices, mathematically derived from cardiac (pressure–volume) data measurements, facilitates the monitoring, assessment, and follow-up of cardiac function.

2.3.1 Indices Characterizing the "Passive" Ventricle

The LV end-diastolic pressure remains the most commonly used clinical parameter to describe its passive elastance. A higher-than-normal filling pressure is considered as an index of LV dilatation, stiffness, and diastolic failure. This parameter is easily measured by catheterization.

However, elevated filling pressure does not distinguish between overfilling, vasoconstriction, absence of atrial contraction, or a changed compliance of the ventricle. Therefore, we need to develop some other indices to describe the function and dysfunction of the passive LV.

In this regard, LV chamber stiffness and myocardial stiffness have been investigated [28–32]. Chamber stiffness is derived from the relationship between pressure and volume during diastole. The operation stiffness at any point along a given pressure–volume curve is equal to the slope of a tangent drawn on the curve at that point. Thus, the shape and position of the entire pressure–volume relation can be used to determine the overall chamber stiffness. As shown in Figure 2.3, the operating chamber stiffness changes throughout the filling phase; stiffness (dP/dV) is less at a smaller volume (point "a") and greater at a larger volume (point "b"). Since diastolic pressure–volume data can be expressed by an exponential relationship, a chamber stiffness parameter (k_c) can thus be derived as the slope of the linear relation between dP/dV and pressure [32]. When the overall chamber stiffness increases, the pressure–volume curve shifts to the left, the slope of the dP/dV versus pressure relation becomes steeper, and the chamber stiffness k_c increases. In order to decrease the complexity, Lisauskas et al. [33] developed the average and passive ventricular diastolic stiffness from transmitral flow, by using a simple formula ($\Delta P/\Delta V)_{avg}$.

Corresponding with chamber stiffness, the myocardial muscle of the LV behaves as an elastic material, developing a resisting force as it is stretched by ventricular filling. The greater the change in muscle length (strain), the greater the increase in the force (wall stress) that resists this deformation and the stiffer the myocardium becomes. Myocardial stiffness can be estimated by examining the relation between LV wall stress (σ) and strain (ε) during diastole. At any given strain throughout filling, myocardial stiffness is equal to the slope ($d\sigma/d\varepsilon$) of a tangent drawn to the stress–strain curve at that strain.

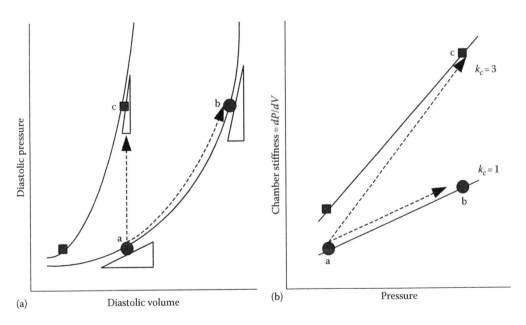

FIGURE 2.3
Schematic diagram of LV diastolic pressure–volume relation. (a) A progressive increase in volume will increase chamber stiffness (dP/dV). (b) A leftward shift of the pressure–volume relation will also increase chamber stiffness. As the pressure–volume relation is assumed exponential, the relation between dP/dV and pressure is linear; the slope of this relation represents the chamber stiffness constant (k_c).

Most investigators have considered the diastolic pressure–volume relation and stress–strain relation as curvilinear and exponential, hence the relationships between dP/dV versus pressure and between $d\sigma/d\varepsilon$ versus stress can be linear [30]. It is a common practice to curve-fit diastolic P–V or stress–strain data from minimum pressure (and stress) to end-diastole in exponential or power form, and then use the exponent as an index of chamber or myocardial stiffness. Such approaches are however limited for several reasons, namely, (1) the data are sparse and often scattered in the clinical setting, particularly when angiographic measurements are used; (2) the exponent used is often size-dependent and therefore not always suitable for patient-to-patient comparisons; and (3) events that occur during the early rapid filling phase are ignored in the analysis [31].

2.3.2 Indices Characterizing LV Contractility

Many cardiac models have dealt with the formulation and measurement of contractility [12,13,34–38]. So then what is the meaning of contractility? Conceptually, cardiac contractility is the potential for contraction that cardiac muscle possesses by virtue of its physicochemical environment, for example, calcium handling and contractile proteins. It is what the muscle (heart) is capable of doing [39]. But how does one measure the total physicochemical environment of the cell in order to measure contractility, which can be difficult? Thus, to use the concept of contractility in evaluating LV performance, we need an operational definition of contractility, which we will now examine.

2.3.2.1 V_{max} as a Measure of Cardiac Muscle Contractility

Based on Hill's theory of the activated muscle, Sonnenblick [40,41] extended this study to the cardiac muscle. He suggested that a hyperbolic relation existed between the velocity of shortening of the contractile element and the developed force in it. In particular, the results indicated that V_{max} (the contractile element shortening velocity at zero load) was independent of the initial muscle length or preload, and seemed as a good contractility index.

As shown in Figure 2.4, as afterload is reduced, the velocity of shortening increases. When afterload is zero, the velocity of shortening is maximal (V_{max}). This V_{max} does not depend on the length of the muscle from which contraction is initiated (left part). Also, V_{max} (velocity at zero afterload) increases with an increase in inotropic state (i.e., increased contractility) even when initial length (preload) is unchanged. Hence, V_{max} is proposed as a measure of contractility [42–44].

However, Mirsky and Ghista [45] gave a summary review of the existing formulae available for conducting force–velocity analyses derived from animal experimental studies and the development of indices for the assessment of heart muscle function. On the basis of this study, it is concluded that V_{max} is sensitive to the relatively high preloads and may not be a reliable index of contractility. A more reliable index for assessing cardiac muscle function can be proposed as $(dP/dt/kP)_{max}$ wherein P is LV pressure and k is its stiffness constant.

2.3.2.2 dP/dt_{max} as a Measure of Cardiac Contractility

The dP/dt means the rate of development of the LV intracavitary pressure with respect to time. The dP/dt record is generated by computer differentiation of the pressure curve, to obtain a record of the rate of ventricular pressure. Figure 2.5 illustrates two separate recordings of the ventricular intracavitary pressure wave as well as the computed curve of dP/dt for normal and isoproterenol stimulated hearts.

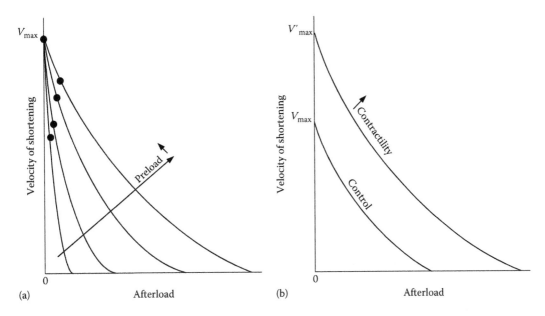

FIGURE 2.4
(a) Force (afterload)-velocity-of-shortening relationship under different preload conditions. (b) Force (afterload)-velocity-of-shortening relationship in control and enhanced contractility states.

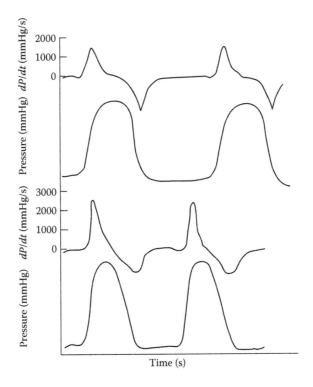

FIGURE 2.5
Simultaneous recordings of ventricular pressure and dP/dt. The upper part shows results from a normal heart, and the below part shows results from a heart stimulated by isoproterenol.

For the past four decades, dP/dt_{max} has arguably been the most sensitive ventricular index of inotropicity and the current "gold standard" [46,47]. Unfortunately, aside from it requiring invasive measurement, the value of dP/dt_{max} is affected by other factors such as preload and afterload [54]. Therefore, it is difficult to use dP/dt_{max} as a measure of contractility in comparing ventricles from one person to another. For this reason, other quantitative measures have also been used in attempts to assess cardiac contractility. So Mirsky and Ghista proposed to employ dP/dt divided by the instantaneous pressure in the ventricle, or $(dP/dt)/kP_{max}$, as a more reliable measure of cardiac contractility [45].

2.3.2.3 E_{max} as a Measure of Cardiac Contractility

Conceivably, LV elastance based on LV pressure–volume relationship reflects LV contractile function quite accurately [3,47–51]. Suga and Sagawa [49] formalized this concept as the time-varying elastance of the ventricle, by defining elastance, E, as: $E(t) = P(t)/(V(t) - V_d)$, where $P(t)$ and $V(t)$ are ventricular pressure and volume that vary with time t, respectively. Therein, V_d is the LV volume corresponding to zero LV pressure, obtained by drawing a tangent to the pressure–volume curves at end-ejection, as shown in Figure 2.6.

It has been shown that the end-systolic pressure–volume (ESPV) relationship, which is the loci of pressure and volume points at end-systole (Figure 2.6), is insensitive to variations of both the end-diastolic volume (preload) and the mean arterial pressure (afterload). The ESPV relationship is usually a straight line, with a slope of E_{max} as the maximal elastance. The value of E_{max} remains essentially constant if the preload and afterload are allowed to vary within the physiological range, but is sensitive to inotropic agents and ischemia. Hence, E_{max} has been proposed as a "load-independent" index of contractility of the ventricle [47]. However, the loading conditions do affect E_{max} if ventricular pressure and volume are made to vary over a wider range [52,53]. Under these conditions, the ESPV relation becomes curvilinear, concave toward the volume axis. A simple calculation of the elastance of a ventricle for different arterial loads reveals that the elastance changes and is load-dependent. Hence, derived indices such as E_{max} and ESPV relationship loose their

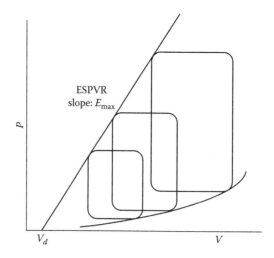

FIGURE 2.6

Defining the concept of ESPVR as a measure of LV contractility (corresponding to zero pressure) is obtained by drawing a tangent to P–V curves at end ejection.

clinical applicability [54]. Elastance measurement also requires cardiac catheterization for measurement of pressure, which further reduces its utility.

An additional limitation of E_{max} is that it is not easy to change afterload and obtain multiple pressure–volume data points in a given subject, while maintaining a constant contractility. Hence, it is impractical to use E_{max} clinically, for patient-specific LV catheterization-ventriculography data.

2.3.2.4 Preload-Adjusted Maximal Power as a Measure of Cardiac Contractility

The maximal value of power is calculated by analyzing the instantaneous values of pressure and flow and their product during ventricular ejection [55]. The preload-adjusted maximal power, obtained by dividing maximum power by end-diastolic volume squared, has been shown to be relatively independent of preload, afterload, and resistance [56,57]. However, more recently, Lester et al. [58] found that preload-adjusted maximal power was not preload-independent in anesthetized humans. In order to get a more accurate value of power, the ventricular intracavitary pressure is needed by catheterization. So then, by combining arterial (aortic) pressure tracing and flow (measured as velocity), obtained with continuous wave Doppler echocardiography through the aortic valve, it is possible to acquire all the data necessary for power estimation.

Although preload-adjusted maximal power has these appealing characteristics, there is still an important limitation to its use in clinical practice. This limitation is mainly of practical in nature, as a series of off-line, time-consuming analyses are necessary to obtain it. Another limitation is that the ventricular intracavitary pressure is replaced by arterial pressure. Due to damping and resonance in the arterial waveform, the peripheral pressure can be a poor estimate of true ventricular intracavitary pressure.

2.3.2.5 Myocardial Strain Rate as a Measure of Cardiac Contractility

Recently, with the advent of new technology, noninvasive index characterizing contractility, myocardial fiber strain rate, obtained by tissue Doppler echocardiography (TDE) and strain rate imaging (SRI), have been proposed by Greenberg et al. [37] and Costa et al. [59], respectively. Myocardial strain reflects the deformation of tissue in response to an applied force. The first temporal derivative of strain, namely, strain rate, is the velocity change in myocardial length. One limitation of TDE, however, is that regional TDE velocities are affected by heart translation and tethering of adjacent myocardial segments. The method of SRI has eliminated the tethering effect as a powerful tool for assessing segmental LV dysfunction such as coronary disease.

2.4 Our Works: Intra-Cardiac Blood Flow, Passive and Active Elastances

2.4.1 Intra-Cardiac Blood-Flow Velocity and Pressure Distributions

Ultimately, cardiac diastolic and systolic function (and the associated indices) result in intra-cardiac blood-flow velocity and pressure distributions. With the advent of FEM, Subbaraj and Ghista [60] were able to provide instantaneous distributions of intra-LV flow and differential pressure during the ejection phases, and in turn derive an intrinsic index of contractility in terms of the intra-LV pressure gradient field. This can be termed as a major contribution to quantitative cardiology. A uniform pressure gradient toward the aortic outflow tract will contribute to an efficient LV pumping. On the other hand, a non-uniform pressure gradient, caused by asynchronous myocardium contraction due to coronary lesions or infarcts, would give rise to poor pumping performance of the LV.

As seen in Figure 2.7, the computed intra-cardiac blood-flow velocity and distributions for a typical Patient Turn are visually so convenient to be interpreted by cardiologists, and to facilitate their decision-making.

2.4.2 Passive and Active Elastances of the Left Ventricle

As an alternative to the P–V loop as a measure of ventricular function, a new paradigm for quantifying ventricular performance is proposed. Herein, we have come up with a new concept of dual passive and active elastances operating throughout the cardiac cycle [12].

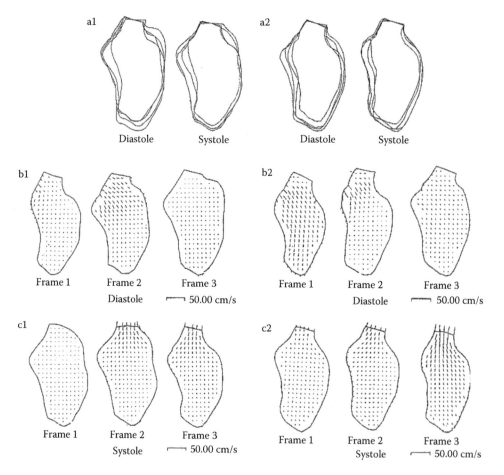

FIGURE 2.7
Patient Turn: (a) Superimposed sequential diastolic and systolic endocardial frames (whose aortic valves centers and the long axis are matched) before (a1) and after (a2) administration of nitroglycerin. (b) Instantaneous intra-LV distributions of velocity during diastole, before (b1) and after (b2) administration of nitroglycerin. (c) Instantaneous intra-LV distributions of velocity during the ejection phase, before (c1) and after (c2) administration of nitroglycerin.

(Continued)

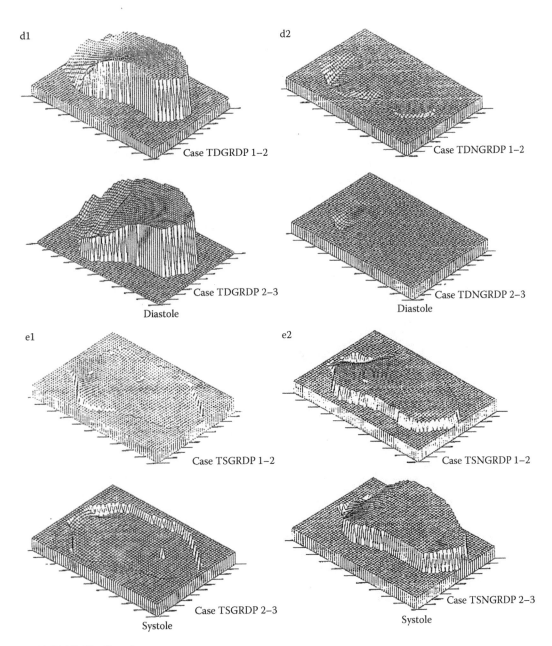

FIGURE 2.7 (Continued)
Patient Turn: (d) Instantaneous intra-LV distributions of pressure-differentials during diastole, before (d1) and after (d2) administration of nitroglycerin. (e) Instantaneous intra-LV distributions of pressure-differentials during the ejection phase, before (e1) and after (e2) administration of nitroglycerin. (Adapted from Subbaraj, K. et al., *J. Biomed. Eng.*, 9, 206, 1987).

The passive elastance (E_p) represents the LV pressure response to LV volume change (i.e., to LV volume increase during the LV filling phase and to LV volume decrease during the LV ejection phase). Additionally, we also have active elastance (E_a) representing the contraction of the left ventricle due to its sarcomeric activation (and the development of force between the sarcomere actin–myosin units) and relaxation (due to disengagement of the actin–myosin units). The passive E_p governs LV stiffness variation due to volume increase during filling phase and due to volume decrease during the ejection phase, and active E_a governs LV pressure increase in the systolic phase due to LV myocardial contraction.

Now, LV E_a develops at the start of isovolumic contraction, becomes maximum some time during late ejection, and thereafter decreases and becomes zero during diastolic filling. On the other hand, LV E_p starts increasing after the start of LV filling as the LV volume increases. It reaches its maximum value at the end-of-filling phase, remains constant during isovolumic contraction, and thereafter decreases during ejection (as the LV volume decreases). The generation (and increase) of E_a helps us to explain the development of the LV pressure increase during isovolumic contraction, while the decrease of E_a during diastole helps us to explain the decrease in LV pressure during early filling to create LV suction of the blood (even before the onset of LA contraction). The incorporation of both E_p and E_a helps us to explain the LV pressure changes during the filling and ejection phases. Now, we will derive expressions for E_a and E_p in terms of LV pressure and volume data.

2.4.2.1 Bioengineering Definition of Passive and Active Elastances of the LV

At the start of the diastolic-filling phase, the LV incremental pressure dP_{LV} is the response (1) to LV E_a continuing to decrease due to the sarcomere continuing to relax well into the filling phase and (2) to the rapid inflow of blood and the corresponding increase in LV volume, along with the associated increase in LV E_p. The corresponding governing differential equation, relating LV pressure and volume, can be put down by referring to our work [12] for its derivation:

$$M(d\dot{V}) + d(EV) = M(d\dot{V}) + V\,dE + E\,dV = dP_{LV} \tag{2.1}$$

where
   V represents the volume of LV (mL), whose derivation with respect to time (t) is expressed
      in seconds (s) from the start of the filling phase
   P_{LV} represents pressure of the LV, in mmHg (hereafter symbolized by P) (mmHg)
   M represents the inertia term = [LV wall-density (ρ)/(LV surface-area/wall-thickness)] =
      $\rho h/4\pi R^2$, for a spherical LV model (in mmHg/(mL/s^2))
   E represents LV elastance (mmHg/mL)

Likewise during ejection, the LV pressure variation (dP_{LV}) is caused by both E_a variation as well as by E_p decrease (due to LV volume decrease). The instantaneous time-varying ventricular elastance (E) is the sum of (1) the volume-dependent passive elastance (E_p) and (2) the active elastance (E_a) due to the activation of the LV sarcomere. Hence,

$$E = E_a + E_p \tag{2.2}$$

We now provide the expressions for E_p and E_a.

2.4.2.2 Expression for Passive Elastance (E_p) of the LV

The passive (unactivated) myocardium exhibits properties of an elastic material, developing an increasing stress as strain increases, as occurs during ventricular filling. The passive stress–strain relation of myocardial muscle strip is nonlinear and follows an exponential relationship [31,61,62]. Likewise, the relation between LV passive pressure and volume is adopted to be exponential, as

$$P = P_0 e^{z_p V} \tag{2.3}$$

so that,

$$E_p = \left(\frac{dP}{dV} \right) = E_{p0} e^{z_p V} \tag{2.4}$$

where
   E_{p0} is the passive elastance coefficient ($= P_0 z_p$)
   z_p is the passive elastance exponent parameter
   V is the LV volume

Its evaluation for a clinical case is provided in a subsequent section. During the latter part of the diastolic phase, we use Equation 2.3 to fit the LV pressure–volume relation to determine the corresponding parameters, P_0 and z_p (or E_{p0} and z_p), and hence obtain the passive elastance E_p.

2.4.2.3 Expression for Active Elastance (E_a) of the LV

During isovolumic contraction, $dV = 0$. Hence $d\dot{V} = 0$, and E_p is constant and equal to E_{ped} (the value of E_p at end-diastole). As a result, the governing Equation 2.1 becomes $VdE = dP_{LV}$, which can be discretized as

$$V_i(E_i - E_{i-1}) = V_i[(E_{a,i} + E_{p,i}) - (E_{a,i-1} + E_{p,i-1})]$$

$$= V_i(E_{a,i} + E_{ped} - E_{a,i-1} - E_{ped})$$

$$= dP_{LV,i} = P_i - P_{i-1}$$

Hence,

$$E_{a,i} = \frac{(P_i - P_{i-1})}{V_i} + E_{a,i-1} \tag{2.5}$$

where
   i is a time instant during the isovolumic contraction and relaxation
   V_i and $P_{LV,i}$ are the monitored LV volume and pressure at this instant
   E_{ped} is the passive elastance at the end-diastolic phase

During the ejection phase, the governing Equation 2.1 can be discretized as:

$$E_{a,i} = \frac{(P_i - P_{i-1}) - M(\dot{V}_i - \dot{V}_{i-1}) - V_i(E_{p,i} - E_{p,i-1})}{2V_i - V_{i-1}} \frac{- E_{p,i}(V_i - V_{i-1}) + V_i E_{a,i-1}}{} \tag{2.6}$$

Also, during isovolumic relaxation, because $dV = 0$, $d\dot{V} = 0$ and E_p is constant and equal to its end-systolic value of E_{pes}. Hence, the governing Equation 2.1 again becomes $VdE = dP_{LV}$, which can be represented as

$$V_i[(E_{a,i} + E_{p,i}) - (E_{a,i-1} + E_{p,i-1})] = V_i(E_{a,i} + E_{pes} - E_{a,i-1} - E_{pes}) = dP_{LV,i} = P_i - P_{i-1}$$

Therefore,

$$E_{a,i} = \frac{P_i - P_{i-1}}{V_i} + E_{a,i-1} \qquad (2.7)$$

where E_{pes} is the passive elastance at the end of systole.

During the diastolic phase, the formula for computing active elastance is the same as Equation 2.6. Hence, from Equations 2.5 through 2.7, we can calculate the values of active elastance from LV pressure–volume data during the cardiac cycle. After calculating the values of active elastance (E_a), we adopt the following expression for E_a [13]:

$$E_a = E_{a0}\left[1 - e^{-(t/\tau_c)^{Z_c}}\right]\left[e^{-(((t-d)u(t-d))/\tau_r)^{Z_r}}\right] \qquad (2.8)$$

where
  t is measured from the start of isovolumic contraction
  E_{a0} is the active elastance coefficient parameter
  (τ_c) is the time-coefficient that describes the rate of elastance rise during the contraction phase,
  (τ_r) describes the rate of elastance fall during the relaxation phase
  "Z_c" and "Z_r" are exponents introduced to smoothen the curvatures of the E_a curve during isovolumic contraction and relaxation phases
  d is a time constant parameter
  $u(t-d)$ is the unit step function, so that $u(t-d) = 0$ for $t < d$

The rationale for the formulation of Equation 2.8 is based on E_a incorporating (1) parameters (Z_c and τ_c) reflecting the generation of LV pressure during isovolumic contraction, (2) parameters (Z_R and τ_R) reflecting the decrease of LV pressure during isovolumic relaxation and early filling, and (3) all of these parameters (Z_c, τ_c, Z_R, and τ_R) representing the LV pressure–volume relationship during filling and ejection phases.

We can then determine the values of these parameters by fitting Equation 2.8 to the computed values of E_a (from Equations 2.5 through 2.7), and employing the parameter-identification procedure to evaluate these aforementioned parameters.

2.5 Clinical Study: LV Passive and Active Elastances

2.5.1 Data Measurements

The subjects in this study (satisfying appropriate ethics procedures by Dr. Lim Soo Teik) were studied in a resting recumbent (baseline) state, after premedication with 100–500 mg of sodium pentobarbital by retrograde aortic catheterization. Angiography was performed by injecting 30–36 mL of 75% sodium diatrizoate into the LV at 10–12 mL/s. During ventriculography, LV chamber pressure was measured by a pigtail catheter and Statham P23Eb pressure transducer. From biplane angiocardiograms, it is seen that the orthogonal chamber diameters are nearly identical [63]. These findings are used to justify the use of single-plane cine techniques, which allow for beat-to-beat analysis of the chamber dimensions.

For our study, monoplane cineangiocardiograms were recorded in a RAO 30° projection from a 9 in image intensifier using 35 mm film at 50 fps, using INTEGRIS Allura 9 system at the Nation Heart Centre (NHC), Singapore. Therefrom, automated analysis was carried out to calculate LV volume and myocardial wall thickness. The LV data consist of measured volume and myocardial thickness of the chamber as well as the corresponding pressure (Figure 2.8). All measurements were corrected for geometric distortion due to the respective recordings systems. A typical subject's LV pressure versus volume data are displayed in Figure 2.9.

From the data in Figure 2.9, we can now compute E_p and E_a, by employing Equations 2.4 and 2.8.

2.5.2 Evaluation of Passive Elastance E_p

By fitting Equation 2.3 to the pressure and volume data during the filling phase, as shown in Figure 2.10, we obtain the values of the parameters P_0 and z_p, as

$$z_p = 0.040 \text{ mL}^{-1}, \quad P_0 = 0.080 \text{ mmHg} \tag{2.9}$$

and the E_p function (corresponding to its expression given by Equation 2.3) as follows:

$$E_p = 3.20 \times 10^{-3} e^{0.040V} \tag{2.10}$$

We now propose E_p as a measure of LV resistance-to-filling. During ejection and filling phases, E_p can be calculated at any time using Equation 2.10.

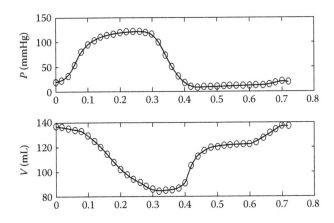

FIGURE 2.8
An example of a patient's measured LV pressure and volume during a cardiac cycle; $t = 0$–0.08 s is the isovolumic contraction phase, $t = 0.08$–0.32 s is the ejection phase, $t = 0.32$–0.40 s is the isovolumic relaxation phase, and $t = 0.40$–0.72 s is the filling phase. (Adapted from Zhong, L. et al., *Biomed. Eng. Online*, 4, 10, 2005.)

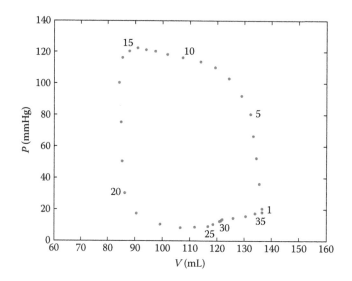

FIGURE 2.9

Relationship between LV volume and pressure for one sample data. Points (21–36) constitute the filling phase, (1–5) constitute the isovolumic contraction phase, (5–17) constitute the ejection phase, and (17–21) constitute the isovolumic relaxation phase. Note that after point 21 (the start of LV filling), the LV pressure decreases; this characterizes LV suction effect. The area enclosed by this loop represents LV work done. (Adapted from Zhong, L. et al., *Biomed. Eng. Online*, 4, 10, 2005.)

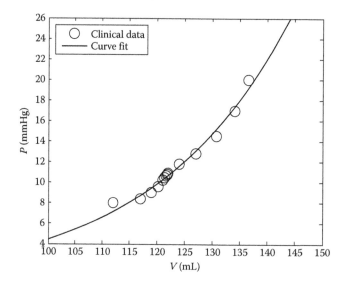

FIGURE 2.10

Using Equation 2.3 to fit the pressure–volume data during the filling phase. The volume 100 mL corresponds to the start of the filling phase, and the volume 150 mL corresponds to the end of the filling phase. (Adapted from Zhong, L. et al., *Biomed. Eng. Online*, 4, 10, 2005.)

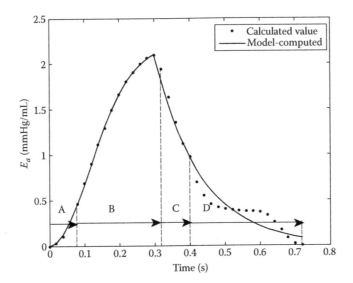

FIGURE 2.11
Calculated values of active elastance E_a during cardiac cycle. Using Equation 2.8 to fit the calculated values, we have: $E_{a0} = 2.20$ mmHg/mL, $\tau_c = 0.17$ s; $Z_c = 1.96$; $d = 0.3$ s, $\tau_R = 0.12$ s; $Z_R = 0.96$. A, isovolumic contraction phase; B, ejection phase; C, isovolumic relaxation phase; D, filling phase. (Adapted from Zhong, L. et al., *Biomed. Eng. Online*, 4, 10, 2005.)

2.5.3 Evaluation of Active Elastance E_a

Using Equations 2.5 through 2.7, we can calculate the active elastance E_a during isovolumic contraction, ejection, isovolumic relaxation, and diastolic-filling phases, respectively. The values of E_a during a cardiac cycle are shown in Figure 2.11. Then, the parameters in Equation 2.8 can be determined by fitting the computed values of E_a; these values are listed in Figure 2.11 caption as well as in Table 2.1.

Upon substituting these computed values of the parameters (E_{a0}, τ_c, Z_c, τ_R, Z_R) into Equation 2.8, we obtain the $E_a(t)$ function as follows:

$$E_a = 2.20\left[1 - e^{-(t/0.17)^{1.96}}\right]\left[e^{-((t-0.3)u(t-0.3)/0.12)^{0.96}}\right] \tag{2.11}$$

TABLE 2.1

Computed Values of Parameters in E_a Expression (Equation 2.8), for Subject in Figure 2.9

Parameter	Value	Units
E_{a0}	2.20	mmHg/mL
τ_c	0.17	s
Z_c	1.96	Nondimensional
d	0.30	s
τ_R	0.12	s
Z_R	0.96	Nondimensional

2.5.4 How Elastances E_p and E_a Can Explain LV Pressure–Volume Dynamics during Filling and Ejection Phases

2.5.4.1 Pressure Dynamics during the Filling Phase

The pressure variation during filling is a combination of pressure changes due to the action of both active elastance (E_a) and passive elastance (E_p) response to blood filling caused by LA contraction. In Equation 2.1, by neglecting the term ($Md\dot{V}$) because it is small [13], the pressure dynamics is expressed as

$$P_i - P_{i-1} = (E_{p,i} + E_{a,i})(V_i - V_{i-1}) + V_i(E_{a,i} - E_{a,i-1} + E_{p,i} - E_{p,i-1}) \qquad (2.12)$$

By employing the monitored LV volume values and the computed values of E_p and E_a, we can compute the values of LV pressure. In other words, if we obtain the LV volume values, and if somehow the E_p and E_a functions (as given by Equations 2.10 and 2.11) are known as intrinsic properties of the LV, then we can compute the LV pressure variation from Equation 2.12. So, let us take typical values of E_a and E_p, and V_i and V_{i-1} during early filling, and compute ($P_{22}-P_{21}$) as follows:

$$P_{22} - P_{21} = (E_{p,22} + E_{a,22})(V_{22} - V_{21}) + V_{22}(E_{a,22} - E_{a,21} + E_{p,22} - E_{p,21}) = -6.7 \text{ mmHg} \qquad (2.13)$$

We can see that ($P_{22}-P_{21}$) is negative, thereby demonstrating the suction effect. We have thus been able to provide a bioengineering basis and explanation of the suction effect.

Now, we take typical values of elastances and LV volumes during late filling and compute ($P_{34}-P_{33}$) as follows:

$$P_{34} - P_{33} = (E_{p,34} + E_{a,34})(V_{34} - V_{33}) + V_{34}(E_{a,34} - E_{a,33} + E_{p,34} - E_{p,33}) = 1.7 \text{ mmHg} \qquad (2.14)$$

We note that ($P_{34}-P_{33}$) is positive and is associated with atrial contraction.

In Figure 2.12, these pressure differences are plotted from the beginning of the filling phase (with respect to P_{21}, the LV pressure at the start of the filling phase). It can be seen that the computed pressure differences closely approximate the monitored LV pressure differences.

2.5.4.2 Pressure Dynamics during the Ejection Phase

We can likewise determine the pressure variation during the ejection phase, by neglecting the term ($Md\dot{V}$) because it is small [13], as

$$P_i - P_{i-1} = (E_{p,i} + E_{a,i})(V_i - V_{i-1}) + V_i(E_{a,i} - E_{a,i-1} + E_{p,i} - E_{p,i-1}) \qquad (2.15)$$

Let us take typical values of (E_p and E_a, V_i and V_{i-1}) during early and late ejection, and compute (P_7-P_6) and ($P_{16}-P_{15}$), as follows:

$$P_7 - P_6 = (E_{p,7} + E_{a,7})(V_7 - V_6) + V_7(E_{a,7} - E_{a,6} + E_{p,7} - E_{p,6}) = 9 \text{ mmHg} \qquad (2.16)$$

$$P_{16} - P_{15} = (E_{p,16} + E_{a,16})(V_{16} - V_{15}) + V_{16}(E_{a,16} - E_{a,15} + E_{p,16} - E_{p,15}) = -4 \text{ mmHg} \qquad (2.17)$$

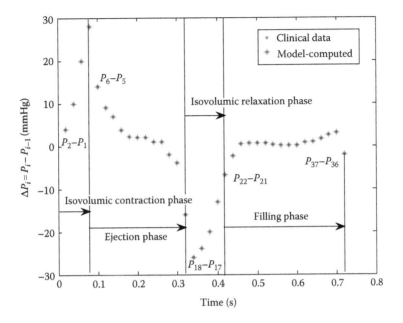

FIGURE 2.12
Pressure dynamics during ejection and filling phases. Note the pressure decrease (i.e., negative ΔP_i) during early filling (from frames 21 to 23), representing LV suction phenomenon. Also, LV pressure increase keeps decreasing during the first third of the ejection phase, remains constant in the middle third phase of ejection, and becomes negative in the late ejection phase. (Adapted from Zhong, L. et al., *Biomed. Eng. Online*, 4, 10, 2005.)

We note that $(P_7 - P_6)$ is positive, while $(P_{16} - P_{15})$ is negative, indicating that the LV pressure has already started decreasing because of the E_p effect.

In Figure 2.12, these computed pressure differences $(P_i - P_{i-1})$ are plotted. This graph illustrates how (1) E_a increase (due to force development in the myocardial sarcomere) and constant E_p during isovolumic contraction contribute to LV pressure increase, (2) E_a increase during ejection (due to increase in sarcomeric force development) and E_p decrease (due to blood volume decrease) contribute to LV pressure dynamics during the ejection phase, and (3) E_a decrease and E_p increase (due to blood volume increase) contribute to the pressure dynamics during the filling phase.

2.6 Maximum Value of Active Elastance, $E_{a,max}$, as a New Contractility Index

The basis of E_a is that the LV chamber wall is comprised of helically wound myocardial fibers. When these fibers contract at the start of isovolumic contraction, the LV chamber is deformed (and even twisted) and the LV pressure increases. Thus, the operation of the myocardial fiber sarcomeres gives rise to the concept of LV active elastance (E_a). However because $E_a(t)$ is a cyclic time-varying function, we have decided to adopt the maximum value of E_a ($E_{a,max}$) during cardiac cycle to represent a new contractility index. In Figure 2.13, we have depicted the good correlation between the computed $E_{a,max}$ and the traditional contractility index dP/dt_{max} for a number of subjects studied by us.

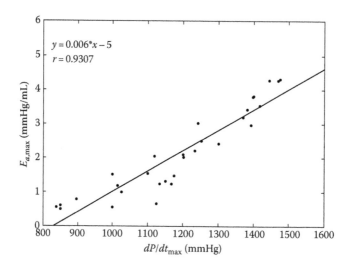

FIGURE 2.13

Relating our contractility index $E_{a,max}$ to the traditional contractility index dP/dt_{max}, with r being the correlation coefficient. (Adapted from Zhong, L. et al., *Biomed. Eng. Online*, 4, 10, 2005.)

It is noted that $E_{a,max}$ has a high degree of correlation with dP/dt_{max}. It is interesting to compare our correlation-coefficient value (0.9307) with the value of 0.89 obtained by Mehmel et al. [64], although the paper by Mehmel et al. computes elastance as an extrinsic property $=[P/(V-V_d)]_{es}$.

2.7 Conclusion

In this chapter, we have provided an elaboration of the existing available indices as well as our new contractility indices for assessing cardiac function in filling and systolic phases. For the new indices, we have provided the theory, methodology, and computation of clinically applied diagnostic measures of LV volume-dependent passive elastance and active elastance to explain the dynamics of LV pressure in filling and systolic phases. We have then proposed maximum value of E_a ($E_{a,max}$) during cardiac cycle to represent a new contractility index and have shown its good correlation with the traditional contractility index dP/dt_{max} in our clinical study.

References

1. Grodins FS. Integrative cardiovascular physiology: A mathematical synthesis of cardiac and blood vessel hemodynamics. *Quart. Rev. Biol.*, 34, 1959, 93–116.
2. Elzinga G, Westerhof N. Pressure and flow generated by the left ventricle against different impedances. *Circ. Res.*, 32, 1972, 178–186.
3. Suga H. Time course of left ventricular pressure–volume relationships under various enddiastolic volume. *Jpn. Heart J.*, 10, 1969, 509–515.

4. Sagawa K. The ventricular pressure-volume diagram revisited. *Circ. Res.*, 43, 1978, 677–687.
5. Vaartjes SR, Boom HBK. Left ventricular internal resistance and unloaded ejection flow assessed from pressure-flow relations: A flow-clamp study on isolated rabbit hearts. *Circ. Res.*, 60, 1987, 727–737.
6. Shoucri RM. The pressure-volume relation and mechanics of left ventricular contraction. *Jpn. Heart J.*, 31, 1990, 713–729.
7. Shoucri RM. Studying the mechanics of left ventricle contraction. *IEEE Eng. Biomed. Eng.*, 17, 1998, 95–101.
8. Shoucri RM. Active and passive stresses in the myocardium. *Am. J. Physiol. Heart Circ. Physiol.*, 279, 2000, H2519–H2528.
9. Palladino JL, Mulier JP, Noordergraaf A. Defining ventricular elastance. *Proceedings of the 20th International Conference of the IEEE Engineering in Medicine and Biology Society*, Hong Kong, China, 1998, pp. 383–386.
10. Kass P, Ding Y-A, Chen CH. Assessment of left ventricular end-systolic elastance from aortic pressure-left ventricular volume relations. *Heart Vessels*, 16, 2002, 99–104.
11. Ishida M, Tomita S, Nakatani T. Acute effects of direct cell implantation into the heart: A pressure-volume study to analyze cardiac function. *J. Heart Lung Transplant.*, 23(7), 2004, 881–888.
12. Zhong L, Ghista DN, Ng EYK, Lim SK. Passive and active ventricular elastance of the left ventricle. *Biomed. Eng. Online*, 4, 2005, 10.
13. Zhong L, Ghista DN, Ng EYK, Lim ST, Chua SJT. Measures and indices for intrinsic characterization of cardiac dysfunction during filling and systolic ejection phase. *J. Mech. Med. Biol.*, 5(2), 2005, 307–332.
14. Ghista DN, Zhong L, Chua LP, Ng EYK, Lim ST, Tan RS, Chua TSJ. Systolic modeling of the left ventricle as a mechatronic system: Determination of myocardial fiber's sarcomere contractile characteristics and new performance indices. *Mol. Cell. Biomech.*, 2(4), 2005, 217–233.
15. Ghista DN, Advani SH, Gaonkar GH, Balachandran K, Brady AJ. Analysis and physiological monitoring of human left ventricle. *J. Basic Eng.*, 93, 1971, 147–161.
16. Ghista DN, Brady AJ, Radhakrishnan S. A three-dimensional analytical (rheological) model of the human left ventricle in passive-active states. *Biophys. J.*, 13, 1973, 832–854.
17. Ghista DN, Sandler H. Elastic modulus of the human intact left ventricle-determination and physiological interpretation. *Med. Biol. Eng.*, 13(2), 1975, 151–160.
18. Brutsaert DL, Rademakers FE, Sys SU. Triple control of relaxation: Implication in cardiac disease. *Circulation*, 69, 1984, 190–196.
19. Gillebert TC, Sys SU. Physiologic control of relaxation in isolated cardiac muscle and intact left ventricle. In: WH Gaasch, MM LeWinter (eds.), *Left Ventricular Diastolic Dysfunction and Heart Failure*, Philadelphia, PA: Lea & Febiger, 1994, pp. 25–42.
20. Arrighi JA, Soufer R. Left ventricular diastolic function: Physiology, methods of assessment, and clinical significance. *J. Nucl. Cardiol.*, 2, 1995, 525–543.
21. Brutsaert DL, Sys SU, Gillebert TC. Diastolic failure: Pathophysiology and therapeutic implications. *J. Am. Coll. Cardiol.*, 22, 1993, 318–325.
22. Rusconi CU, Ghizzoni GL, Sabatini T, Oneglia CA, Faggiano PM. Pathophysiology of diastole and left ventricular filling in humans: Noninvasive evaluation. In: GM Drzewiecki and JKJ Li (eds.), *Analysis and Assessment of Cardiovascular Function*, New York: Springer, 1998, pp. 172–192.
23. Frank O. Zur Dynamik des Herzmuskels. *Z. Biol.*, 32, 1895, 370–447. Translated into English by Chapman CB and Wasserman E. On the dynamics of cardiac muscle. *Am. Heart J.*, 58, 1959, 282–317 and 467–478.
24. Hill AV. The heat of shortening and dynamic constants of muscle. *Proc. R. Soc. Lond., Ser. B*, 1938, 126–136.
25. Huxley AF, Niedergerke R. Structural changes in muscle during contraction. *Nature*, 173, 1954, 971–973.
26. Huxley AF. Muscular contraction: A review lecture. *J. Physiol.*, 243, 1974, 1–43.

27. Suga H. How we view systolic function of the heart: E_{max} and PVA. In: NB Ingels Jr., GT Daughters, J Baan, JW Covell, RS Reneman, FCP Yin (eds.), *Systolic and Diastolic Function of the Heart*, Amsterdam, the Netherlands: IOS Press and Ohmsha, 1994.

28. Gaasch WH, Levine HJ, Quinones MA. Left ventricular compliance: Mechanisms and clinical implications. *Am. J. Cardiol.*, 38, 1976, 645–653.

29. Mirsky I, Rankin JS. The effects of geometry, elasticity and external pressure on the diastolic pressure-volume and stiffness-stress relations. How important is the pericardium? *Circ. Res.*, 44, 1979, 601–611.

30. Mirsky I. Assessment of diastolic function: Suggested methods and future considerations. *Circulation*, 69, 1984, 836–841.

31. Mirsky I, Pasipoularides A. Clinical assessment of diastolic function. *Prog. Cardiovasc. Dis.*, 32, 1990, 291–318.

32. Smith VE, Zile MR. Relaxation and diastolic properties of the heart. In: HA Fozzard (ed.), *The Heart and Cardiovascular System*, New York: Raven Press, 1992, pp. 1353–1367.

33. Lisauskas JB, Singh J, Bowman AW, Kovács SJ. Chamber properties from transmitral flow: Prediction of average and passive left ventricular diastolic stiffness. *J. Appl. Physiol.*, 91, 2001, 154–162.

34. Mason DT. Usefulness and limitations of the rate of rise of intraventricular pressure (dP/dt) in the evaluation of myocardial contractility in man. *Am. J. Cardiol.*, 23, 1969, 516–527.

35. Little WC. Comparison of measures of left ventricular contractile performance derived from pressure-volume loops in conscious dogs. *Circulation*, 71, 1989, 994–1009.

36. Kara S, Okandan M, Usta G, Tezcaner T. Investigation of a new heart contractility power parameter. *Comput. Methods Programs Biomed.*, 76, 2004, 177–180.

37. Greenberg NL, Firstenberg MS, Castro PL, Main M, Travaglini AT. Doppler-derived myocardial systolic strain rate is a strong index of left ventricular contractility. *Circulation*, 105, 2002, 99–105.

38. Xiao SZ, Guo XM, Wang FL, Xiao ZF, Liu GC, Zhan ZF, Sun XB. Evaluating two new indicators of cardiac reserve. *IEEE Eng. Med. Biol.*, 22, 2003, 147–152.

39. Slinker BK. Searching for indices of contractility is counterproductive. In: NB Ingels, Jr., GT Daughters, J Baan, JW Covell, RS Reneman and FCP Yin (eds.), *Systolic and Diastolic Function of the Heart*, Amsterdam, the Netherlands: IOS Press and Ohmsha, 1995.

40. Sonnenblick EH. Force-velocity relations in mammalian heart muscle. *Am. J. Physiol.* 202(5), 1962, 931–939.

41. Sonnenblick EH. The contractile state of the heart as expressed by force-velocity relations. *Am. J. Cardiol.*, 23, 1969, 488–503.

42. Mason DT, Braunwald E, Ross J Jr et al. Diagnostic value of the first and second derivative of the arterial pressure pulse in aortic valve disease and hypertrophic subaortic stenosis. *Circulation*, 30, 1964, 90–100.

43. Mason DT, Spann JF Jr, Zelis R. Quantification of the contractile state of the human heart. Maximal velocity of contractile element shortening determined by the instantaneous relation between the rate of pressure rise and pressure in the left ventricle during isovolumic systole. *Am. J. Cardiol.*, 26, 1970, 248–257.

44. Wolk MJ, Keefe JF, Bing PHL et al. Estimation of V_{max} in auxotonic systoles from the rate of relative increase of isovolumic pressure: dP/dt/KP. *J. Clin. Invest.*, 50, 1971, 1276–1285.

45. Mirsky I, Ghista DN. Assessment of cardiac function: A mathematical and clinical evaluation, part1. Force velocity analyses of isolated and intact heart muscle. *Automedia*, 1, 1974, 83–91.

46. Kass DA, Beyer R. Evaluation of contractile state by maximal ventricular power divided by the square of end-diastolic volume. *Circulation*, 84, 1991, 1698–1708.

47. Kass DA, Maughan WL, Guo ZM, Kono A, Sunagawa K, Sagawa K. Comparative influence of load versus inotropic states on indices of ventricular contractility: Experimental and theoretical analysis based on pressure-volume relationships. *Circulation*, 76, 1987, 1422–1436.

48. Suga H, Sagawa K. Instantaneous pressure volume relationships and their ratio in the excised, supported canine left ventricle. *Circ. Res.*, 35, 1974, 117–126.

49. Suga H, Sagawa K, Shoukas AA. Load independence of the instantaneous pressure-volume ratio of the canine left ventricle and effects of epinephrine and heart rate on the ratio. *Circ. Res.*, 32, 1973, 314–322.

50. Sagawa K. The end-systolic pressure-volume relation of the ventricles: Definition, modification and clinical use. *Circulation*, 63, 1981, 1223–1227.

51. Mirsky I, Tajimi T, Peterson KL. The development of the entire end-systolic pressure-volume and ejection fraction-afterload relations: A new concept of systolic myocardial stiffness. *Circulation*, 76, 1987, 343–356.

52. Burkhoff D, de Tombe PP, Hunter WC. Impact of ejection on magnitude and time course of ventricular pressure-generation capacity. *Am. J. Physiol. Heart Circ. Physiol.*, 265, 1993, H899–H903.

53. Noda T, Cheng CP, de Tombe PP, Little WC. Curvilinearity of LV end-systolic pressure-volume and dP/dt$_{max}$-end-diastolic volume relations. *Am. J. Physiol.*, 34, 1993, H910–H917.

54. Mulier JP. Ventricular pressure as a function of volume and flow, PhD thesis, University of Leuven, Leuven, Belgium, 1994.

55. Schmidt C, Roosens C, Struys M et al. Contractility in humans after coronary artery surgery. Echocardiographic assessment with preload-adjusted maximal power. *Anesthesiology*, 91, 1999, 58–70.

56. Sharir T, Feldman MD, Haber H et al. Ventricular systolic assessment in patients with dilated cardiomyopathy by preload-adjusted maximal power: Validation and noninvasive application. *Circulation*, 89, 1994, 2045–2053.

57. William AM, Michael RP, John G. Assessment of left ventricular contractile state by preload-adjusted maximal power using echocardiographic automated border detection. *J. Am. Coll. Cardiol.*, 31(4), 1998, 861–868.

58. Lester SJ, Shin H, Lambert AS, Miller JP, Cahaland MK, Seeberger MD, Foster E, Schiller NB. Is PA-PWRmax truly a preload-independent index of myocardial contractility in anesthetized humans? *Cardiology*, 102(2), 2004, 77–81.

59. Costa SP, Sam F, Falk RH, Colucci WS, Davidoff R. Strain rate imaging in idiopathic cardiomyopathy: More sensitive than tissue Doppler and potential application as a contractility index (abstract). *J. Am. Coll. Cardiol.*, 6(2), 2004, 416.

60. Subbaraj K, Ghista DN, Fallen EL. Intrinsic indices of the left ventricle as a blood pump in normal and infarcted left ventricles. *J. Biomed. Eng.*, 9, 1987, 206–215.

61. Mirsky I. Assessment of passive elastic stiffness of cardiac muscle: Mathematical concepts, physiologic and clinical consideration, direction of future research. *Prog. Cardiovasc. Dis.*, XVIII, 1976, 277–308.

62. Gibert JC, Glantz SA. Determinants of left ventricular filling and of the diastolic pressure-volume relation. *Circ. Res.*, 64(5), 1989, 827–852.

63. Sandler H, Dodge HT. The use of single plane angiocardiograms for the calculation of left ventricle volume in man. *Am. Heart. J.*, 75, 1968, 325–334.

64. Mehmel HC, Stochins B, Ruffmann K, Olshausen K, Schuler G, Kubler W. The linearity of the end-systolic pressure-volume relationship in man and its sensitivity for assessment of left ventricular function. *Circulation*, 63(6), 1981, 1216–1222.

3

Novel Cardiac Contractility Index and Ventricular-Arterial Matching Index to Serve as Markers of Heart Failure

Liang Zhong, Dhanjoo N. Ghista, Ghassan S. Kassab, and Ru San Tan

CONTENTS

In this chapter, we introduce a new cardiac (left ventricular) contractility index $d\sigma^*/dt_{max}$, which can be determined without the measurement of intra-left ventricular pressure. We have provided its rationale and derivation and demonstrated (1) its good correlation with the traditional contractility index dP/dt_{max}, in patients with varying ejection fractions, and (2) its capacity to diagnose heart failure with normal ejection fraction (HFNEF, or diastolic heart failure) and with reduced ejection fraction (HFREF, or systolic heart failure).

We then incorporate this contractility index in the formulation of a ventricular-arterial matching (VAM) index as the ratio of the contractility index and the aortic arterial elastance. We present a study for the determination of both the ventricular contractility index and the VAM index from echocardiography. Now in heart failure (HFREF), we have reduced cardiac contractility; we can also have aortic arteriosclerosis and hence enhanced arterial elastance requiring more contractile effort by the left ventricle (LV), which it cannot provide due to its impaired contractility; this leads to heart failure (HF), as manifested by reduced value of the VAM index. The study shows the correlation between ventricular-arterial mismatching with elevated N-terminal pro B-type natriuretic peptide (NT-proBNP) as a marker of HF.

3.1 Cardiac Contractility Expressed in Terms of Maximum Rate of Change of Pressure-Normalized LV Wall Stress, $d\sigma^*/dt_{max}$

Cardiac contractility constitutes the prime mechanism by which the intra-LV pressure is increased and made available for ejection of blood into the aorta. Cardiac contractility is affected by myocardial perfusion from the coronary circulatory system. Traditionally, cardiac contractility has been assessed in terms of dP/dt_{max}. However, this measure of contractility is based on the outcome of contractility in generating LV presure for blood ejection. In a way it is an afterthought, aside from it also requiring invasive measurement of LV pressure. The LV pressure increase is caused by the generation of active wall stress due to the contractile stress developed in the myocardial structural unit between the myocardial sarcomer's myosin and actin filaments, as depicted in Figure 3.1. Cardiac contractility can hence be termed as the capacity of the LV to develop intra-myocardial stress, and thereby appropriate intra-cavitary pressure to eject adequate blood volume into the aorta. It is hence rational and appropriate to formulate a LV contractility index on the basis of LV wall stress. The traditional dP/dt_{max} is based on left ventricular intra-cavitary pressure, which is generated by an active myocardial stress. Hence, analogous to dP/dt_{max}, which is based on LV intra-cavitary pressure, we have formulated a new LV contractility index based on LV wall stress, namely the maximum rate of change during systole of LV wall stress normalized to LV intra-cavitary pressure, $d(\sigma/P)/dt_{max}$ or $d\sigma^*/dt_{max}$, where $\sigma^* = \sigma/P$ [1].

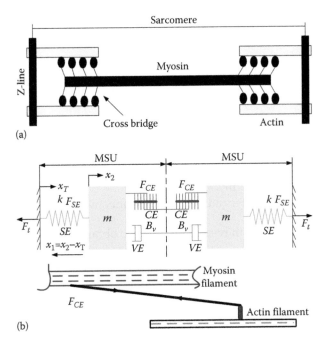

FIGURE 3.1
In this figure, we have linked the anatomical associations of these myocardial model elements with micro-scopic structure of the heart muscle. (a) Illustrates the actin and myosin filaments constituting the contractile components of the myocardial fibril. (b) Illustrates the myocardial fibril model composed of two symmetrical myocardial structural units (MSUs), which are mirror images of each other. Each MSU is composed of (1) an effective mass (m) that is accelerated; (2) connective-tissue series element having parameter k (elastic modulus of the series element) and the force F_{SE}; (3) the parallel viscous element of the sarcolemma having viscous damp-ing parameter B_v and force F_{VE}; (4) the contractile element (CE), which generates contractile force F_{CE} between the myosin (thick) and actin (thin) filaments. When the contractile element shortens (by amount x_2), the series element lengthens (i.e., x_1 increases). During ejection, the MSU x_T decreases, and during filling the MSU x_T increases. (Adapted from Ghista, D.N. et al., *Mol. Cell. Biomech.*, 2(4), 217, 2005.)

3.1.1 Model Analysis and Index Formulation

For mathematical simplicity, we have approximated the LV as a thick-wall spherical shell consisting of incompressible, homogeneous, isotropic, elastic material. The maximum circumferential wall stress ($\sigma\theta$) can be expressed at the endocardium, as

$$\sigma_\theta(r_i) = P\left[\frac{\left(r_i^3/r_e^3\right)+1/2}{1-\left(r_i^3/r_e^3\right)}\right] \tag{3.1}$$

where
r_i and r_e are the inner and outer radii
P is LV intra-cavitary pressure

By normalizing wall stress to LV intra-cavitary pressure (P), we obtain

$$\sigma^*(r) = \frac{\sigma_\theta}{P} = \frac{r_i^3}{r_e^3 - r_i^3}\left(1+\frac{r_e^3}{2r^3}\right) \tag{3.2}$$

The derivation of Equation 3.2 is provided in Appendix 3A [2]. Since the maximum wall stress occurs at the inner endocardial wall, we have

$$\sigma^*(r = r_i) = \left(\frac{V/(V_m + V) + 1/2}{1 - V/(V_m + V)} \right) = \left(\frac{3V + V_m}{2V_m} \right) = \left(\frac{3V}{2V_m} + \frac{1}{2} \right) \tag{3.3}$$

where

P is LV intra-cavitary pressure
σ_θ is the wall stress
$V(= 4\pi r_i^3 / 3)$ denotes LV volume
$V_m(= 4\pi(r_e^3 - r_i^3)/3)$ denotes LV myocardial volume
r_i and r_e are the inner and outer radii of the LV, respectively

Differentiating Equation 3.3 with respect to time, we obtain

$$\frac{d\sigma^*}{dt}_{max} = \left| \frac{d(\sigma_\theta/P)}{dt} \right|_{max} = \frac{3}{2V_m} \left| \frac{dV}{dt} \right|_{max} \tag{3.4}$$

It can be noted that, in contrast to the traditional contractility index of dP/dt_{max}, the $d\sigma^*/dt_{max}$ index can be determined solely from noninvasive assessment of LV myocardial volume and its maximum outflow rate. Normalizing LV wall stress to LV pressure obviates the need for invasive LV pressure measurement.

This LV contractility formulation has been based on the premise that LV wall stress (due to LV myocardial sarcomere contraction) is responsible for the development of LV pressure, as validated by us [3]. Therefore, it provides more rationale to base LV contractile function on LV wall stress normalized with respect to LV pressure. Hence, analogous to dP/dt_{max}, this LV contractility index was formulated as the maximal rate of pressure-normalized wall stress (as given by Equation 3.4), to represent the maximum flow rate out of the ventricle (dV/dt) normalized to myocardial volume (V_m). In a way, this is consistent with the use of LV pressure–volume loop area to represent the total mechanical energy generated by ventricular contraction.*

3.2 Clinical Application to Subjects with Varying Ejection Fractions to Demonstrate Strong Correlation of $d\sigma^*/dt_{max}$ with dP/dt_{max}

The index $d\sigma^*/dt_{max}$ was validated against dP/dt_{max} and $E_{a,max}$ in 30 subjects with disparate ventricular function in Figure 3.2, and demonstrated the index's load independence, albeit under conditions of limited preload and afterload manipulations [1]. A more recent swine study demonstrated a much broader range of load independence [5].

For the clinical study, 30 volunteers (mean 58.1 [range 48–77] year of age, 13:2 male-to-female ratio) with diverse cardiac conditions were recruited. From the LV pressure–volume

---

* Our original work on this novel contractility index has been widely reported in journal publications as well as in our previous book chapter [4].

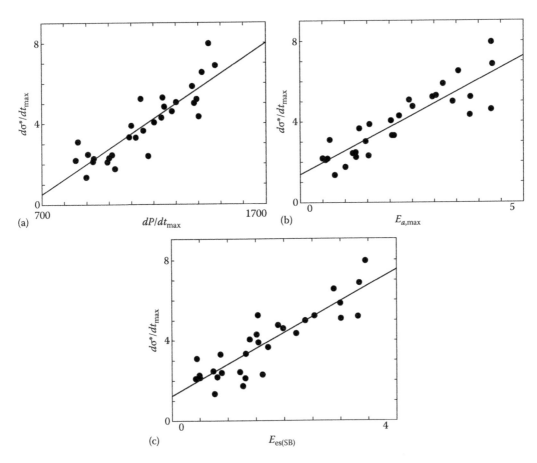

FIGURE 3.2
Linear regression analysis demonstrates good correlation between $d\sigma^*/dt_{max}$ and dP/dt_{max}: ((a) $d\sigma^*/dt_{max}$ = 0.0075 dP/dt_{max}−4.70, r = 0.88), between $d\sigma^*/dt_{max}$ and $E_{a,max}$ ((b) $d\sigma^*/dt_{max}$ = 1.20 $E_{a,max}$+1.40, r = 0.89), and between $d\sigma^*/dt_{max}$ and $E_{es(SB)}$ ((c) $d\sigma^*/dt_{max}$ = 1.60 $E_{es(SB)}$+1.20, r = 0.88). (From Zhong, L. et al., *Am. J. Physiol. Heart Circ. Physiol.*, 292(6), H2764, 2007.)

data, LVEF and dP/dt_{max} were computed directly. The active elastance E_a at various times was also computed from the pressure–volume loops, from the data in Table 3.1, based on earlier work on E_a definition [6]; the $E_{a,max}$ was extrapolated from the peak of the E_a–time curve. The single-beat estimation of end-systolic elastance $E_{es(SB)}$ was determined, by using bilinearly approximated time-varying elastance [7].

The patients were divided into three groups on the basis of tertiles of LVEF, with 10 individuals in each group, as shown in Table 3.2. Intergroup comparisons showed significant differences between the mean values of dP/dt_{max}, $E_{a,max}$, $E_{es(SB)}$, and $d\sigma^*/dt_{max}$ in those in the highest tertile compared with those in lowest and middle tertiles. There is agreement with regard to the new index $d\sigma^*/dt_{max}$ with dP/dt_{max}, $E_{a,max}$, and $E_{es(SB)}$ across the three tertiles of ascending LVEF values, with statistically significant differences in LV contractility indexes among the three groups. The values of dP/dt_{max}, $E_{es(SB)}$, and $d\sigma^*/dt_{max}$ were significantly lower in patients in the lowest and middle tertiles than those in the highest tertile.

TABLE 3.1

Active Elastance E_a Computed at Discrete Time Points during Isovolumic Contraction and Relaxation in a Sample Subject

Frame No. (i)	t (s)	P (mmHg)	V (mL)	E_a (mmHg/mL)
Isovolumic contraction				
1	0	18	136.7	0
2	0.02	22	135.7	0.0295
3	0.04	32	134.6	0.1038
4	0.06	52	133.5	0.2536
5	0.08	80	132.5	0.4636
Isovolumic relaxation				
18	0.34	74	85	0.0590
19	0.36	50	85.5	0.1778
20	0.38	30	86.4	0.3127
21	0.40	17	90.6	0.4636

Sources: Zhong, L. et al., *Am. J. Physiol. Heart Circ. Physiol.*, 292(6), H2764, 2007; Zhong L. et al.,. *Biomed Eng Online*, 4, 10, 2005.

i, time instant in the cardiac cycle (frame number from end-diastole); t, time from start of isovolumic contraction; P, measured left ventricular intra-cavitary pressure; V, measured left ventricular intra-cavitary volume; $E_{a,i}$, calculated active elastance at instant i.

TABLE 3.2

LV Contractility Indexes Classified into Tertiles of LVEF

	Lowest Tertile	Middle Tertile	Highest Tertile
Ejection (fraction)	0.38 ± 0.12[a]	0.49 ± 0.13[a]	0.63 ± 0.05
Age (year)	58.30 ± 8.86	56.10 ± 6.15	59.90 ± 6.17
Heart rate (beats/min)	71.18 ± 10.72	71.77 ± 10.68	71.46 ± 9.09
dP/dt_{max} (mmHg/s)	960 ± 115[a]	1121 ± 113[a]	1360 ± 97
$E_{a,max}$ (mmHg/m)	0.95 ± 0.32	1.85 ± 0.59[a]	3.61 ± 0.62
$E_{es(SB)}$ (mmHg/mL)	0.72 ± 0.26[a]	1.51 ± 0.20[a]	2.81 ± 0.51
$d\sigma^*/dt_{max}$ (s^{-1})	2.30 ± 0.58[a]	3.60 ± 1.06[a]	5.64 ± 1.13

Source: Zhong, L. et al., *Am. J. Physiol. Heart Circ. Physiol.*, 292(6), H2764, 2007.

Left ventricular contractility indices classified into tertiles of left ventricular ejection fraction. Values are expressed as mean ± standard deviation.

[a] Denotes statistically significant difference ($p < 0.05$) when compared with corresponding values in the highest tertile of left ventricular ejection fraction. dP/dt_{max}, peak first time-derivative of the ventricular pressure; $E_{a,max}$, maximum left ventricular elastance; $E_{es(SB)}$, single-beat LV end-systolic elastance; $d\sigma^*/dt_{max}$, left ventricular contractility index.

Figure 3.2 summarizes the correlation between $d\sigma^*/dt_{max}$, dP/dt_{max}, and $E_{a,max}$, as well as $E_{es(SB)}$. Linear regression analysis revealed good correlation between $d\sigma^*/dt_{max}$ and dP/dt_{max}, $E_{a,max}$, and $E_{es(SB)}$, with significant correlation coefficients in each case: $d\sigma^*/dt_{max} = 0.0075\ dP/dt_{max} - 4.70$ ($r = 0.88$, $p < 0.01$), $d\sigma^*/dt_{max} = 1.20\ E_{a,max} + 1.40$ ($r = 0.89$, $p < 0.01$), and $d\sigma^*/dt_{max} = 1.60\ E_{es(SB)} + 1.20$ ($r = 0.88$, $p < 0.01$). In contrast, the correlation between $d\sigma^*/dt_{max}$ and LVEF was less strong ($r = 0.71$), similar to the correlation between $E_{es(SB)}$ and LVEF ($r = 0.78$), underscoring the lack of sensitivity of LVEF as an index of myocardial contractility. This study has validated the use of $d\sigma^*/dt_{max}$ as a valid noninvasively determinable contractility index.

3.3 Use of Cardiac Contractility Index $d\sigma^*/dt_{max}$ to Diagnose Heart Failure with Normal and Reduced Ejection Fractions

The index $d\sigma^*/dt_{max}$ was then used to diagnose HF in another study [8], involving patients with HFNEF and HFREF.

3.3.1 Background Information

Heart failure is a major health care burden as the leading cause of hospitalization in persons older than 65 years [9] and confers an annual mortality of 10% [10]. HF can occur with either normal or reduced LV ejection fraction (EF), depending on different degrees of ventricular remodeling. Both HFNEF and HFREF, also commonly known as diastolic and systolic heart failure, respectively, have equally poor prognosis [11]. Medical therapy targets to reduce load, by using vasodilators and/or to alter contractile strength using inotropic agents. Alternatively, some therapies target to affect cardiac remodeling, such as passive cardiac support devices, surgical restoration of LV shape (i.e., the Dor procedure), and stem cell therapies.

Assessment of LV contractility is important for HF management and evaluation of the heart's response to medical and surgical therapies. Although approaches based on pressure–volume analysis, stress–strain analysis, and dP/dt_{max}–EDV relations [12] can provide assessments of contractile function, these relations generally require invasive data measurements at several chamber loads and thus are difficult to apply in routine or long-term clinical studies. This is an important limitation, because HF often requires longitudinal evaluation. The ideal measure of contractility should have the following characteristics: sensitivity to inotropic changes, independence from loading conditions as well as heart size and mass, ease of application, and proven usefulness in the clinical setting. LVEF is the index overwhelmingly used to assess cardiac function in both clinical and experimental studies, despite the fact that it is highly dependent upon preload and afterload. Based on the National Heart Lung and Blood Institute's Framingham Heart Study, an LVEF 50% as cut-off for the presence of normal LVEF has been used in the present study [13].

3.3.1.1 Utility of $d\sigma^*/dt_{max}$ as a Contractility Index

During LV systolic phase, LV wall stress is generated intrinsically by sarcomere contraction and results in the development of extrinsic LV pressure. We have shown earlier in Section 3.2, that the index $d\sigma^*/dt_{max}$ (maximal change rate of pressure-normalized wall stress) correlates well with LV dP/dt_{max} [1]. From the right-hand side of Equation 3.4, this index is also seen to represent the maximal flow rate from the ventricle (cardiac output) normalized to myocardial volume (or mass). This index is easily measured noninvasively (i.e., from echocardiography or magnetic resonance imaging), sensitive to LV inotropic changes, and has been demonstrated by us to be preload and afterload independent. Importantly, it is measured in a single steady-state condition, as opposed to the multiple variably loaded cardiac cycles required for many of the other indices. Thus, $d\sigma^*/dt_{max}$ has several qualities that make it a useful LV contractility index.

Now, this study [8] has constituted an important step toward also establishing the clinical utility of $d\sigma^*/dt_{max}$ as a tool for diagnosis of HF (both HFNEF and HFREF) as well as for follow-up surveillance of LV function. Hence, there is significant potential for application of this index to evaluate heart function in diverse heart conditions.

3.3.2 Clinical Methodology

Patients with symptoms and signs of HF underwent echocardiography and electrocardiography (ECG). Patients with atrial fibrillation, more than mild mitral or aortic valvular regurgitation, and unsatisfactory echocardiographic images were excluded. Clinical signs of HF were defined as presence of at least one of the following: raised jugular venous pressure, peripheral edema, hepatomegaly, basal inspiratory crepitation, or gallop rhythm. Patients with LVEF ≥ 50% and LVEF < 50% on echocardiography were classified into HFNEF and HFREF, respectively.

3.3.2.1 Echocardiography Study

With the subject in the left lateral decubitus position, 2D examinations, M-mode measurements, and Doppler recordings were made from the standard left parasternal long and short axes and the apical four-chamber view with simultaneous ECG. The LVEF was assessed by using a 2D method by an experienced observer; normal LVEF was defined as greater or equal to 50%. Mitral flow velocities were obtained from the apical four-chamber view using pulsed-wave Doppler technique with the sample volume at the tips of the corresponding valve leaflets. The LV outflow tract (LVOT) velocity was obtained from apical five-chamber view, by using pulsed-wave Doppler technique with the sample volume at the aortic valve level.

The measurements included peak E (peak early transmitral filling velocity during early diastole) and A (peak transmitral atrial filling velocity during late diastole) wave velocities (cm/s). The E/A ratio was calculated along with E wave deceleration time (DT) as the time elapsed between peak E velocity and the point where the extrapolation of the deceleration slope of E velocity crosses the zero baseline measured in milliseconds. The LVOT maximal velocity V_{peak} was measured, and LV mass was calculated by using ASE methods [14,15]. Myocardial tissue Doppler (TDI) velocities were also estimated at the atrioventricular ring, septal positions, in the apical four-chamber view. All measurements were averaged over two or three cardiac cycles.

3.3.2.2 Calculation of $d\sigma^*/dt_{max}$ from Echocardiography

The contractility index was computed by means of Equation 3.4. M-mode echocardiographic measurements of the LV were obtained, and LV mass calculated using standardized methodology [14,15]. Myocardial volume was calculated by dividing LV mass with myocardial density (assumed to be 1.05 g/mL). Furthermore, 2D apical four- and two-chamber views of the LV were acquired, and end-diastolic and -systolic endocardial contours were manually outlined. The corresponding LVEDV were then automatically determined using biplane Simpson's method.

From pulsed-wave echo-Doppler interrogation of the LVOT, we calculated (in the absence of significant mitral regurgitation or aortic valve dysfunction) the maximal LV volume rate (dV/dt_{max}) during ejection: $dV/dt_{max}=V_{peak} * AVA$, where V_{peak} is the peak velocity sampled at the LVOT and AVA is the aortic valve area (= $\pi D^2/4$, where D is the LVOT diameter measured in the 2D parasternal long-axis image of the heart), as shown in Figure 3.3. Upon substituting values of myocardial volume and dV/dt_{max} into Equation 3.4, we determined the value of $d\sigma^*/dt_{max}$.

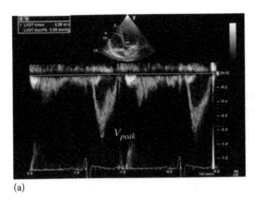
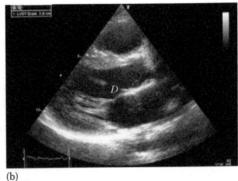

(a)   (b)

FIGURE 3.3
Echocardiographic measurement on (a) peak velocity V_{peak} sampled at the LVOT and (b) LVOT diameter D measured in the 2D parasternal long-axis image of the heart. (Adapted from Zhong, L. et al., *Ann. Acad. Med. Singapore*, 40(4), 179, April 2011.)

3.3.3 Clinical Studies

The study included 26 age- and sex-matched subjects in each of the groups of normal controls, HFNEF, and HFREF. The characteristics of 78 subjects are shown in Table 3.3, which summarizes the subjects' age, BSA, LVEF, peak E, peak A, E/A ratio, DT, heart rate (HR), septal E/E', lateral E/E', and our index $d\sigma^*/dt_{max}$. The mean $d\sigma^*/dt_{max}$ was 3.91 s^{-1} (95% CI, 3.56–4.26 s^{-1}) in control subjects; it reduced in HF, HFNEF to 2.90 s^{-1} (95% CI, 2.56–3.24 s^{-1}) and in HFREF to 1.84 (95% CI, 1.60–2.07 s^{-1}).

There was no significant difference between the average values of LVEF, peak E, peak A, E/A ratio, DT, HR, septal E/E', and lateral E/E' in HENEF compared to normal controls,

TABLE 3.3

Patients Characteristics and Echocardiographic Measurements in Group 1 (Controls), Group 2 (HFNEF), and Group 3 (HFREF)

	Controls (*n* = 26)	**HFNEF (*n* = 26)**	**HFREF (*n* = 26)**
Age (years)	72 ± 8	70 ± 8	70 ± 8
Gender (male:female)	16:10	16:10	16:10
BSA (m^2)	1.69 ± 0.20	1.71 ± 0.20	1.61 ± 0.20
LVEF (%)	68.3 ± 5.1	66.5 ± 4.9	33 ± 13.7^{ab}
E/A ratio	0.96 ± 0.38	0.78 ± 0.24	1.26 ± 0.90^{b}
DT (ms)	214 ± 47	214 ± 67	157 ± 41^{ab}
HR (beats/min)	66 ± 10	72 ± 16	80 ± 11^{a}
Septal E/E'	8.48 ± 2.10	9.79 ± 3.29	13.68 ± 4.78^{ab}
Lateral E/E'	6.64 ± 1.55	8.39 ± 2.76	10.28 ± 3.40^{ab}
$d\sigma^*/dt_{max}$ (s^{-1})	3.91 ± 0.87	2.90 ± 0.84^{ab}	1.84 ± 0.59^{ab}

Source: Zhong, L. et al., *Ann Acad Med*, Singapore, 40(4), 179, April 2011.
The values are expressed as mean ± SD.
[a] and [b] Denote statistically significant difference of HF compared to controls, and HFREF compared to HFNEF patients, respectively (Bonferroni pairwise test, $p < 0.05$).
A, mitral atrial flow velocity on echo-Doppler; BSA, body surface area; DT, mitral *E* deceleration time; *E*, mitral early velocity; *E'*, septal mitral annular myocardial velocity on tissue Doppler imaging; HR, heart rate, LVEF, left ventricular ejection fraction.

except $d\sigma^*/dt_{max}$ (2.90 ± 0.84 vs. 3.91 ± 0.87, $p < 0.001$). There was a significant difference, however, between the average values of LVEF, peak E, peak A, E/A ratio, DT, septal E/E', lateral E/E', and $d\sigma^*/dt_{max}$ in HEREF compared to HFNEF.

3.3.3.1 Assessment of Heart Failure with Normal Ejection Fraction and Reduced Ejection Fraction

Heart failure may be viewed as a progressive disorder that is initiated after an "index event" with a concomitant loss of myocyte function that prevents the heart from contracting normally. HF can occur with either normal or reduced LVEF, depending on different degree of ventricular remodeling. Perhaps 50% of patients with HF have a normal or minimally impaired LVEF (HFNEF), which by definition cannot be diagnosed with LVEF [16,17].

Although mechanisms for HFNEF remain incompletely understood, diastolic dysfunction is said to play a dominant role: impaired relaxation, increased passive stiffness, and raised end-diastolic pressure (EDP) [18]. The diagnostic standard for HFNEF is cardiac catheterization, which demonstrates increased EDP. A more practical noninvasive alternative, however, may be echocardiography. Parameters based on transmitral Doppler have been validated in patients with an impaired systolic function and HFREF but have demonstrated shortcoming in patients with a normal LVEF. Our study has demonstrated that E/A ratio (1.26 ± 0.90 vs. 0.96 ± 0.38, $p < 0.05$) and DT (157 ± 41 ms vs. 214 ± 47 ms, $p < 0.05$) are significantly different between HFREF and normal controls, but not so between HFNEF and normal subjects (Table 3.3).

The contractility index, $d\sigma^*/dt_{max}$, is only dependent on lumen and wall volume of LV chamber and represents an integrated assessment of LV systolic performance [1]. As shown in Table 3.4, we find that there exists significant difference in dV/dt_{max} between HFREF compared to HFNEF (233 ± 48 mL/s vs. 355 ± 65 mL/s, $p < 0.05$), while there exists no difference between HFNEF and normal controls (355 ± 65 mL/s vs. 353 ± 80 mL/s, NS). Similarly, there exists significant difference in LV mass between normal controls compared to HFNEF (147 ± 41 g vs. 202 ± 47 g, $p < 0.05$), while there is no difference between HFREF and HFNEF (213 ± 60 g vs. 202 ± 47 g, NS).

It is clearly seen that $d\sigma^*/dt_{max}$, dV/dt_{max} normalized to LV mass, can differentiate HFREF, HFNEF, and normal controls ($p < 0.05$) (Table 3.4). The average value of $d\sigma^*/dt_{max}$

TABLE 3.4

Comparison of the Maximal Flow Rate dV/dt_{max}, V_{peak}, LV Mass, and $d\sigma^*/dt_{max}$ in Group 1 (Controls), Group 2 (HFNEF), and Group 3 (HFREF)

	Controls (95% CI)	HFNEF (95% CI)	HFREF (95% CI)
dV/dt_{max} (mL/s)	353 (320, 385)	355 (329, 381)	233 (213, 252)[ab]
V_{peak} (cm/s)	106 (98, 115)	112 (104, 119)	73 (68, 78)[ab]
LV mass (g)	147 (131, 164)	202 (183, 221)[a]	213 (189, 297)[a]
$d\sigma^*/dt_{max}$ (s⁻¹)	3.91 (3.56, 4.26)	2.90 (2.56, 3.24)[ab]	1.84 (1.60, 2.07)[ab]

Source: Shishido, T. et al., *Circulation*, 102, 1983, 2000.

[a] and [b] denote statistically significant difference of HF compared to controls, and HFREF compared to HFNEF patients, respectively.

decreases in HFNEF and HFREF, in relation to that for normal controls. The mean value of $d\sigma^*/dt_{max}$ was found to be 3.91 s^{-1} (95% CI, 3.56–4.26 s^{-1}) in control subjects; the index was reduced in HF patients to: HFNEF, 2.90 s^{-1} (95% CI, 2.56–3.24 s^{-1}) and HFREF, 1.84 (95% CI, 1.60–2.07 s^{-1}). This suggests that poor systolic function of LV is associated with lower $d\sigma^*/dt_{max}$ values. Therefore, we can conclude that $d\sigma^*/dt_{max}$ is an appropriate index for representing assessment of LV contractile function in HF with/without preserved LVEF.

3.4 Formulation of Ventricular-Arterial Matching Index, and Study Showing Decreased Left Ventricular Contractility and Ventricular-Arterial Matching Index Correlation with N-Terminal Pro B-Type Natriuretic Peptide in Heart Failure

3.4.1 Introduction

Patients with heart failure with preserved ejection fraction (HFPEF) generally have concentric LV remodeling with increased wall thickness (due to increased cardiomyocyte diameter and extracellular matrix collagen), whereas patients with HFREF often exhibit eccentric remodeling with an increase in end-diastolic volume (due to increased cardiomyocyte length) [19]. Both HFPEF and HFREF, also commonly known as diastolic and systolic HF, respectively, have equally poor prognosis [11]. Several studies have reported that various systolic function indices are mildly depressed in patients with HFPEF [20,21]. The demonstrated abnormalities include a reduction in long-axis contractile shortening [22], a decline in systolic velocity of basal myocardial and mitral valve annular motion [23], and abnormalities of both ventricular endocardial strain and strain rate [24]. Indeed, it is well recognized that impairments in myocardial contractility may coexist with HFPEF [25].

Our LV contractility index, $d\sigma^*/dt_{max}$ (maximal rate of change of pressure-normalized wall stress) has been clinically validated in studies related to HF [1] and also been ventricular restoration of LV contractility [26].

We now study the interaction of the left ventricle with the arterial system, in terms of a VAM index. We then employ ventricular-arterial mismatching in patients with NT-proBNP, as a marker of HF. For this purpose, we have formulated the ventricular-arterial matching index, as the ratio of the cardiac contractility index and the arterial elastance (Ea). We have carried out a study [27] to determine both the LV contractility index and the VAM index from echocardiography. Also, in our study, venous blood samples were taken from the HF patients and tested in the laboratory for NT-proBNP. The NT-proBNP is secreted by the heart ventricles in response to excessive stretching of heart muscle cells (cardiomyocytes), and is a strong predictor of mortality among patients with acute coronary syndromes and a strong prognostic marker in patients with chronic coronary heart disease as well [28].

We have been able to see a strong a relationship between the VAM index and NT-proBNP. In patients with elevated NT-proBNP levels, the VAM index is shown to decrease due to impaired LV contractility (as caused by LV myocardial infarct) as well as due to elevated arterial elastance. Hence, the VAM index can serve as a strong marker of HF. Our study has shown the association of (1) ventricular-arterial mismatching with impaired cardiac performance and (2) ventricular-arterial mismatching with elevated N-terminal pro B-type natriuretic peptide (NT-proBNP), which is a proven marker of HF. This then confirms the validity of the use of VAM index as a marker of HF [27].

3.4.1.1 Subjects

Normal subjects ($n = 81$) with no signs of cardiovascular disorder and HF patients ($n = 80$) who presented and were hospitalized for HF symptoms were recruited in this study. Both normal subjects and HF patients underwent echocardiography examination, and their brachial blood pressure was taken by using sphygmomanometer. Venous blood samples were taken from the HF patients and sent to the laboratory for NT-proBNP testing; the NT-proBNP was analyzed immediately for optimal results.

3.4.1.2 Echocardiography

Echocardiography was performed by using ALOKA 10 with a 2.5 MHz transducer in the left lateral decubitus position. Standard 2D echocardiographic evaluation for left ventricular size, volume, and function was performed. Left ventricular ejection fraction (LVEF) was measured from the apical four-chamber and two-chamber view, by using modified biplane Simpson's method [29]. In each subject, the color flow Doppler velocity (V_{peak}) was measured in the LVOT.

The cuff blood pressure, systolic blood pressure (SBP), and diastolic blood pressure (DBP) were measured with standardized automated mercury cuff sphygmomanometer, after the patients were at rest for at least 5 min.

3.4.1.3 Formulation of the Ventricular-Arterial Matching Index

The arterial stiffness or elastance (E_a) is determined as 0.9*SBP/SV (SV is the stroke volume) [30].

The LV contractility index ($d\sigma^*/dt_{max}$) is calculated from Equation 3.4, as $3 \times V_{peak} \times [\pi D^2/4]/(2V_m)$, where V_{peak} is the peak velocity sampled at the LVOT and D is the LVOT diameter [8], as shown in Figure 3.4.

The VAM index is formulated as the ratio of ventricular contractile parameter $d\sigma^*/dt_{max}$ and arterial elastance E_a, as

$$\text{VAM index} = \frac{d\sigma^*/dt_{max}}{E_a} \tag{3.5}$$

3.4.1.4 Statistical Analysis

Continuous variables are presented as mean ± standard deviation (SD), and dichotomous variables as number, n and percentage, %. Comparisons of patient baseline characteristics and echocardiographic measurements between the normal subjects and HF patient were analyzed by using *T*-test and independent-sample test. The NT-proBNP values were log-transformed to normalize the distribution in this analysis. Scatterplot and spearman are used to analyze the relationship between the continuous variables. The p value <0.05 is defined to be statistically significant. Statistical analyses were performed by using the

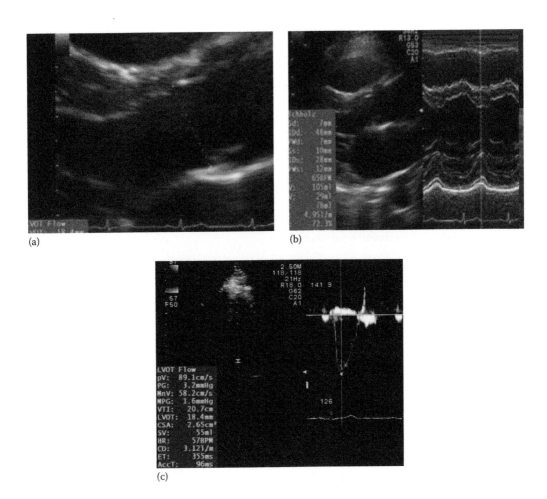

FIGURE 3.4

Echocardiographic parameters were measured in a normal volunteer. (a) LVOT diameter from 2D echocardiography in a parasternal long-axis view (LVOT diameter = 1.94 cm). (b) M-mode-derived LV mass (LV mass = 96 g). (c) LVOT peak velocity was measured from pulsed-wave Doppler echocardiography (V_{peak} = 89.1 cm/s). The computed LV contractility index $d\sigma^*/dt_{max}$ = 4.32 s^{-1}. (From Zhong, L. et al., *J. Mech. Med. Biol.*, 15(2), 1540016-1 - 1540016-9, 2015.)

Statistical Package for the Social Sciences (SPSS) Version 21 (IBM SPSS Statistics, IBM Corporation, Armonk, New York).

3.4.2 Results

3.4.2.1 Patient Characteristics

For this study, 81 normal subjects and 80 HF patients were recruited. The patient baseline characteristics, medical history, and laboratory findings are listed in Table 3.5. Subjects with atrial fibrillation and unsatisfactory echocardiography images were excluded. Heart failure patients were older (less female), with a high prevalence of hypertension, hyperlipidemia, and diabetes.

TABLE 3.5

Patients' Baseline Characteristics, Medical History, and Echocardiographic Measurements

	Normal (*n* = 81)	HF (*n* = 80)	*p*
Age (years)	56 ± 9	63 ± 11	<0.05
Female, *n* (%)	51 (63)	31 (39)	0.003
Height (cm)	161 ± 8	161 ± 11	0.918
Weight (kg)	63 ± 11	69 ± 16	0.002
Systolic blood pressure (mmHg)	126 ± 14	122 ± 22	0.225
Medical history			
Hypertension, *n* (%)		59 (75)	—
Hyperlipidemia, *n* (%)		59 (75)	—
Peripheral vascular disease, *n* (%)		11 (15)	—
Previous hospitalization for chronic heart failure, *n* (%)		41 (50)	—
Diabetes, *n* (%)		47 (59)	—
Chronic renal insufficiency, *n* (%)		24 (30)	—
Log NT-proBNP (pg/mL)		3.72 ± 0.59	—
Echocardiography			
LV mass (g)	129 ± 27	250 ± 98	<0.001
LVOT, V_{peak} (cm/s)	101 ± 16	65 ± 20	<0.001
LVOT diameter, D (cm)	2.01 ± 0.10	2.02 ± 0.18	0.581
Stroke volume (mL)	64 ± 12	42 ± 15	<0.001
$d\sigma^*/dt_{max}$ (s^{-1})	4.06 ± 1.06	1.46 ± 0.73	<0.001
E_a (mmHg/mL)	1.80 ± 0.38	2.90 ± 0.87	<0.001
VAM index (mL/mmHg·s)	2.38 ± 0.91	0.66 ± 0.57	<0.001

3.4.2.1.1 Echocardiography Findings and Computation of LV Contractility Index and VAM Index

Compared to normal subjects, HF patients were seen to have significantly (1) higher LV mass (HF: 250 ± 98 g vs. normal: 125 ± 32 g, *p* < 0.001), (2) lower stroke volume (HF: 42 ± 15 mL, normal: 63 ± 12 mL, *p* < 0.001), (3) lower blood velocity at LVOT (HF: 65 ± 20 cm/s, normal: 99 ± 14 cm/s, *p* < 0.001), (4) comparable LVOT diameter (HF: 2.02 ± 0.18 cm vs. normal: 2.02 ± 0.14 cm, *p* = 0.989), (5) lower LV contractility index value (HF: 1.46 ± 0.73 s^{-1} vs. normal: 4.22 ± 1.09 s^{-1}, 0.001), and (6) higher arterial stiffness (HF: 2.90 ± 0.87 mmHg/mL, normal: 1.80 ± 0.37 mmHg/mL, *p* < 0.001), as shown in Table 3.5. As a result, HF patients were found to have a lower VAM index value (HF: 0.66 ± 0.57 mL/mmHg·s vs. Normal: 2.46 ± 0.90 mL/mmHg·s, *p* < 0.001).

Figure 3.5 shows that the VAM index is well correlated inversely with NT-proBNP (*r* = −0.32) and positively with the stroke volume (*r* = 0.85, *p* < 0.001). Based on ROC analysis, the VAM index value of <1.51 was able to differentiate a failing heart from a normal heart (AUC = 0.959, sensitivity = 0.911, specificity = 0.905).

3.4.3 Discussion

The main finding of this study is that HF patients are found to have lower VAM index value, compared to the normal subjects. This is likely caused by decreased LV contractility ($d\sigma^*/dt_{max}$ index value) and arterial stiffening (i.e., increased E_a value) in HF. The attenuated ventricular arterial matching index is associated with elevated NT-proBNP and lower cardiac output.

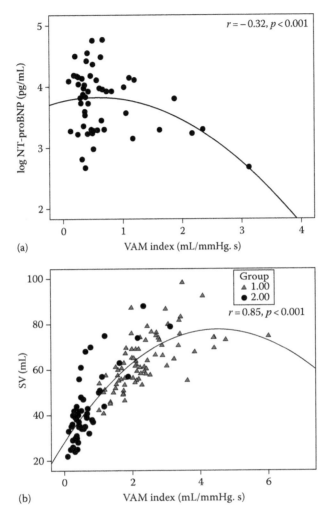

FIGURE 3.5
(a) Correlation between ventricular-arterial matching (VAM) index and log NT-proBNP. (b) Correlation between VAM index and stroke volume (SV). Group 1: Normal; Group 2: Heart failure. The VAM index value of <1.51 is associated with heart failure, and bears close correlation with NT-proBNP as a marker of HF. (From Zhong, L. et al., *J. Mech. Med. Biol.*, 15(2), 1540016-1 - 1540016-9, 2015.)

3.4.3.1 Ventricular Contractility Index

Heart failure may be viewed as a progressive disorder that is initiated after an "index event" with a resultant loss of functioning cardiac myocytes, thereby preventing the heart from contracting normally. Although approaches based on pressure–volume, stress–strain, and dP/dt_{max}–EDV [12] relations can provide assessment of contractile function, these relations generally require invasive data measured at several chamber loads, and thus are difficult to apply in routine or long-term clinical studies. This is an important limitation, because HF often requires longitudinal evaluation. Clearly, there is a clinical need for a LV contractility index that is easy to apply and reproducible. Further, it should be load-independent and within the physiologic limits encountered in clinical practice; even established invasive LV contractility indices like dP/dt_{max} [31] and ESPVR [32] become load-dependent at wider loading conditions.

Our $d\sigma^*/dt_{max}$ contractility index has several qualities that make it a useful LV contractility index. It is easily measured noninvasively, is sensitive to LV inotropic changes, and has been demonstrated by us to be relatively preload- and afterload-independent [1,5]. Several studies have reported close association between this index and cardiovascular events, like HF [8,26,33–37]. This study constitutes an important step toward establishing the clinical utility of LV contractility index ($d\sigma^*/dt_{max}$) and VAM index ($d\sigma^*/dt_{max}/E_a$), as reliable tools for assessing ventricular performance in HF (both HFPEF and HFREF) as well as for follow-up surveillance of LV function. Hence we see a great potential for application of these novel indexes to evaluate heart function in diverse heart conditions.

3.4.3.2 *Ventricular-Arterial Matching Index*

The VAM index governs the coupling between the ventricle and arterial system during the systolic phase. The ratio of LV contractility index to arterial elastance (E_a) is deployed in this index. In affirming the importance of this ventriculo-arterial coupling measure, our current study has confirmed that (1) LV contractility decreases in HF patients, and (2) arterial elastance is enhanced in HF patients compared to normal subjects. Hence their ratio, as given by the VAM index, is reduced in HF patients.

Often, older patients display arterial stiffening condition known as arteriosclerosis. Calcification within the aorta may result in arterial stiffening, and hence a higher systolic pressure is needed to eject the blood from the LV to the aorta. The greater the aortic elastance (stiffening), the higher is the aortic pressure generated, thereby requiring a greater LV contractile force to eject the blood into the aorta. Now, when under this circumstances, the LV has decreased contractility, this results in heart faiure.

3.4.3.3 *Relationship between Ventricular-Arterial Matching Index and NT-proBNP*

In chronic HF, natriuretic peptides are secreted by heart ventricles in response to myocardial stretching. The NT-proBNP measurement has been known to be one of the strong stand alone diagnostic tests for HF, as patients with elevated NT-proBNP levels are more likely to have HF. Increased plasma levels of brain natriuretic peptide are observed in patients with acute myocardial infarction [38]. The NT-proBNP increase is associated with alteration in LV contractility, resulting in the decrease of the VAM index. This relationship has showed correspondence with studies by Palazzuoli et al. [39] about elevated BNP levels correlating well with the severity of LV systolic function, filling alterations, and pressure. Also, Mak et al. [40] have shown that NT-proBNP correlates well with E/E' (ratio of mitral peak velocity of early filling E to early diastolic mitral annular velocity E'), which is a simple and effective measure for assessing cardiac risk due to diastolic dysfunction. This can explain why (1) the correlation between VAM index and NT-proBNP is justified, and (2) we can effectively associate reduction of VAM index value to be a marker of HF.

HF patients have demonstrated impaired ventricular contractility, arterial stiffening (i.e., increased arterial elastance), and hence attenuated VAM index. This attenuated

VAM or ventricular-arterial mismatching is associated with elevated NT-proBNP and lower cardiac output, as a marker of HF.

3.5 Conclusion

The hearts of myocardial infarct patients undergo substantial remodeling and loss of contractility, and can progress to HF. Echocardiographic texture analysis enables us to determine the percentage volume of the infarcted segments in the ventricular volume.

Herein, we have provided the theory of the new contractility index $d\sigma^*/dt_{max}$. The utility of this contractility index is that it can be evaluated without monitoring LV pressure. As shown in Figure 3.1, this noninvasive index was shown to correlate strongly with the traditional invasively determined contractility index dP/dt_{max}. Further, as depicted in Tables 3.3 and 3.4, this index was also found to characterize and diagnose both diastolic and systolic HF.

We have then formulated the VAM index as the ratio of ventricular contractile parameter $d\sigma^*/dt_{max}$ and arterial elastance E_a, as $[d\sigma^*/dt_{max}]/E_a$. This VAM index governs the coupling between the ventricle and arterial systems during the systolic phase. We have shown that (1) LV contractility decreases in HF patients, (2) arterial elastance is enhanced in HF patients compared to normal subjects, and (3) the VAM index is reduced in HF patients.

There is a relationship between the VAM index and NT-proBNP. Patients with elevated NT-proBNP levels are more likely to have HF. The NT-proBNP increase is associated with decrease in LV contractility, resulting in the decrease of the VAM index. This is why we can effectively employ the reduction of VAM index value to be a marker of HF.

3A Appendix: Analysis of Wall Stress in a Thick-Walled Spherical LV Model

This analysis of wall stress in a thick-walled spherical LV model is based on the theory of elasticity [2]. We have modeled the LV as a pressurized thick-walled spherical shell.

If u_r represents the radial displacement of a spherical surface element in the LV wall at radius r, then at the outer surface of radius $r + \Delta r$, the corresponding radial displacement can be expressed as $u_r + (\partial u_r/\partial r)dr$. The strain ε_r in the radial direction is then given by

$$\varepsilon_r = \frac{(u_r + (\partial u_r/\partial r)dr) - u_r}{dr} = \frac{\partial u_r}{\partial r} \tag{3A.1}$$

Now, spherical symmetry implies that the strains ε_ϕ and ε_θ in the orthogonal circumferential axes are identical. Therefore, the strain ε_ϕ in the circumferential direction is

$$\varepsilon_\phi = \frac{2\pi(r + u_r) - 2\pi r}{2\pi r} = \frac{u_r}{r} = \varepsilon_\theta \tag{3A.2}$$

The strains along the three orthogonal axes are

$$\varepsilon_r = \frac{\partial u_r}{\partial r}, \quad \varepsilon_\theta = \frac{u_r}{r}, \quad \varepsilon_\phi = \frac{u_r}{r} \tag{3A.3}$$

Similarly, $\sigma_\theta = \sigma_\phi$. For equilibrium in the radial direction, we have

$$-\sigma_r(2\theta r)(2\theta r) + (\sigma_r + \Delta\sigma_r)(r + \Delta r)2\theta(r + \Delta r)2\theta$$
$$- 2\left(r + \frac{\Delta r}{2}\right)2\theta\Delta r\sigma_\phi \sin\theta - 2\left(r + \frac{\Delta r}{2}\right)2\theta\Delta r\sigma_\theta \sin\theta = 0 \tag{3A.4}$$

Since $\sigma_\theta = \sigma_\phi$ and $d\sigma_r = (\partial\sigma_r/\partial r)\Delta r$, Equation 3A.4 reduces in the limit to

$$\frac{1}{r^2}\frac{d}{dr}(r^2\sigma_r) = \frac{2}{r}\sigma_\phi \tag{3A.5}$$

Based on Hooke's law, we can express the constitutive equation as

$$\varepsilon_r = \frac{1}{E}[\sigma_r - v(\sigma_\theta + \sigma_\phi)] = \frac{\partial u_r}{\partial r} \quad \text{or} \quad \frac{du_r}{dr} = \frac{1}{E}[\sigma_r - 2v\sigma_\phi] \tag{3A.6}$$

where
  E is the elastic modulus
  v is Poisson's ratio

Likewise, from Equation 3A.2:

$$\varepsilon_\phi = \frac{1}{E}[\sigma_\phi - v(\sigma_\theta - \sigma_r)] = \frac{u_r}{r} \quad \text{or} \quad \frac{u_r}{r} = \frac{1}{E}[(1-v)\sigma_\phi - v\sigma_r] \tag{3A.7}$$

Differentiating Equation 3A.7 with respect to r, we obtain

$$\frac{du_r}{dr} = \frac{1}{E}\left[(1-v)\frac{\partial(r\sigma_\phi)}{\partial r} - v\frac{\partial(r\sigma_r)}{\partial r}\right] \tag{3A.8}$$

Equations 3A.6 and 3A.8 can be combined as

$$(1-v)\frac{d(r\sigma_\phi)}{dr} - v\frac{d(r\sigma_r)}{dr} - (\sigma_r - 2v\sigma_\phi) = 0 \tag{3A.9}$$

If we combine σ_ϕ (Equation 3A.5) into Equation 3A.9, we obtain

$$\frac{1-v}{2}\frac{d^2(r^2\sigma_r)}{dr^2} - v\frac{d(r\sigma_r)}{dr} - \sigma_r + \frac{v}{r}\frac{d(r^2\sigma_r)}{dr} = 0 \tag{3A.10}$$

If we substitute $r^2\sigma_r = y$, Equation 3A.10 becomes

$$\frac{1}{2}(1-v)\frac{d^2y}{dr^2} - \frac{v}{r}\frac{dy}{dr} + \frac{vy}{r^2} - \frac{y}{r^2} + \frac{v}{r}\frac{dy}{dr} = 0 \quad \text{or} \quad \frac{d^2y}{dr^2} - 2\frac{y}{r^2} = 0 \qquad (3A.11)$$

This yields a homogeneous linear equation with the solution:

$$y = Ar^2 + \frac{B}{r} \quad \text{and} \quad \sigma_r = \frac{y}{r^2} = A + \frac{B}{r^3} \qquad (3A.12)$$

where A and B are constants. From Equations 3A.5 and 3A.12, we find

$$\sigma_\phi = A - \frac{B}{2r^3} \qquad (3A.13)$$

For a thick-walled spherical shell with internal and external radii r_i and r_e, respectively, which is subjected to internal pressure P_i and zero external pressure, the boundary conditions are $\sigma_r = -P_i$ when $r = r_i$; and $\sigma_r = 0$ when $r = r_e$. Hence, from Equation 3A.12, we obtain

$$A + \frac{B}{r_i^3} = -P_i \quad \text{and} \quad A + \frac{B}{r_e^3} = 0 \qquad (3A.14)$$

Hence, we can determine the constants of integration as

$$A = \frac{r_i^3 P_i}{r_e^3 - r_i^3}; \quad B = \frac{r_e^3 r_i^3 P_i}{r_e^3 - r_i^3} \qquad (3A.15)$$

Now, from Equations 3A.12 through 3A.14, the expressions for radial and circumferential stresses are obtained as

$$\sigma_r = P_i \frac{r_i^3}{r_e^3 - r_i^3}\left(1 - \frac{r_e^3}{r^3}\right) \qquad (3A.16)$$

$$\sigma_\phi = \sigma_\theta = P_i \frac{r_i^3}{r_e^3 - r_i^3}\left(1 + \frac{r_e^3}{2r^3}\right) \qquad (3A.17)$$

For the LV model, this circumferential stress is larger in magnitude and opposite in sign (tensile) as compared to the radial stress (compressive).

References

1. Zhong L, Tan RS, Ghista DN, Ng EYK, Chua LP, Kassab GS. Validation of a novel noninvasive index of left ventricular contractility in patients. *Am J Physiol Heart Circ Physiol*, 292(6): H2764–H2772, 2007.

2. Srinath LS. *Advanced Mechanics of Solids*. New Delhi, India: McGraw-Hill, Chapter 8, pp. 264–295, 2001.

3. Ghista DN, Li L, Chua LP, Tan RS, Tan YS. Mechanism of left ventricular pressure increase during isovolumic contraction, and determination of its equivalent myocardial fibres orientation. *J Mech Med Biol*, 9(2): 177–198, 2009.

4. Ghista DN, Zhong L, Chua LP, Kassab GS, Su Y, Tan RS. Cardiac myocardial disease states cause left ventricular remodelling with decreased contractility and lead to heart failure; Interventions by coronary arterial bypass grafting and surgical ventricular restoration can reverse LV remodeling with improved contractility. *Biomed Sci Eng Technol.*, Ghista DN, ed., InTech 2011, pp. 831–850.

5. Jia X, Choy S, Zhang ZD, Svendson M, Zhong L, Tan RS, Kassab GS. Extent of load independence of pressure-normalized stress in swine. *Exp Biol Med*, 238(7): 821–829, 2013.

6. Zhong L, Ghista DN, Ng EYK, Lim ST. Passive and active ventricular elastances of the left ventricle. *Biomed Eng Online*, 4: 10, 2005.

7. Shishido T, Hayashi K, Shigemi K, Sato T, Sugimachi M, Sunagawa K. Single-beat estimation of end-systolic elastance using bilinearly approximated time-varying elastance. *Circulation*, 102: 1983–1989, 2000.

8. Zhong L, Poh KK, Lee LC, Le TT, Tan RS. Attenuation of stress-based ventricular contractility in patients with heart failure and normal ejection fraction. *Ann Acad Med, Singapore*, 40(4), 179–185, April 2011.

9. Krumholz HM, Chen YT, Wang Y, Caccarino V, Radford MJ, Horwita RI. Predictors of readmission among elderly survivors of admission with heart failure. *Am Heart J*, 139: 72–77, 2000.

10. Stefan N. The failing heart—An engine out of fuel. *N Engl J Med*, 356: 1140–1151, 2007.

11. Hogg K, Swedberg K, McMurray J. Heart failure with preserved left ventricular systolic function: Epidemiology, clinical characteristics, and prognosis. *J Am Coll Cardiol*, 43: 317–327, 2004.

12. Little WC. The left ventricular (dP/dt)$_{max}$-end-diastolic volume relation in closed-chest dogs. *Circ Res*, 56: 808–815, 1985.

13. Vasan RS, Levy D. Defining diastolic heart failure: A call for standardized diagnostic criteria. *Circulation*, 101: 2118–2121, 2000.

14. Devereux RB, Alonso DR, Lutas EM, Gottlieb GJ, Campo E, Sachs I, Reichek N. Echocardiographic assessment of left ventricular hypertrophy: Comparison to necropsy findings. *Am J Cardiol*, 57: 450–458, 1986.

15. Lang RM, Bierig M, Devereux RB, Flachskampf FA, Foster E. Recommendations for chamber quantification. *J Am Soc Echocardiogr*, 18: 1440–1463, 2005.

16. Kitzman DW, Gardin JM, Gottdiener JS et al. Importance of heart failure with preserved systolic function in patients > or =65 years of age. CHS Research Group Cardiovascular Health Study. *Am J Cardiol*, 87: 413–419, 2001.

17. Banerjee P, Banerjee T, Khand A et al. Diastolic heart failure: Neglected or misdiagnosed? *J Am Coll Cardiol*, 39: 138–141, 2002.

18. Burkhoff D, Maurer MS, Packer M. Heart failure with a normal ejection fraction: Is it really a disorder of diastolic function? *Circulation*, 107: 656–658, 2003.

19. Aurigemma GP, Zile MR, Gaasch WH. Contractile behavior of the left ventricle in diastolic heart failure: With emphasis on regional systolic function. *Circulation*, 113: 296–304, 2006.

20. Yip G, Wang M, Fung JWH. Left ventricular long axis function in diastolic heart failure is reduced in both diastole and systole: Time for redefinition? *Heart*, 87: 12–15, 2002.

21. Garcia EH, Perna ER, Farias EF. Reduced systolic performance by tissue Doppler in patients with preserved and abnormal ejection fraction: New insight in chronic heart failure. *Int J Cardiol*, 108: 181–188, 2006.

22. Petrie MC, Caruana L, Berry C. Diastolic heart failure or heart failure caused by subtle left ventricular systolic function? *Heart*, 87: 29–31, 2002.

23. Bruch C, Gradaus R, Gunia S. Doppler tissue analysis of mitral annular velocities: Evidence for systolic abnormalities in patients with diastolic heart failure. *J Am Soc Echocardiogr*, 16: 1031–1036, 2003.

24. Pellerin D, Sharma R, Elliott P. Tissue Doppler, strain, and strain rate echocardiography for the assessment of left and right systolic ventricular function. *Heart*, 89: iii9–iii17, 2003.

25. Borlaug BA, Lam CS, Roger VL, Rodeheffer RJ, Redfield MM. Contractility and ventricular systolic stiffening in hypertensive heart disease: Insights into the pathogenesis of heart failure with preserved ejection fraction. *J Am Coll Cardiol*, 54: 410–418, 2009.

26. Zhong L, Sola S, Tan RS, Le TT, Ghista DN, Kurra V, Navia JL, Kassab G. Effects of surgical ventricular restoration on LV contractility assessed by a novel contractility index. *Am J Cardiol*, 103: 674–679, 2009.

27. Zhong L, Wang YJ, Huang FQ, Ghista DN, Tan RS. Decreased left ventricular contractility and ventricular-arterial matching index correlation with N-terminal pro B-type natriuretic peptide in heart failure. *J Mech Med Biol* 15(2), 1540016-1 - 1540016-9, 2015.

28. Kragelund C, Grønning B, Køber L, Hildebrandt P, Steffensen R. N-terminal pro–B-type natriuretic peptide and long-term mortality in stable coronary heart disease. *N Engl J Med*, 352: 666–675, 2005.

29. Lang RM, Bierig M, Devereux RB et al. Chamber Quantification Writing Group: American Society of Echocardiography's Guideline and Standards Committee: European Association of Echocardiography. Recommendations for chamber quantification: A report from American Society of Echocardiography's Guideline and Standards Committee and the Chamber Quantification Writing Group, developed in conjunction with the European Association of Echocardiography, a Branch of the European Society of Cardiology. *Eur J Echocardiogr*, 7: 79–108, 2006.

30. Chen CH, Fetics B, Nevo E et al. Noninvasive single-beat determination of left ventricular end-systolic elastance in humans. *J Am Coll Cardiol*, 38: 2028–2034, 2001.

31. Mulier JP. Ventricular pressure as a function of volume and flow. PhD thesis, University of Leuven, Belgium, 1994.

32. Noda T, Cheng CP, de Tombe PP, Little WC. Curvilinearty of LV end-systolic pressure-volume and dP/dtmax-end-diastolic volume relations. *Am J Physiol*, 34: H910–H917, 1993.

33. Zhong L, Su Y, Gobeawan L, Sola S, Tan RS, Navia JL, Ghista DN, Chua T, Guccione J, Kassab G. Impact of surgical ventricular restoration on ventricular shape, wall stress and function in heart failure patients. *Am J Physiol Heart Circ Physiol*, 300: H1653–H1660, 2011.

34. Zhong L, Ng KK, Sim L et al. Myocardial contractile dysfunction associated with increased 3-month and 1-year mortality in hospitalized patients with heart failure and preserved ejection fraction. *Int J Cardiol*, 168: 1975–1980, 2013.

35. Zhong L, Huang FQ, Tan LK, Allen JC, Ding ZP, Tan RS. Age and gender—Specific changes in left ventricular systolic function in human volunteers. *Int J Cardiol*, 172: e102–e105, 2014.

36. Hummel SL, Seymour EM, Brook RD. Low-sodium DASH Diet improves diastolic function and ventricular-arterial coupling in hypertensive heart failure with preserved ejection fraction. *Circ Heart Failure*, 6(6): 1165–1171, 2013.

37. Svendsen M, Prinzen FW, Das MK, Berwick Z, Rybka M, Tune JD, Combs W, Berbari E, Kassab G. Bi-ventricular pacing improves pump function only with adequate myocardial perfusion in canine hearts with pseudo-left bundle branch block. *Exp Biol Med*, 237: 644–651, 2012.

38. Morita E, Yasue H, Yoshimura M, Ogawa H, Jougasaki M, Matsumura T, Mukoyama M, Nakao K. Increased plasma levels of brain natriuretic peptide in patients with acute myocardial infarction. *Circulation*, 88: 82–91, 1993.

39. Palazzuoli A, Gallotta M, Quatrini I, Nuti R. Natriuretic peptides (BNP and NT-proBNP): Measurement and relevance in heart failure. *Dove Press*, 6: 411–418, 2010.

40. Mak GS, DeMaria A, Clopton P, Maisel AS. Utility of B-natriuretic peptide in the evaluation of left ventricular diastolic function: Comparison with tissue Doppler imaging recordings. *Am Heart J*, 148: 895–902, 2004.

4

Cardiomyopathy Effect on Left Ventricle Function (Shape and Contractility) and Improvement after Surgical Ventricular Restoration

Dhanjoo N. Ghista, Yi Su, Liang Zhong, Ru San Tan, and Ghassan S. Kassab

CONTENTS

Acronyms

C	Curvedness
C_{ED}	Curvedness at end-diastole
C_{ES}	Curvedness at end-systole
CI	Indexed cardiac output
CMR	Cardiac magnetic resonance
E_a	Effective arterial elastance
EDVI	Indexed end-diastolic volume
EF	Ejection fraction
ESVI	Indexed end-systolic volume
HR	Heart rate
IDCM	Ischemic dilated cardiomyopathy
LV	Left ventricle
MRI	Magnetic resonance imaging
R	Wall radius
R_{ED}	Wall radius at end-diastole
R_{ES}	Wall radius at end-systole
S	Surface area
S_{ED}	Surface area at end-diastole

S_{ES}	Surface area at end-systole
SI	Sphericity index
SLv	Normalized shape index
SW	Stroke work
T	Wall thickness
T_{ED}	Wall thickness at end-diastole
T_{ES}	Wall thickness at end-systole
WS	Wall stress
WT	Wall thickening
σ/P	Pressure-normalized stress
$(\sigma/P)_{ED}$	Pressure-normalized stress at end-diastole
$(\sigma/P)_{ES}$	Pressure-normalized stress at end-systole
ΔC	Percentage curvedness change
$(d\sigma^*/dt)_{max}$	Left ventricular contractility index $(=1.5(dV/dt_{max})/V_m)$
ΔS	Percentage change in surface area
2DLR	Two-dimensional radius in the long-axis plane
2DLT	Two-dimensional wall thickness in the long-axis plane
2DLWS	Wall stress in the long-axis plane
2DLWT	Wall thickening in the long-axis plane
2DSR	Two-dimensional radius in the short-axis plane
2DST	Two-dimensional wall thickness in the short-axis plane
2DSWS	Wall stress in the short-axis plane
2DSWT	Wall thickening in the short-axis plane
3DR	Three-dimensional radius accounting for 3D curvature
3DT	Three-dimensional wall thickness accounting for 3D curvature
3DWS	Three-dimensional wall stress
3DWT	Three-dimensional wall thickening

4.1 Introduction

Cardiomyopathy refers to diseases of the heart muscle. These diseases enlarge the heart muscle or make it thicker and more rigid than normal. In some cases, scar tissue replaces the muscle tissue. Myocardial ischemia and infarction can cause cardiomyopathy. Cardiomyopathy causes measurable deterioration of myocardial function and can lead to heart failure (HF).

Heart failure is generally defined as the inability of the heart to supply sufficient blood flow to meet the body's needs. The term *heart failure* is often incorrectly used to describe other cardiac-related illnesses, such as myocardial infarction (MI) (heart attack) or cardiac arrest. Common causes of HF include MI and other forms of ischemic heart diseases and cardiomyopathy.

Some people live long, healthy lives with cardiomyopathy. In others, however, it can make the heart less able to pump blood throughout the body. This can cause serious complications, including HF and abnormal heart rhythms. Ischemic dilated cardiomyopathy (IDCM) is caused by coronary artery disease and heart attack.

In IDCM, the heart's ability to pump blood is decreased, because the heart's main pumping chamber, the left ventricle (LV), is enlarged, dilated, and weak. This is caused by ischemia, the lack of blood supply to the heart muscle caused by coronary artery disease and heart attacks.

IDCM is diagnosed based on medical history (symptoms and family medical history), physical examination, and other tests. Specific tests may include blood tests, electrocardiogram (ECG), chest x-ray, exercise stress test, cardiac catheterization, computed tomography (CT) scan, magnetic resonance imaging (MRI) scan, and radionuclide studies.

Treatment of ischemic cardiomyopathy is aimed at treating coronary artery disease, improving cardiac function and reducing HF symptoms. Patients usually take medications to improve cardiac function, to treat symptoms and prevent complications; to manage HF, most people take a beta-blocker and angiotensin-converting enzyme (ACE) inhibitor. In addition, devices and surgical ventricular restoration (SVR) may be advised and employed to reduce risk to HF in IDCM patients.

MI can cause IDCM and associated changes in left ventricular shape (regional curvatures), myocardial wall stress, and contractility. In this chapter, we have quantified heart dysfunction caused by IDCM by studying 10 IDCM patients and 10 normal subjects. In these subjects, the 3D LV reconstructions were carried out using MRI. The IDCM patients also underwent delayed gadolinium-enhancement imaging to delineate the extent of myocardial infarct. The LV shape change was characterized in terms of LV regional curvedness (C), local radii-of-curvature and wall thickness were calculated, along with percentage curvedness change (ΔC) between end-diastole and end-systole.

The LV shape in IDCM patients differed from those in normal subjects in several ways. First, the LV had a more spherical shape (sphericity index, 0.62 ± 0.08 vs. 0.52 ± 0.06, $p < 0.05$). Second, the curvedness at ED (mean for 16 segments, 0.034 ± 0.0056 mm^{-1} vs. 0.040 ± 0.0071 mm^{-1} $p < 0.001$) and ES (mean for 16 segments, 0.037 ± 0.0068 mm^{-1} vs. 0.067 ± 0.020 mm^{-1} $p < 0.001$) was reduced by IDCM. In normal hearts, the short-axis and long-axis 2D analyses showed $41\% \pm 11\%$ and $45\% \pm 12\%$ increase in the mean of peak systolic wall stress between basal and apical sections, respectively. The peak systolic wall stress was significantly increased at each of the anterior, inferior, and apical segments in patients with IDCM, implying increased oxygen demand. However, cardiac contractility, measured by the index $(d\sigma^*/dt)_{max}$, decreased from a mean value of 5.7 s^{-1} in normal subjects to 2.4 s^{-1} in IDCM patients.

Surgical ventricular restoration is carried out to treat patients with aneurysms or large akinetic walls and dilated ventricles. So, in this chapter, we present the effect of SVR in restoring LV function, based on a study to quantify the efficacy of SVR, based on LV regional shape in terms of curvedness (C), regional wall stress, and ventricular systolic function. In our study, 40 patients underwent MRI before and after SVR. Both short-axis and long-axis MRI were used to reconstruct end-diastolic (ED) and end-systolic (ES) 3D LV geometry. The regional shape in terms of surface curvedness, regional wall thickness, and wall stress indices were determined for the entire LV. The infarct zone (IZ), border zone (BZ), and remote zone (RZ) were defined in terms of ED wall thickness. The LV global systolic function was examined in terms of global ejection fraction (EF), the ratio between stroke work (SW) and end-diastolic volume (EDV), LV contractility index $((d\sigma^*/dt)_{max})$, and regional function in terms of surface area change (ΔS).

Following SVR, it is noted that (1) the LV EDV and end-systolic volume (ESV) indices were significantly reduced from 156 ± 39 to 110 ± 33 and from 117 ± 39 to 77 ± 31 mL/m^2, respectively, and (2) the global systolic function was improved in terms of EF from 26 ± 7 to 31 ± 10, SW/EDV from 21.76 ± 8.25 to 25.64 ± 7.40 mmHg, and the contractility index $((d\sigma^*/dt)_{max})$ value from 2.69 ± 0.74 to 3.23 ± 0.73 s^{-1}.

In addition, the ES stresses in all the three zones (IZ, BZ, RZ) were reduced: from 43 ± 12 to 23 ± 6 kPa in the IZ; from 29 ± 7 to 20 ± 6 kPa in the BZ; and from 22 ± 6 to 17 ± 5 kPa in the RZ. The SVR reduced regional wall stress along with improved global LV systolic function. However, the regional LV shape did not improve significantly; there was only a slight increase in regional curvedness (C) in each zone.

4.2 Ischemic Dilated Cardiomyopathy Effect on Left Ventricle: Shape (Regional Wall Curvedness), Regional Wall Stress, Global Contractility

4.2.1 Introduction

Ischemic dilated cardiomyopathy (IDCM) is a degenerative disease of the myocardial tissue, following MI (or a heart attack), accompanied by LV remodeling [38]. LV remodeling is a multistep process, which involves acute dilation of the ischemic/infarcted area, increase of LV volume, lengthening of LV perimeter, and decrease of LV curvature [12,46].

The elevation of LV wall stress in IDCM is associated with morphological changes in the myocardium which may cause regional hypokinesis [23–25]. The LV wall stress is in part determined by the local curvature of the ventricular wall, that is, decreased curvature will increase wall stress [26]. In addition to increasing LV size, IDCM can alter the passive and active stiffness (or elastance) property of the myocardium and the LV shape curvature. The BZ around a myocardial infarct will have a higher stress, which makes it more susceptible to ischemia and extension of infarction (due to decreased myocardial perfusion and myocardial oxygen supply-demand mismatch); this can further accentuate the remodeling process [47]. Therefore, therapeutic approaches for IDCM include LV size reduction by SVR, to disrupt the downward spiral cycle toward HF [16].

The geometry of the remodeled LV in IDCM is complicated, and a 3D approach is employed to characterize the ventricular regional-shape changes during the cardiac cycle as well as the ventricular mechanics of contractility [44,54]. MRI is the most comprehensive approach to quantify the 3D ventricular structure and function [3,32], in comparison with echocardiography [21], ventriculography [20,52], angiography [43], and indicator-dilution methods [15].

End-systolic wall stress, which is governed by the systolic pressure and shape of the LV [22,26,51], is an important effect-parameter of the remodeled shape of the LV. Several types of mathematical models have been used to calculate the wall stress (WS) [51]. Some models are for idealized LV geometry for spherical or ellipsoidal shapes, and hence only allow calculation of the global WS. Other models are applicable to estimation of the local myocardial stress [26], based on measurement of the local thickness of the LV wall and local radius-of-curvature [4].

Herein, we have determined the effect of IDCM on (1) the regional variation in the 3D shape of the LV (i.e., in terms of surface curvedness), (2) left ventricular (cardiac) contractility index, (3) the 3D regional variations of WS (incorporating the regional wall curvature), and (4) the relationship between peak systolic wall stress and the regional extent of myocardial infarct.

4.2.2 Methodology

4.2.2.1 Subjects Involved in the Study

Our analysis of how IDCM affects the LV is based on the study of 10 normal subjects and 10 IDCM patients [54]. All of these subjects underwent diagnostic MRI scan. None of the normal subjects had: (1) significant valvular or congenital cardiac disease, (2) history of MI, (3) coronary artery lesions, or (4) abnormal left ventricular pressure, EDV or ejection fraction.

4.2.2.2 MRI Scanning for Acquisition of LV Geometry

MRI scanning was performed by using steady-state free precession cine gradient echo sequences. The subjects were imaged on a 1.5T Siemens scanner (Avanto, Siemens Medical Solutions, Erlangen). TrueFISP (fast imaging with steady-state precession) MR pulse sequence, with segmented k-space and retrospective electrocardiographic gating, was used to acquire a parallel stack of 2D cine images of the LV in the short-axis planes, from the LV base to apex (of 8 mm inter-slice thickness, with no inter-slice gap). The field of view was typically 320 mm with an in-plane spatial resolution of less than 1.5 mm. Each slice was acquired in a single breath hold, with 25 temporal phases per heart cycle.

From the MRI scans, LV short-axis image acquisitions are used to (1) locate the planes passing through the mitral and aortic valves and hence (2) designate the oblique long-axis plane of the LV, orthogonal to the short-axis planes and passing through the mitral valve, apex, and aortic valve. In addition, from the short-axis plane images, the vertical long-axis planes (connecting the short-axis planes) were constructed.

Figure 4.1 depicts the MR short- and long-axes plane image slices, during end-diastole and end-systole phases [54]. By using customized software, these MRI derived short- and long-axis planes are utilized to carry out 3D LV reconstruction (at end-diastole and end-systole), as depicted in Figure 4.2.

4.2.2.3 Delayed Gadolinium Enhancement Imaging

For evaluation of myocardial viability, 25 contiguous short-axis views were acquired with 2D MR imaging. For this purpose, standard extracellular MR contrast agents were injected intravenously at a dose of 0.2 mmol gadolinium/Kg (gadoterate dimeglumine, Schering, Berlin, Germany). All images were acquired during end-expiratory breath holds at 5–15 min, after injection. T1 weighting was achieved with an inversion-recovery fast low-angle shot (IR-FLASH) pulse sequence. Typical parameters were TE = 2 ms, TR = 6 ms, voxel size = $1 \times 1 \times 6$ mm, 300 ms inversion delay, k-space data segmented over 4 cardiac cycle (32 lines/cycle), with data acquired every cardiac cycle. Images were acquired at mid-diastole during breath-hold (8 s).

A commercially available image analysis software (Syngo 3D; Siemens Medical Solution) was employed to designate the regions of interest in the viable myocardium (dark) and in the nonviable myocardium (highly enhanced), for each image frame in the short-axis cine DE series. The thickness of the hyperenhancement was planimetered on all short-axis images from base to apex.

Each 3D reconstructed LV model was then divided into 16 segments, as illustrated in Figure 4.3. The myocardial contrast in each of these segments was then quantified in terms of scar scores. Next, a scar extent score was assigned to each region, based on scores of 0 (i.e., no scarring), 1 (1%–25% scarring), 2 (26%–50% scarring), 3 (51%–75% scarring), 4 (76%–99% scarring), and 5 (100% scarring).

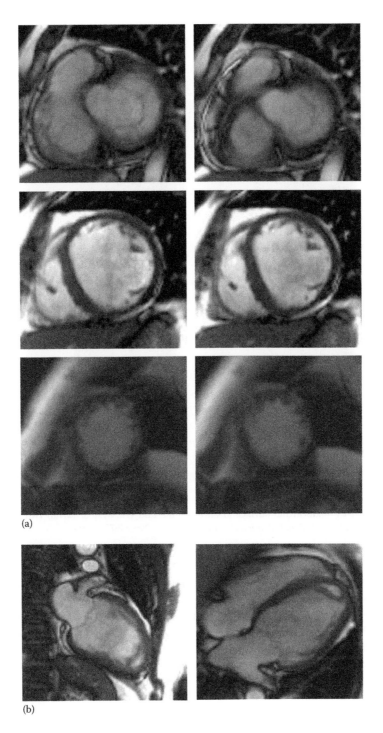

FIGURE 4.1

Sample segmented trueFISP 2D cine MR images of (a) short-axis slices acquired at the base, middle, and apex (from top to bottom, respectively) and (b) long-axis of the left ventricle. The end-diastolic and end-systolic phases are depicted in the left and right columns, respectively. (Adapted from Zhong, L. et al., *Am. J. Physiol. Heart Circ. Physiol.*, 296, H573, 2009.)

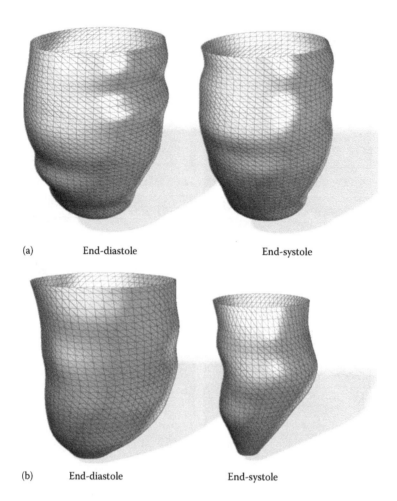

(a)   End-diastole   End-systole

(b)   End-diastole   End-systole

FIGURE 4.2
3D reconstruction of LV endocardial surface at end-diastole and end-systole for (a) DCM and (b) normal. (Adapted from Zhong, L. et al., *Am. J. Physiol. Heart Circ. Physiol.*, 296, H573, 2009.)

4.2.3 Data Processing and LV Geometry Reconstruction

The MRI data were processed by using a semi-automatic technique provided in the CMRtools suite (Cardiovascular Solution, UK). Short- and long-axis images were displayed simultaneously, so that segmentation in the two planes could be carried out interactively [39]. For each phase, every control point on the endocardium was constrained to lie on the intersection of the short- and long-axis views.

The construction of long-axis planes (orthogonal to the short-axis planes oriented at regular angular intervals) enabled the fitting of a series of B-spline curves to represent the contours of the endocardial surface. This allowed the addition or manipulation of control points to obtain the desired boundary locations. The papillary muscles and trabeculae were included in the chamber volume to obtain smooth endocardial contours suitable for shape analysis. The 3D reconstructions of a typical IDCM and normal LV during ED and ES are shown in Figure 4.2.

From the reconstructed LV, the chamber volume, wall mass, stroke volumes (SV), and EF were determined [54].

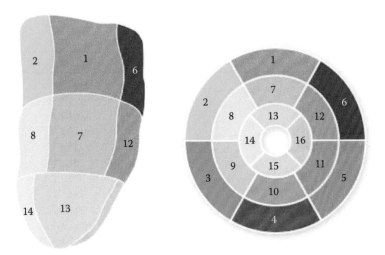

FIGURE 4.3
Standardized myocardial segmentation and nomenclature. (Adapted from Zhong, L. et al., *Am. J. Physiol. Heart Circ. Physiol.*, 296, H573, 2009.)

4.2.3.1 Contractility and Shape Indices

Based on our reported work [53], the contractility index $(d\sigma^*/dt)_{max}$ is calculated by using the formula:

$$\left(\frac{d\sigma^*}{dt}\right)_{max} = 1.5 \times \frac{(dV/dt)_{max}}{V_m} \tag{4.1}$$

wherein (1) V_m is the myocardial volume at the ED phase, and (2) the volume-change rate (dV/dt) was obtained by means of a six-order polynomial function used to curve-fit the volume–time data. The derivation of this formula given in Equation 4.1 is provided in Appendix 4A.

The global LV shape is assessed by calculating the Sphericity Index (SI) in diastole, using the formula SI = AP/BA, where BA is measured in four-chamber view from the apex to the mid-point of the mitral valve and AP is measured as the axis that perpendicularly intersects the mid-point of the long-axis. A small SI value implies an ellipsoidal LV, whereas SI values approaching the value of 1 suggests a more spherical LV.

Table 4.1 provides the characteristics of subjects studied, including the mean values (and variations) of their diastolic and systolic pressures, heart rate, cardiac index, end-diastolic volume index (EDVI), end-systolic volume index (ESVI), EF, SI, and contractility index.

Ischemic dilated cardiomyopathy; cardiac contractility index $(=1.5 \times (dV/dt)_{max}/V_m)$, where $(dV/dt)_{max}$ is the maximum volume rate, and V_m is the myocardial volume.

4.2.3.2 Computation of 3D Surface Shape Descriptors

An in-house developed software was used to reconstruct the LV endocardial meshes at ED and ES and the LV surface shape descriptors, expressed in terms of local normal curvature and curvedness. The formulations for these descriptors are shown in Appendix 4B [54].

TABLE 4.1

Characteristics of Normal Control and IDCM Patients

	Control ($n = 10$)	IDCM ($n = 10$)	p value
Age (years)	39 ± 17	52 ± 9	.05
Weight (kg)	67 ± 15	71 ± 16	0.57
Height (cm)	169 ± 8	164 ± 8	0.18
Diastolic pressure (mmHg)	73 ± 12	70 ± 9	0.54
Systolic pressure (mmHg)	122 ± 17	113 ± 12	0.19
Heart rate, HR (beats/min)	70 ± 9	81 ± 18	0.10
Cardiac index, CI (mL/m²)	3.3 ± 0.4	2.3 ± 0.4	<0.001
End-diastolic volume index, EDVI (mL/m²)	73 ± 10	144 ± 27	<0.001
End-systolic volume index, ESVI (mL/m²)	26 ± 6	114 ± 32	<0.001
Ejection fraction, EF (%)	65 ± 5	22 ± 9	<0.001
Sphericity index, SI	0.52 ± 0.06	0.62 ± 0.08	<0.05
Cardiac contractility index, $(d\sigma^*/dt)_{max}$ (s^{-1})	5.7 ± 1.3	2.4 ± 0.9	<0.001

Source: Zhong, L. et al., *Am. J. Physiol. Heart Circ. Physiol.*, 296, H573, 2009.
IDCM, ischemic dilated cardiomyopathy; cardiac contractility index ($=1.5 \times (dV/dt)_{max}/V_m$), where $(dV/dt)_{max}$ is the maximum volume rate, and V_m is the myocardial volume.

To evaluate the shape at a particular point on the mesh, a local surface geometry was fitted to the region. The normal curvature at that point is then calculated as

$$\kappa(\lambda) = \frac{L + 2M\lambda + N\lambda^2}{E + 2F\lambda + G\lambda^2} \tag{4.2}$$

where
$\lambda = dv/du$ such that u and v are the parameters of the underlying geometry, and
$\{E, F, G\}$ and $\{L, M, N\}$ are components of the first and second fundamental forms, respectively

The extreme values κ_1 and κ_2 of $\kappa(\lambda)$ are the maximum and minimum principal curvatures, respectively. These are obtained from the roots of the equation:

$$\det = \begin{bmatrix} L - \kappa E & M - \kappa F \\ M - \kappa F & N - \kappa G \end{bmatrix} = 0 \tag{4.3}$$

The corresponding directions of κ_1 and κ_2 are the principal directions and are orthogonal to each other. Figure 4.4 depicts typical principal curvatures on the endocardial wall of the LV in IDCM and normal heart. The arrowheads represent the directions of the principal curvature on the surface of the endocardium.

The LV wall shape descriptor is characterized in terms of the curvedness value (C), as presented by Koenderink [30]. It is a measure of the degree of regional curvature and is defined as

$$C = \sqrt{\frac{\kappa_1^2 + \kappa_2^2}{2}} \tag{4.4}$$

The derivation of this formula is provided in Appendix 4B.1. The value of C indicates the magnitude of the curvedness at a point, which is a measure of how much a region deviates from flatness. A normal LV will exhibit a larger value of C.

The percentage curvedness change (ΔC) between ED and ES phases is defined as

$$\Delta C = \frac{C_{ED} - C_{ES}}{C_{ES}} \times 100\% \qquad (4.5)$$

where C_{ED} and C_{ES} are curvedness at end-diastole and end-systole, respectively. Positive values of ΔC indicate LV wall regions of increasing curvature during systole while negative values of ΔC indicate wall regions of decreasing curvature.

4.2.3.3 Regional Wall Thickening

In addition to the evaluation of curvature measures at each point of the surface mesh, the LV radius (R) and wall thickness (T) were deduced from the 3D geometry of the LV.

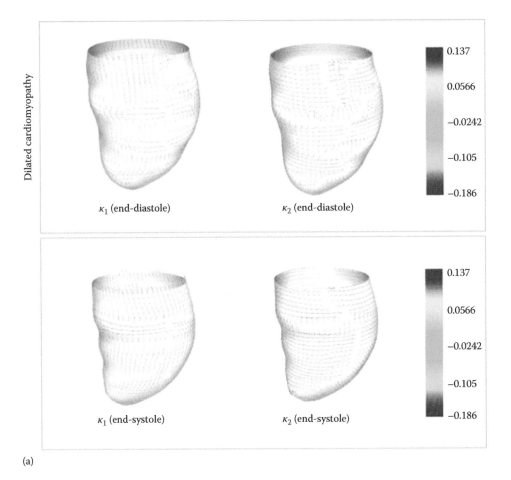

(a)

FIGURE 4.4
The plots represent principal curvature analysis done on the endocardial wall of the left ventricle. The arrowheads represent directions of maximum principal curvature (left panel) and minimum principal curvature (right panel) of the endocardial surface of (a) DCM. *(Continued)*

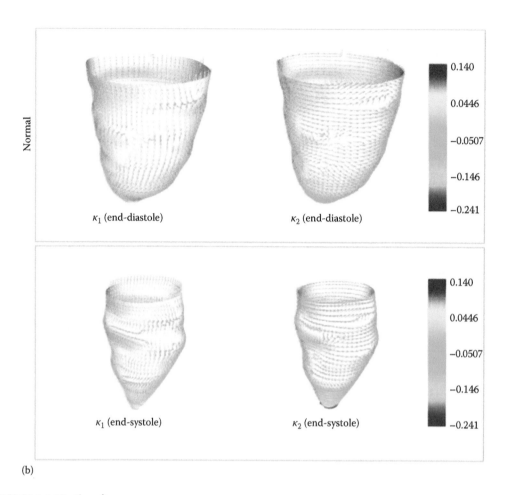

(b)

FIGURE 4.4 (Continued)
The plots represent principal curvature analysis done on the endocardial wall of the left ventricle. The arrow-heads represent directions of maximum principal curvature (left panel) and minimum principal curvature (right panel) of the endocardial surface of (b) Normal subjects. (Adapted from Zhong, L. et al., *Am. J. Physiol. Heart Circ. Physiol.*, 296, H573, 2009.)

The steps of the computation of wall radius-of-curvature and thickness are summarized in Appendix 4C [54]. The wall thickening (WT) is expressed at each segment, by means of the following formula:

$$WT = \frac{T_{ES} - T_{ED}}{T_{ED}} \tag{4.6}$$

where T_{ES} and T_{ED} are wall thickness at end-systole and end-diastole, respectively.

4.2.3.4 Regional Peak Systolic Wall Stress

The regional wall stress is obtained by the equilibrium of forces due to stresses in the wall and blood pressure acting on the wall. Following the work of Grossman [22], the regional peak systolic wall stress (WS) is determined from the inner radius of curvature (R) and wall thickness (T) at end-systole by means of the formula:

$$WS = 0.133 \times SP \times \frac{R}{2T \times (1 + (T/2R))} \qquad (4.7)$$

where SP is the peak systolic ventricular blood pressure in mmHg, assessed from the systolic noninvasive blood pressure [40]; a conversion factor of 0.133 was used to express the final results in 1000 Pa (or N/m²).

From this formula, WS is calculated by using the wall radius of curvature and wall thickness values. The WS determination, by using Equation 4.7, is illustrated in Figure 4.12 in the circumferential and longitudinal (or meridional) directions in (1) 2D as 2DSWS and 2DLWS, and (2) 3D as 3DWS. In the 2D case, the wall radius of curvature is the inverse of the curvature computed from Equation 4.4; in the 3D case, the wall radius of curvature is the inverse of the curvature computed from Equation 4.4. The derivations of the curvatures and their corresponding wall thickness values are provided in Appendix 4C.

To determine the regional LV properties of curvedness, WS, and WT, the LV is divided into a 16-segment model [9] from apex to base (as illustrated in Figure 4.3). The average values (and variations) of parameters of (1) curvedness and curvedness difference are provided in Table 4.2, (2) systolic wall stress and WT for each region are provided in Figure 4.5 and Table 4.3.

TABLE 4.2

Left Ventricular Regional Curvedness Analysis in Normal and IDCM

Segment	Normal ($n = 10$)			IDCM ($n = 10$)		
	C_{ED} (mm⁻¹)	C_{ES} (mm⁻¹)	ΔC (%)	C_{ED} (mm⁻¹)	C_{ES} (mm⁻¹)	ΔC (%)
1. Basal anterior	0.040 ± 0.0098	0.054 ± 0.0064	25 ± 21	0.031 ± 0.0073^a	0.036 ± 0.0079^b	12 ± 13
2. Basal anterior septal	0.037 ± 0.0058	0.058 ± 0.010	33 ± 13	0.032 ± 0.0064^a	0.034 ± 0.0063^b	8 ± 7^b
3. Basal inferior septal	0.030 ± 0.0036	0.047 ± 0.0062	36 ± 7	0.030 ± 0.0084	0.033 ± 0.0096^c	8 ± 17^b
4. Basal inferior	0.038 ± 0.0053	0.056 ± 0.0079	31 ± 10	0.032 ± 0.0074^a	0.036 ± 0.011^b	8 ± 17^c
5. Basal inferior lateral	0.035 ± 0.0040	0.055 ± 0.0096	36 ± 8	0.031 ± 0.0070	0.033 ± 0.0079^c	5 ± 15^b
6. Basal anterior lateral	0.036 ± 0.0063	0.050 ± 0.0065	27 ± 16	0.031 ± 0.0057	0.035 ± 0.0062^b	8 ± 16^a
7. Middle anterior	0.034 ± 0.0035	0.057 ± 0.010	39 ± 10	0.029 ± 0.0054^a	0.032 ± 0.0056^b	6 ± 12^b
8. Middle anterior septal	0.043 ± 0.0057	0.070 ± 0.016	38 ± 8	0.031 ± 0.0042^b	0.033 ± 0.0050^b	6 ± 8^b
9. Middle inferior septal	0.037 ± 0.0059	0.056 ± 0.0096	34 ± 7	0.031 ± 0.0044^a	0.031 ± 0.0048^b	-1 ± 8^b
10. Middle inferior	0.043 ± 0.0044	0.060 ± 0.010	28 ± 10	0.033 ± 0.0042^b	0.034 ± 0.0056^b	2 ± 7^b
11. Middle inferior lateral	0.037 ± 0.0025	0.063 ± 0.011	39 ± 10	0.032 ± 0.0052^a	0.034 ± 0.0059^b	4 ± 13^b
12. Middle anterior lateral	0.033 ± 0.0029	0.052 ± 0.011	34 ± 11	0.030 ± 0.0078	0.030 ± 0.0042^b	-1 ± 16^b
13. Apical anterior	0.043 ± 0.0061	0.083 ± 0.016	47 ± 9	0.043 ± 0.017	0.049 ± 0.016^b	11 ± 12^b
14. Apical septal	0.052 ± 0.0092	0.10 ± 0.024	47 ± 12	0.040 ± 0.010^c	0.042 ± 0.012^b	6 ± 8^b
15. Apical inferior	0.056 ± 0.0077	0.10 ± 0.030	43 ± 14	0.047 ± 0.0045^c	0.050 ± 0.0087^b	3 ± 16^b
16. Apical lateral	0.048 ± 0.0091	0.10 ± 0.026	50 ± 13	0.045 ± 0.0093	0.051 ± 0.014^b	10 ± 14^b

Source: Zhong, L. et al., *Am. J. Physiol. Heart Circ. Physiol.,* 296, H573, 2009.

IDCM, ischemic dilated cardiomyopathy; C_{ED}, curvedness at end-diastole; C_{ES}, curvedness at end-systole; ΔC, % curvedness change between end-diastole and end-systole.

[a] $p < 0.05$, [b] $p < 0.001$, [c] $p < 0.01$, for regional segments that are significantly different in IDCM compared to normal.

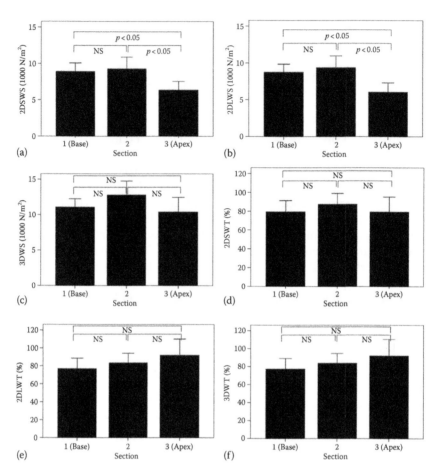

FIGURE 4.5
Variation of LV systolic wall stress and wall thickening from base to apex in normal subjects. (a) Wall stress 2DSWS in short-axis direction. (b) Wall stress 2DLWS in long-axis direction. (c) Wall stress 3DWS by taking 3D wall curvature. (d) Wall thickening 2DSWT in short-axis direction. (e) Wall thickening 2DLWT in long-axis direction. (f) Wall thickening 3DWT by taking 3D wall curvature. Values are means ± SD; *p*, two-tailed significance of paired differences; N.S., not significant. (Adapted from Zhong, L. et al., *Am. J. Physiol. Heart Circ. Physiol.*, 296, H573, 2009.)

4.2.4 Results

4.2.4.1 Global Left Ventricular Function

The hemodynamic and volumetric parameters of the subjects are summarized in Table 4.1. It can be noted that in IDCM patients, the cardiac contractility index $(d\sigma^*/dt)_{max}$ and LV EF are significantly lower than that in the control normal subjects. It can also be noted that the LV EDV and ESV in IDCM patients are greater than those in control subjects. As can be seen from Figures 4.2 and 4.4, the LV in IDCM patients has a broader apex compared to that of normal subjects. The increase in dilated volume in the LV with IDCM is accompanied by a corresponding increase in sphericity. Consequently, the LVs with IDCM are significantly more spherical than those in control subjects.

TABLE 4.3

Left Ventricular End-Systolic Wall Stress that Takes Account of Curvature in Normal Heart

Segment	3DWS, (N·1000/m2)	2DLWS, (N·1000/m2)	2DSWS, (N·1000/m2)	p value, 3DWS vs. 2DSWS	p value, 3DWS vs. 2DLWS	p value, 2DSWS vs. 2DLWS
1. Basal anterior	10.9 ± 3.92	8.19 ± 3.55	10.1 ± 4.99	0.01	0.030	NS
2. Basal anterior septal	10.1 ± 3.96	7.99 ± 4.38	8.81 ± 2.62	0.006	NS	NS
3. Basal inferior septal	12.4 ± 3.21	12.1 ± 5.56	7.54 ± 2.81	NS	<0.0001	NS
4. Basal inferior	10.3 ± 4.07	8.00 ± 2.67	8.08 ± 3.26	0.009	0.03	NS
5. Basal inferior lateral	10.4 ± 4.69	7.80 ± 3.46	8.73 ± 3.83	0.003	0.021	NS
6. Basal anterior lateral	12.5 ± 5.50	9.50 ± 4.68	9.39 ± 5.80	<0.001	0.003	NS
7. Middle anterior	13.7 ± 4.52	9.10 ± 3.88	10.0 ± 3.93	<0.0001	<0.0001	NS
8. Middle anterior septal	10.2 ± 3.85	7.41 ± 4.02	9.85 ± 3.33	0.024	NS	0.048
9. Middle inferior septal	11.9 ± 4.69	10.5 ± 6.60	7.41 ± 3.44	NS	<0.0001	NS
10. Middle inferior	11.1 ± 5.77	8.35 ± 3.91	8.05 ± 5.74	0.039	<0.0001	NS
11. Middle inferior lateral	12.6 ± 9.63	8.00 ± 5.89	10.8 ± 9.49	0.021	<0.0001	NS
12. Middle anterior lateral	17.3 ± 11.12	12.4 ± 9.20	10.2 ± 7.31	<0.0001	0.006	NS
13. Apical anterior	12.5 ± 6.02	6.27 ± 3.38	7.15 ± 3.49	<0.0001	<0.0001	NS
14. Apical septal	8.50 ± 4.23	6.07 ± 3.79	5.53 ± 2.54	NS	0.015	NS
15. Apical inferior	10.0 ± 6.40	7.16 ± 4.13	5.08 ± 3.88	NS	0.003	NS
16. Apical lateral	10.7 ± 7.40	5.87 ± 3.14	10.7 ± 7.40	0.045	0.006	NS

Source: Zhong, L. et al., *Am. J. Physiol. Heart Circ. Physiol.*, 296, H573, 2009.

4.2.4.2 Variation of Curvedness, Peak Systolic Wall Stress, and Wall Thickening from Base to Apex in Normal Subjects

The calculated regional values for curvedness at end-diastole (ED) and end-systole (ES) in normal and IDCM are summarized in Table 4.2. It can be seen that generally in normal hearts, the curvedness is highest at the apex, and the inferior regions have larger curvedness than the lateral regions (among the four circumferential zones), especially at ED. In IDCM patients, the curvedness is also highest at the apex, but there is not much significant difference among the six circumferential zones.

Wall thickness and radius of the LV cavity were measured in the short-axis plane, long-axis plane (perpendicular to the short-axis), and 3D surface. For normal subjects, the WSs calculated with these data are shown in Figure 4.5a (2DSWS), Figure 4.5b (2DLWS), and Figure 4.5c (3DWS). The peak systolic wall stress in the short-axis plane (Figure 4.5a) and long-axis plane (Figure 4.5b) has significant variation from base to apex (ANOVA, $p < 0.0001$). The short-axis and long-axis wall stress show 41% ± 11% and 45% ± 12% increase of peak systolic wall stress between basal and apical sections, respectively. When wall thickness and radius of the cavity were calculated in the 3D space, the variation of the wall stress (3DWS) from the base to apex was not observed (Figure 4.5c). The differences between 2DSWS and 3DWS, 2DLWS and 3DWS are reduced more at the basal level. The 3DWS values tend to be highest at the anterior and lowest at the inferior region (Table 4.3).

The WT values determined in the short-axis plane, long-axis plane, and 3D surface are shown in Figure 4.5d (2DSWT), Figure 4.5e (2DLWT), and Figure 4.5f (3DWT). There is no significant difference in WT from the base to apex. The comparison between 3DWT and a 2D assessment of WT (i.e., 2DSWT and 2DLWT) does not reveal significant differences at the basal and mid-zone, anterior, septal, and lateral regions.

4.2.4.3 Comparison of Curvedness, Radius-to-Thickness Ratio, Peak Systolic Wall Stress, and Wall Thickening in IDCM Patients and Normal Subjects

In order to highlight the regional variations of the LV curvature, the curvedness values from base to apex in normal and IDCM patients are given in Table 4.2. There is significant reduction in percentage curvedness change (ΔC) from end-diastole to end-systole in most segments for IDCM patients compared to normal subjects. This demonstrates the effect of LV remodeling on LV shape change from end-diastole to end-systole. The ΔC reduction in IDCM patients can be related to decreased regional contractility (due to ischemic and infarcted segments), which also corresponds to the significant reduction in the value of the overall contractility index in IDCM patients (Table 4.1).

Table 4.4 shows pronounced increase in the values of ED radius-to-thickness, $(R/T)_{ED}$, in 9 out of 16 segments. On the other hand, significant differences in ES radius-to-thickness, $(R/T)_{ES}$, can be noted in all the regions between normal and IDCM groups.

Figure 4.6 compares the end-systolic wall stress in normal subjects with IDCM patients. It can be seen that in IDCM patients, the 3DWS is significantly increased, and the 3DWT is decreased compared with those of normal subjects (Figure 4.6a). It can also be observed that in the IDCM patients, the 3DWS is highest at the apex, and the 3DWT is significantly decreased in all regions compared with normal values (Figure 4.6b). Additionally, 3DWT

TABLE 4.4

Left Ventricular Radius-to-Thickness, Taking into Account 3D Curvature in Normal and IDCM

Segment	Normal (*n* = 10)		IDCM (*n* = 10)	
	$(R/T)_{ED}$	$(R/T)_{ES}$	$(R/T)_{ED}$	$(R/T)_{ES}$
1. Basal anterior	5.04 ± 1.35	1.86 ± 0.65	5.64 ± 1.63	4.35 ± 1.03[c]
2. Basal anterior septal	4.22 ± 1.26	1.66 ± 0.58	5.62 ± 1.43[a]	4.64 ± 1.29[c]
3. Basal inferior septal	4.59 ± 1.06	2.01 ± 0.53	6.13 ± 2.06[a]	4.84 ± 1.62[c]
4. Basal inferior	3.90 ± 0.60	1.72 ± 0.61	5.00 ± 1.07[a]	3.98 ± 1.14[c]
5. Basal inferior lateral	4.95 ± 1.19	1.84 ± 0.80	5.30 ± 1.30	4.42 ± 1.72[c]
6. Basal anterior lateral	5.65 ± 1.83	2.15 ± 0.96	5.31 ± 1.38	4.50 ± 1.60[c]
7. Middle anterior	6.98 ± 3.17	2.10 ± 0.70	8.79 ± 2.16[a]	7.02 ± 1.77[c]
8. Middle anterior septal	4.77 ± 1.20	1.65 ± 0.55	8.04 ± 1.56[c]	6.55 ± 1.57[c]
9. Middle inferior septal	4.74 ± 1.25	1.94 ± 0.69	6.18 ± 1.51[a]	5.72 ± 1.37[c]
10. Middle inferior	4.18 ± 0.83	1.83 ± 0.84	5.27 ± 1.10[a]	4.84 ± 1.33[c]
11. Middle inferior lateral	5.15 ± 1.00	2.03 ± 1.34	5.56 ± 1.44[a]	5.26 ± 1.96[c]
12. Middle anterior lateral	6.26 ± 1.87	2.57 ± 1.53	7.06 ± 2.49	6.10 ± 1.84[c]
13. Apical anterior	5.86 ± 1.67	1.97 ± 0.86	7.51 ± 3.27	6.23 ± 2.65[c]
14. Apical septal	4.55 ± 0.83	1.41 ± 0.59	7.59 ± 2.64[b]	6.37 ± 2.22[c]
15. Apical inferior	4.78 ± 1.15	1.59 ± 0.89	5.74 ± 1.24	4.90 ± 1.45[c]
16. Apical lateral	5.67 ± 2.42	1.72 ± 1.01	6.10 ± 2.03	5.17 ± 2.02[c]

Source: Zhong, L. et al., *Am. J. Physiol. Heart Circ. Physiol.*, 296, H573, H584, 2009.

IDCM, ischemic dilated cardiomyopathy; C_{ED}, curvedness in end-diastole; C_{ES}, curvedness in end-systole.

[a] $p < 0.05$, [b] $p < 0.01$, [c] $p < 0.001$ for regional segments that are significantly different in IDCM compared to normal.

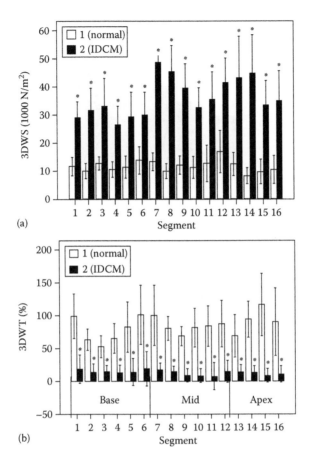

FIGURE 4.6
Variation of end-systolic wall stress, 3DWS, of the left ventricle in normal subjects and in patients with ischemic dilated cardiomyopathy (IDCM). (a) 3DWS assessment from 3D curvature; (b) 3DWT assessment from 3D curvature. Values are mean ± SD. *Significant difference between IDCM versus normal subjects. (Adapted from Zhong, L. et al., *Am. J. Physiol. Heart Circ. Physiol.*, 296, H573, 2009.)

is smallest in the inferior segments and highest in the anterior segments. There is also significant variation among the four circumferential regions (ANOVA, $p < 0.001$) and from base to apex (ANOVA, $p < 0.001$).

4.2.4.4 Analysis of Segment Scar Extent in IDCM Patients

The correlation of mean values of WS and WT with the extent of segment scar is shown in Figure 4.7a and b. A total of 160 segments were analyzed in the IDCM patients. As expected, there is a positive correlation between the extent of myocardial infarct and peak systolic wall stress 3DWS ($r = 0.652$, $p < 0.0001$) in Figure 4.7a. Likewise, a negative correlation can be seen between the extent of myocardial infarct and wall thickening 3DWT ($r = -0.622$, $p < 0.0001$) in Figure 4.7b.

4.2.5 Discussion

This study gives us an idea of what MI and IDCM does to (1) the LV 3D shape, (2) decreased regional curvedness change from end-diastole to end-systole, which can also serve as

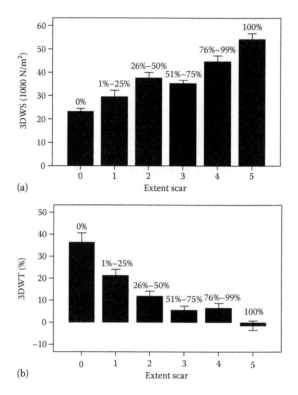

(a)

(b)

FIGURE 4.7

Distribution of (a) peak systolic wall stress, 3DWS, and (b) wall thickening, 3DWT, based on different segment scar extent in patients with IDCM. Values are mean ± SD. (Adapted from Zhong, L. et al., *Am. J. Physiol. Heart Circ. Physiol.*, 296, H573, 2009.)

a measure of decreased regional contractility, (3) increased regional wall stress, due to increase in the value of wall R/T, as a measure of increased oxygen demand and enhanced oxygen supply-demand mismatch, and (4) decreased global contractility.

4.2.5.1 In Normal Hearts

The WS values, derived from both short-axis and long-axis methods, tend to vary from base to apex, with the smallest WS value at the apex. However, the 3DWS is fairly uniform, from the base to apex (ANOVA analysis, $p = 0.298$) among the four circumferential regions (ANOVA analysis, $p > 0.05$). It is also observed that 3DWS is about 10% lower at the apex, and 20% lower at the inferior region than elsewhere. These modest variations in the WS are in agreement with the relatively uniform radius-to-thickness ratio from base to apex (Table 4.4).

4.2.5.2 In IDCM Hearts

LV remodeling in IDCM is a multistep process, which has been investigated in numerous studies [9,38,41]. The loss of contractile function following coronary occlusion and MI is accompanied by acute dilatation of the infarction area, increase in the LV volume, lengthening of the LV perimeter, and blunting of the normal curvature.

Geometrically, there is increase of LV EDV and ESV, SI, and the local R/T ratios. The development of IDCM is also accompanied by a decrease of LV function, as represented by decreased LVEF and the contractility index $(d\sigma^*/dt)_{max}$. The increase in local wall stress (due to increase in local R/T values) gives rise to enhanced oxygen supply-demand mismatch, and hence, in the spread of the myocardial infarcted region.

4.2.5.3 End-Systolic Curvedness and Wall Stress

Herein, we have provided a framework for the analysis of LV regional curvature, WS, and WT for normal subjects and patients with IDCM. The methodology is based on MR anatomical data and local surface fitting techniques to construct 3D LV shapes, and then interrogate LV geometry at end-diastole and end-systole.

In patients with IDCM, there is a decrease of ES curvedness and associated increase of peak systolic wall stress in segments, in comparison with normal subjects, as noted in Tables 4.2 and 4.3 and Figure 4.5a. This increased end-systolic wall stress in segments will cause increased oxygen demand in the ischemic regions, thereby making them prone to becoming infarcted and thereby causing the spread of the infarcted region which can lead to HF.

4.3 Effect of Surgical Ventricular Restoration on Ventricular Shape, Wall Stress, and Function in IDCM Patients

4.3.1 Introduction

SVR has been used to treat patients with LV dysfunction and akinetic or dyskinetic segments from prior anterior MI. Several studies have documented that this procedure can be performed with reasonably low operative mortality and results in good patient outcomes [2,34,35,42]. The recent result of the STICH (The Surgical Treatment for Ischemic Heart Failure) trial, however, showed that SVR did not improve survival, hospitalization, and quality of life over coronary artery bypass graft (CABG) alone after 4 years of follow-up [27]. The underlying reasons of this failure have been speculated as: (1) progressive LV dilation and distortion occurring after SVR [19], and (2) the long-term effects of SVR on LV diastolic dysfunction contributing to worsening of HF [8].

An additional issue is whether SVR can produce an optimal ventricular shape and size. Buckberg and colleague [7] endorsed the concept that the creation of an elliptical shape (from the pre-surgical spherical shape) may provide an optimal LV deformation for favorable EF. Furthermore, LV regional wall stress reduction after surgery has been believed to reverse adverse ventricular remodeling. Finite element analysis studies in animals [14,32,51] have shown decreased LV wall stress in remote, border, and infarct zones. So this study was undertaken to analyze the effects of SVR on LV regional shape and regional wall stress in humans.

In Section 4.2, we have determined the LV regional shape along with curvedness and WS, based on 3D LV models reconstructed from MRI. It is shown therein that IDCM patients had significantly smaller LV regional curvedness (in particular at the apex region) and higher systolic wall stress in all segments compared to normal healthy subjects [54]. We are now documenting the results of SVR on the 40 patients studied, in terms of LV regional shape, WS, and systolic function [56].

4.3.2 Methodology

4.3.2.1 Study Population

A retrospective analysis was carried out on the prospectively consecutively acquired MRI data of 40 patients with ischemic cardiomyopathy, who had undergone CABG combined with SVR. Some of these patients had concomitant mitral regurgitation that required mitral valve repair surgery (MVS) by means of restrictive mitral annuloplasty. In each case, the SVR procedure was performed by means of endoventricular circular patch plasty, as previously described by Dor and associates [18]. All patients underwent full pre- and post-SVR MRI protocol. The study was carried out at the Cleveland Clinic. The patient characteristics are listed in Table 4.5.

4.3.2.2 MRI Image Acquisition

MRI studies were performed 1–2 weeks before surgery and 1–2 weeks after surgery on a 1.5 T MRI scanner (Siemens Somatom, Erlangen, Germany) equipped with fast gradients (23 mT/m amplitude, 105 mT/m per ms slew rate) and a dedicated cardiac phased-array surface coil. ECG-gated consecutive cine short-axis views were acquired to cover the LV, using breath-held steady-state free-precession technique (echo-time, 1.4 ms; repetition time, 2.9 ms; slice thickness, 8 mm; flip angle, 60°; spatial resolution, 1.4×1.2 mm^2, and temporal resolution, 42 ms). Both long-axis and short-axis were obtained to determine the 3D LV shape.

TABLE 4.5

Patients' Characteristics and Clinical Data

Variables	Value
Male: female	36:4
Age (years)	69 ± 9
Body surface area (m^2)	1.98 ± 0.18
Left ventricular ejection fraction (%)	26 ± 7
Coronary artery disease	39 (98%)
Congestive heart failure	28 (70%)
New York Heart Association class	
I–II	26 (65%)
III–IV	14 (35%)
Surgery	
SVR + CABG	21 (52%)
SVR + CABG + MVS	19 (48%)

Source: Zhong, L. et al., *Am. J. Physiol. Heart Circ. Physiol.*, 300(5), H1653, 2011.
Values are mean ± SD or numbers of patients (percentages).
SVR, surgical ventricular restoration; CABG, coronary artery bypass graft; MVS, mitral valve surgery.

4.3.2.3 Determination of LV Geometry

The MRI images were reviewed on a commercially available computer workstation, by using a commercially available software (CMRtools, Cardiovascular Imaging Solution, UK). Manual tracing of the epicardial and endocardial borders of contiguous short-axis slices enabled reconstruction of the LV 3D shape, and allowed calculation of LV EDV, ESV, SV, EF, and LV mass. The LV mass (g) was derived from the product of myocardial volume and specific density of the myocardium (1.05 g/cm^3) [28]. Papillary muscles were included in the mass but excluded from the volumes.

The global shape of the LV was characterized by means of the SI, which (as defined earlier) is the ratio of the short-axis to the long-axis; SI was calculated in systole and diastole [31]. A normalized measure of the SI was also calculated in terms of the volume ratio of the LV volume and a theoretical sphere volume of $1/6\pi \times L^3$ (where L is the long-axis of the LV), as defined by Kono et al. [31]. Figure 4.8 shows MRI samples in short-axis views and four-chamber long-axis views, along with the reconstructed LV shape before and after SVR.

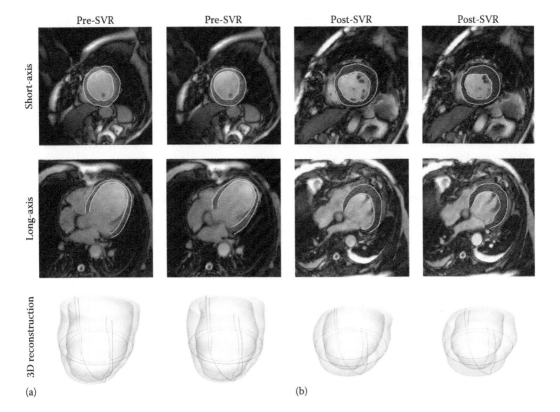

FIGURE 4.8

Magnetic resonance image showing a short-axis slice (top) at the level of the equator and long-axis slice (middle) at end-diastole and end-systole, with the left ventricular endocardial and epicardial surfaces denoted by yellow lines. Its corresponding 3D reconstructed left ventricular shape (below) at end-diastole and end-systole are shown before (a) and after (b) surgical ventricular restoration (SVR). (Adapted from Zhong, L. et al., *Am. J. Physiol. Heart Circ. Physiol.*, 300(5), H1653, 2011.)

4.3.2.4 Determination of LV Regional Shape and Geometric Parameters: Curvedness, LV Radius and Wall Thickness, Endocardial Surface Area

A validated triangulation algorithm was used to reconstruct the 3D model of the LV endocardial surface for each patient from the aforementioned steady-state free-precession short-axis and long-axis cine images [50]. The LV surface properties were computed via an analytical approach, using a surface fitting method from the reconstructed 3D model of the LV (Figure 4.8), as described earlier [54]. An in-house algorithm was used to calculate the maximum and minimum principal curvatures for each point on the surface, and the local curvedness was calculated as the root mean square of these principal curvatures [50], as shown in Equation 4.4. The regional LV radius (R) and wall thickness (T) were deduced from the 3D geometry of the LV. The endocardial surface area (S) was determined, and its change ($\Delta S = (S_{ED} - S_{ES})/S_{ED} \times 100\%$) from end-diastole to end-systole was calculated.

4.3.2.5 Determination of Left Ventricular Systolic Function and Vascular Function

The LV systolic properties were assessed by determination of LV performance and systolic function indices [6,53]. These LV systolic properties are (1) LV systolic performance in terms of SW, calculated as the product of SV and mean arterial pressure [6]; (2) LV systolic function in terms of the EF, the SW index of the ratio of SW and EDV; (3) LV contractility index $(d\sigma^*/dt)_{max}$ (given, in Equation 4.1, by $1.5 \times (dV/dt)_{max}/V_m$, where dV/dt is the first derivative of the volume and V_m is the myocardium volume at end-diastole); and (4) LV regional systolic function in terms of ΔS.

Vascular function was assessed in terms of (1) effective arterial elastance (E_a), estimated as the ES pressure divided by the SV [27]; (2) total arterial compliance, estimated by ratio of SV and pulse-pressure [10]; and (3) systolic vascular resistance index, given by the mean arterial pressure divided by the cardiac index times a conversion factor (80 dyn/cm²/mmHg).

4.3.2.6 Determination of Wall Stress Indices at End-Diastole and End-Systole

The pressure-normalized stress (σ/P), based on Equation 4.7, was used as an index of WS. Since it is a pure geometric parameter, it represents the physical response of the LV to the loading and allows comparison between ventricles at different pressures and for different regions of the same ventricle [33]. Accordingly, based on Equation 4.7, the pressure-normalized stress (σ/P) and end-systolic wall stress (σ_{ES}) are calculated (in terms of R and T) as follows:

$$\frac{\sigma}{P} = \frac{R}{2T \times (1 + (T/2R))} \tag{4.8}$$

$$\sigma_{ES} = 0.133 \times P_{ES} \frac{R_{ES}}{2T_{ES}(1 + T_{ES}/2R_{ES})} \tag{4.9}$$

where the ES pressure P_{ES} is estimated as the systolic pressure (SP) multiplied by a factor of 0.9, as previously validated [11,29]. Herein, SP was assessed from the systolic noninvasive blood pressure and a conversion of 0.133 was used to express the final results in kPa [54].

4.3.2.7 Definition of Border Zone and Remote Zones

We have identified the BZ from the MR images as the region where the LV wall thickness at end-diastole varied between normal (8–12 mm) and thin (<5 mm) [32]. In other words, the BZ was identified as the transition zone between normally thick myocardium (RZ) and the infarcted myocardium (IZ). Thus, IZ, BZ, and RZ were anatomically specified throughout the ventricle, as illustrated in Figure 4.9.

4.3.3 Results

4.3.3.1 Subject Characteristics

All the 40 patients studied were treated with CABG and SVR (endoventricular circular patch plasty) (Table 4.5). The age of the patients averaged 69 years old (range, 52–84 years old). Among them, 19 patients had severe mitral regurgitation and received additional mitral valve surgery (MVS) and 28 patients had congestive heart failure (CHF).

4.3.3.2 LV Geometry

After SVR, there was a significant decrease in the dimensions of both the long- and short-axes of the LV. The long-axis dimension of the LV decreased more than the short-axis dimension, which resulted in an increase of SI after SVR, as seen in Table 4.6: SI at diastole: 0.65 ± 0.087 versus 0.81 ± 0.11, $p < 0.001$; SI at systole: 0.57 ± 0.094 versus 0.67 ± 0.13, $p < 0.001$;

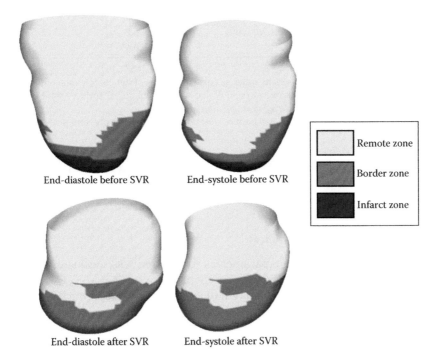

FIGURE 4.9
3D geometry of the left ventricle before and after SVR. Surface was classified into three regions (remote zone, border zone, and infarct zone). (Adapted from Zhong, L. et al., *Am. J. Physiol. Heart Circ. Physiol.*, 300(5), H1653, 2011.)

TABLE 4.6

Measures of Ventricular Structure and Function

	Pre-SVR ($n = 40$)	Post-SVR ($n = 40$)
LV Structure		
End-diastolic volume index (mL/m²)	156 ± 39	110 ± 33[a]
End-systolic volume index (mL/m²)	117 ± 39	77 ± 31[a]
Stroke volume index (mL/m²)	39 ± 9	33 ± 8[a]
Cardiac index (L/min/m²)	2.84 ± 0.74	2.59 ± 0.74[b]
LV mass index (g/m²)	112 ± 25	101 ± 23[a]
Sphericity index_ed	0.65 ± 0.087	0.81 ± 0.11[a]
Sphericity index_es	0.57 ± 0.094	0.67 ± 0.13[a]
SLv_ed	0.47 ± 0.14	0.74 ± 0.21[a]
SLv_es	0.41 ± 0.14	0.61 ± 0.20[a]
LV Systolic function		
Stroke work (mmHg·L)	6.61 ± 1.96	5.46 ± 1.64[a]
SW/EDV (mmHg)	21.76 ± 8.25	25.64 ± 7.40
Ejection fraction (%)	26 ± 7	31 ± 10[a]
$(d\sigma^*/dt)_{max}$ (s⁻¹)	2.69 ± 0.74	3.23 ± 0.73[a]
End-diastolic infarct surface area (%)	27 ± 14	3 ± 4[a]
End-diastolic surface area, S_{ED} (cm²)	184 ± 30	140 ± 36[a]
End-systolic surface area, S_{ES} (cm²)	155 ± 32	117 ± 33[a]
Surface area change, ΔS (%)	16 ± 7	18 ± 9
Vascular Function		
E_a (mmHg/mL)	1.41 ± 0.37	1.66 ± 0.40[c]
Systemic vascular resistance index (dyn·s·m²/cm⁵)	2488 ± 624	2759 ± 773[b]
Arterial compliance (mL/mmHg)	1.84 ± 0.63	1.51 ± 0.36[c]

Source: Zhong, L. et al., *Am. J. Physiol. Heart Circ. Physiol.*, 300(5), H1653, 2011.

SLv, A normalized measure of the sphericity index calculated in terms of the volume ratio of the LV volume and a theoretical sphere volume; SW, stroke work; EDV, end-diastolic volume; S, surface area; ΔS, surface area change from end-diastolic to end-systole; E_a, effective arterial elastance.

[a] $p < 0.001$, [b] $p < 0.05$; [c] $p < 0.01$; for two-tail paired t-test used in comparing pre- and post-SVR values.

SLv at diastole: 0.47 ± 0.14 versus 0.74 ± 0.21, $p < 0.001$; SLv at systole: 0.41 ± 0.14 versus 0.61 ± 0.20, $p < 0.001$. Also, as seen in Table 4.6, there were also significant reductions in EDVI, ESVI, LV stroke volume index, and LV mass index after SVR.

4.3.3.3 Regional Geometric Parameters

The calculated regional geometric parameters for curvedness, radius-of-curvature, and ratio of radius versus wall thickness (R/T) in patients before and after SVR are summarized in Table 4.7. Before SVR, the curvedness is small in all regions, averaging 0.033 mm⁻¹ at end-diastole (compared with 0.043 mm⁻¹ in normal heart) and 0.037 mm⁻¹ at end-systole (compared with normal value of 0.075 mm⁻¹). The highest curvedness values are found in the infarct zone (≈0.039 mm⁻¹), whereas the smallest curvedness values are found in RZ. There are increases of both $(R/T)_{ED}$ and $(R/T)_{ES}$ from remote to infarct zones. There was a slight increase in curvedness in RZ, BZ, and IZ (7%, 18%, and 8%, respectively) at end-diastole and (9%, 5%, and 3%, respectively) at end-systole after SVR (Figure 4.10 and Table 4.7),

TABLE 4.7

Comparison of Characteristic Local Parameters in Three Zones (IZ, BZ, and RZ) Pre- and Post-SVR

	Pre-SVR			Post-SVR		
	RZ	BZ	IZ	RZ	BZ	IZ
C_{ED} (mm^{-1})	0.030 ± 0.006	0.032 ± 0.005	0.036 ± 0.006	0.032 ± 0.005	0.038 ± 0.01^a	0.039 ± 0.010
C_{ES} (mm^{-1})	0.035 ± 0.006	0.037 ± 0.006	0.039 ± 0.007	0.038 ± 0.008	0.039 ± 0.01	0.040 ± 0.011
R_{ED} (mm)	38 ± 5	36 ± 5	32 ± 5	36 ± 5	31 ± 6^a	28 ± 7
R_{ES} (mm)	33 ± 4	31 ± 5	30 ± 5	31 ± 5	29 ± 6	28 ± 8
R/T_{ED}	4.31 ± 0.88	5.92 ± 0.87	8.29 ± 1.56	3.82 ± 0.74^b	4.84 ± 1.10^c	6.28 ± 1.38^c
R/T_{ES}	3.49 ± 0.91	4.50 ± 0.95	6.48 ± 1.75	2.91 ± 0.80^b	3.33 ± 1.04^c	3.90 ± 1.01^c
S_{ED} (cm^2)	79 ± 44	57 ± 25	50 ± 24	109 ± 35^b	28 ± 30^c	7 ± 8^c
S_{ES} (cm^2)	66 ± 40	47 ± 22	43 ± 22	91 ± 33^b	23 ± 27^c	6 ± 7^c
ΔS (%)	16 ± 8	17 ± 8	14 ± 7	17 ± 9	21 ± 14	14 ± 4
$(\sigma/P)_{ED}$	1.98 ± 0.42	2.76 ± 0.44	4.04 ± 0.88	1.72 ± 0.37^b	2.20 ± 0.55^c	2.94 ± 0.71^c
$(\sigma/P)_{ES}$	1.62 ± 0.44	2.14 ± 0.50	3.22 ± 0.97	1.28 ± 0.41^c	1.47 ± 0.53^c	1.76 ± 0.50^c
σ_{ES} (kPa)	22 ± 6	29 ± 7	43 ± 12	17 ± 5^c	20 ± 6^c	23 ± 6^c

Source: Zhong, L. et al., *Am. J. Physiol. Heart Circ. Physiol.*, 300(5), H1653, 2011.

C_{ED}, ventricular wall curvedness at end-diastole; C_{ES}, ventricular wall curvedness at end-systole; R_{ED}, ventricular chamber radius of curvedness at end-diastole; R_{ES}, ventricular chamber radius of curvedness at end-systole; T_{ED}, ventricular wall thickness at end-diastole; T_{ES}, ventricular wall thickness at end-systole; S_{ED}, ventricular surface area at end-diastole; S_{ES}, ventricular surface area at end-systole; ΔS, ventricular surface area change from end-diastole to end-systole; $(\sigma/P)_{ED}$, normalized wall stress at end-diastole; $(\sigma/P)_{ES}$, normalized wall stress at end-diastole; σ_{ES}, ventricular wall stress at end-systole.

[a] $p < 0.05$, [b] $p < 0.01$, [c] $p < 0.001$ for two-tail paired t-test used in comparing pre- and post-SVR values.

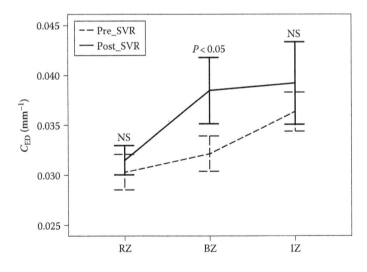

FIGURE 4.10

Left ventricular regional curvedness at end-diastole (C_{ED}) and end-systole (C_{ES}) in RZ, BZ, and IZ before and after SVR. There is no significant change in curvedness in each zone. *$p < 0.05$, NS, not significant pre- versus post-SVR. (Adapted from Zhong, L. et al., *Am. J. Physiol. Heart Circ. Physiol.*, 300(5), H1653, 2011.)

but the change was not statistically significantly. However, there were significant decreases in $(R/T)_{ED}$ and $(R/T)_{ES}$ in all zones.

4.3.3.4 Left Ventricular Function and Vascular Function

As shown in Table 4.6, there was a decrease in EDVI from 156 ± 39 to 110 ± 33 mL/m^2 and ESVI from 117 ± 39 to 77 ± 31 mL/m^2 postoperatively. The mean EF increased significantly from 26 ± 7 to 31 ± 10%. Similarly, there was an increase in SW/EDV from 21.76 ± 8.25 to 25.64 ± 7.40 mmHg. Particularly noteworthy was the increase in contractility index value from 2.69 ± 0.74 to 3.23 ± 0.73 mL/m^2 after SVR.

Surprisingly, there were significant decreases in cardiac index from 2.84 ± 0.74 to 2.59 ± 0.74 L/min/m^2 and SW from 6.61 ± 1.96 to 5.46 ± 1.64 mmHg·L post-SVR. In addition, arterial elastance (E_a) and systemic vascular resistance index were increased, and arterial compliance was decreased significantly, mainly because SV had decreased. Although there was slight improvement in ΔS, the change was not significant.

4.3.3.5 Regional Wall Stress Indices at End-Diastole and End-Systole

As seen in Table 4.7 and Figure 4.11, there were decreases in σ/P at both end-diastole (ED) and end-systole after surgery. The $(\sigma/P)_{ED}$ decreased by 27% from 4.04 ± 0.88 to 2.94 ± 0.71 ($p < 0.001$) in the infarct zone, by 20% in the BZ from 2.76 ± 0.44 to 2.20 ± 0.55 ($p < 0.001$) and by 9% in the RZ from 1.90 ± 0.42 to 1.72 ± 0.37 ($p < 0.05$). At end-systole, $(\sigma/P)_{ES}$ decreased by 45% in the infarct zone from 3.22 ± 0.97 to 1.76 ± 0.50 ($p < 0.0001$), by 31% in the BZ from 2.14 ± 0.50 to 1.47 ± 0.53 ($p < 0.001$) and by 21% in the RZ from 1.62 ± 0.44 to 1.28 ± 0.41 ($p < 0.05$). Similarly, the end-systolic wall stress decreased at each zone, respectively (IZ: pre-SVR = 43 ± 12 kPa, post-SVR = 23 ± 6 kPa; BZ: pre-SVR = 29 ± 7 kPa, post-SVR = 20 ± 6 kPa; RZ: pre-SVR = 22 ± 6 kPa, post-SVR = 17 ± 5 kPa, all $p < 0.001$).

4.3.4 Discussion

In our analysis of 3D LV regional shape for patients pre- and post-SVR, it can be noted that SVR reduces WSs, improves LV global systolic function, but fails to improve regional shape. This failure to restore LV shape to optimal (e.g., normal elliptical ventricle) may contribute to diastolic dysfunction in the long term.

4.3.4.1 Effect of Surgical Ventricular Restoration on LV Shape

Myocardial infarction can result in a spectrum of LV shape abnormalities, related to the extent of myocardial damage [5,36,37]. SVR aims to reshape the LV, rebuild a more physiological LV chamber, and improve cardiac pump function [7]. The introduction of the curvedness index can help to better identify 3D LV regional shape changes after MI and post-surgery. A decrease of curvedness is observed in post-MI patients, in particular at the apex zone [54].

In this study, SVR did not change LV regional shape significantly in all zones (see Table 4.7). In Section 4.2, we have reported that ES curvedness in normal heart is approximately 0.05, 0.06, and 0.10 mm^{-1} in the basal, middle, and apical regions, respectively. It should be noted that SVR slightly increases ES curvedness to 0.038, 0.039, and 0.040 mm^{-1} in the remote, border, and infarct zones, respectively, but is not optimizing the

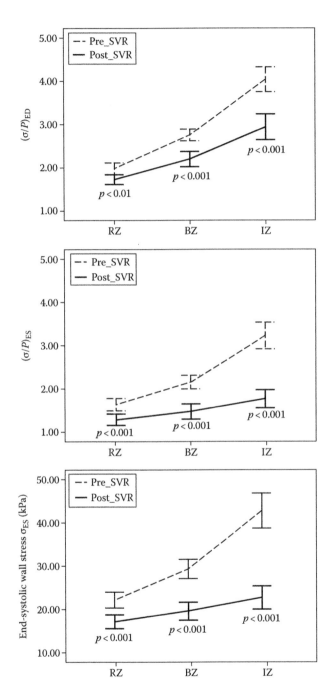

FIGURE 4.11
Left ventricular regional wall stress indices at end-diastole $(\sigma/P)_{ED}$, end-systole $(\sigma/P)_{ES}$ and end-systolic wall stress σ_{ES} in RZ, BZ, and IZ before and after SVR. End-diastolic wall stress index decreased significantly in each zone. *$p < 0.05$ pre- versus post-SVR. (Adapted from Zhong, L. et al., *Am. J. Physiol. Heart Circ. Physiol.*, 300(5), H1653, 2011.)

ventricular shape. This remaining distortion may cause non-optimal filling and diastolic dysfunction of the LV. Our observation is consistent with the findings of a recent study which used a combination of computational fluid dynamics (CFD) and cardiac MR techniques [17]. It was found that post-SVR shape, while being less spherical compared to pre-SVR shape, is nevertheless more spherical than pre-operative and healthy heart. Indeed, "ball"-shaped ventricles have impaired fluid dynamics and fluid washout [17].

4.3.4.2 Effect of Surgical Ventricular Restoration on LV Wall Stress

Studies of LV wall stress have provided substantial insights into cardiac remodeling [12,13]. The inability of the remaining viable myocardium to compensate for the increased WS associated with LV dilatation and thinning is a trigger for LV enlargement after MI [1]. The primary effect of SVR is to reduce LV wall stress and hence oxygen demand, and there is evidence for this occurrence [14,48,49,51,55]. Despite its obvious importance, however, WS is difficult to measure after MI because of the heterogeneous deformation of the LV chamber.

Our 3D MRI-based methodology for 3D reconstruction (accompanied by local radius-of-curvature and thickness determination) and use of Equation 4.1 is much more efficient computationally and easier to implement. Our 3D approach [54] is found to be more accurate than existing 2D approaches for precise evaluation of the regional wall stress. In this study, the LV end-systolic wall stress was reduced to 17 ± 5, 20 ± 6, and 23 ± 6 kPa at remote, border, and infarct zones, respectively. In Section 4.2, we have reported that peak systolic stress in normal heart is of the order of 10 kPa (Table 4.3). Hence, it should be noted that while SVR reduces end-systolic wall stress, it does not succeed in restoring the stress to normal values.

4.3.4.3 Effect of Surgical Ventricular Restoration on Ventricular Systolic Function

The effect of SVR on LV systolic function has been documented in terms of EF [1,34,35,42]. In this study, we have measured several indices to assess LV systolic function. It is hypothesized that if multiple indices are employed and if the results are generally in agreement and viewed in aggregate, it should be possible to determine and conclude whether patients after SVR have significant improvement in LV systolic function. Our results have shown that there were significant improvements in LV systolic function after SVR (Table 4.6).

Particularly noteworthy is the increase in contractility index value from 2.69 ± 0.74 to 3.23 ± 0.73 mL/m^2 after SVR.

Previously, LV systolic function improvement after SVR has also been demonstrated in terms of some loading-independent LV contractile indices such as ES elastance from invasive pressure–volume measurements [48]. These improvements of systolic function after SVR, however, may be due to concurrent CABG. It is well known that viable but dysfunctional myocardium exists in about 50% of patients undergoing CABG and revascularization can lead to striking changes in the LV parameters due to functional recovery. The viability analysis and the potential contribution of CABG, as opposed to SVR, is a logical next step.

4.3.4.4 Implications and Significance

Compared to CABG alone, SVR confers additional effects on LV volume reduction and wall stress [14,49,51]. However, the recent results of the STICH trial showed that SVR did not improve survival, hospitalization, and quality of life over CABG alone after 4 years of follow-up [27]. One possible explanation is that SVR disrupts the 3D helical structure of the myocardium [19], which impairs LV diastolic function [48] and LV contractility [45] to the extent that the benefits of reduced WS and improved LV systolic function are negated. Furthermore, some or most of the improvements in systolic function are due to CABG, as revascularization is well known to improve contractility.

Finally, some potential negative consequences of the SVR procedure are suture line or patch dehiscence, excessive LV volume reduction, and remaining distorted shape with resulting pathophysiology. The clinical advantage of SVR may be neutral [27] because regional LV shape and function (as assessed with surface area change, ΔS) do not improve significantly.

4A Appendix: Derivation of the Cardiac Contractility Index, Equation 4.1

For mathematical simplicity, we have approximated the LV as a thick-wall spherical shell, consisting of incompressible, homogeneous, isotropic, elastic material.

For a thick-walled spherically shaped LV, the maximum circumferential wall stress (σ_θ), occurring at the endocardial wall at $r = r_i$, is given as

$$\sigma_\theta(r_i) = P\left[\frac{r_i^3/r_e^3 + 1/2}{1 - r_i^3/r_e^3}\right] \tag{4A.1}$$

where

r_i and r_e are the inner and outer radii
P is the LV intra-cavitary pressure

By normalizing the circumferential wall stress (σ_θ) with respect to LV intra-cavitary pressure (P), we obtain

$$\sigma^*(r) = \frac{\sigma_\theta}{P} = \frac{r_i^3}{r_e^3 - r_i^3}\left(1 + \frac{r_e^3}{2r^3}\right) \tag{4A.2}$$

Since the maximum wall stress occurs at the inner endocardial wall, we have from Equations 4A.1 and 4A.2:

$$\sigma^*(r = r_i) = \left(\frac{V/(V_m + V) + 1/2}{1 - V/(V_m + V)}\right) = \left(\frac{3V + V_m}{2V_m}\right) = \left(\frac{3V}{2V_m} + \frac{1}{2}\right) \tag{4A.3}$$

where

P is the LV intra-cavitary pressure
σ_θ is the wall stress
$V(= 4\pi r_i^3/3)$ denotes LV volume
$V_m(= 4\pi(r_e^3 - r_i^3)/3)$ denotes LV myocardial volume
r_i and r_e are the inner and outer radii of the LV, respectively

By differentiating Equation 4A.3 with respect to time, we get

$$\left(\frac{d\sigma^*}{dt}\right)_{max} = \left|\frac{d(\sigma_\theta/P)}{dt}\right|_{max} = \left(\frac{3}{2V_m}\right)\left|\frac{dV}{dt}\right|_{max} \tag{4A.4}$$

It can be thus noted that in contrast to the traditional contractility index of $(dP/dt)_{max}$, our new $(d\sigma^*/dt)_{max}$ contractility index can be determined solely from noninvasive assessment of LV geometry and flow.

4B Appendix: Computation of 3D Shape Descriptors

We compute the LV surface curvatures via an analytic approach using a local surface patch fitting method.

4B.1 Local Surface Patch Fitting

A surface in 3D space can be expressed in the parametric form

$$\mathbf{s}(u,v) = \left[x(u,v),\ y(u,v),\ z(u,v)\right]^T \tag{4B.1}$$

where u and v are the parameters of the surface. For the implicit representation of the quadric patch

$$z = ax^2 + bxy + cy^2 + dx + ey \tag{4B.2}$$

a suitable parameterization is to choose $u = x$ and $v = y$, leading to

$$\mathbf{s}(u,v) = \begin{bmatrix} u \\ v \\ au^2 + buv + cv^2 + du + ev \end{bmatrix} \tag{4B.3}$$

In differential geometry, the curvature of a surface $\mathbf{s}(u,v)$ at a point $\mathbf{p}(u(t),v(t))$ is evaluated with respect to a normal section. This is done by constructing a plane π such that it passes through the unit surface normal $\hat{\mathbf{n}}$ and unit tangent vector in the direction of $\dot{\mathbf{u}}$ (where $\dot{\mathbf{u}} = [\dot{u}, \dot{v}]^T$). The intersection of π with $\mathbf{s}$ results in a curve called the "normal section." The curvature of the normal section at $\mathbf{x}$ is the *normal curvature* of the surface along the direction of $\dot{\mathbf{u}}$.

The normal curvature κ can be evaluated by the equation

$$\kappa(\dot{\mathbf{u}}) = \frac{\dot{\mathbf{u}}^T \mathbf{D} \dot{\mathbf{u}}}{\dot{\mathbf{u}}^T \mathbf{G} \dot{\mathbf{u}}} \tag{4B.4}$$

where $\mathbf{G} = \begin{bmatrix} \mathbf{s}_u \cdot \mathbf{s}_u & \mathbf{s}_u \cdot \mathbf{s}_v \\ \mathbf{s}_u \cdot \mathbf{s}_v & \mathbf{s}_v \cdot \mathbf{s}_v \end{bmatrix} = \begin{bmatrix} E & F \\ F & G \end{bmatrix}$ and $\mathbf{D} = \begin{bmatrix} \mathbf{s}_{uu} \cdot \hat{\mathbf{n}} & \mathbf{s}_{uv} \cdot \hat{\mathbf{n}} \\ \mathbf{s}_{uv} \cdot \hat{\mathbf{n}} & \mathbf{s}_{vv} \cdot \hat{\mathbf{n}} \end{bmatrix} = \begin{bmatrix} L & M \\ M & N \end{bmatrix}$ are the first and second fundamental matrices of the surface, respectively.

The unit surface normal can be calculated by

$$\hat{\mathbf{n}} = \frac{\mathbf{s}_u \times \mathbf{s}_v}{|\mathbf{s}_u \times \mathbf{s}_v|} \tag{4B.5}$$

In the case of the quadric patch, the components of the first and second fundamental matrices evaluated at the origin of the local coordinate frame (i.e., $u = 0$ and $v = 0$) are

$$E = \mathbf{s}_u \cdot \mathbf{s}_u = 1 + d^2$$
$$F = \mathbf{s}_u \cdot \mathbf{s}_v = de$$
$$G = \mathbf{s}_v \cdot \mathbf{s}_v = 1 + e^2 \tag{4B.6}$$

$$\hat{\mathbf{n}} = \frac{\begin{bmatrix} -d & -e & 1 \end{bmatrix}^T}{A}$$

$$L = \mathbf{s}_{uu} \cdot \hat{\mathbf{n}} = \frac{2a}{A}$$

$$M = \mathbf{s}_{uv} \cdot \hat{\mathbf{n}} = \frac{b}{A}$$

$$N = \mathbf{s}_{vv} \cdot \hat{\mathbf{n}} = \frac{2c}{A} \tag{4B.7}$$

where $A = \sqrt{d^2 + e^2 + 1}$.

The values of κ change and its extreme values are known as the principal curvatures κ_1 and κ_2. Their values are the roots of the following equation

$$\det \begin{bmatrix} \kappa E - L & \kappa F - M \\ \kappa F - M & \kappa G - N \end{bmatrix} = 0$$

$$\det \begin{bmatrix} \dfrac{2a}{A} - \kappa(1 + d^2) & \dfrac{b}{A} - \kappa de \\ \dfrac{b}{A} - \kappa de & \dfrac{2c}{A} - \kappa(1 + e^2) \end{bmatrix} = 0$$

$$\kappa_1 = \frac{B + \sqrt{B^2 - A^2(4ac - b^2)}}{A^3}$$

$$\kappa_2 = \frac{B - \sqrt{B^2 - A^2(4ac - b^2)}}{A^3} \tag{4B.8}$$

where $B = a + ae^2 + c + cd^2 - bde$.

Finally, we can then determine the shape descriptor, which is based on the curvedness C, presented by Koenderink [30] as the curvedness of a surface is used to measure the intensity of the degree a surface is curved. It is simply the root mean square of κ_1 and κ_2 and is calculated as

$$C = \sqrt{\frac{\kappa_1^2 + \kappa_2^2}{2}} = \frac{1}{A^3} \sqrt{2B^2 - A^2(4ac - b^2)} \tag{4B.9}$$

4C Appendix: Computation of Wall Radius of Curvature and Wall Thickness using Short-Axis and Long-Axis Approach and 3D Approach

To enable the calculations of 2DSR and 2DLR, we need to determine the properties of the intersection curve between the quadric surface and the intersecting plane, be it the short-axis plane (see Figure 4.12b) or the long-axis plane (see Figure 4.12c). The objective is to find the curvature of the intersection curve, as well as the vector defining the direction to measure the wall thickness. The wall radius is then the inverse of the curvature. The direction vector will be used to perform a ray-triangle intersection with the epicardial surface mesh to determine the wall thickness.

The calculation is carried out in the local frame of the quadric surface obtained during the patch fitting. As the intersection plane passes through the origin of the quadric surface, the implicit form in the local frame is given by

$$px + qy + rz = 0 \qquad\qquad (4C.1)$$

If we put the quadric equation into the plane equation, we obtain

$$px + qy + r(ax^2 + bxy + cy^2 + dx + ey) = 0$$

$$arx^2 + brxy + cry^2 + (dr + p)x + (er + q)y = 0 \qquad\qquad (4C.2)$$

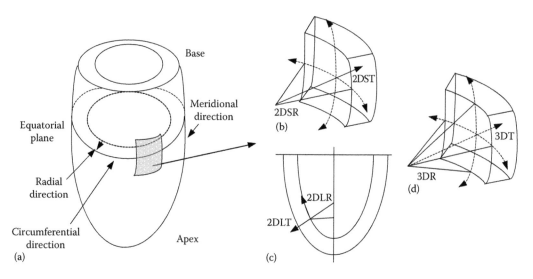

FIGURE 4.12

(a) Illustration of the LV geometry. (b) Schematics of 2DSR and 2DST in short-axis plane; R and T are radius of cavity and wall thickness. (c) Schematics of 2DLR and 2DLT in long-axis plane. (d) Schematics of 3DR and 3DT accounting for 3D curvature. (Adapted from Zhong, L. et al., *Am. J. Physiol. Heart Circ. Physiol.*, 296, H573, 2009.)

The parametric curve which describes the intersection between the quadric and the plane is then given by

$$\mathbf{r}(\alpha) = \begin{bmatrix} x \\ y \\ z \end{bmatrix} = \begin{bmatrix} x \\ y \\ ax^2 + bxy + cy^2 + dx + ey \end{bmatrix} \tag{4C.3}$$

where α is the curve parameter. A suitable parameterization is to take $\alpha = x$. Based on differential geometry, the curvature κ of $\mathbf{r}$ at the origin is

$$\kappa = \frac{|\dot{\mathbf{r}}(0) \times \ddot{\mathbf{r}}(0)|}{|\dot{\mathbf{r}}(0)|^3} \tag{4C.4}$$

where $\dot{\mathbf{r}}(0)$ and $\ddot{\mathbf{r}}(0)$ are the first and second derivative of $\mathbf{r}$ with respect to the curve parameter, respectively.

To calculate these derivatives, we evaluate the y-component of $\mathbf{r}$. The derivative of Equation 4C.2 with respect to x gives

$$2arx + bry + 2cry\frac{dy}{dx} + (dr + p) + (er + q)\frac{dy}{dx} = 0 \tag{4C.5}$$

$$\frac{dy}{dx} = \frac{-2arx - bry - dr - p}{2cry + er + q} \tag{4C.6}$$

Differentiating Equation 4C.5 again with respect to x yields

$$2ar + br\frac{dy}{dx} + 2cr\frac{dy}{dx} + 2cry\frac{d^2y}{dx^2} + (er + q)\frac{d^2y}{dx^2} = 0$$

$$\frac{d^2y}{dx^2} = \frac{-2ar - (br + 2cr)dy/dx}{2cry + er + q} \tag{4C.7}$$

Next, we evaluate the z-component of $\mathbf{r}$ by differentiating the quadric equation $z = ax^2 + bxy + cy^2 + dx + ey$ with respect to x gives

$$\frac{dz}{dx} = 2ax + by + bx\frac{dy}{dx} + 2cy\frac{dy}{dx} + d + e\frac{dy}{dx} \tag{4C.8}$$

If we differentiate Equation 4C.8 with respect to x, we obtain

$$\frac{d^2z}{dx^2} = 2a + 2b\frac{dy}{dx} + 2c\left(\frac{dy}{dx}\right)^2 + (bx + 2cy + e)\frac{d^2y}{dx^2} \tag{4C.9}$$

At $\alpha = 0$, $x = y = 0$. Using the results in Equations 4C.6 and 4C.8, we obtain

$$\dot{r}(\alpha = 0) = \begin{bmatrix} \dfrac{dx}{d\alpha} \\[2mm] \dfrac{dy}{d\alpha} \\[2mm] \dfrac{dz}{d\alpha} \end{bmatrix} = \begin{bmatrix} \dfrac{dx}{dx} \\[2mm] \dfrac{dy}{dx} \\[2mm] \dfrac{dz}{dx} \end{bmatrix} = \begin{bmatrix} 1 \\[2mm] \dfrac{-2arx - bry - dr - p}{2cry + er + q} \\[2mm] 2ax + by + bx\dfrac{dy}{dx} + 2cy\dfrac{dy}{dx} + d + e\dfrac{dy}{dx} \end{bmatrix}$$

$$\dot{r}(\alpha = 0) = \begin{bmatrix} 1 \\ m \\ d + em \end{bmatrix} \tag{4C.10}$$

where $m = (-dr - p)/(er + q)$

Furthermore, using the results in Equations 4C.7 and 4C.9, we obtain

$$\ddot{r}(\alpha = 0) = \begin{bmatrix} \dfrac{d^2x}{d\alpha^2} \\[2mm] \dfrac{d^2y}{d\alpha^2} \\[2mm] \dfrac{d^2z}{d\alpha^2} \end{bmatrix} = \begin{bmatrix} \dfrac{d^2x}{dx^2} \\[2mm] \dfrac{d^2y}{dx^2} \\[2mm] \dfrac{d^2z}{dx^2} \end{bmatrix}$$

$$= \begin{bmatrix} 0 \\[2mm] \dfrac{-2ar - (br + 2cr)\dfrac{dy}{dx}}{2cry + er + q} \\[4mm] 2a + 2b\dfrac{dy}{dx} + 2c\left(\dfrac{dy}{dx}\right)^2 + (bx + 2cy + e)\dfrac{d^2y}{dx^2} \end{bmatrix}$$

$$\ddot{r}(\alpha = 0) = \begin{bmatrix} 0 \\ n \\ 2a + 2bm + 2cm^2 + en \end{bmatrix} \tag{4C.11}$$

where

$$n = \frac{d^2y}{dx^2} = \frac{-2ar - (br + 2cr)m}{er + q}.$$

Using Equations 4C.10 and 4C.11, the curvature κ of the intersection curve r can then be determined by Equation 4C.4. The tangent of the curve $\hat{t}$ at the origin was calculated using $\hat{t} = \dot{r}(0)/|\dot{r}(0)|$. The direction of the wall thickness was then taken as the cross-product of

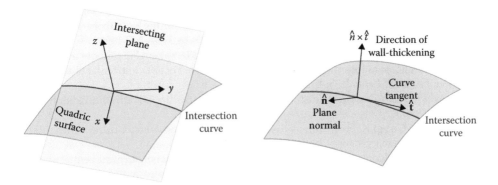

FIGURE 4.13
The normal at the endocardial surface used in subsequent curvature and wall stress calculation. (Adapted from Zhong, L. et al., *Am. J. Physiol. Heart Circ. Physiol.*, 296, H573, 2009.)

the plane normal $\hat{\mathbf{n}}$ and the curve tangent $\hat{\mathbf{t}}$ (in the global coordinate space), as illustrated in Figure 4.13.

To calculate the wall thickness, a ray was defined with origin at the point of interest **o** and direction $\hat{\mathbf{t}}$. An intersection was then performed between the ray and the epicardial surface to yield the intersection point $\mathbf{x}_{\text{intersect}}$. The wall thickness was then taken as the distance between the point of interest and the point of ray–surface intersection, i.e.,

$$t = \left\| \mathbf{o} - \mathbf{x}_{\text{intersect}} \right\| \tag{4C.12}$$

However, for the 3DR method (see Figure 4.12d) that employs the surface fitting method, the direction of the ray is the normal of the quadric surface at the origin, and is given by

$$\hat{\mathbf{n}} = \frac{1}{\sqrt{d^2 + e^2 + 1}} \begin{bmatrix} -d \\ -e \\ 1 \end{bmatrix} \tag{4C.13}$$

References

1. Aikawa Y, Rohde L, Plehn J, Greaves SC, Menapace F, Arnold MO, Rouleau JL, Pfeffer MA, Lee RT, Solomon SD. Regional wall stress predicts LV remodeling after anteroseptal myocardial infarction in the healing and early afterload reducing trial (HEART): An echocardiography-based structural analysis. *Am Heart J*, 141: 234–242, 2001.
2. Athanasuleas CL, Stanley AW Jr, Buckberg GD, Dor V, DiDonato M, Blackstone EH. Surgical anterior ventricular endocardial restoration (SAVER) in the dilated remodeled ventricle after anterior myocardial infarction. RESTORE group. Reconstructive Endoventricular Surgery, returning Torsion Original Radius Elliptical Shape to the LV. *J Am Coll Cardiol*, 37: 1199–1209, 2001.
3. Bellenger NG, Francis JM, Davies CL, Coats A, Pennell DJ. Establishment and performance of a magnetic resonance cardiac function clinic. *J Cardiovasc Magn Reson*, 2: 15–22, 2000.

4. Beyar R, Shapiro E, Graves W, Guier W, Carey G, Soulen R, Zerhouni E, Weisfeldt M, Weiss J. Quantification and validation of left ventricular wall thickening by a three-dimensional element magnetic resonance imaging approach. *Circulation,* 81: 297–307, 1990.

5. Bogaert J, Bosmans H, Maes A, Suetens P, Marchal G, Rademakers FE. Remote myocardial dysfunction after acute anterior myocardial infarction: Impact of left ventricular shape in regional function. *J Am Coll Cardiol,* 35: 1525–1534, 2000.

6. Braunwald E. *Heart Disease: A Textbook of Cardiovascular Disease,* 5th edn. Philadelphia, PA: WB Saunders, 1997.

7. Burkberg GD, Group R. Form versus disease: Optimizing geometry during ventricular restoration. *Eur J Cardiothorac Surg,* 29(Suppl 1): S238–S244, 2006.

8. Castelvecchio S, Menicanti L, Ranucci M, Di Donato M. Impact of surgical ventricular restoration on diastolic function: Implications of shape and residual ventricular size. *Ann Thorac Surg,* 86: 1849–1855, 2008.

9. Cerqueira MD, Weissman NJ, Dilsizian V, Jacobs AK, Kaul S, Laskey WK, Pennell DJ, Rumberger JA, Ryan T, Verani MS. Standardized myocardial segmentation and nomenclature for tomographic imaging of the heart. A statement for healthcare professionals from the Cardiac Imaging Committee of the Council on Clinical Cardiology of the American Heart Association. *Circulation,* 105: 539–542, 2002.

10. Chemla D, Hebert JL, Coirault C, Zamani K, Suard I, Colin P, Lecarpentier Y. Total arterial compliance estimated by stroke volume-to-aortic pulse pressure ratio in humans. *Am J Physiol Heart Circ Physiol,* 274: H500–H505, 1998.

11. Chen CH, Fetics B, Nevo E, Rochitte CE, Chiou KR, Ding PA, Kawaguchi M, Kass DA. Noninvasive single-beat determination of left ventricular end-systolic elastance in humans. *J Am Coll Cardiol,* 38: 2028–2034, 2001.

12. Cohn JN, Ferrari R, Sharpe N. Cardiac remodeling-concepts and clinical implications: A consensus paper from an international forum on cardiac remodeling. *J Am Coll Cardiol,* 35(3): 569–582, 2000.

13. Cohn JN. New therapeutic strategies for heart failure: Left ventricular remodeling as a target. *J Card Fail,* 10: S200–S201, 2004.

14. Dang AB, Guccione JM, Zhang P, Wallace AW, Gorman RC, Gorman JH 3rd, Ratcliffe MB. Effect of ventricular size and patch stiffness in surgical anterior ventricular restoration: A finite element study. *Ann Thorac Surg,* 79: 185–193, 2005.

15. Debatin J, Nadel SN, Sostman HD, Spritzer CE, Evans AJ, Grist TM. Magnetic resonance imaging-cardiac ejection fraction measurements. Phantom study comparing four different methods. *Invest Radiol,* 27: 198–204, 1992.

16. Di Donato M, Toso A, Dor V, Sabatier M, Barletta G, Menicanti L, Fantini F, the RESTORE Group. Surgical ventricular restoration improves mechanical intraventricular dyssynchrony in ischemic cardiomyopathy. *Circulation,* 109: 2536–2543, 2004.

17. Doenst T, Spiegel K, Reik M, Markl M, Hennig J, Nitzsche S, Beyersdorf F, Oertel H. Fluid-dynamic modeling of the human left ventricle: Methodology and application to surgical ventricular reconstruction. *Ann Thorac Surg,* 87: 1187–1195, 2009.

18. Dor V, Sabatier M, Di Donato M, Montiglio F, Toso A, Maioli M, Pasque MK, Mickleborough LL. Efficacy of endoventricular patch plasty in large postinfarction akinetic scar and severe left ventricular dysfunction: Comparison with a series of large dyskinetic scars. *J Thorac Cardiovasc Surg,* 116: 50–59, 1998.

19. Eisen HJ. Surgical ventricular reconstruction for heart failure. *N Engl J Med,* 360: 17, 2009.

20. Gaudio C, Tanzilli G, Mazzarotto P, Motolese M, Romeo F, Marino B, Reale A. Comparison of left ventricular ejection fraction by magnetic resonance imaging and radionuclide ventriculography in idiopathic dilated cardiomyopathy. *Am J Cardiol,* 67: 411–415, 1991.

21. Germain P, Roul G, Kastler B, Mossard J, Bareiss P, Sacrez A. Inter-study variability in left ventricular mass measurement. Comparison between M-mode echocardiography and MRI. *Eur Heart J,* 13: 1011–1019, 1992.

22. Grossman W, Braunwald E, Mann T, McLaurin L, Green L. Contractile state of the left ventricle in man as evaluated from end-systolic pressure-volume relations. *Circulation*, 56: 845–852, 1977.
23. Hayashida W, Kumada T, Nohara R, Tanio H, kambayashi M, Ishikawa N, Nakamura Y. Left ventricular regional wall stress in dilated cardiomyopathy. *Circulation*, 82: 2075–2083, 1990.
24. Hirota Y, Shimizu G, Kaku K, Saito T, Kino M, Kawamura K. Mechanisms of compensation and decompensation in dilated cardiomyopathy. *Am J Cardiol*, 54: 1033–1038, 1984.
25. Jackson BM, Parish LM, Gorman JH 3rd, Enomoto Y, Sakamoto H, Plappert T, St John Sutton MG, Salgo I, Gorman RC. Borderzone geometry after acute myocardial infarction: A three-dimensional contrast enhanced echocardiographic study. *Ann Thorac Surg*, 80(6): 2250–2255, 2005.
26. Janz R. Estimation of local myocardial stress. *Am J Physiol Heart Circ Physiol*, 242: H875–H881, 1982.
27. Jones BH, Velazquez EJ, Michler RE, Sopko G, Oh JK, O'Connor CM, Hill JA et al., for the STICH Hypothesis 2 Investigators. Coronary bypass surgery with or without surgical ventricular reconstruction. *N Engl J Med*, 360: 1705–1717, 2009.
28. Katz J, Milliken MC, Stray-Gundersen J, Buji LM, Parkley RW, Mitchell JH, Peshock RM. Estimation of human myocardial mass with MR imaging. *Radiology*, 169: 495–498, 1998.
29. Kelly RP, Ting C-T, Yang T-M, Liu C-P, Maughan WL, Chang M-S, Kass DA. Effective arterial elastance as index of arterial vascular load in humans. *Circulation*, 86: 513–521, 1992.
30. Koenderink JJ, Van Doom AJ. Surface shape and curvature scales. *Image Vision Comput*, 10(8): 557–565, 1992.
31. Kono T, Sabbah HN, Steain PD, Brymer JF, Khaja F. Left ventricular shape as a determinant of mitral regurgitation in patients with several heart failure secondary to either coronary artery disease or idiopathic dilated cardiomyopathy. *Am J Cardiol*, 68: 355–359, 1991.
32. Lessick J, Sideman S, Azhari H, Marcus M, Grenadier E, Beyar R. Regional three-dimensional geometry and function of left ventricles with fibrous aneurysms. A cine-computed tomography study. *Circulation*, 84(3): 1072–1086, 1991.
33. Lessick J, Sideman S, Azhari H, Shapiro E, Weiss JL, Beyar R. Evaluation of regional load in acute ischemia by three-dimensional curvature analysis of the left ventricle. *Ann Biomed Eng*, 21(2): 147–161, 1993.
34. Menicanti L, Castelvecchio S, Ranucci M, Frigiola A, Santambrogio C, de Vincentiis C, Brankovic J, Di Donato M. Surgical therapy for ischemic heart failure: Experience from one single-center with surgical ventricular restoration. *J Thorac Cardiovasc Surg*, 134: 433–441, 2007.
35. Mickleborough LL, Merchant N, Ivanov J, Rao V, Carson S. Left ventricular reconstruction: Early and late results. *J Thorac Cardiovasc Surg*, 128: 27–37, 2004.
36. Mitchell GF, Lamas GA, Vaughan DE, Pfeffer MA. Left ventricular remodeling in the year after first anterior myocardial infarction: A quantitative analysis of contractile segment lengths and ventricular shape. *J Am Coll Cardiol*, 19: 1136–1144, 1992.
37. Moustakidis P, Maniar HS, Cupps BP, Absi T, Zheng J, Guccione JM, Sundt TM, Pasque MK. Altered left ventricular geometry changes the border zone temporal distribution of stress in an experimental model of left ventricular aneurysm: A finite element model study. *Circulation*, 106: I168–I175, 2002.
38. Nakayama Y, Shimizu G, Hirota Y, Saito T, Kino M, Kitaura Y, Kawamura K. Functional and histopathologic correlation in patients with dilated cardiomyopathy: An integrated evaluation by multivariate analysis. *J Am Coll Cardiol*, 10: 186–192, 1987.
39. Niggel TJ, Borowski DT, LeWinter MM. Relation between left ventricular shape and exercise capacity in patients with left ventricular dysfunction. *J Am Coll Cardiol*, 22: 751–757, 1993.
40. Reichek N, Wilson J, St. John Sutton M, Plappert TA, Goldberg S, Hirshfeld JW. Noninvasive determination of left ventricular end-systolic stress: Validation of the method and initial application. *Circulation*, 65: 99–108, 1982.
41. Sabbah HN, Kono T, Stein PD, Mancini GB, Goldstein S. Left ventricular shape changes during the course of evolving heart failure. *Am J Physiol Heart Circ Physiol*, 263: H266–H270, 1992.
42. Sartipy U, Albage A, Lindblom D. The Dor procedure for left ventricular reconstruction. Ten-year clinical experience. *Eur J Cardiothorac Surg*, 27: 1005–1010, 2005.

43. Semelka R, Tomei E, Wagners S, Mayo J, Kondo C, Suzuki J, Caputo G, Higgins C. Normal left ventricular dimensions and function: Reproducibility of measurements with cine MR imaging. *Radiology,* 174: 763–768, 1990.

44. Su Y, Zhong L, Lim CW, Ghista DN, Chua T, Tan RS. A geometrical approach for evaluating left ventricular remodeling in myocardial infarct patients. *Comput Methods Programs Biomed,* 108(2): 500–510, 2012.

45. Sun K, Zhang ZH, Suzuki T, Wenk JF, Stander N, Einstein DR, Saloner DA, Wallace AW, Guccione JM, Ratcliffe BM. Dor procedure for dyskinetic anteroapical myocardial infarction fails to improve contractility in the border zone Original Research Article. *J Thorac Cardiovasc Surg,* 140(1): 233–239, 2010.

46. Swynghedauw B. Molecular mechanisms of myocardial remodeling. *Physiol Rev,* 79(1): 215–262, 1999.

47. Tibayan FA, Lai DT, Timek TA, Dagum P, Liang D, Zasio MK, Daughter GT, Miller DC, Ingels NB Jr. Alteration in left ventricular curvature and principal strains in dilated cardiomyopathy with functional mitral regurgitation. *J Heart Valve Dis,* 12(3): 292–299, 2003.

48. Tulner SA, Steendijk P, Klautz RJ, Bax JJ, Schalij MJ, van der Wall EE, Dion RAE. Surgical ventricular restoration in patients with ischemic dilated cardiomyopathy: Evaluation of systolic and diastolic ventricular function, wall stress, dyssynchrony, and mechanical efficiency by pressure-volume loops. *J Thorac Cardiovasc Surg,* 132: 610–620, 2006.

49. Walker JC, Ratcliffe MB, Zhang P, Wallace AW, Hsu EW, Saloner DA, Guccione JM. Magnetic resonance imaging-based finite element stress analysis after linear repair of left ventricular aneurysm. *J Thorac Cardiovasc Surg,* 135: 1094–1102, 2008.

50. Yeo SY, Zhong L, Su Y, Tan RS, Ghista DN. A Curvature-based approach for left ventricular shape analysis from cardiac magnetic resonance imaging. *Med Biol Eng Comput,* 47: 313–322, 2009.

51. Yin FC. Ventricular wall stress. *Circ Res,* 49: 829–842, 1981.

52. Zhang P, Guccione JM, Nicholas SI, Walker JC, Crawford PC, Shamal A, Saloner DA, Wallace AW, Ratcliffe MB. Left ventricular volume and function after endoventricular patch plasty for dyskinetic anteroapical left ventricular aneurysm in sheep. *J Thorac Cardiovasc Surg,* 130: 1032–1038, 2005.

53. Zhong L, Tan RS, Ghista DN, Ng EYK, Chua LP, Kassab GS. Validation of a novel noninvasive cardiac index of left ventricular contractility in patients. *Am J Physiol Heart Circ Physiol,* 292(6): H2764–H2772, 2007.

54. Zhong L, Su Y, Yeo SY, Tan RS, Ghista DN, Kassab GS. Left ventricular regional wall curvedness and wall stress in patients with ischemic dilated cardiomyopathy. *Am J Physiol Heart Circ Physiol,* 296: H573–H584, 2009.

55. Zhong L, Sola S, Tan RS, Ghista DN, Kurra V, Navia JL, Kassab GS. Effects of surgical ventricular restoration on left ventricular contractility assessed by a novel contractility index in patients with ischemic cardiomyopathy. *Am J Cardiol,* 103: 674–679, 2009.

56. Zhong L, Su Y, Gobeawan L, Sola S, Tan RS, Navia JL, Ghista DN, Chua T, Guccione J, Kassab GS. Impact of surgical ventricular restoration on ventricular shape, wall stress and function in heart failure patients. *Am J Physiol Heart Circ Physiol,* 300(5): H1653–H1660, 2011.

5

Cardiac Contractility Measures for Left Ventricular Systolic Functional Assessment in Normal and Diseased Hearts

Dhanjoo N. Ghista, Liang Zhong, Thu-Thao Le, and Ru San Tan

CONTENTS

Glossary

B_v	Viscous damping parameter of VE, N·s/cm
CE, SE, VE	Contractile, series, and viscous elements in MSU model
CFD	Computational fluid dynamics
dP/dt_{max}	Maximal first time-derivative of LV pressure, mmHg/s
$d\sigma^*/dt_{max}$	Maximal change rate of pressure-normalized wall stress, $\sigma^* = \sigma/P$, s^{-1}
E_a	Active elastance, mmHg/mL
$E_{a,max}$	Maximum active elastance, mmHg/mL
E_{es}	End-systolic elastance, mmHg/mL
EF	Ejection fraction, %
Elastance	Change of pressure per change in volume, dP/dV
E_p (mmHg/mL)	Passive elastance, mmHg/mL
ESPVR	End-systolic pressure–volume relationship
F_{CE}, F_{SE}	Force of contractile element, force of series element $(=kx_1)$, N
k	Elastic modulus of SE, N/cm
MSPI	Myocardial sarcomere power index, W/mL
MSU	Myocardial structural unit
P	Left ventricular pressure, mmHg
PAMP	Preload-adjusted maximal power, W/mL^2
SR	Strain rate, that is, rate of change of strain, s^{-1}
Stiffness	Pressure per volume change (dP/dV) of the LV as a whole, mmHg/mL
Strain	Length change in percent of initial length; two definitions are used: Lagrangian strain $e = (l - lo)/lo$; and natural strain $e = \ln(l/lo)$
Stress	Force per area, dyn/cm^2
V	Left ventricular volume, mL
V_m	Myocardial volume, mL
ϕ	Velocity potential in finite element analysis
∇^2	Laplacian operator
x_1, x_2, x_T	Displacement relative to centerline of series element, viscous element, and MSU, respectively, cm
$\dot{x}_1, \dot{x}_2, \dot{x}_T$	First time-derivative of x_1, x_2, x_T, cm/s
$\ddot{x}_1, \ddot{x}_2, \ddot{x}_3$	Second time-derivative of x_1, x_2, x_T, cm/s^2

5.1 Introduction and Objective

Left ventricular (LV) contraction is the basis of LV pumping function, impairment of which underlies heart failure pathophysiology. Its scientific quantification is vital for the diagnosis and surveillance of patients with heart failure. To garner clinical applicability, these LV contractility indices must be derived from LV bioengineering models based on clinically measurable data and be easily adapted for clinical assessment. In this chapter, we provide LV models for detailed formulations and formulae of intrinsic LV indices, and examine their medical applications. Herein we analyze LV contractile performance in terms of LV contractility indices at different physiological organizational levels: from sarcomere dynamics to LV myocardial properties (such as elastic modulus and elastance), and from LV wall contractile stress development to the generation of intra-LV blood flow velocities and pressure distributions. Using techniques for measuring ventricular pressure, geometry, and volume, we show how these indices have become more amenable for clinical usage to obtain more reliable patient assessment. The purport of this chapter is to present a comprehensive coverage of LV contraction physiology, indices to qualify LV contraction, formulation, and medical applications of some major intrinsic LV contractility indices so as to provide the basis of functional assessment of normal versus diseased hearts in cardiology practice.*

5.2 LV Contractility: Global Indices Governing LV Pressure–Volume Data, Based on LV Chamber Modeling

As per our listed categories of intrinsic contractility indices (in Section 5.1), we now present some approaches and indices to quantify LV contractility, based on modeling of LV elastance [26] and LV chamber wall stress [28], LV myocardial elastic modulus [9], myocardial sarcomere contractile dynamics [10], and intra-LV blood flow mechanics [22,23].

5.2.1 Passive and Active LV Elastance, E_p and E_a

We offer a new concept of dual passive and active elastances, operating in tandem throughout the cardiac cycle. The passive elastance (E_p) represents the LV pressure response to LV volume changes—LV volume increase during LV filling phase and decrease during LV ejection phase—and is a measure of LV stiffness [26]. Additionally, we have also designated active elastance (E_a) to represent LV contraction and relaxation, both of which can be traced to LV sarcomeric units activation and of the actin–myosin units disengagement, respectively [10].

5.2.1.1 Model Analysis and Index Formulation

In order to determine these passive and active elastances, we adopt a spherically shaped LV model with radius, R; wall thickness, h. The governing differential equation, relating LV pressure and volume, is [26]

$$Md\dot{V} + d(EV) = MdV + V\,dE + E\,dV = dP \qquad (5.1)$$

where
  V represents the volume of LV
  $\dot{V}$ is the first time-derivative of V
  P denotes *LV* pressure in mmHg
  M is the inertia term $= \rho h/4\pi R^2$
  E is the LV elastance $= E_p + E_a$ [16]

---

* This chapter is based on Cardiac contractility measures of left ventricular systolic functional assessment of normal and diseased hearts, DN Ghista, L Zhong, T-T Le, and R-S Tan, *J Mech Med Biol*, 9(40), 2009.

The first term in Equation 5.1 is of a much smaller order of magnitude relative to the other terms, and can hence be safely omitted. We, hence, rewrite Equation 5.1 as

$$V\,dE + E\,dV = dP \tag{5.2}$$

wherein the volume V is expressed in mL and dP in mmHg, so that the elastance E can be expressed in mmHg/mL.

E_p constitutes an intrinsic LV volume-dependent stiffness property of the LV. The expression for E_p is obtained from LV late-diastolic pressure–volume data as

$$P = P_0 e^{Z_p V}; \quad E_P = \frac{dP}{dV} = E_{P0} e^{Z_p V} \tag{5.3}$$

This expression is then employed to simulate LV pressure–volume data during the later half of filling phase, in order to evaluate E_{P0} and Z_p parameters.

During isovolumic contraction phase, Equations 5.1 and 5.2 are modified to

$$V\,dE = dP \tag{5.4}$$

and discretized to correspond to time instants i and $(i-1)$ as

$$E_{a,i} = \frac{(P_i - P_{i-1})}{V_i + E_{a,i-1}} \tag{5.5}$$

As per Equation 5.3, E_p represents the intrinsic property of the LV in terms of how its pressure changes in response to its volume changes. On the other hand, E_a, as per Equation 5.4, varies in relation to LV pressure changes at a given volume, due to LV contraction.

Equation 5.5 can be employed to evaluate $E_{a,i}$ during the isovolumic contraction phase; then, Equations 5.1 through 5.5 can be employed, to simulate LV pressure and volume during the ejection phase, for determining the values of $E_{a,i}$. Similarly, in isovolumic relaxation phase, we can adopt Equation 5.5 to determine $E_{a,i}$ values; then, Equations 5.1 through 5.5 can be employed to determine $E_{a,i}$ values during the early part of diastolic phase.

Upon determining these instantaneous values of active elastance, we can represent the cyclic variation of E_a as

$$E_a = E_{a0}\left[1 - e^{-(t/\tau_C)^{ZC}}\right]\left[e^{-(((t-d)u(t-d))/\tau_R)^{ZR}}\right] \tag{5.6}$$

where
  t is measured from the start of isovolumic contraction
  the parameter E_{a0} is the active elastance coefficient
  the time coefficient (τ_C) describes the rate of elastance rise during the contraction phase, while (τ_R) describes the rate of elastance fall during the relaxation phase
  the exponents "Z_C" and "Z_R" are parameters of the E_a curve during isovolumic contraction and relaxation phases
  the parameter d is a time constant
  $u(t-d)$ is the unit step function, so that $u(t-d) = 0$ for $t < d$

These parameters are determined by fitting Equation 5.6 to the computed instantaneous values of E_a during a cardiac cycle.

5.2.1.2 Medical Application

The above analysis is now applied to clinical data. Figure 5.1a depicts a sample LV pressure–volume data during the filling phase, from which the passive elastance function can be obtained, from Equation 5.3. Figure 5.1b depicts the computed cyclic variation of active elastance, based on Equation 5.6.

Then, Figure 5.1c and d provide the model-derived E_p and E_a functions for two subjects (subject HEL and DDM). Subject HEL serves as a sample patient with myocardial infarct, and sample subject DDM has double vessel disease and hypertension. The E_p versus LV volume plots, in Figure 5.1c, clearly reveal that E_p increases exponentially with increase LV volume. It is seen that the passive elastance curve is steeper for the stiffer myocardium of patient HEL, with a corresponding bigger value of the exponential coefficient Z_p (subject HEL).

The "E_a versus normalized time" plot in Figure 5.1d reveals the development and decrease of E_a during systole, which in turn governs the generation of LV pressure. It is evident that the active elastance of patient DDM is greater than that of patient HEL with myocardial infarct.

As validation of our advocating $E_{a,max}$ as a contractility index, we have depicted its good correlation with the traditional dP/dt_{max} index ($E_{a,max} = 0.006 \, dP/dt_{max} - 5$, $r = 0.93$, $p < 0.0001$) in 30 characterized patients with different tertiles of LV ejection fraction [26], in Figure 5.1e.

Knowing E_p and E_a, we can reconstruct the LV pressure data from LV volume data. An interesting outcome of this study (as depicted in Figure 5.1b) is that while E_a develops at the start of isovolumic contraction and becomes maximum during late ejection, it becomes zero only during diastolic filling. Thus, the retention and operation of E_a during diastole helps to explain the phenomenon of LV suction, that is, LV filling before the onset of LV atrial contraction [27]. This clinical application is based on invasive measurement of pressure and volume data, which is somewhat limited in clinical setting.

5.2.2 Maximum Rate of Change of Pressure-Normalized LV Wall Stress, $d\sigma^*/dt_{max}$

LV contractility can be termed as the capacity of the LV to contract and develop intramyocardial stress, and thereby intracavitary pressure, to eject blood volume as rapidly as possible [25]. It is hence rational and appropriate to formulate a LV contractility index on the basis of LV wall stress generated by LV contraction [1,3,14]. Hence, analogous to the traditional contractility index dP/dt_{max} which is based on LV intracavitary pressure, we propose a novel LV contractility index based on LV wall stress, namely, the maximum rate of change during systole of LV wall stress normalized to LV intracavitary pressure, $d(\sigma_\theta/P)/dt_{max}$ or $d\sigma^*/dt_{max}$ where $\sigma^* = \sigma_\theta/P$ [25,28].

5.2.2.1 Model Analysis and Index Formulation

Numerous methods abound for LV wall stress determination from LV geometrical models [2,20,24]. Herein, we have employed a thick-walled spherical LV model with radius r, and express LV pressure-normalized wall stress (σ^*) as [25,28]

$$\sigma^*(r) = \frac{\sigma_\theta}{P} = \frac{r_i^3}{r_e^3 - r_i^3}\left(1 + \frac{r_e^3}{2r^3}\right)$$

$$\sigma^*(r = r_i) = \left(\frac{V/(V_m + V) + 1/2}{1 - V/(V_m + V)}\right) = \left(\frac{3V + V_m}{2V_m}\right) = \left(\frac{3V}{2V_m} + \frac{1}{2}\right) \tag{5.7}$$

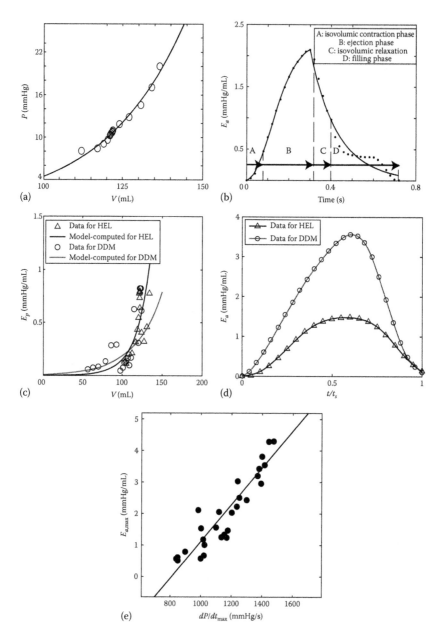

FIGURE 5.1

(a) Pressure–volume data of a sample patient: By using Equation 5.3 to fit this pressure–volume data during the filling phase, we obtain: $P = 8.00 \times 10^{-2}e^{0.040V}$, and $E_p = 3.20 \times 10^{-3}e^{0.040V}$. The volume 100 mL corresponds to the start of filling phase, and the volume 150 mL corresponds to the end of filling phase. (b) The calculated values of active elastance E_a during a cardiac cycle are shown dotted. Then using Equation 5.6 to fit the calculated values, we obtain $E_{a0} = 2.20$ mmHg/mL, $\tau_c = 0.17$ s; $Z_c = 1.96$; $d = 0.3$ s, $\tau_R = 0.12$ s; $Z_R = 0.96$. It is noted (from the figure) that the active elastance E_a continues into the filling phase, as LV myocardial contraction decreases and ends during the filling phase. (Adapted from Figures 4 and 5 of Zhong, L. et al., *Proc. Inst. Mech. Eng. Part H: J. Eng. Med.*, 220, 647, 2006.) (c) LV volume and corresponding volume-dependent passive elastance for subjects HEL and DDM. (d) Active elastance versus normalized time for subjects HEL and DDM. Herein, t_s is the duration from start-of-isovolumic contraction phase to end-of-isovolumic relaxation. (e) Correlation between $E_{a,max}$ and dP/dt_{max} ($r = 0.93$, $p < 0.0001$). (Adapted from Figures 9 and 11 of Zhong, L. et al., *Biomed. Eng. Online*, 4, 10, 2005.)

where

    P is LV intra-cavitary pressure

    σ_θ is the wall stress

    $V(= 4\pi r_i^3/3)$ denotes LV volume

    $V_m(= 4\pi(r_e^3 - r_i^3)/3)$ denotes LV myocardial volume

    r_i and r_e are the inner and outer radii of the LV, respectively

Differentiating with respect to time, we get

$$\frac{d\sigma^*}{dt_{max}} = \left|\frac{d(\sigma_\theta/P)}{dt}\right|_{max} = \frac{3}{2V_m}\left|\left(\frac{dV}{dt}\right)\right|_{max} \tag{5.8}$$

It can be thus noted that in contrast to the indices of dP/dt_{max}, E_{es}, and $E_{a,max}$, our $d\sigma^*/dt_{max}$ index can be determined solely from noninvasive assessment of LV geometry and flow. Normalizing LV wall stress to LV pressure has obviated the need for invasive LV pressure measurement.

5.2.2.2 Medical Application

We have validated $d\sigma^*/dt_{max}$ against dP/dt_{max} and $E_{a,max}$ in 30 subjects with disparate ventricular function in Figure 5.2, and demonstrated the index's load independence, albeit under conditions of limited preload and afterload manipulations [28].

We have also recently evaluated the changes of LV contractile function, using $d\sigma^*/dt_{max}$ (determined from noninvasive cine MRI images), in patients who had undergone CABG with surgical ventricular restoration (SVR) [29]. In these patients, SVR was performed, in addition to revascularization, to exclude akinetic and dyskinetic wall segments in patients with anterior myocardial infarction. Our study has shown considerable improvement in LV contractile function, as indicated by increased $d\sigma^*/dt_{max}$, albeit unfavorable spherical LV shape after SVR procedure [29], as depicted in Table 5.1. This improvement may be due to improved contractility of the remote myocardium, as a result of decreased myocardial stress and revascularization [19].

5.2.3 Elasticity Model of LV to Determine Its Stress, Strain, and Elastic Modulus Parameters

LV myocardial property can be expressed in terms of the diastolic and systolic elastic modulus of the LV myocardial wall. Many early 3D LV models are based on shell theory, such as the ellipsoidal shell [24] and large-strain models [13]. In a departure from shell models, Ghista and Sandler developed the ellipsoidal-shaped elasticity-theory model (Figure 5.3) [4,5,8].

5.2.3.1 Model Analysis and Index Formulation

This model comprises of (1) a Line Dilatation system, over a length "a" along the longitudinal axis of LV, of amplitude parameter A, (2) superimposed on a hydrostatic stress system, of amplitude parameter B. Incorporating invasively monitored LV pressure and

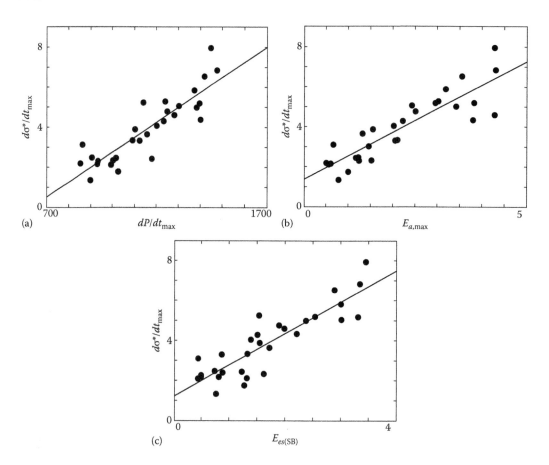

FIGURE 5.2
Linear regression analysis demonstrates good correlation between $d\sigma^*/dt_{max}$ and dP/dt_{max}: [(a) $d\sigma^*/dt_{max}$ = 0.0075 dP/dt_{max} − 4.70, r = 0.88], between $d\sigma^*/dt_{max}$ and $E_{a,max}$ [(b) $d\sigma^*/dt_{max}$ = 1.20 $E_{a,max}$ + 1.40, r = 0.89], and between $d\sigma^*/dt_{max}$ and $E_{es(SB)}$ [(c) $d\sigma^*/dt_{max}$ =1.60 $E_{es(SB)}$ + 1.20, r = 0.88].

geometry data in patients, this model yields (1) the expression for LV wall stress (whose variation across the wall is depicted in Figure 5.3c), (2) the principle stress-trajectory surfaces (shown in Figure 5.3a), having approximately ellipsoidal LV geometry, and (3) the expressions for the displacements at these stress-trajectory surfaces.

The model is then matched with the monitored instantaneous LV geometries, to obtain the value of the size parameter "*a.*" At each instant, two stress-trajectory surfaces of the model are selected, and scaled to represent the shape and size of the LV (Figure 5.3a). Then, the stress states in the equatorial elements on the endocardial and epicardial surfaces of the LV model are made to satisfy the LV chamber pressure boundary conditions (*P* on the endocardial surface, and zero pressure on the epicardial surface), to evaluate the parameters *A* and *B*. Therefrom, we can determine the wall stress variation (Figure 5.3c).

Then, the derived formulations for hoop and meridional strains at the equatorial wall element (expressed in terms of the elastic modulus *E*) are matched to the instantaneous strains computed from LV instantaneous geometries, in order to calculate the value of the effective elastic modulus (*E*) of the LV [9].

TABLE 5.1

Patients' Data Pre- and Post-SVR

Variables	Pre-SVR ($n = 40$)	Post-SVR ($n = 40$)
Cardiac index (L/min/m²)	2.84 ± 0.74	2.59 ± 0.74
Mean arterial pressure (mmHg)	85 ± 14	84 ± 8
Systolic blood pressure (mmHg)	115 ± 20	113 ± 10
Diastolic blood pressure (mmHg)	71 ± 12	70 ± 8
End-diastolic volume index (mL/m²)	156 ± 39	110 ± 33[a]
End-systolic volume index (mL/m²)	117 ± 39	77 ± 31[a]
Stroke volume index (mL/m²)	39 ± 9	33 ± 8[a]
Left ventricular ejection fraction (%)	26 ± 7	31 ± 10[a]
LV mass index (g/m²)	112 ± 25	101 ± 23[a]
End-diastolic long axis, BA_{ed} (cm)	10.89 ± 1.16	8.31 ± 1.00[a]
End-diastolic short axis, AP_{ed} (cm)	7.00 ± 0.80	6.64 ± 0.78[a]
End-systolic long axis, BA_{es} (cm)	10.37 ± 1.20	7.87 ± 1.05[a]
End-systolic short axis, AP_{es} (cm)	5.86 ± 0.98	5.23 ± 1.06[a]
End-diastolic sphericity index, SI_{ed}	0.65 ± 0.087	0.81 ± 0.11[a]
End-systolic sphericity index, SI_{es}	0.57 ± 0.094	0.67 ± 0.13[a]
Difference between end-diastolic and end-systolic sphericity index, $SI_{ed} - SI_{es}$	0.077 ± 0.043	0.14 ± 0.059[a]
Long-axis shortening (%)	4.8 ± 3.6	5.4 ± 4.4
Short-axis shortening (%)	16.4 ± 6.8	22 ± 9.7[a]
dV/dt_{max} (mL/s)	364 ± 83	401 ± 81[a]
Pressure normalized wall stress	4.30 ± 0.95	3.31 ± 0.75[a]
Stroke work (mmHg·L)	6.61 ± 1.96	5.46 ± 1.64[a]
$d\sigma^*/dt_{max}$ (s⁻¹)	2.69 ± 0.74	3.23 ± 0.73[a]

Source: Zhong, L. et al., *Am. J. Cardiol.*, 103, 674, 2009.
Values are mean ± SD.
[a] $p < 0.05$.

The expressions for model strains (with reference to Figure 5.3) are [8]

$$\varepsilon_{M_{ww'equator}} = \frac{P(1-2\upsilon)}{EK_2} + \frac{4P(1+\upsilon)}{EK(W_c/a)^2[(W_c/a)^2 + 1]^{1/2}}$$

$$\varepsilon_{M_{\beta\beta'equator}} = \frac{P(1-2\upsilon)}{EK_2} + \frac{4P(1+\upsilon)}{EK_1[(W_c/a)^2 + 1]^{3/2}} \qquad (5.9)$$

where K_1 and K_2 are dimensional functions of the model's geometric parameters.

For the purpose of calculating the strain in the LV at an instant i, we characterize the instantaneous geometry of the LV by a thick-walled ellipsoid with wall thickness, internal major and minor axes H_i, L_i, and W_i, respectively (Figure 5.3b). The experimentally obtained instantaneous strains for a central element in the equatorial plane of the LV are determined as follows:

$$\varepsilon_{V_{ww\,equator}} = \frac{(W_c)_i - (W_c)@P_{min}}{(W_c)@P_{min}}, \quad \text{during diastole}$$

$$= \frac{(W_c)_i - (W_c)_{min}}{(W_c)_{min}}, \quad \text{during systole} \qquad (5.10)$$

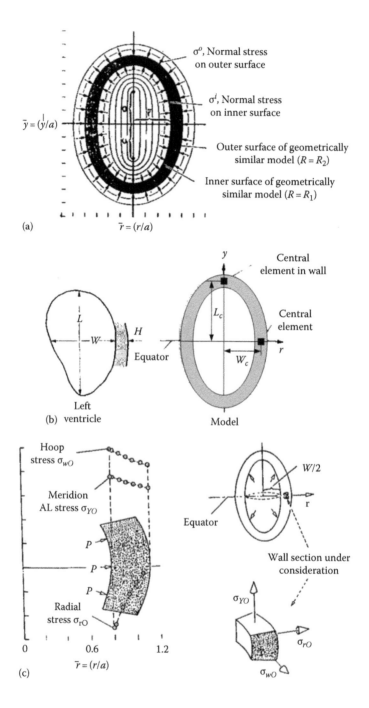

FIGURE 5.3
(a) Stress trajectories for the analytical LV model (in Section 5.2.3): the equatorial stress in the LV medium is made to satisfy the LV pressure loading, to evaluate the stress parameters. (b) Comparison of actual left ventricle geometry with corresponding model geometry: The LV model expressions for hoop and meridional strains at the central equatorial element (in terms of the modulus E) are made to match the computed strains (based on LV geometry data), to evaluate E of the LV. (c) 3D stress distribution across the left ventricular wall. These figures are based on the Ghista–Sandler model. (Adapted from Figures 7 through 9 in Ghista, D.N. and Sandler, H., *Med. Biol. Eng.*, 13(2), 151, 1975.)

$$\varepsilon_{V_{\beta\beta}\,equator} = \frac{(W_c)\,@\,P_{min}\left[(W_c)_i - (W_c)\,@\,P_{min}\right]}{\left(L_c^2\right)@\,Q_{min}}, \quad \text{during diastole}$$

$$= \frac{(W_c)_{min}\left[(W_c)_i - (W_c)_{min}\right]}{\left(L_c^2\right)_{min}}, \quad \text{during systole}$$

(5.11)

Equating the model expressions ε_{ww}^M or $\varepsilon_{\beta\beta}^M$, as functions of the elastic modulus E (Equation 5.9), to their numerical values ε_{ww}^V or $\varepsilon_{\beta\beta}^V$ (Equations 5.10 and 5.11), we solve for the unknown instantaneous value of the LV elastic modulus, E. A cyclic continuous time-variation of the elastic modulus E is thereby created. We interpret the instantaneous systolic effective modulus as a representation of the effort put in by the LV myocardium to perform its pumping function. This is the first known connotation and index of LV contractility based on LV functional modeling, expressed in terms of the systolic elastic modulus of the LV myocardial wall.

The stress variation across the wall is depicted in Figure 5.3c. LV geometry has had considerable influence on effects on wall stresses in these early LV shell and elasticity-theory models. This has provided the impetus for development of finite element models of LV, in order to incorporate the effects of LV's irregular wall geometry. Among the earliest finite-element models of the LV was the model developed by Ghista and Hamid [6], to incorporate the irregular geometry of the LV and compute LV regional wall stress and modulus.

5.2.3.2 Medical Application

The clinical application of the LV elasticity model [9] has enabled us to determine the cyclic variation of effective elastic modulus of the LV. The maximum value of this elastic modulus during the systolic phase, E_s, index can represent the maximal contractile effort required to eject the blood; this was the first known LV contractility index, obtained from LV functional modeling. Table 5.2 provides us the summary of the clinical results applied to subjects with valvular disorders and idiopathic myocardial hypertrophy. This clinical application of the LV elastic modulus opened the doors to LV property-based indices of LV contractility [4–6]. The clinical remarks, provided in the last column, indicate whether or not (based on the maximum value of systolic modulus E) (1) the contractile effort (or contractility) of the LV is normal, (2) there is adequate compensatory hypertrophy, and (3) there is adequate reserve contractile effort capacity. This was the first such clinical application of the LV contractility index (represented by the LV effective modulus).

5.2.4 LV myocardial Sarcomere Biomechatronic Modeling: Contractile Force, Shortening Velocity, and Myocardial Contractile Power

The heart is truly a mechatronic organ. Ghista et al. have modeled the heart muscle as a mechatronic system [10]. The LV is assumed to be a thick-walled cylinder with internal and external radii, R_i and R_o; length, L, and wall thickness, h (Figure 5.4a). The LV myocardial (V_M) and intracavitary (V) volumes are given by

$$V_M = \pi\left(R_o^2 - R_i^2\right), \quad L = \pi(2R_i + h)hL$$

(5.12)

$$V = \pi R_i^2 L$$

(5.13)

TABLE 5.2

Effective Elastic Modulus for Patients

Subject	Disease	LVP (mmHg)	LVM (g)	H, ED (mm)	H/W ED	EDV (mL)	Hoop strain (%)	Peak hoop stress ($\times 102$ N/m2)	Modulus, S/D ($\times 102$ N/m^2)	Remarks (LV muscle state)
1	MS	102/10	90	5.4	0.11	89	30	310	600/70	Normal
2	MS, MI	105/8	430	13	0.26	290	20	150	800/160	Normal C.E.
3	MS, MI	116/9	180	6	0.09	191	48	398	450/70	High dispensability
4	MS, MI, AI	162/10	190	9	0.17	168	26	430	1500/210	Low R.C.E.C.
5	MS, MI, AI	140/8	300	10	0.15	257	22	350	1800/1000	Low R.C.E.C.
6	AS	198/25	270	8.5	0.13	263	16	550	4000/1100	Low R.C.E.C.

Source: Ghista, D.N. et al., *Biophys. J.*, 13, 832, 1973.

MS, mitral stenosis; AS, aortic stenosis; MI, mitral insufficiency; AI, aortic insufficiency; LVP, left ventricular pressure; EDV, end-diastolic volume; SV, stroke volume; LVM, left ventricular myocardium mass (from ventriculography); C.E., contractile effort; R.C.E.C., reserve contractile effort capacity.

Inputting the values of V_M, V, and h obtained by cine-ventriculography, the instantaneous R_i (t) and length $L(t)$ at any time instant t can be calculated as

$$R_i = \frac{2Vh/V_M + \sqrt{(2Vh/V_M)^2 + 4Vh^2/V_M}}{2}, \quad L = \frac{V}{\pi R_i^2} \tag{5.14}$$

5.2.4.1 Model Analysis and Index Formulation

Now, let us suppose that there are N number of myocardial fibers, located helically within the model's wall: one set of fibers ($N/2$) oriented clockwise, and the other set ($N/2$), counter-clockwise (Figure 5.4a). Each myocardial fiber comprises two myocardial structural units (MSU)—including the core sarcomeric contractile element (CE)—in series, that are mirror images of each other (Figure 5.4c). The vertical components of the fiber forces exert pressure on the top and bottom surfaces of the LV chamber. Their horizontal components produce a torque (T_t) in the LV (Figure 5.4b), that is given by

$$T_t = \left(\frac{N}{2}\right) F_t \cos \alpha_t = \frac{(N/2)\pi R_i^2 P_t \cos \alpha_t}{(N/2)\sin \alpha_t} = \pi R_j^2 P_t ctg\alpha_t \tag{5.15}$$

where
F_t is the force within each fiber
α_t is the instantaneous fiber angle

N is determined by the cross-sectional area of the cylindrical model myocardium divided by the cross-section area of MSU, the latter being approximately 7.85×10^{-5} cm^2 [15]. For analysis of this cylindrical LV mechatronic model, a constant fiber angle α of $35.26°$ (determined by considering the equilibrium of the fiber forces and LV chamber pressure) has been adopted, as per the analysis of Pietrabissa et al. [18].

In turn, this torque T_t results in a twist of the LV by angle θ_t:

$$\theta_t = \frac{T_t L_t}{JG} = \frac{\pi R_j^2 P_t L_t ctg\alpha}{JG} \tag{5.16}$$

where
L_t is the instantaneous length at time t of the LV cylindrical model
$\alpha_t (= \alpha) = 35.26°$
J is the polar moment of inertia
G is the shear modulus of LV myocardium ≈ 100 GPa [12]

Inputting nominal values of $R_i = 2$ cm, $R_o = 3$ cm, and $L = 14$ cm into the LV model, a $10°$ twist will evince an approximate 60 mmHg pressure rise during isovolumic contraction, and a $15°$ twist will give rise to peak LV systolic pressure. Then, as the LV untwists, the LV pressure drops. These calculated twist angles correspond to monitored values by 2D speckle tracking echocardiography [17], thereby lending some credibility to our model.

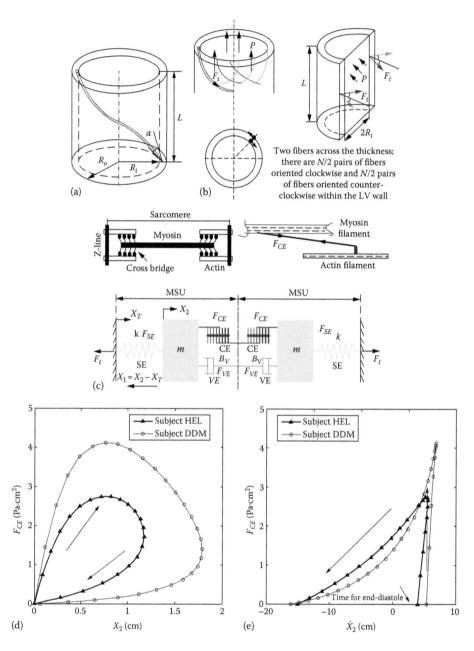

FIGURE 5.4

(a) LV cylindrical model, depicting a typical myocardial fiber arranged as a helix within the LV model wall; L, R_i, and R_o are the length, inner, and outer radii of the LV cylindrical model. (b) Equilibrium of fiber forces and LV pressure of the LV cylindrical model at the top circular cross-section plane and across the longitudinal plane in the circumferential direction. (c) Myocardial fibril model, composed of two symmetrical myocardial structural units (MSUs), which are mirror images of each other. Each MSU is composed of (1) an effective mass (m) that is accelerated, (2) connective-tissue series element. (3) the parallel viscous element of the sarcolemma, (4) the contractile element (CE), which generates contractile force between the myosin (thick) and actin (thin) filaments. When the contractile element shortens, the series element lengthens. (d) Relationship between contractile element force (F_{CE}) and displacement (x_2). (e) Relationship between contractile element force (F_{CE}) and shortening velocity ($\dot{x}_2$). (Adapted from Figures 1, 2, 3, 13 and 14 of Ghista, D.N., *Mol. Cell. Biomech.*, 2, 217, 2005.)

While we have assumed a fixed fiber angle α above, it does vary slightly in reality [21]. From Equation 5.16, it is evident that instantaneous values of α_t can be calculated if we simultaneously measure LV pressure and geometry, as well as the time-varying twist angle θ_t of the LV apex with respect to the base by using techniques like echocardiographic speckle tracking or magnetic resonance tagging. Conversely, for certain instantaneous dimensions R_i and L_i, the in vivo values of θ_t during the cardiac cycle influences the value of P_t generated. Hence, from the monitored LV pressure generated, LV geometry, and LV deformations (including the twist angle), we can determine the stress distribution in the LV, the principal stress trajectories, and the fiber orientations (deemed to be oriented along the stress trajectories). We have recently carried out this analysis, and have shown that the monitored LV twist angle of 5° during isovolumic contraction is due to the contraction of its helically wound myocardial fibers from an angle of 38° at the start of isovolumic contraction to 33° at the end of isovolumic contraction [7].

Let us now put down the governing differential equation for MSU dynamics and the generated MSU contractile force (F_{CE}), expressed as

$$m\ddot{x}_2 + B_v\dot{x}_2 - F_{CE} + kx_1 = 0 \tag{5.17}$$

or

$$m\ddot{x}_1 + B_v\dot{x}_1 + kx_1 = F_{CE} - B_v\dot{x}_T - m\ddot{x}_T \tag{5.18}$$

Rearranging the terms, we obtain

$$F_{CE} = m\ddot{x}_2 + B_v\dot{x}_2 + kx_1, \quad F_{CE} = m(\ddot{x}_1 + \ddot{x}_T) + B_v(\dot{x}_1 + \dot{x}_T) + kx_1 \tag{5.19}$$

where
   F_{CE} is the applied force exerted by the CE of MSU
   m is the muscle mass per unit cross-sectional area ($= \pi(R_o^2 - R_i^2)L\rho/(2N)$)
   B_v is the viscous damping parameter of the parallel viscous element (VE)
   k is the elastic stiffness (or modulus) of the series elastic element (SE)
   x_T is the shortening displacement of the myocardial fiber unit relative to its centerline (determined from LV dimension changes)
   x_1 is the stretch of the SE ($= x_2 - x_T$)
   x_2 is the displacement of m relative to centerline due to CE contraction ($= x_1 + x_T$)

The term $m\ddot{x}_2$ is of a small order of magnitude compared to the other two terms and is hence neglected in the analysis [10].

The MSU shortening velocity ($\dot{x}_2$) is given by

$$\dot{x}_2 = \dot{x}_1 + \dot{x}_T \tag{5.20}$$

where
   x_1 is determined from monitored LV pressure and dimensions
   $\dot{x}_1$ is its first time-derivative of x_1
   x_T is determined from LV dimensional change during isovolumic contraction and ejection phases, $\dot{x}_T$ is its first time-derivative

Using instantaneous LV pressure and dimensional data obtained during ventriculography, the sarcomere force F_{CE} and the shortening velocity $\dot{x}_2$ can be determined [10]. In this procedure, initially x_T is monitored during the cardiac cycle (for α assumed to be 35.26°), as

$$x_T = \frac{(L_{t+1} - L_t)}{2\sin\alpha} \tag{5.21}$$

F_{CE} is then expressed as a time-varying cyclic expression:

$$F_{CE} = F_{CE0}\sin(\omega_{ce}t)e^{-Z_{ce}t} \tag{5.22}$$

where
F_{CE0}, ω_{ce}, and Z_{ce} are the additional parameters to be determined
$t = 0$ corresponds to the start of isovolumic contraction phase

Upon substituting Equations 5.21 and 5.22 into the governing Equation 5.19, we obtain the differential equation:

$$B_v\dot{x}_1 + kx_1 = F_{CE0}\sin(\omega_{ce}t)e^{-(Z_{ce}t)} - B_v\dot{x}_T \tag{5.23}$$

which, on solving, yields an expression for

$$x_1 = f(m, k, B_v, F_{CE0}, w_{ce}, Z_{ce}, t) \tag{5.24}$$

Now, the parallel series element force, F_{SE}, is given by

$$F_{SE} = k \times (\text{total SE deformation}) = k \times x_1 = \frac{2\pi R_i^2 P_i}{N\sin\alpha} \tag{5.25}$$

Matching this expression for kx_1 (Equation 5.24) with the value of $2\pi R_i^2 P_i/(N\sin\alpha)$ calculated by means of Equation 5.25 from monitored P_i and R_i data, and carrying out parameter identification, the parameters k, B_v, F_{CE0}, ω_{ce}, and Z_{ce} can be determined. Substituting the values of these parameters into Equations 5.23 through 5.25, we determine F_{CE} and x_1. The myocardial fiber shortening $x_2 (= x_1 + x_T)$ and velocity of shortening $\dot{x}_2 (= \dot{x}_1 + \dot{x}_T)$ can then be obtained from the values of x_1 and x_T, as per Equation 5.20.

Now, by linking the MSU's sarcomere contractile force, F_{CE}, and shortening velocity, $\dot{x}_2$, to the monitored LV pressure and volume, a power index for LV contractility can be derived [10], expressed as

$$\text{Power} = N(F_{CE} \times \dot{x}_2) \tag{5.26}$$

and the myocardial sarcomere power index (MSPI) expressed as

$$\text{MSPI} = \frac{\text{Power}_{\text{max}}}{V_m} \tag{5.27}$$

where $\text{Power}_{\text{max}}$ is the maximal value of power (Equation 5.26).

5.2.4.2 Medical Application

The "force versus shortening displacement" characteristics during systole (based on the above analysis) is determined for the same earlier mentioned two subjects HEL and DDM, and shown in Figure 5.4d. It is noted that the CE shortening reaches its maximum value late in the ejection phase. The area encircled by contractile force–displacement curve and the x-axis represents the CE energy input. Figure 5.4e shows the computed CE force–shortening velocity relationship, for these two subjects HEL and DDM with different heart diseases. Subject HEL serves as a representative of a patient with myocardial infarct. Subject DDM is an example of a patient with double vessel disease and hypertension. It is seen that the CE force (F_{CE})–shortening velocity ($\dot{x}_2$) curve follows the same trend for both the subjects. The CE force (F_{CE}) and shortening velocity ($\dot{x}_2$) both reach their maximal values at about one-third ejection. However, the loop made by subject HEL has a lesser area encircled within it, and correspondingly has lower contractile power input of the two subjects. This is because subject HEL has myocardial infarct, and hence has a weaker contracting myocardium. This is manifested by a lower contractile element maximal force (F_{CE}) and shortening velocity ($\dot{x}_2$), in comparison with subject DDM.

Correspondingly, HEL subject's values of maximum power generated by CE (Equation 5.26) and MSPI the contractility index (Equation 5.27) are lower than for DDM. These results help to quantify how myocardial infarct impairs the LV performance, in terms of our model's contractile power-generated and MSPI contractility index.

5.2.5 Intra-LV Blood Flow Modeling-Based Intra-LV Blood Velocity and Pressure-Gradient Distributions

Many interrelated factors and events from sarcomere to chamber level influence LV function. All of these events ultimately contribute to the generation of intra-LV flow velocity and pressure gradients. A detailed investigation of intra-LV flow patterns, obtained by FEM analysis of blood flow within the LV, can provide practical insight into how the LV is functioning. Very early computational models were confined to 2D flow patterns, pressure waveforms, and transmitral flow in simplified geometries [11].

In 1985, Subbaraj and Ghista [22,23] employed FEM for computational fluid dynamics (CFD) analysis of intra-LV blood flow, to compute the instantaneous distributions of intra-LV flow and differential pressure during the filling and ejection phases, using actual instantaneous cine-ventriculographic LV geometry data.

5.2.5.1 Model Analysis and Index Formulation

The data required for FEM analysis of blood flow inside the LV chamber [22,23] consists of (1) LV 2D long-axis frames geometries during LV diastolic and systolic phases and (2) computation of LV instantaneous wall-motion velocities as well as instantaneous velocity of blood entering the LV during the filling phase and leaving the LV during the ejection phase. Using FEM, the computational solution of the potential equation

$$\nabla^2 \phi = 0 \tag{5.28}$$

where
   ϕ is the velocity potential
   $\nabla\phi$ is the velocity vector

For 2D planar flow domain, $\nabla^2\phi = 0$. Equation 5.28 is transformed into a finite element form and solved for ϕ at nodal points in the flow domain, by specifying (1) $\partial\phi/\partial n$ ($=V_n$) along the endocardial boundary, and (2) ϕ to be constant along the open boundary (so as to constrain the flow to be normal to that boundary); since the value of this constant ϕ along the open boundary is arbitrary, $\phi = 0$ is specified along the open boundary. From the computed values of ϕ at each internal point, the velocity components at each internal point of the LV chamber are determined, hence yielding instantaneous maps of intra-LV blood flow velocity patterns.

The intra-cardiac pressure distribution at any point inside the LV chamber can then be obtained, by using the Bernoulli equation for unsteady potential flow:

$$p + \frac{1}{2}\rho V^2 + \rho\frac{\partial\phi}{\partial t} = C(t) \tag{5.29}$$

wherein
   p is the pressure
   $1/2\rho V^2$ is the dynamic pressure
   ρ is the blood density
   V is the blood velocity
   $\rho\,\partial\phi/\partial t$ represents the effect due to acceleration
   $C(t)$ represents the total pressure sensed by a pressure probe facing the oncoming fluid,
       and is a constant
   The gravitational or hydrostatic effects are neglected.

The partial derivative, $\partial\phi/\partial t$, is computed from the value of ϕ at the same point at successive instants, using the finite different scheme.

The need for invasive catheter pressure measurement can be obviated by obtaining the pressure distribution relative to a reference point in the chamber, say at the center of the aortic or mitral orifice. The differential pressure field at a point s, in terms of the pressure p_o at the inlet (during diastole) or outlet (during the ejection phase) of the LV, is given by

$$p_s - p_o = \frac{1}{2}\rho\left(V_o^2 - V_s^2\right) + \rho\left(\left.\frac{\partial\phi}{\partial t}\right|_o - \left.\frac{\partial\phi}{\partial t}\right|_s\right) \tag{5.30}$$

where V_o and V_s are, respectively, the velocities of blood flow at the center of the valve orifice (i.e., aortic orifice during systole and mitral orifice during diastole) and at a point s inside the LV chamber.

The differential pressure $(p_s - p_o)$ can then be expressed and displayed, in nondimensional form, as

$$C_p = \frac{p_s - p_o}{(1/2)\rho V_o^2} \tag{5.31}$$

where C_p is the nondimensional pressure coefficient.

This instantaneous graphical display of the relative pressure distribution in the LV provides an indication of the resistance to filling as well as the effectiveness of LV contraction in setting up the appropriate pressure distribution in the chamber to promote adequate emptying.

In this way, computational solutions are obtained for the instantaneous distributions of intra-LV blood flow velocities and differential pressures during filling and ejection phases, thereby intrinsically characterizing LV resistance-to-filling and LV contractility, respectively [22,23]. A uniform and adequate intra-LV pressure gradient generated toward the aortic outflow tract implies efficient LV contraction and efficient pumping. In contrast, a non-uniform and inadequate pressure gradient, caused by asynchronous myocardium contraction due to myocardial ischemia or infarct, connotes poor pump performance.

5.2.5.2 Medical Application

Figure 5.5 presents for a patient (with a myocardial infarct), superimposed LV outlines during diastole and systole, before (Figure 5.5a1) and after (Figure 5.5a2) nitroglycerin administration. Figure 5.5b1 and c1 depict maps of diastolic and systolic intra-LV blood flow velocities, respectively, before nitroglycerin administration; then, Figure 5.5b2 and c2 depict diastolic and systolic intra-LV blood flow velocities, respectively, after nitroglycerin administration.

Similarly, Figure 5.5d1 and e1 depict maps of diastolic and systolic intra-LV blood pressure-gradient distributions, respectively, before nitroglycerin administration; then, Figure 5.5d2 and e2 depict maps of diastolic and systolic intra-LV blood pressure-gradient distributions, respectively, after nitroglycerin administration.

We can interpret this phenomenon as if the LV wall stiffness was providing the resistance to wall motion during diastole, and the contracting LV was facilitating emptying of the LV during systole, thereby setting up the requisite intra-LV pressure gradients and velocity distributions. The maximum pressure gradient (at the aortic valve outlet) is of the order of 3 mmHg/cm, after the administration of nitroglycerin.

For this patient, Figure 5.5d1 and e1 demonstrate high resistance-to-filling and poor LV contractility, in terms of adverse intra-LV blood pressure gradients during filling and ejection phases, respectively. However, following the administration of nitroglycerin, these filling and ejection phases' pressure gradients (and hence LV resistance-to-filling and LV contractility) are improved (Figure 5.5d2 and e2), thereby providing the basis for advocating coronary revascularization for this patient. These graphic and visual maps of intra-LV pressure variation are obtained from noninvasive measurements. In fact, these maps constitute perhaps the most direct and legible outcome-based index of impaired LV contractility (due to myocardial infarct).

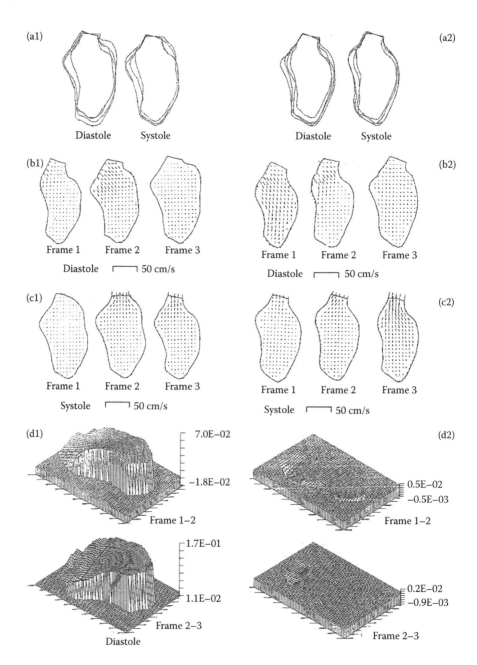

FIGURE 5.5
Construction of intra-LV blood flow velocity and pressure-gradient distributions for a patient with myocardial infarct: (a) Superimposed sequential diastolic and systolic endocardial frames (whose aortic valves centers and the long axis are matched), before (a1) and after (a2) administration of nitroglycerin. (b) Instantaneous intra-LV distributions of velocity during diastole, before (b1) and after (b2) administration of nitroglycerin. (c) Instantaneous intra-LV distributions of velocity during ejection phase, before (c1) and after (c2) administration of nitroglycerin. (d) Instantaneous intra-LV distributions of pressure-differentials during diastole, before (d1) and after (d2) administration of nitroglycerin.   *(Continued)*

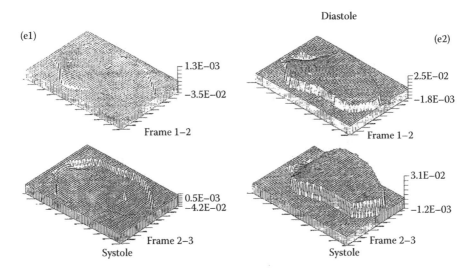

FIGURE 5.5 (*Continued*)
Construction of intra-LV blood flow velocity and pressure-gradient distributions for a patient with myocardial infarct: (e) Instantaneous intra-LV distributions of pressure-differential during ejection phase, before (e1) and after (e2) administration of nitroglycerin. (Adapted from Figure 5 of Subbaraj, K. et al., *J. Biomed. Eng.*, 9, 206, 1987.)

5.3 Conclusion

The science of cardiology has evolved parallel to most medical sciences: first emphasizing anatomy, then physiology, and now molecular biology. From 1960s onwards, when it had become obvious that effective medical and surgical therapies were available for cardiac diseases, there developed a heightened interest in measuring cardiac contractile function and associated LV contractility indices, as a way of evaluating the heart's condition and as a marker of heart failure, as well as for assessing the heart's response to medical therapies.

5.3.1 Usefulness of Cardiac Left Ventricular Contractility Indices

Because the heart is an electrically activated muscle pump, it is logical that determination and quantification of LV (myocardial function and) contractility can provide diagnostic indication of heart failure and prognostic indication of the success or failure of a given therapy. In the patient care setting, the evaluation of cardiac contractility (with data obtained with echo or MRI or even catheterization procedure) constitutes an essential component of clinical cardiology.

We have shown herein the modeling and formulation of relevant contractility indices at different LV physiological levels, in terms of sarcomere dynamics, LV mechanics, LV myocardial properties, and intra-LV blood flow profile. We have shown how these indices can be employed to assess patients with different types of cardiac disorders.

The LV contraction mechanism is based on the LV sarcomere contractile force versus shortening displacement and velocity characteristics, which enables us to distinguish a poorly contracting LV, as evinced by Figure 5.4d and e. As shown in Section 5.2.1, the LV active elastance index enables us to reconstruct the variation of LV pressure from

LV volume data during filling and ejection phases; it also provides an explanation of LV suction phenomenon as a mechanism of LV filling during the early diastolic phase.

The contractility index maximum rate-of-increase of normalized wall stress $d\sigma^*/dt_{max}$ of LV has enabled us to recognize decreased LV contraction in cardiomyopathy, and some improvement of contractility following surgical ventricular restoration of LVs with aneurysmic myocardial infarcted segments [29]. Then, the maximum value of the effective elastic modulus has been shown (in Table 5.2) to determine how well LVs with valvular diseases have compensated by hypertrophy, such that their systolic modulus value is restored to the normal range so that there is adequate reserve contractile capacity.

Then in Section 5.2.4, we have modeled the heart as a mechatronic organ. The LV is assumed to be a thick-walled cylinder, with its myocardial fibers located helically (oriented both clockwise and counterclockwise) within the model wall. As illustrated in Figure 5.4, each myocardial fiber comprises two MSU in series. The vertical components of the fiber forces exert pressure on the top and bottom surfaces of the LV chamber, and their horizontal components produce a torque (T_t) in the LV. We have put down the governing differential equation for MSU dynamics and derived expressions for MSU contractile force, shortening velocity, and power index as a measure of cardiac contractility. It is seen that the CE force (F_{CE})–shortening velocity ($\dot{x}_2$) curve loop area is lesser and the MSPI the contractility index value is lower for patient HEL with myocardial infarct.

Finally, we come to the outcome of LV contraction process, in terms of the setting up of favorable intra-ventricular maps of blood-flow velocity and pressure gradients (Figure 5.5), that are conducive to effective ejection of adequate blood volume. These illustrative maps provide to the cardiologist a graphic picture of the severity of heart failure. Further, by noting improvement in these intra-LV blood-flow pressure gradients following the administration of coronary vasculature's vaso-dilating agents, it enables the cardiologist to assess the viability of this LV to have improved performance following coronary bypass surgery.

5.3.2 Employment of Indices in Clinical Practice

This chapter can now promote the employment of these contractility indices into routine cardiology practice, by clinical applications of these indices in a large pool of patients with varied etiology of cardiac disorders. In this way, we can develop the range of values of these contractility indices for normal patients and for cardiac disease states, so that they can be effectively employed in differential diagnosis.

References

1. DeAnda A Jr., Komeda M, Moon MR, Green GR, Bolger AF, Nikolic SD, Daughters GT, Miller DC (1988) Estimation of regional left ventricular wall stresses in intact canine hearts. *Am J Physiol*, 275:H1879–H1885.
2. Falsetti HL, Mates RE, Grant C, Greene DG, Bunnell IL (1970) Left ventricular wall stress calculated from one-plane cineangiography. *Circ Res*, 26:71–83.
3. Fifer MA, Gunther S, Grossman W, Mirsky I, Carabello B, Barry W (1979) Myocardial contractile function in aortic stenosis as determined from the rate of stress development during isovolumic systole. *Am J Cardiol*, 44:1318–1325.

4. Ghista DN, Advani SH, Gaonkar GH, Balachandran K, Brady AJ (1971) Analysis and physiological monitoring of human left ventricle. *J Basic Eng*, 93:147–161.

5. Ghista DN, Brady AJ, Radhakrishnan S (1973) A three-dimensional analytical (rheological) model of the human left ventricle in passive-active states. *Biophys J*, 13:832–854.

6. Ghista DN, Hamid S (1977) Finite element stress analysis of the human left ventricle whose irregular shape is developed from single plane cineangiocardiogram. *Comput Methods Programs Biomed*, 7(3):219–231.

7. Ghista DN, Liu L, Chua LP, Zhong L, Tan RS, Tan YS (2009) Mechanism of left ventricular pressure increase during isovolumic contraction, and determination of its equivalent myocardial fiber orientation. *J Mech Med Biol*, (in press).

8. Ghista DN, Sandler H (1969) An analytical elastic-viscoelastic model for the shape and forces of the left ventricle. *J Biomech*, 2(1):35–47.

9. Ghista DN, Sandler H, Vayo WH (1975) Elastic modulus of the human intact left ventricle—Determination and physiological interpretation. *Med Biol Eng*, 13(2):151–160.

10. Ghista DN, Zhong L, Chua LP, Ng EYK, Lim ST, Tan RS, Chua TSJ (2005) Systolic modelling of the left ventricle as a mechatronic system: Determination of myocardial fiber's sarcomere contractile characteristics and new performance indices. *Mol Cell Biomech*, 2(4):217–233.

11. Gordon DG (1976) The physics of left ventricular ejection and its implications for muscle mechanics. *Eur J Cardiol*, 4:87–95.

12. Ionescu I, Guilkey J, Berzins M, Kirby RM, Weiss J (2005) Computational simulation of penetrating trauma in biological soft tissues using the material point method. *Stud Health Technol Inform*, 111:213–218.

13. Mirsky I (1973) Ventricular and arterial wall stresses based on large deformations analyses. *Biophys J*, 13:1141–1159.

14. Nakano K, Sugawara M, Ishihara K, Kanazawa S, Corin WJ, Denslow S, Biederman RWW, Carabello BA (1990) Myocardial stiffness derived from end-systolic wall stress and logarithm of reciprocal of wall thickness: Contractility index independent of ventricular size. *Circulation*, 82:1352–1361.

15. Paladino JL, Noordergraff A (1997) Muscle contraction mechanism from ultra-structural dynamics. In: Drzewiecki GM, Li JKJ (eds.), *Analysis and Assessment of Cardiovascular Function*, Springer, New York, pp. 33–57.

16. Paladino JL, Noordergraff A (2002) A paradigm for quantifying ventricular contraction. *Cell Mol Biol Lett*, 7(2):331–335.

17. Park SJ, Miyazaki C, Bruce CJ, Ommen S, Miller FA, Oh JK (2008) Left ventricular torsion by two-dimensional speckle tracking echocardiography in patients with diastolic dysfunction and normal ejection fraction. *J Am Soc Echocardiogr*, 21:1129–1137.

18. Pietrabissa R, Montevecchi FM, Funero R. Ventricular mechanics based on sarcomere and fibre models. In: Spilker RL, Simon BR (eds.), *Computational Methods in Bioengineering*, ASME, New York, BED 9, pp. 399–410.

19. Schreuder JJ, Castiglioni A, Maisano F, Steendijk P, Donelli A, Baan J, Alfieri O (2005) Acute decrease of left ventricular mechanical dyssynchrony and improvement of contractile state and energy efficiency after left ventricular restoration. *J Thorac Cardiovasc Surg*, 129:138–145.

20. Segar DS, Moran M, Ryan T (1991) End-systolic regional wall stress-length and stress-shortening relations in an experimental model of normal, ischemic and reperfused myocardium. *J Am Coll Cardiol*, 17:1651–1660.

21. Streeter DD, Hanna WT (1973) Engineering mechanics for successive state in canine left ventricular myocardium: II Fiber angle and sarcomere length. *Circ Res*, 33:656–664.

22. Subbaraj K, Ghista DN, Fallen EL (1987) Intrinsic indices of the left ventricle as a blood pump in normal and infarcted left ventricles. *J Biomed Eng*, 9:206–215.

23. Subbaraj K, Ghista DN, Fallen DN (1985) Determination of intra-cardiac pressure and flow distributions from cineangiograms. *Automedica* 6(3):137–141.

24. Wong AYK, Rautaharju PM (1968) Stress distribution within the left ventricular wall approximated as a thick ellipsoidal shell. *Am Heart J*, 75:649–662.

25. Zhong L (2005) Biomechanical engineering indices for cardiac function and dysfunction during filling and ejection phase. PhD thesis, Nanyang Technological University, Singapore.
26. Zhong L, Ghista DN, Ng EYK, Lim SK (2005) Passive and active ventricular elastance of the left ventricle. *Biomed Eng Online*, 4:10.
27. Zhong L, Ghista DN, Ng EYK, Lim ST, Tan RS, Chua LP (2006) Explaining left ventricular pressure dynamic in terms of LV passive and active elastances. *Proc Inst Mech Eng H*, 220(5):647–655.
28. Zhong L, Tan RS, Ghista DN, Ng EYK, Chua LP, Kassab GS (2007) Validation of a novel noninvasive cardiac index of left ventricular contractility in patients. *Am J Physiol Heart Circ Physiol*, 292(6):H2764–H2772.
29. Zhong L, Sola S, Tan RS, Ghista DN, Kurra V, Navia JL, Kassab G (2009) Effect of surgical ventricular restoration on left ventricular contractility by a novel contractility index in patients with ischemic cardiomyopathy. *Am J Cardiol*, 103:674–679.

6

Analysis for Left Ventricular Pressure Increase during Isovolumic Contraction Phase due to Active Stress Development in Myocardial Fibers

Dhanjoo N. Ghista, Li Liu, and Foad Kabinejadian

CONTENTS

6.1 Introduction and Preview of the Analysis Procedure

During diastolic filling, the left ventricular (LV) wall stress builds due to the LV chamber pressure passively acting on the LV wall. This constitutes the development of passive stress. When this happens, the LV starts contracting as the myocardium is electrically activated, which in turn activates the excitation–contraction coupling mechanism of the myocardial sarcomere, resulting in contraction and stress development in the myocardial fibers. The contraction and force development in the myocardial fibers causes development of what might be termed as "active stress" in the myocardium, which in turn deforms the LV (including causing its twisting) and thereby decreases its chamber volume. This resultant high value of the bulk modulus of blood causes a substantial rise in LV pressure from the start of isovolumic contraction. However, during the isovolumic contraction phase, it is the active stress developed in the LV myocardial wall that causes LV chamber pressure rise.

The LV deforms due to the activation and contraction of its myocardial fibers, which caused by the formation of the sarcomere actin–myosin cross-bridges, resulting in the development of sarcomere contractile force and sarcomere shortening. This contraction of the helically wound myocardial fibers and the stresses (and forces) thus developed cause shortening and twisting of the LV cylindrical model and reduction in its chamber volume, and hence a sharp increase in the LV pressure. By way of analogy, let us simulate the contracted LV by a thick-walled cylinder, with a coiled muscle fiber spring located within its wall. If this spring is twisted (due to its contraction), it will shorten and squeeze the encased LV cylinder, causing substantial increase in its pressure because of the high value of the blood's bulk modulus.

For this purpose, we present a LV thick-walled cylindrical-shaped model (illustrated in Figure 6.1) and carry out an inverse analysis by employing the monitored LV pressure and its dimensions (expressed in terms of the initially monitored LV volume and myocardial volume). The deformation of this LV cylindrical model due to the monitored rise in its chamber pressure (Δp) is simulated by a decrease in its chamber volume (ΔV) in terms of its bulk modulus (K). The resulting changes in the length and radius of the LV cylindrical model are expressed in terms of this chamber volume decrease (ΔV). These changes in the LV cylindrical length and radius along with the LV twist angle (whose reasonable values are assumed in this analysis) constitute LV deformations.

By employing finite elasticity and large-deformation analysis, we then express (1) the stretches and strains within the LV cylinder wall in terms of these deformations and (2) the LV wall stresses in terms of these stretches and strains, by means of the strain energy density function and its material parameters. We then carry out the equilibrium analysis of wall stress in terms of the monitored chamber pressure. By solving these equilibrium equations, we determine the values of (1) the myocardial material parameters of the strain energy density function, (2) the stretches and strains, and (3) the stresses.

We then proceed to determine and compute the principal stresses and the principal angle. We then associate (1) the principal compressive stress with that of the contractile stress in the myocardial fibers and (2) the principal angle with the myocardial fiber angle. Thus, by means of this inverse analysis, we determine the stresses and the orientation of the activated and contracted myocardial fibers, which cause LV deformation

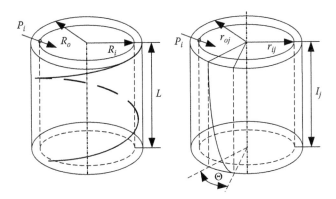

FIGURE 6.1
Schematic of fiber orientation and twisting of a left ventricle (LV) cylindrical model that simulate LV contraction and account for LV pressure rise during the isovolumic contraction phase.

(shortening and twisting) and rapid chamber pressure rise during the (0.04–0.06 s of) isovolumic contraction phase.

Finally, we determine the torque and the axial compressive force induced in the LV due to its contraction and the activation of the helically wound myocardial fibers. This induced torque, causing the twisting of the LV and the resulting chamber pressure increase, is an important aspect of the LV contraction process.

In this chapter, we determine that the LV pressure generated during isovolumic contraction and the LV twist angle are caused by the active stress in the LV wall (equivalent to LV twisting and compression), due to contractile stress in the helically wound myocardial fibers (depicted in Figure 6.1). This mechanism of LV pressure generation during isovolumic contraction is of great significance to LV systolic function, LV contractility, and LV ejection. In the process, we also obtain the constitutive properties of the myocardium, the LV active wall stresses, and most importantly the equivalent myocardial fiber orientation responsible for the LV pressure increase during isovolumic contraction.

Several studies [1–6] have shown that the architecture and orientation of myocardial fibers have significant effects on the mechanical properties of the myocardium. Based on experimental studies, myocardial fibers are found to be helically wound, at an angle varying from −60° to 60° across the LV wall [7–10]. However, there is no way this fiber orientation can be measured. Hence, in this chapter we determine the equivalent myocardial fiber orientation (averaged across the LV wall) from the orientation of the principal stresses obtained from the computed stresses in the LV wall based on the monitored LV deformation and pressure increase.

In other words, we adopt the principal stresses in the LV wall to be the stresses in the myocardial fibers. From the orientation of the principal compressive stresses, we determine the myocardial fibers orientation during isovolumic contraction. Conversely, it is intended to thereby indicate that the active stress developed in the myocardial fibers during the isovolumic contraction phase induces torque in the LV and causes LV deformation (including its twisting); this results in the compression of the LV chamber and LV pressure increase. Thereby, our model offers insight into how the myocardial fiber orientation and the stress developed in the myocardial fibers can cause LV deformation and the observed rapid LV pressure rise during the isovolumic contraction phase.

Hence, the important determinants and outcomes of our model analysis are (1) the orientation of the myocardial fibers and (2) the determination of the *LV torque versus twist angle* relationship. We deem this LV equivalent myocardial fibers orientation (EMFO) to be an intrinsic property of the LV, which governs how effectively the LV can develop pressure to effect adequate stroke volume ejection. The *LV torque versus twist angle* relationship can be employed as an additional index of contractility. In this regard, both EMFO and the *LV torque versus twist angle* relationship can come to be regarded as LV diagnostic properties characterizing LV contraction.*

6.2 LV Thick-Walled Cylindrical Model Development and Analysis

6.2.1 Monitoring of LV Chamber Pressure

Although the chapter presents a theoretical model for the mechanism of development of LV pressure during the isovolumic contraction phase, we have employed some relevant clinical data from the literature in order to develop and elucidate the model.

The subject in this study was examined in a resting recumbent (baseline) state after premedication with 100–500 mg of sodium pentobarbital by retrograde aortic catheterization. For this LV model, the chamber pressure was measured by a pigtail catheter and a Statham P23Eb pressure transducer; the pressure was recorded during ventriculography. Angiography was performed by injecting 30–36 mL of 75% sodium diatrizoate in the LV at 10–12 mL/s. Then, monoplane cineangiocardiograms were recorded in a RAO 30° projection from a 9 in. image intensifier on a 35 mm film at 50 fps using the Intergris Allura 9 system at the National Heart Centre Singapore.

Automated LV analysis was carried out to calculate LV volume and myocardial wall thickness. The LV data, derived from the cineangiographic films, consist of measured chamber volume and myocardial thickness of the chamber and the corresponding pressure. All measurements were corrected for geometric distortion due to the respective recording systems.

6.2.2 LV Cylindrical Model Dimensions

The LV data, derived from the cineangiocardiographic (cineventriculographic) measurements, consisted of LV pressure, LV volume (V), LV wall thickness (h), and LV myocardial volume (V_M). The geometrical parameters of the LV cylindrical model are defined in Figure 6.1.

The volumes of myocardial wall (V_M) and of the LV are given as

$$V_M = \pi\left(R_o^2 - R_i^2\right)L = \pi(2R_i + h)hL \tag{6.1}$$

---

* This chapter is based on our paper: Mechanism of left ventricular pressure increase during isovolumic contraction, and determination of its equivalent myocardial fibers orientation, by DN Ghista, L Li, LP Chua, L Zhong, RS Tan, and YS Tan, *Journal of Mechanics in Medicine and Biology*, 9(2), 177–198, 2009 (published by World Scientific Publishers).

$$V = \pi R_i^2 L \tag{6.2}$$

where
    V_M is the myocardial volume
    V is the ventricular chamber volume
    R_o is the outer radius
    R_i is the inner radius
    h is the wall thickness
    L is the length

Here, the LV volume (V), wall thickness (h), and myocardial volume (V_M) are obtained by cineventriculography.

Using Equations 6.1 and 6.2, we can calculate the model's instantaneous radii $R_i(t)$ and length $L(t)$ (or any time instant t) in terms of the measured V, V_M, and h, as

$$R_i = \frac{2Vh/V_M + \sqrt{(2Vh/V_M)^2 + 4Vh^2/V_M}}{2} \tag{6.3}$$

$$V = \pi R_i^2 L$$

$$L = \frac{V}{\pi R_i^2} \tag{6.4}$$

Then, $R_o = R_i + h$ and $R_m = (R_o + R_i)/2$.

As can be noted from Equations 6.3 and 6.4, the LV model length L is obtained from V, V_M, and h.

6.2.3 LV Model Mechanics Description

The LV is modeled as a thick-walled fluid-filled cylindrical elastic shell, closed at both ends, and attached to the aorta at its top base. This LV model is constrained in the longitudinal direction at its base (as depicted in Figure 6.2). The LV wall is taken to be made up of an incompressible transversely isotropic, hyperelastic material. In this model, we have simulated the phenomenon of LV isovolumic contraction (which causes the intra-LV pressure to rise very fast during 0.04–0.06 s of isovolumic contraction) by means of a finite-elasticity analysis of the thick-walled LV cylindrical shell under incremental pressure.

From the LV (radial, longitudinal, and twist) deformation and pressure increase, we have obtained the stress state in the LV wall. From the wall stress state, we determine the principal stresses, which are considered as the fiber stresses. Then from the orientation of the principal compressive stress, we determine the myocardial fibers orientation during isovolumic contraction. Conversely, it is intended to thereby indicate that it is the active stress developed in the myocardial fibers that in fact causes LV pressure increase and LV deformation (including LV twist).

In other words, the LV wall is reckoned to be made up of helically oriented myocardial fibers (as depicted in Figure 6.1), whose contraction causes compression and twisting of the LV, resulting in the rapid increase of its internal pressure. Thus, we have inversely shown

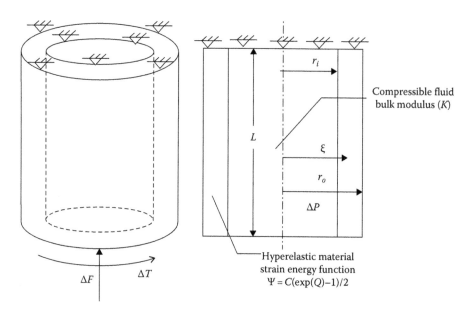

FIGURE 6.2
The fluid-filled LV cylindrical shell model: (1) geometry, (2) material property, and (3) equivalent compression and torsion associated with its internal active stress state due to the contraction of its myocardial fibers, resulting in the rapid rise of its internal pressure.

that the LV pressure generated during isovolumic contraction and the LV torque and twist angle are caused by the stress developed in the LV wall (causing LV twisting and compression), due to contractile stresses in the helically wound myocardial fibers (depicted in Figure 6.1).

6.2.4 Summary of LV Model Analysis Procedure

We approximate the LV during isovolumic contraction as a fluid-filled, thick-walled cylindrical shell that is closed at both ends and constrained in the longitudinal direction at the base (as depicted in Figure 6.2). We further consider that the LV wall behaves as an incompressible, transversely isotropic, hyperelastic material. Here is a summary of the steps involved in the model analysis:

Step 1: Starting with monitored LV dynamic geometry and LV pressure increase, we determine the corresponding LV internal volume change, based on the bulk modulus of blood. From this volume change, we characterize the radial and longitudinal deformations of the LV cylindrical model; herein, we also adopt a reasonable value of LV twist deformation (which is expected to be determinable from the current technology).

Step 2: From these deformations, we determine the corresponding stretches and therefore the strains in the LV wall using finite-elasticity formulations.

Step 3: Next, we express the LV wall stresses in terms of the LV wall strains to represent the LV wall material's constitutive property.

Step 4: We now impose the boundary conditions involving equilibrating the LV stress in the inner wall to the LV internal blood pressure. In these equations, the LV constitutive properties are unknown. By computationally solving these equations, we determine the best values of these myocardial constitute property parameters.

Step 5: Once the LV constitutive property parameters are determined, we can go back to the expressions for the LV wall stresses and evaluate the LV wall stress state. We then continue to determine the principal stresses from the obtained stress state.

Step 6: We designate the relevant principal stresses and accompanying principal stress directions to correspond to the LV myocardial fiber stress and orientations, respectively. By so doing, we can estimate the equivalent myocardial fiber angle.

Step 7: From the LV wall stress state, we can also determine the equivalent torsion (T) and compression (F) applied at the apical end of the cylindrical model (which is taken to be fixed at the base of the upper end, as illustrated in Figures 6.1 and 6.2) by active contraction of the myocardium.

6.3 LV Cylindrical Finite-Elasticity Active Stress Model Analysis: Simulation of Isovolumic Contraction Phenomenon due to Myocardial Fibers' Contraction

6.3.1 LV Deformed State Dimensions

We model the LV as an incompressible thick-walled cylindrical shell, which is constrained in the long-axis direction at one end to represent the suspension of the LV by the aorta at its base. Considering the LV at ED to be in the unloaded reference configuration, the cylindrical model in its undeformed state is represented geometrically in terms of cylindrical coordinates (R, Θ, Z) by

$$R_i \leq R \leq R_o, \quad 0 \leq \Theta \leq 2\pi, \quad 0 \leq Z \leq L \tag{6.5}$$

where R_i, R_o, and L denote the inner and outer radii and the length of the undeformed LV model, respectively. The LV model in its deformed state can then be defined in terms of cylindrical coordinates (r, θ, z) as

$$r_i \leq r \leq r_o, \quad 0 \leq \theta \leq 2\pi, \quad 0 \leq z \leq l \tag{6.6}$$

where r_i, r_o, and l denote the inner and outer radii and the length of the deformed cylindrical model, respectively.

We consider the incompressible LV model in its deformed state (r, θ, l) to be subjected to twisting and radial and axial deformations in the radial and long-axis directions during isovolumic contraction such that, based on incompressibility criterion of

$$\pi\left(R^2 - R_i^2\right)L = \pi\left(r^2 - r_i^2\right)l = \pi\left(r^2 - r_i^2\right)\lambda_z L$$

we have

$$r = \sqrt{\frac{R^2 - R_i^2}{\lambda_z} + r_i^2}, \quad \theta = \Theta + Z\frac{\Phi}{L}, \quad z = \lambda_z Z \tag{6.7}$$

where
   R_i, R, L represent the undeformed state
   r_i, r, l represent the deformed state
   λ_z is the axial stretch per unit of unloaded length
   Φ is the angle of twist measured at the apex (relative to the base)

We consider the blood in the LV cavity to be slightly compressible, based on the value of its bulk modulus ($K = 2.0 \times 10^9$ Pa). By doing so, we are allowing a small change in the LV cavity volume, as a result of the substantial pressure change during isovolumic contraction. The instantaneous change in the cavity volume (ΔV) can thus be expressed in terms of the instantaneous pressure change (Δp) and the bulk modulus (K) of blood. Hence, starting with monitored LV dynamic geometry (and hence LV volume V and myocardial volume VM) along with the LV pressure increase, we determine the corresponding LV internal volume change (based on the bulk modulus of blood) as

$$\frac{\Delta V}{V} = \frac{\Delta p}{K}; \quad K = 2 \times 10^9 \, \text{Pa} \tag{6.8}$$

From this volume change, we characterize the radial and longitudinal deformations of the LV cylindrical model as follows:

$$\Delta l = \left(1 - \sqrt[3]{1 - \frac{\Delta p}{K}}\right)L, \quad \Delta r_i = \left(1 - \sqrt[3]{1 - \frac{\Delta p}{K}}\right)R \tag{6.9}$$

$$l_j = l'_j - \Delta l_j \quad \text{and} \quad r_{ij} = r'_{ij} - \Delta r_{ij} \tag{6.10}$$

$$h_j = \sqrt{\frac{V_M/l_j + \pi r_{ij}^2}{\pi}} - r_{ij} \tag{6.11}$$

Let $\Delta\Phi$ denote the relative angle of twist measured at the apex, at each of the three stages of isovolumic contraction phase, obtained by magnetic resonance imaging (MRI). At this stage, we were unable to simultaneously measure the pressure and twist angle at different stages of the isovolumic contraction phase. Hence, we have adopted a reasonable value of LV twist deformation $\Delta\Phi$ (which can be obtained from MRI) during the isovolumic contraction phase, which is equal to 0.67°, 1.33°, and 2° at 0.02, 0.04, and 0.06 s from the start of isovolumic contraction [11,12].

Table 6.1 shows a sample patient and model data, including pressure, volume, and model deformations for the cylindrical LV model. The pressure is obtained by catheterization for different time instants. The volume (V), myocardial volume (V_M), and wall thickness (h) are measured by ventriculography at the beginning of isovolumic contraction ($t = 0$).

The cylindrical model radius R_i, R_o, and L are calculated using Equations 6.3 and 6.4. Then the ΔV_j, Δr_{ij}, and Δl_j are calculated using Equations 6.8 and 6.9 for the time instants ($t = 0.02$, 0.04, 0.06); therefrom, the V, r_{ij}, and l_j are obtained. The wall thickness h_j for the cylindrical model is calculated using Equation 6.11. The outer radius r_{oj} is then obtained ($= r_{ij} + h_j$).

6.3.2 Large Deformation Stretches and Strains

From these deformations, we determine the corresponding stretches and therefore the strains in the LV wall using finite-elasticity formulations [13]:

$$\lambda_z(R) = \frac{l}{L}, \quad \lambda_r(R) = \frac{\partial r}{\partial R} = \frac{R}{r\lambda_z}, \quad \lambda_\theta(R) = \frac{r\partial\theta}{R\partial\Theta} = \frac{r}{R} \tag{6.12}$$

$$\lambda_\Phi(r) = \gamma = \frac{r\partial\theta}{\partial z} = \frac{r\Delta\Phi}{l} \tag{6.13}$$

The components of the Green–Lagrange strain tensor (E_{ij}) can thus be expressed in terms of the stretches and deformations [13]:

$$E_{rr} = \frac{1}{2}\left(\lambda_r^2 - 1\right), \quad E_{\theta\theta} = \frac{1}{2}\left(\lambda_\theta^2 - 1\right), \quad E_{zz} = \frac{1}{2}\left(\lambda_z^2(1+\gamma^2) - 1\right), \quad E_{\theta z} = \frac{\gamma\lambda_z\lambda_\theta}{2} \tag{6.14}$$

6.3.3 LV Myocardial Constitutive Property

The LV myocardial constitutive property is expressed as the strain energy density function in terms of the LV wall strains. For the myocardium material, we assume a Fung-type exponential strain energy density function Ψ of the form [14]

$$\Psi = \frac{C(\exp(Q) - 1)}{2} \tag{6.15}$$

where Q characterizes the material's transverse isotropy in the cylindrical polar coordinate system and is given by [15]

$$Q = b_1 E_{\theta\theta}^2 + b_2 E_{zz}^2 + b_3 E_{rr}^2 + 2b_4 E_{\theta\theta}E_{zz} + 2b_5 E_{rr}E_{zz} + 2b_6 E_{\theta\theta}E_{rr} + 2b_7 E_{\theta z}^2 + 2b_8 E_{rz}^2 + 2b_9 E_{\theta r}^2 \tag{6.16}$$

where
  b_i ($i = 1, 2, \ldots, 9$) are the nondimensional material parameters
  $E_{i,j}$ ($i, j = R, \Theta, Z$) are components of the modified Green–Lagrange strain tensor referred
    to as the cylindrical polar coordinates (R, Θ, Z)

TABLE 6.1

Pressure–Volume and Model Deformation for a Sample Subject with $VM = 185$ mL

t (s)	P (mmHg)	ΔP (mmHg)	V (mL)	ΔV (mL)	r_{ij} (cm)	Δr_{ij} (cm)	l_j (cm)	Δl_j (cm)	h_j (cm)	r_{oj} (cm)	$\Delta \Phi$ (°)
0	18		1.3670000E +02		2.03208400E +00 (=R_i)		1.053745000E + 01 (=L)		1.085247000E + 00	3.117331000E + 00 (R_o)	0
0.02	43	25	1.36699773E +02	2.27263750E − 04	2.032083992E + 00	8.46701669E − 09	1.053744996E + 01	4.39060418E − 08	1.085246679E + 00	3.117330670E + 00	0.667
0.04	63	45	1.36699591E +02	4.09074750E − 04	2.032083985E + 00	1.52406301E − 08	1.053744992E + 01	7.90308757E − 08	1.085246684E + 00	3.117330669E + 00	1.333
0.06	81	63	1.3669427E +02	5.72704650E − 04	2.032083979E + 00	2.13368822E − 08	1.053744989E + 01	1.10643226E − 07	1.085246689E + 00	3.117330667E + 00	2.00

6.3.4 Expressions for LV Wall Stresses

We now express the LV Cauchy stress tensor (and the wall stresses) in terms of the strain energy density function Ψ, and hence in terms of the LV wall stretches and strains.

$$\sigma_{\theta\theta} = \lambda_\theta^2 \frac{\partial \Psi}{\partial E_{\theta\theta}} + 2\gamma\lambda_z\lambda_\theta \frac{\partial \Psi}{\partial E_{\theta z}} + \gamma^2\lambda_z^2 \frac{\partial \Psi}{\partial E_{zz}} - \bar{p}$$

$$\sigma_{rr} = \lambda_r^2 \frac{\partial \Psi}{\partial E_{rr}} - \bar{p}, \quad \sigma_{zz} = \lambda_z^2 \frac{\partial \Psi}{\partial E_{zz}} - \bar{p}, \quad \sigma_{\theta z} = \lambda_z\lambda_\theta \frac{\partial \Psi}{\partial E_{\theta z}} + \gamma\lambda_z^2 \frac{\partial \Psi}{\partial E_{zz}} \tag{6.17}$$

where
  $\bar{p}$ denotes the hydrostatic pressure
  Ψ is defined in Equations 6.15 and 6.16

In order to reduce the mathematical complexity of the problem, we assume negligible transverse shear strains during isovolumic contraction. Thus, the strains E_{rz} and $E_{\theta r}$ in Equation 6.16 and their corresponding stress components (i.e., σ_{rz} and $\sigma_{\theta r}$) are neglected in the analysis.

6.3.5 Stress Equilibrium Relation and Boundary Conditions

The stress equilibrium relation (in the cylindrical coordinate system) is given by

$$\frac{d\sigma_{rr}}{dr} + \frac{(\sigma_{rr} - \sigma_{\theta\theta})}{r} = 0 \tag{6.18}$$

where σ_{rr} and $\sigma_{\theta\theta}$ denote the radial and circumferential stresses, respectively.
  We now impose the boundary conditions, involving equilibrating the LV radial stress in the inner wall to the LV internal blood pressure:

$$\sigma_{rr}(r = r_0) = 0; \quad \sigma_{rr}(r = r_i) = -p_i \tag{6.19}$$

where p_i denotes the internal or cavity blood pressure acting on the inner surface of the LV model.
  By integrating Equation 6.18, we obtain the Cauchy radial stress σ_{rr} as

$$\sigma_{rr}(r) = \int_{r_i}^{r_0} (\sigma_{rr} - \sigma_{\theta\theta}) \frac{dr}{r}, \quad sr_i \leq r \leq r_0 \tag{6.20}$$

Substituting this into the boundary condition in Equation 6.19, the internal pressure p_i can be denoted as

$$p_i = -\int_{r_i}^{r_0} (\sigma_{rr} - \sigma_{\theta\theta}) \frac{dr}{r} \tag{6.21}$$

Since both the LV valves are closed during isovolumic contraction, we impose a set of boundary conditions at both the top and bottom of the internal LV surface, giving

$$\sigma_{zz}\pi\left(r_o^2 - r_i^2\right) = p_i\left(\pi r_{si}^2\right) \tag{6.22}$$

where σ_{zz} denotes the axial component of the Cauchy stresses.

6.3.6 Determination of Myocardial Constitutive Property and Wall Stresses

By integrating Equation 6.21 along with the boundary condition described in Equation 6.22, we can determine the (best values of the) myocardial constitutive property parameters b_i, $(i = 1, 2, ..., 9)$ and $\bar{p}$, by using a nonlinear least squares method. For the sample case shown in Table 6.1, the myocardial material property parameters are determined and shown in Table 6.2 ($b_1 = 5{,}946.2278$, $b_2 = 15{,}690.58158$, $b_3 = 422.514993$, $b_4 = 16{,}157.10454$, $b_5 = 16{,}360.53744$, $b_6 = 33{,}299.28998$, $b_7 = 680.7385218$, $b_8 = 0$, $b_9 = 0$).

After the LV constitutive property parameters are determined (as in Table 6.2), we determine (1) the stretches from Equations 6.12 and 6.13, as shown in Table 6.3, and therefrom (2) the strains $E_{i,j}$ from Equation 6.14 and the strain energy density function Ψ from Equations 6.15 and 6.16.

Then, by substituting the computed strain components (E_{ij}) and the strain energy density function (Ψ) into Equation 6.17, we determine the LV wall stress components (as shown in Tables 6.4 and 6.5).

6.3.7 Principal Stresses, Strains, and Angle

We now continue to determine the principal stresses, strains, and angles from the obtained stress state as follows:

$$\sigma_{1,2} = \frac{\sigma_{zz} + \sigma_{\theta\theta}}{2} \pm \sqrt{\left(\frac{\sigma_{zz} - \sigma_{\theta\theta}}{2}\right)^2 + \sigma_{\theta z}^2} \tag{6.23}$$

$$E_{1,2} = \frac{E_{zz} + E_{\theta\theta}}{2} \pm \sqrt{\left(\frac{E_{zz} - E_{\theta\theta}}{2}\right)^2 + E_{\theta z}^2} \tag{6.24}$$

$$\tan 2\phi = \frac{2\sigma_{\theta z}}{\sigma_{\theta\theta} - \sigma_{zz}} = \frac{2E_{\theta z}}{E_{\theta\theta} - E_{zz}} \tag{6.25}$$

The computed wall stresses and the principal stresses are also shown in Table 6.5. We designate the compressive principal stresses and the corresponding principal stress directions to correspond to the LV myocardial fiber stress and orientations, respectively. By so doing, we can estimate the equivalent myocardial fiber angle (found to vary from 38° to 33° during the isovolumic contraction phase). The estimated fiber angles' values correspond to those obtained from experimental studies [1–3]. Also, it is shown later on that the computed magnitude of the compressive principal stress at the end of the isovolumic contraction phase is found to be in the same range as the maximum isometric tension value, which lends credibility to our analysis.

TABLE 6.2

Parameters of the Strain Energy Function for the Sample Case Shown in Table 6.1

Parameter	b_1	b_2	b_3	b_4	b_5	b_6	b_7	b_8	b_9
Value	5,946.2278	15,690.58158	422.514993	16,157.10454	16,360.53744	33,299.28998	680.7385218	0	0

TABLE 6.3

Stretches Calculated from Equations 6.10 and 6.11 for the Sample Case Shown in Table 6.1

T	λ_z	λ_r	$\lambda\theta$	$\lambda\phi (= \gamma)$
0				
0.02	0.9999999958	1.000000008E+00	9.9999996E-01	1.28626948E-01
0.04	0.9999999925	1.000000015E+00	9.9999993E-01	2.56482520E-01
0.06	0.9999999895	1.000000021E+00	9.9999990E-01	3.85688000E-01

TABLE 6.4

Radial Stress Distributions (in pa) Along the LV Wall from the Endocardium to the Epicardium

t (s)	Endocardium									Epicardium
0	0	1.99E−02	1.02E−01	2.37E−01	4.08E−01	0.591715	0.762765	0.89833	0.98014	1
0.02	−24.0809	−23.4615	−17.2801	−12.9839	−8.73378	−4.9888	−2.11726	−0.41173	−0.2144	0
0.04	−44.2917	−43.1341	−31.6543	−23.7482	−15.9694	−9.13029	−3.88098	−0.75569	−0.3542	0
0.06	−6.21E+01	−6.05E+01	−5.43E+01	−4.48E+01	−3.39E+01	−2.31E+01	−1.34E+01	−5.75E+00	−1.13E+00	0

TABLE 6.5

Results for the Sample Subject at Different Time Instants

	Results								
t (s)	Circumferential Stress (Pa)	Radial Stress (Pa)	Axial Force (N)	Torque (Nm)	Axis Stress (Pa)	Shear Stress (Pa)	Principal Stress–Tension (Pa)	Principal Stress–Compression (Pa)	Principal Direction (°)
0	0.00	0.00	0.00	0.00	0.00E+00	0.00E+00	0.00	0.00	
0.02	3358.33	−2844.53	−13.51	0.38	−1.35E+04	3.29E+04	28,221.68	−38,395.38	37.82
0.04	5318.61	−5956.38	−46.06	0.89	−4.70E+04	8.21E+04	63,836.28	−105,547.96	36.18
0.06	4481.83	−8530.94	−102.38	1.30	−1.04E+05	1.22E+05	81,673.18	−180,897.35	33.02

6.3.8 Equivalent Torsion (ΔT) and Axial Compression (ΔF) Applied at the Apical End (Due to LV Contraction)

From the LV wall stress state, we can also determine the equivalent torsion (*T*) and compression (*F*) applied at the apical end of the cylindrical model (which is taken to be fixed at the base of the upper end) by the active contraction of the myocardium. We can hence obtain the relationship between LV torsion and twist angle, which is a key determinant of this work.

$$\Delta F = 2\pi \int_{r_i}^{r_o} \sigma_{zz} r \, dr \tag{6.26}$$

$$\Delta T = 2\pi \int_{r_i}^{r_o} \sigma_{\theta z} r^2 \, dr \tag{6.27}$$

6.4 Results

6.4.1 Flowchart of Procedure to Compute Principal Stresses

Figure 6.3 provides the methodology to compute the principal stresses and their orientation from the measurements data obtained through the analysis in Section 6.3.

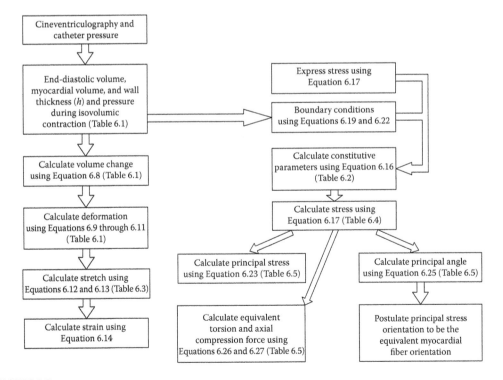

FIGURE 6.3
Flowchart shows how we determine the principal stresses in the LV cylindrical wall and assign these stresses to be the myocardial fiber stresses.

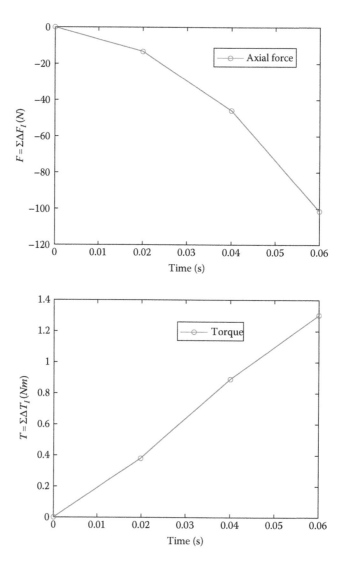

FIGURE 6.4
Variations of axial force and torque induced within the LV as functions of time during the isovolumic contraction phase.

6.4.2 Active Torque and Axial Compressive Force Induced in the LV

The variations of the induced equivalent active torque ΔT and axial compressive force ΔF (Equations 6.26 and 6.27) during the isovolumic contraction phase are calculated and shown in Figure 6.4. This demonstrates that the large increment of internal pressure in the LV cavity during the isovolumic phase is caused by the corresponding torque and axial force developed within the LV, due to the contraction of the LV myocardial fibers.

6.4.3 LV Myocardial Wall Stresses

The variations in the LV wall radial and circumferential stresses (σ_{rr}, $\sigma\theta\theta$) and axial and shear stresses (σ_{zz}, $\sigma\theta_z$) are shown in Table 6.5 and Figure 6.5. It can be seen that all the

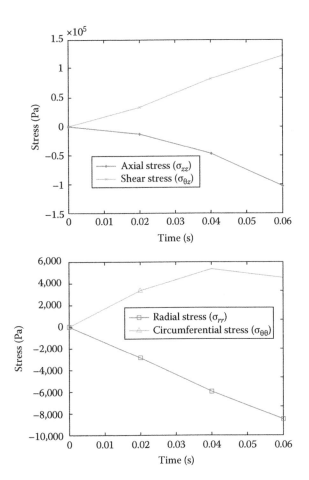

FIGURE 6.5
Variations of axial, shear, radial, and circumferential stresses as functions of time during the isovolumic contraction phase.

stresses increase in magnitude during the isovolumic contraction phase; the axial and shear stresses are much greater in magnitude than the circumferential and radial stresses in the LV wall.

The radial stress distribution along the thickness of the LV wall at different times is shown in Table 6.4 and Figure 6.6. The radial stress also increases in magnitude during the isovolumic contraction phase; it has its maximum magnitude at the endocardium (equal to the LV internal pressure) and is zero at the epicardium.

6.4.4 Principal Stresses and Principal Angle

We then display the time variations of the principal stress and the corresponding angle during the isovolumic phase (whose values are given in Table 6.3) in Figure 6.7. The notable result from Figure 6.7 is that both the principal stresses and their orientation angle keep changing during the isovolumic phase. At the end of the isovolumic phase, the magnitude of the compressive principal stress is around 1.75×10^5 Pa, which is in good agreement with the isometric tension value of 1.45×10^5 Pa achieved under maximal activation [16].

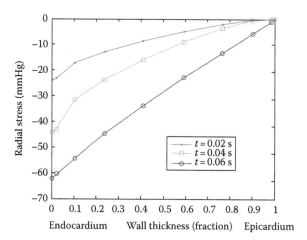

FIGURE 6.6
Radial stress distributions along the LV wall.

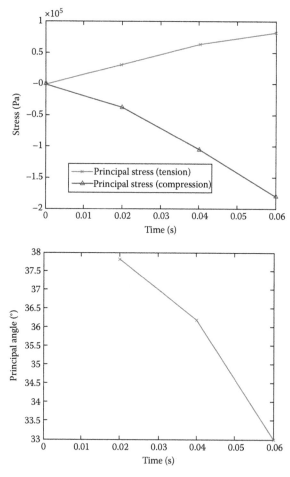

FIGURE 6.7
Variations of the principal stresses and the corresponding angle as functions of time during the isovolumic contraction phase.

It is seen from Figure 6.7 that the equivalent myocardial fiber orientation is 38° at the start of isovolumic contraction, and as the LV twists it becomes 33° at the end of the isovolumic phase. In other words, the monitored internal pressure increase during isovolumic phase from 25 to 45 to 63 mmHg is attributed to the active contraction of the helically woven myocardial fibers from 38° to 33°, which causes increasing torque as depicted in Figures 6.4 and 6.10a. It is noteworthy that the computed equivalent myocardial fiber orientation is in the range of the values determined experimentally [17,18].

The variations of principal stresses and the corresponding principal angle, along the LV wall thickness during isovolumic phase are shown in Figure 6.8. The principal stresses (tension and compression) do not vary much from the endocardium to the epicardium. However, the principal angle increases slightly from the endocardium to the epicardium during the isovolumic contraction phase.

6.4.5 Principal Stress versus Principal Strain: Constitutive Relationship of the Myocardial Fibers

We now compute the principal stress and principal strain during the three stages of isovolumic contraction, based on Equations 6.23 and 6.24. The results of principal stress versus principal strain are plotted and depicted in Figure 6.9.

This principal stress versus principal strain variation (in Figure 6.9) represents the constitutive relationship of the "activated" (or contracted) myocardial fiber. This relationship can be expressed by the constitutive property:

Principal stress (σ_1) = Initial (or pre-contraction) stress (σ_0) + Elastic modulus (E_m)·Strain (ε)

$$(6.28)$$

where
  σ_0 represents the stress in the fiber at the start of isovolumic contraction (or at the end of the filling phase)
  E_m represents the elastic modulus of the activated fiber

The values of σ_0 and E_m are computed to be σ_0 = 30,000 Pa and E_m = 10^6 Pa. In other words, at the end of the filling phase, the principal stress has a magnitude of 30,000 Pa, due to the LV filling pressure. Then with the contraction of the LV and the activation of the myocardial fibers, the fibers undergo compressive strain and develop the corresponding active (compressive) stress.

This constitutive relationship can enable us to characterize the LV myocardial fibers in terms of their constitutive relationship. Down the road, when we determine this fiber constitutive property for various patients, we will be able to indicate the normal ranges of constitutive properties and (based on that) their pathological ranges for cardiomyopathic LVs. We expect that in cardiomyopathic LVs, the values of myocardial fiber modulus (E) and the fiber angle will diminish, indicating reduced contractility of the LV.

6.4.6 Induced Torque versus Twist Angle and Principal Angle versus Twist Angle

The projected relationship between the torque induced in the LV and the twist angle is shown in Figure 6.10a. In other words, based on the myocardial fiber constitutive relationship displayed in Figure 6.9, if we increase the rotate or twist angle (beyond 2°), then the corresponding torque causing this twist is shown by this relationship. This shows that with increased contraction

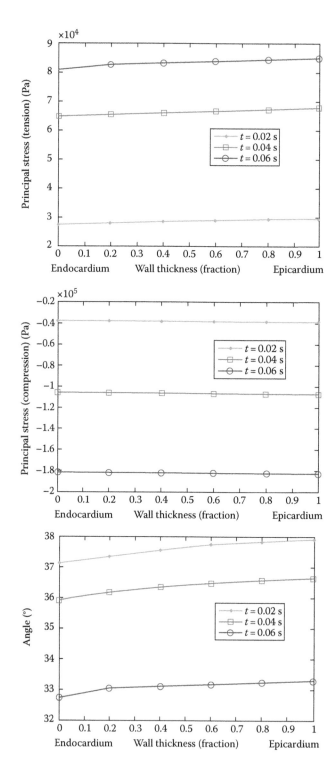

FIGURE 6.8
Variations of the principal stresses and the corresponding principal angle along LV wall thickness during the isovolumic contraction phase.

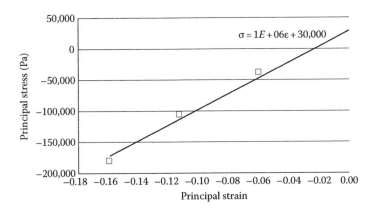

FIGURE 6.9
Principal stress versus principal strain.

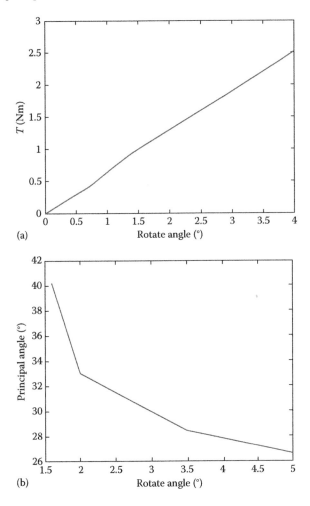

FIGURE 6.10
Relation between (a) the torque induced in the LV and the rotate (or twist) angle, and (b) between the principal stress angle and the rotate (or twist) angle during the isovolumic contraction phase.

the torque induced in the LV increases and consequently the twist angle also increases. This "torque versus twist angle" relationship can be considered a contractile property of the LV.

Likewise, the projected relationship between the principal stress angle and the twist (or rotate) angle is also shown in Figure 6.10b. It is seen that as the twist angle increases from 2° to 3.5° to 5°, the principal angle decreases from 33° to 28.5° to 26.5°. In other words, with increasing contraction and induced torque in the LV, the myocardial fibers become less inclined and the LV twist angle increases.

6.5 Concluding Comments

By determining the compressive principal stress or the fiber stress from the LV pressure and deformations data, we have indirectly demonstrated that the LV pressure buildup is due to the contraction of the LV spiral-wound myocardial fibers. This work also enables us to provide a measure of the equivalent LV myocardial fiber orientation (taken to be equal to the compressive principal stress angle). In other words, what is implied is that for known LV pressure rise and twist angle, we can determine the LV myocardial fiber orientations and stresses that cause this LV deformed state.

We can now postulate that this equivalent myocardial fiber orientation of the LV constitutes an intrinsic property of the LV that governs its contractility. Taking into consideration that it is not possible to measure the in vivo wall fiber orientation, the determination of this equivalent fiber orientation is an important outcome of this work, because it provides us an important clue as to why some persons' LVs are not able to effectively raise the pressure and are more prone to impaired contractility and hence reduced cardiac output and stroke volume.

We have shown that the incremental intra-LV pressures (Δp_i) and LV deformations during isovolumic contraction are associated with and result in the development of incremental torsion, axial compression, and incremental principal stresses in the LV. The compressive principal stress corresponds to the active contractile stress generated in the myocardial fibers, while the angle of the compressive principal stress corresponds to the myocardial fiber helical angle, which is in agreement with the experimental data on the fiber angle.

Conversely, we have been able to analytically demonstrate how the contraction of the helically wound and specifically oriented myocardial fibers causes deformation and twisting of the LV, and thereby results in substantial increase in LV pressure during the isovolumic contraction phase.

References

1. Streeter Jr. DD, Basset DL, An engineering analysis of myocardial fiber orientation in pig's left ventricle in systole, *Anat Rec*, 155:503–511, 1966.
2. Streeter Jr. DD, Hanna WT, Engineering mechanics for successive states in canine left ventricular myocardium: I. Cavity and wall geometry, *Circ Res*, 33:639–655, 1973.
3. Streeter Jr. DD, Hanna WT, Engineering mechanics for successive states in canine left ventricular myocardium: II, Fiber angle and sarcomere length, *Circ Res*, 33:656–664, 1973.

4. Yin FCP, Strumpf RK, Chew PH, Zeger SL, Quantification of the mechanical properties of noncontracting canine myocardium under simultaneous biaxial loading, *J Biomech*, 20:577–589, 1987.

5. Nielsen PMF, LeGrice IJ, Smail BH, Hunter PJ, A mathematical model of the geometry and fibrous structure of the heart, *Am J Physiol*, 260:H1365–H1378, 1991.

6. Costa KD, Holmes JW, McCulloch AD, Modeling cardiac mechanical properties in three dimensions, *Philos Trans R Soc Lond A*, 359:1233–1250, June 2001.

7. Mirsky I, Basic terminology and formulae for left ventricular wall stress, in *Cardiac Mechanics: Physiological, Clinical, and Mathematical Considerations*, Mirsky I, Ghista DN, and Sandler H (eds.), Wiley, New York, pp. 3–10, 1974.

8. Moriarty TF, The law of Laplace, its limitations as a relation for diastolic pressure, volume or wall stress of the left ventricle, *Circ Res*, 46:321–331, 1980.

9. Wong AYK, Rautaharju PM, Stress distribution within the left ventricular wall approximated as a thick ellipsoidal shell, *Am Heart J*, 75:649–662, 1968.

10. Mirsky I, Ventricular and arterial wall stresses based on large deformations analyses, *Biophysical J*, 13:1141–1159, 1973.

11. Nagel E, Stuber M, Burkhard B, Fischer SE, Scheidegger MB, Boesiger P, Hess OM, Cardiac rotation and relaxation in patients with aortic valve stenosis, *Eur Heart J*, 21:582–589, 2000.

12. Henson RE, Song SK, Pastorek JS, Ackerman JJH, Lorenz CH, Left ventricular torsion is equal in mice and humans, *Am J Physiol Circ Physiol*, 278:1117–1123, 2000.

13. Holzapfel GA, Gasser T, A new constitutive framework for arterial wall mechanics and a comparative study of material models, *J Elas*, 61:1–48, 2000.

14. Guccoine JM, McCulloch AD, Waldman LK, Passive material properties of the intact ventricular myocardium determined from a cylindrical model, *ASME J Biomech Eng*, 113:42–55, 1991.

15. Azhari H, Buchalter M, Sideman S, Shapiro E, Beyar R, A conical model to describe the nonuniformity of the left ventricular twisting motion, *Ann Biomed Eng*, 20:149–165, 1992.

16. Arts T, Reneman RS, Veenstra PC, A model of the mechanics of the left ventricle, *Ann Biomed Eng*, 7:299–318, 1979.

17. Streeter Jr. DD, Hanna WT, Engineering mechanics for successive states in canine left ventricular myocardium: I. Cavity and wall geometry, *Circ Res*, 33:639–655, 1973.

18. Streeter Jr. DD, Hanna WT, Engineering mechanics for successive states in canine left ventricular myocardium: II. Fiber angle and sarcomere length, *Circ Res*, 33:656–664, 1973.

7

Left Ventricular Remodeling due to Myocardial Infarction and its Surgical Ventricular Restoration

Dhanjoo N. Ghista, Yi Su, Liang Zhong, Ghassan S. Kassab, and Ru San Tan

CONTENTS

7.1 Introduction

In this chapter, we present the course of (1) left ventricular (LV) cardiomyopathy (with myocardial infarcts) progressing to heart failure (HF) through cardiac remodeling and decreased contractility, and (2) recovery of LV through surgical ventricular restoration (SVR), by restoration of myocardial ischemic segments, reversal of remodeling, and improvement in contractility.*

---

* This chapter is based on Cardiac myocardial disease states cause left ventricular remodeling with decreased contractility and lead to heart failure; Interventions by coronary arterial bypass grafting and surgical ventricular restoration can reverse LV remodeling with improved contractility, D Ghista et al., *Biomedical Science, Engineering and Technology*, DN Ghista, ed., InTech, 2011, ISBN 978-953-307-471-9.

For this purpose, we first provide a methodology for the detection of myocardial infarcts. Then, we characterize LV remodeling of cardiomyopathy (with myocardial infarcts) in terms of reduced change in curvedness from end-diastole to end-systole. We provide clinical studies of remodeled LV cardiomyopathy, in terms of reduced values of curvedness and contractility indices. In regards to the contractility index, in Chapter 3 we have presented a new index for cardiac contractility, in terms of maximal rate-of-change of normalized wall stress, and have demonstrated its effectiveness as a marker of HF.

Then, by way of therapeutic interventions, we show that SVR, in conjunction with CABG, is seen to benefit the ischemic-infarcted heart, by (1) restoration of cardiac remodeling index of "end-diastolic to end-systolic curvedness change," (2) reduction of regional wall stresses, and (3) augmentation of the cardiac contractility index value.

In Sections 7.2 and 7.3, we provide the myocardial sarcomere contraction model and detection of infarcted myocardial segments as highly reflectile echo zones (HREZs) in 2D B-scan echocardiograms. Now myocardial infarction (MI) reduces the contractile capacity of the LV, and hence the LV is unable to attain its tight contracted curved shape in systole. In other words, the LV undergoes remodeling and its systolic shape curvedness decreases. So in Section 7.4, we provide indices to quantify this remodeling phenomenon, in terms of local curvedness index and diastole-to-systole change in curvedness (%ΔC). Then, we present a study involving 10 normal subjects and 11 patients after MI. It is seen that the diastole-to-systole change in curvedness (%ΔC) is significantly lower in MI patients compared to the normal group, which characterizes or quantifies LV remodeling following myocardial infarct.

Then in Section 7.5, we present a study showing how SVR, combined with CABG is able to increase (1) the diastolic–systolic change in sphericity index SI (i.e., $SI_{ED}-SI_{ES}$), as well as (2) the value of the contractility index $d\sigma^*/dt_{max}$.

So in this chapter, we are showing how the LV undergoes remodeling and its curvedness index decreases due to increase in the amount of MI segments. As MI progresses into HF, the LV size increases, LV function deteriorates, and symptoms of HF become evident. Thus, cardiac remodeling (expressed in terms of the regional curvedness of the LV) constitutes a measure of the progression of HF after MI. It is seen that intervention by SVR combined with CABG causes some reversal of this LV remodeling process and improved mortality in patients with HF. Hence in this chapter we demonstrate how the three indices of percentage volume of MI segments, curvedness index, and contractility index enable us to track and assess LV progression to HF, and its recovery following CABG and SVR intervention.

7.2 Myocardial Infarction: What it Entails

In approximately two-thirds of congestive heart failure (CHF) cases, the etiology is coronary artery disease that may be accompanied with myocardial infarcts. The infarcted myocardial wall compromises adequate contraction of the wall. The end result of an infarcted LV is poor LV motion and intra-LV pressure-gradient distribution which causes impaired outflow into the aorta.

In the infarcted myocardial segments, the infrastructure of actin and myosin filaments (and their cross-bridges) is disrupted, and hence there is no contraction within these

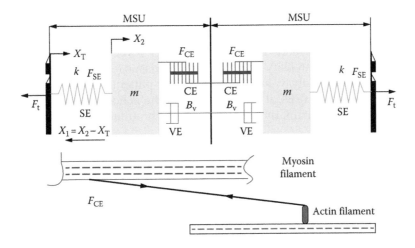

FIGURE 7.1
Based on the conventional Hill three-element model and Huxley cross-bridge theory, we have developed a myocardial model involving the LV myocardial mass, series-elastic element (CE). In this figure, we have linked the anatomical associations of these myocardial model elements with microscopic structure of the heart muscle. The sarcomere element contractile model is illustrated, involving the effective mass (m) of the muscle tissue that is accelerated, elastic parameter k of the series element stress σ_{SE} (k = elastic modulus of the sarcomere), viscous damping parameter B of the stress σ_{VE} in the parallel viscous element VE, the generated contractile stress σ_{CE} between myosin (thick) and actin (thin) filaments.

infarcted regions. Figure 7.1 illustrates a myocardial sarcomere model, composed of two symmetrical myocardial structural units (MSUs). In these MSUs, the contractile elements represent the actin–myosin contractile components of the sarcomere segment. The disruptions of these contractile elements impair the contractile capability of that sarcomere segment. Hence, a LV with infarcted myocardial segments will have diminished contractility, inadequate intra-LV flow, and poor ejection.

7.3 Detection of Myocardial Infarcted Segments

Infarcted myocardial segments can be detected as HREZs in 2D B-scan echocardiograms. In this context, we have shown how infarcted myocardial segments can be detected (in shape and size), by echo-texture analysis, as HREZs. Each myocardial tissue component of the heart generates a gray scale pattern or texture related to the tissue density and fibrous content. In diseased states (such as myocardial ischemia, myocardial fibrosis, and infiltrative diseases), changes in myocardial tissue density have been recognized by employing echo intensity and mean gray level of pixel as the basis for recognition of such myocardial disorders. It is found that hyper-reflectile echoes (HREs) correlated well with diseased cardiac muscle, and that myocardial tissue containing HREs corresponded with foci of sub-endocardial necrosis and even calcification.

In our study [1], echocardiograms were recorded, and each image was made up of 256 × 256 pixels, with each pixel having a resolution of 0–256 gray scales to determine HREZs. The echocardiographic images were digitized into 256 gray scales and the echo-intensity levels from normal infants were used to delineate the range of echo intensities for normal tissues. The upper bound of the echo intensity was set to 100% in each normal infant, and the intensities from the rest of the image were referenced to this level. Normally, the pericardium had the highest intensity level, and it was found that the upper bound of the echo-intensity value for healthy tissue (expressed as a percentage of the pericardial echo-intensity value) was 54.2%. For patients whose echo-texture analysis showed presence of HREs, it was found that the echocardiographic of the HREs from these patients were distinctly higher than the echo-intensity range of normal tissue (as depicted in Table 7.1).

Myocardial tissue pixels having echo-intensity values greater than 200 are generally noted to be infarcted. This infarcted region's echo-intensity values can remain unaffected

TABLE 7.1

Echo-Intensity Values for Various Anatomic Regions of Diseased Pediatric Hearts (Based on Long-Axis View)

Patient (sex)	Region A	Region B	Region C	Region D	HRE and its location
B (M)	M: 167.44	54.76	51.02	82.20	105.74
	SD: 25.00	28.2	17.71	24.68	30.88
	N: 65	84	75	31	65
	P: 100	32.7	30.5	49.1	63.1
					Septum
P (F)	148.76	61.73	79.81	61.7	108.18
	26.78	23.02	22.05	24.2	13.03
	50	75	47	49	40
	100	41.5	53.8	41.5	72.6
					Septum
Br (M)	141.65	68.3	69.3	33.93	89.412
	29.56	26.8	24.8	24.4	28.0
	40	40	49	44	79
	100	41.5	53.8	41.5	73.1
					Septum
F (F)	157.34	50.1	60.8	53.8	112.1
	30.0	29.5	18.8	22.7	10.3
	35	45	49	44	31
	100	31.8	38.6	34.2	71.2
					R. ventricle
HI (M)	168.1	54.7	58.2	62.4	96.4
	21.35	21.8	16.9	20.0	14.7
	47	36	35	37	49
	100	32.5	34.6	37.1	57.3
					L. ventricle
G (M)	117.7	46.9	45.5	42.7	85.3
	20.6	19.0	20.6	19.1	22.6
	45	44	40	49	37
	100	39.8	38.7	36.2	72.5
					R. ventricle

Source: Kamath, M.V. et al., *Eng. Med.*, 15(3), 137, 1986.
The numbers in the four rows represent mean (M), standard deviation (SD), number of pixels (N), percentage of posterior pericardial intensity (P).
A, posterior pericardium; B, anterior myocardium; C, posterior myocardium; D, septum.

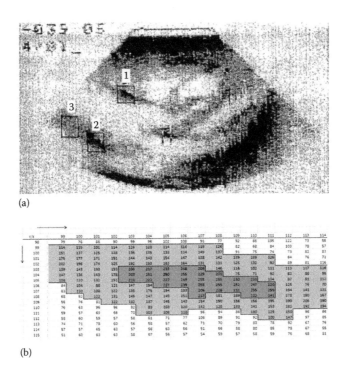

(a)

(b)

FIGURE 7.2

(a) Long-axis view of a pediatric patient's heart showing HRE regions 1 and 2 and a healthy region 3 [1]. (b) Pixel values corresponding to highly reflectile echo region 1. The central region having echo-intensity values greater than 200 is infarcted, while the immediately surrounding region shown in lighter shade is ischemic.

by administration of a myocardial perfusing agent. This infarcted subregion is seen to be surrounded by an ischemic subregion whose pixels are noted to have echo-intensity values between 100 and 200. This ischemic region's echo intensity can be reduced by the administration of a myocardial perfusion agent. The surrounding healthy tissue has echo-intensity value less than 100. Figure 7.2a depicts an echo image of an infant with visible scars regions 1 and 2, while Figure 7.2b depicts printouts of the echo intensities from these two regions, wherein the infarcted segments are depicted in dark color and the surrounding ischemic segments are depicted in a lighter shade.

In this way, in each HREZ made up of, for example, N number of pixels, we can determine the number (I) of infarcted pixels. The ratio I/N represents the infarcted potion of that HREZ myocardial segment. The total number of all the infarcted pixels in all the HREZs provides an indication of the amount of infarcted myocardium of the heart or of the LV.

7.4 Cardiac Remodeling following Myocardial Infarction and Progression to Heart Failure

Myocardial infarction reduces the amount of contractile myocardium, which in turn reduces the LV contractile capacity for pumping adequate cardiac output (CO). As MI extends, it may progress into HF. A manifestation of MI and its decreased contractile capacity is the inability of the LV to retain its compact systolic curved shape. In other words, in MI-induced HF, the LV undergoes remodeling and its curvedness index decreases. As MI progresses into HF, LV size increases, LV function deteriorates, and symptoms of HF become evident. Thus, cardiac remodeling (expressed in terms of regional curvedness of the LV) constitutes a measure of the progression of HF after MI, and interventions causing some reversal of this LV remodeling process have been shown to improve mortality in patients with HF. Therefore, reversal of LV remodeling (through medical or surgical treatment) has been emerging as a therapeutic target in HF of all etiologies.

The challenge is now to develop specific measures of LV remodeling that can be incorporated into the clinical management pathway. For patients with HF after MI, the LV shape is more spherical in terms of the global sphericity index. Focus on global sphericity index may be misleading, however, since the simple plane ratio reflects a linear alteration in the two axes of the LV chamber. Hence, regional curvedness index, determined from 3D magnetic resonance imaging (MRI)-based LV model, is proposed as a measure of LV shape. The curvedness value describes the magnitude of the curvature at a surface point (a measure of degree of curvature at a point) and the regional curvedness describes the curvedness of the segment of the LV. In MI patients, the regional curvedness index value does not increase significantly from end-diastole to end-systole (due to decreased LV contractile capacity), as in the case of normal subjects.

Since the LV cannot generate adequate contractile force in HF following MI, the overall LV contractility index of maximal rate-of-change of normalized systolic wall stress $d\sigma^*/dt_{max}$ is decreased, and the LV ejection force is also diminished. LV regional wall stress is proportional to the wall surface radius-of-curvature and inversely proportional to the wall thickness. Hence, for patients with HF after MI, the inability of the remaining viable myocardium to compensate for the increased wall stress associated with LV dilatation and thinning may be a trigger for LV enlargement.

7.4.1 Remodeling Quantification in Terms of Local Curvedness Indices and Regional Curvedness Index

7.4.1.1 Overall Approach

The remodeling is quantified in terms of the *Regional Curvedness* index of the 16 segments of the LV endocardial surface. The method entails generation of the LV endocardial shape and its compartmentalization into 16 segments or regions (as explained later on). Each segment is discretized into triangular meshes, so that a point on the endocardial surface is a vertex of a triangular mesh. At each vertex point, we determine the *Local Curvedness* index [2], by employing its surrounding neighboring vertices in the form of n-rings around the local point. To ensure accurate curvedness computation without over smoothing, the optimal number of n-rings is determined to be 5. For each segment, we then determine the *Regional Curvedness* index as the mean of the *Local Curvedness* indices in the segment.

The values of *Regional Curvedness* are determined for normal and MI patients, at end-diastolic and end-systolic instants. For normal patients, the *Regional Curvedness* index changes significantly from diastole to systole, as given by the *Diastole-to-Systole Change in Curvedness* (%ΔC) [2]

$$\%\Delta C = \frac{C_{ED} - C_{ES}}{C_{ED}} \times 100 \qquad (7.1)$$

TABLE 7.2

Characteristics of Normal Control and Patients after MI, Involved in the Study

	Control (*n* = 10)	MI (*n* = 11)	*p* value
Age (years)	41 ± 16	60 ± 6	0.003
Weight (kg)	67 ± 15	65 ± 14	0.30
Height (cm)	169 ± 8	165 ± 10	0.86
Diastolic pressure (mmHg)	73 ± 12	74 ± 18	0.79
Systolic pressure (mmHg)	122 ± 17	116 ± 20	0.50
Heart rate (beats/min)	70 ± 9	84 ± 13	0.012
Cardiac index (L/min/m²)	3.3 ± 0.4	2.2 ± 0.5	<0.001
End-diastolic volume index (mL/m²)	73 ± 10	148 ± 40	<0.001
End-systolic volume index (mL/m²)	26 ± 6	122 ± 38	<0.001
Ejection fraction (%)	65 ± 5	18 ± 5	<0.001
Sphericity index[a]	0.52 ± 0.06	0.62 ± 0.08	0.01
LV mass index	56 ± 12	83 ± 13	0.004

[a] Defined in Equation 7.6.

where C_{ED} and C_{ES} are end-diastolic and end-systolic curvedness, as defined later by Equation 7.2. The mean alteration in regional curvedness index value of %ΔC can be determined for all the segments, for normal subjects and MI patients (that are summarized in Table 7.2). It can be seen from Table 7.3 that the *Diastole-to-Systole Change in Curvedness* (%ΔC) for MI patients is not significant in comparison with normal subjects. We now proceed to the further elaboration of this Regional Curvedness Index and its clinical application.

7.4.1.2 Clinical Application Methodology

Our study involved 10 normal subjects and 11 patients after MI. The hemodynamic and volumetric parameters of the subjects are summarized in Table 7.2.

7.4.1.2.1 Human Subjects and MRI Scans

The study to characterize regional curvedness index or (%ΔC) involved 10 normal subjects and 11 patients after MI [2]. All subjects underwent diagnostic MRI scans. For each subject, short-axis MRI images were taken along the plane that passes through the mitral and aortic valves of the heart at an interval of 8 mm thickness. Each image had a spatial resolution of 1.5 mm, acquired in a single breath hold, with 25 temporal phases per heart cycle. Of these images, the set of images corresponding to the cardiac cycle at end-diastole and end-systole were then used for the study.

7.4.1.2.2 LV Endocardial Surface Reconstruction and Segmentation

The MRI images were processed, by using a semi-automatic technique that is included in the CMRtools suite (Cardiovascular Solution, UK). The contours demarcating the myocardium and the LV chamber were defined by means of B-spline curves. The endocardial surface of the LV was reconstructed by joining the series of contours to form a triangle mesh. In order to facilitate quantification of the LV segmental regional curvedness, the endocardial surface was partitioned into 16 segments; the method of segmentation of the LV endocardial surface is provided in Reference 2.

TABLE 7.3

Curvedness Indices of MI Patients Compared to Normal Patients

Segment	Controls (n = 10)			MI (n = 11)		
	C_{ED} (× 10⁻² mm⁻¹)	C_{ES} (× 10⁻² mm⁻¹)	ΔC (%)	C_{ED} (× 10⁻² mm⁻¹)	C_{ES} (× 10⁻² mm⁻¹)	ΔC (%)
1. Basal anterior	4.1 ± 0.8	5.6 ± 0.7	38 ± 22	3.4 ± 0.5[a]	3.7 ± 0.5[b]	7 ± 17[c]
2. Basal anterior septal	3.4 ± 0.6	5.3 ± 1.1	57 ± 30	3.7 ± 1.0	3.7 ± 0.9[a]	4 ± 26[b]
3. Basal inferior septal	3.1 ± 0.5	4.8 ± 0.6	61 ± 25	3.6 ± 0.9	4.0 ± 1.0[a]	12 ± 23[b]
4. Basal inferior	4.0 ± 0.5	5.8 ± 1.0	45 ± 27	3.7 ± 1.0	4.1 ± 1.0[a]	13 ± 21[a]
5. Basal inferior lateral	3.5 ± 0.5	5.3 ± 0.9	50 ± 22	3.0 ± 0.6[a]	3.3 ± 0.9[b]	13 ± 25[a]
6. Basal anterior lateral	3.6 ± 0.8	5.0 ± 0.7	46 ± 26	3.1 ± 0.8	3.2 ± 0.8[b]	8 ± 24[a]
7. Middle anterior	3.9 ± 0.5	6.0 ± 0.1	56 ± 20	3.4 ± 0.2[a]	3.6 ± 0.3[b]	6 ± 12[b]
8. Middle anterior septal	3.9 ± 0.4	0.6 ± 1.4	55 ± 26	3.3 ± 0.6[a]	3.4 ± 0.4[b]	5 ± 17[b]
9. Middle inferior septal	3.6 ± 0.6	5.2 ± 1.1	44 ± 18	3.5 ± 0.7	3.4 ± 0.5[b]	1 ± 16[b]
10. Middle inferior	4.1 ± 0.5	6.0 ± 1.2	51 ± 31	3.8 ± 0.7	4.0 ± 0.7[b]	7 ± 17[a]
11. Middle inferior lateral	3.6 ± 0.3	5.5 ± 0.8	52 ± 25	3.1 ± 0.6[a]	3.4 ± 0.6[b]	10 ± 14[b]
12. Middle anterior lateral	3.2 ± 0.3	4.7 ± 0.9	45 ± 19	2.9 ± 0.5	3.0 ± 0.3[b]	4 ± 14[b]
13. Apical anterior	4.8 ± 1.0	9.3 ± 2.0	96 ± 33	3.8 ± 0.7[a]	4.1 ± 1.0[b]	6 ± 15[b]
14. Apical septal	4.9 ± 0.6	9.0 ± 1.9	83 ± 34	4.4 ± 0.7	4.6 ± 0.9[b]	4 ± 14[b]
15. Apical inferior	5.7 ± 0.9	11 ± 2.8	90 ± 44	4.7 ± 1.0[a]	4.9 ± 1.0[b]	5 ± 14[b]
16. Apical lateral	4.4 ± 0.7	8.8 ± 2.2	103 ± 65	3.8 ± 0.4	4.0 ± 0.7[b]	2 ± 12[b]
Mean	4.0 ± 0.4	6.5 ± 1.0	61 ± 18	3.6 ± 0.5[a]	3.8 ± 0.5[b]	7 ± 9[b]
Coefficient of variation of curvedness (%)	21 ± 5	31 ± 8	51 ± 14	19 ± 5	18 ± 4[b]	392 ± 501[a]

Note: (1) Left ventricular regional curvedness (C), as defined by Equation 7.2; (2) diastole-to-systole change in curvedness (%ΔC), as defined by Equation 7.1; (3) coefficient of variation of curvedness (CV_C), as defined by Equation 7.3.

[a] $p < 0.05$
[b] $p < 0.001$
[c] $p < 0.01$

7.4.1.2.3 Left Ventricular Shape Analysis

To quantify LV remodeling, we first define a measure known as the *Local Curvedness* index [2]. This is essentially a shape descriptor used to quantify how curved the surface is in the vicinity of a vertex on the LV endocardial surface. This is done by using the 3D mesh of the LV endocardial surface as an input. Each vertex of the mesh is processed by fitting a quadric surface over a local region around the vertex as described in our paper [2]. The extent of this local region is determined by the *n*-ring parameter. Next, the *Local Curvedness* index of each vertex can be calculated from the coefficients of the fitted quadric surface by [2]:

$$C = \sqrt{\frac{\kappa_1^2 + \kappa_2^2}{2}} = \frac{1}{A^2}\sqrt{\frac{2B^2 + A^2(4ac - b^2)}{A}} \tag{7.2}$$

such that

$$A = \sqrt{d^2 + e^2 + 1}$$

$$B = a + ae^2 + c + cd^2 - bde$$

where *a*, *b*, *c*, *d*, and *e* are the coefficients of the fitted quadric surface at the vertex.

In order to derive the *Regional Curvedness*, the endocardial surface is partitioned into 16 segments (Figure 7.3). The *Regional Curvedness* for the each segment is the mean of the *Local Curvedness* indices in the segment. The flowchart of the overall workflow for the regional LV shape analysis is shown in Figure 7.4.

7.4.1.3 Clinical Study Results

In our clinical studies, it was found that (1) MI patients exhibit decreased curvedness and %ΔC, (2) MI patients exhibit increased variation of curvedness and variation of %ΔC, and (3) LV ejection fraction is positively correlated with curvedness and %ΔC, and inversely correlated with variation of %ΔC.

The *Diastole-to-Systole Change in Curvedness* (%ΔC), as defined by Equation 7.1, is a measure of regional deformity due to contraction. Positive values of %ΔC indicate regions of increasing inward concavity of the LV wall during systole, while negative values of %ΔC indicate wall regions of decreasing inward concavity. The %ΔC measure can be employed to relate the regional differences in hypokinesis due to MI.

7.4.1.3.1 Variation of Curvedness

The extent of LV surface inhomogeneity is characterized by a coefficient of variation of curvedness at end-diastole (CV_C)$_{ED}$ and a coefficient of variation of curvedness at end-systole (CV_C)$_{ES}$, such that

$$CV\_C = \frac{\sigma(C)}{\mu(C)} \tag{7.3}$$

where
   $\sigma(C)$ is the standard deviation of the regional curvedness
   $\mu(C)$ is the mean of the regional curvedness of the segments of the LV mesh

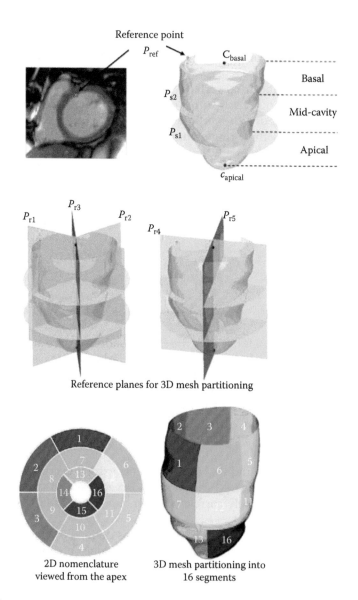

FIGURE 7.3
Partitioning of LV mesh into 16 segments. (Based on Su, Y. et al., *Comput. Methods Programs Biomed.*, 108(2), 500, 2012.)

To evaluate the extent of functional non-uniformity of LV regions, we have developed the index $\Delta(CV\_C)$ to quantify the proportional change in coefficient of variation of curvedness from end-diastole $(CV\_C)_{ED}$ to end-systole $(CV\_C)_{ES}$. This index is given by [2]

$$\Delta(CV\_C) = \frac{(CV\_C)_{ED} - (CV\_C)_{ES}}{(CV\_C)_{ED}} \times 100 \tag{7.4}$$

In general, the larger the values of $(CV\_C)_{ED}$ and $(CV\_C)_{ES}$, the more inhomogeneous the LV endocardial surface appears. Hence, the larger the value of index $\Delta(CV\_C)$, the more functionally non-uniform are the LV shape changes due to LV contraction.

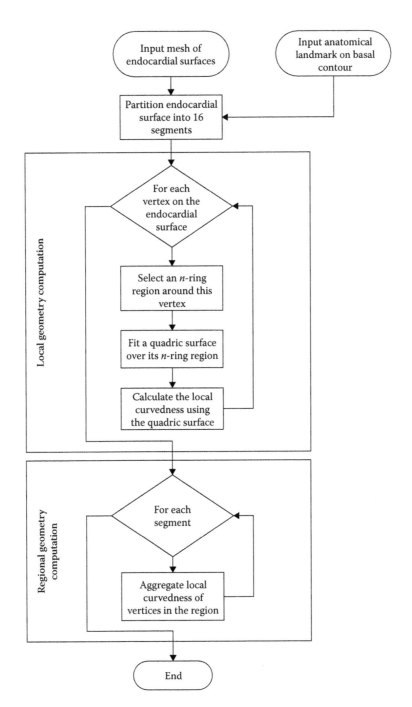

FIGURE 7.4
Flowchart of the overall workflow for the regional LV shape analysis. (Based on Su, Y. et al., *Comput. Methods Programs Biomed.*, 108(2), 500, 2012.)

7.4.1.3.2 *Curvedness, Variation of Curvedness, and Diastole-to-Systole Change %ΔC in* MI *Patients Compared to Normal Subjects*

The hemodynamic and volumetric parameters of the subjects are summarized in Table 7.2. For patients after MI, the LV ejection fraction was significantly lower than that in the control subjects. In addition, their LV end-diastolic and end-systolic indexed volumes were greater than those in the control subjects.

The values of regional curvedness from apex to base in MI patients and normal subjects are given in Table 7.3 and Figure 7.5, to highlight the regional variations of the LV curvature.

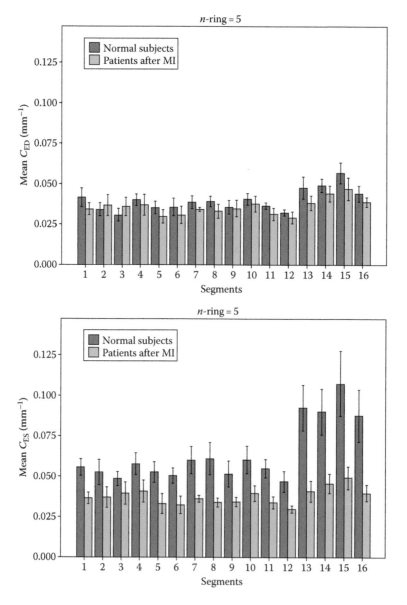

FIGURE 7.5

Comparison of regional curvedness (five-ring selection) in normal subjects and patients after myocardial infarction. (Based on Su, Y. et al., *Comput. Methods Programs Biomed.*, 108(2), 500, 2012.)

In the normal group, there was a significant increase in the curvedness at the apex from diastole to systole. In MI patients, however, there was no significant difference in curvedness in all segments. Significant differences in end-diastolic curvedness C_{ED} and end-systolic curvedness C_{ES} were noted between MI and normal groups. Among the 16 segments of the LV, the variation coefficient of C_{ES} (i.e., $(CV\_C)_{ES}$) was significantly lower in MI patients than in the normal group (18% ± 4% in MI vs. 31% ± 8% in normal, $p < 0.0001$), indicating homogeneity of LV shape in MI at end-systole. Correspondingly, the diastole-to-systole change in curvedness (%ΔC) was significantly lower, and the variation of %ΔC was higher in MI patients compared to normal group, indicating ventricular functional non-homogeneity due to the pathologic state.

7.5 Surgical Ventricular Restoration, Combined with CABG, Restores LV Shape and Improves Cardiac Contractility

Ischemic heart disease is one of the most widely spread, progressive, and prognostically unfavorable diseases of the cardiovascular system. In ischemic dilated cardiomyopathy (IDC) patients, the remodeling process involves a lesser systolic LV curved shape, increase of peak wall stress, and decrease of contractile functional index, compared with normal subjects. Surgical ventricular restoration is performed in chronic ischemic heart disease patients with large non-aneurysmal or aneurysmal post-MI zones. It involves operative methods that reduce LV volume and "restore" ventricular ellipsoidal shape, by exclusion of anteroseptal, apical, and anterolateral LV scarred segments by means of intra-cardiac patch or direct closure.

For patients in HF resulting from serious myocardial diseases of ischemic dilated cardiomyopathy and MI, SVR was designed to restore the LV to its normal shape (reversal of LV remodeling), which is typically performed in conjunction with CABG. In our study [3] of 40 IDC patients who underwent SVR and CABG, there was found to be (1) a decrease in end-diastolic volume from 318 ± 63 to 206 ± 59 mL ($p < 0.01$) and in end-systolic volume from 228 ± 58 mL to 133 ± 61 mL ($p < 0.01$), (2) an increase in LV ejection fraction from 26% ± 7% to 31% ± 8% ($p < 0.01$), (3) a decrease in LV mass (from 204 ± 49 g to 187 ± 53 g, $p < 0.01$), (4) a decrease in peak normalized wall stress (PNWS) (from 4.30 ± 0.95 to 3.31 ± 0.75, $p < 0.01$), (5) an increase in end-systolic sphericity index (SI) (from 0.57 ± 0.094 to 0.67 ± 0.13, $p < 0.01$), (6) an increased value of shape index (S) (from 0.44 ± 0.085 to 0.54 ± 0.089, $p < 0.01$) during end-systole indicating that LV became more spherical after SVR, and most importantly (7) an improvement in LV contractility index $d\sigma^*/dt_{max}$ (from 2.69 ± 0.74 to 3.23 ± 0.73 s^{-1}, $p < 0.01$).

In summary, SVR (in combination with CABG) has been shown to (1) improve ventricular function and decrease wall stress, along with making a more curved apex, and (2) improve cardiac contractility. It is not the LV shape alone that defines LV contractility. Rather, a complex interaction of the rate of change of shape factor (dS/dt_{max}) along with LV maximal flow rate and LV mass may explain the improvement in LV contractility.

7.5.1 Clinical Study

The study was carried out to retrospectively evaluate (with cardiac MRI) the changes on systolic function and LV wall stress; the relationships between LV geometry (shape) and dimensions; and systolic function after SVR performed in chronic ischemic heart disease patients with aneurismal post-MI zones. The study consisted of 40 patients (age averaged 69 years with range of 52–84 years) with ischemic dilated cardiomyopathy who had SVR. MRI scans were performed 2 weeks before surgery (pre-surgery) and 1 week after the surgery; the details of the MRI procedure are reported in an earlier work [3].

Cardiac MRI provides the means to study heart structure and function. The ventricular systolic and diastolic volumes (and hence ejection fraction) are easily assessed reproducibly and accurately. The regional wall motion of the asynergy area and the remote myocardium can also be measured by myocardial tagging while the presence or absence of nonviable, irreversible scar can be detected with gadolinium-based interstitial contrast agents.

7.5.1.1 Data Analysis, 3D Modeling of LV

For analysis, the images were displayed on a computer monitor in a cine-loop mode using CMRtools, to reconstruct the 3D model of the LV. The LV epicardial and endocardial borders were outlined, and all the frames were delineated to produce a volume curve from end-diastolic and end-systolic phases. These measurements were used to determine the end-diastolic volume (EDV), end-systolic volume (ESV), stroke volume (SV), ejection fraction (EF), and LV mass.

7.5.1.1.1 *Ellipsoidal Shape Factor, Eccentricity (E) and Sphericity Index, and Normalized Wall Stress*

The LV is modeled as a prolate spheroid, truncated 50% of the distance from equator to base, as shown in Figure 7.6 [4,5]. Then, the LV cavity wall volume is calculated, from the endocardial anterior–posterior (AP) and base–apex (BA) lengths [4], as

$$V_m = \frac{9}{8}\left[\left(\frac{BA}{1.5}+h\right)\left(\frac{AP}{2}+h\right)^2 - \left(\frac{BA}{1.5}\right)\left(\frac{AP}{2}\right)^2\right] \tag{7.5}$$

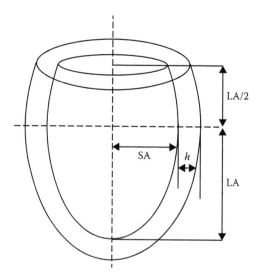

FIGURE 7.6

LV model geometry, showing the major and minor radii of the inner surface of the LV (i.e., LA and SA, respectively) and the wall thickness (*h*).

where BA and AP dimensions are identified in Figure 7.7. The mean wall thickness (h) is calculated at each cavity volume, from the above equation, by assuming that myocardial wall volume (V_m) remains constant throughout the cardiac cycle. The endocardial minor axis dimension (SA) and major axis dimension (LA), shape factor (S), eccentricity (E), and sphericity index (SI) were then calculated as follows (refer Figures 7.6 and 7.7):

$$\text{SA} = \frac{\text{AP}}{2}; \quad \text{LA} = \frac{\text{BA}}{1.5}; \quad S = \frac{\text{SA}}{\text{LA}}; \quad E = \left(\frac{\text{BA}^2 - \text{AP}^2}{\text{BA}^2} \right)^{0.5}; \quad \text{SI} = \frac{\text{AP}}{\text{BA}} \tag{7.6}$$

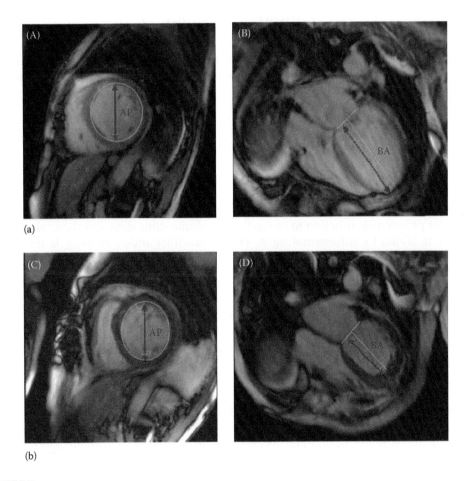

FIGURE 7.7
Short-axis (panels A and C) and long-axis (panels B and D) magnetic resonance images of patients: (a) pre-SVR (panels A and B) and (b) post-SVR (panels C and D). Multiple short-axis cines from the apex to the base of the heart (or orientated axial) and long-axis cines are used to quantify LV function. Anterior–posterior (AP) (panels A and C) and base–apex (BA) (panels B and D) were measured from 2D CMR imaging before (panels A and B) and after (panels C and D) SVR during cardiac cycle. The shape factor (S), eccentricity index, and sphericity index (SI) were calculated from Equation 7.6. It can be noted that the long-axis decreased more dramatically compared with the short-axis dimension, thereby producing a more spherical ventricle. (Adapted from Zhong, L. et al., *Am. J. Cardiol.*, 103(5), 674, 2009.)

where BA (the LV long axis) is defined as the longest distance from the apex to the base of the LV (defined as the mitral annular plane), as measured on the four-chamber cine MRI view of the heart; AP is defined as the widest LV minor axis (Figure 7.7). A small value of SI implies an ellipsoidal LV, whereas values approaching "1" suggest a more spherical LV. The SI at end-diastole (SI_{ED}) and end-systole (SI_{ES}), the percentage shortening of the long and minor axes, as well as the difference between end-diastolic and end-systolic values of SI (i.e., $SI_{ED} - SI_{ES}$) were calculated and are tabulated in Table 7.6.

The time-varying circumferential normalized wall stress, NWS(t), is calculated from the instantaneous measurements of LV dimensions and wall thickness, by treating the LV as a prolate spheroid model truncated 50% of the distance from equator to base [4,5]

$$NWS(t) = \frac{AP(t)}{2h(t)}\left[1 - \frac{(9AP(t)/32h(t))(SI)^2}{(AP(t)/h(t)) + 1}\right] \tag{7.7}$$

The LV wall thickness, $h(t)$, is calculated from the following formula (based on Equation 7.5), by assuming that the myocardial wall volume (V_m) remains constant throughout the cardiac cycle:

$$\frac{9}{8}\left[\left(\frac{BA(t)}{1.5} + h(t)\right)\left(\frac{AP(t)}{2} + h(t)\right)^2\right] = V_m(t) + \left(\frac{BA(t)}{1.5}\right)\left(\frac{AP(t)}{2}\right)^2 \tag{7.8}$$

7.5.1.1.2 Cardiac Contractility $d\sigma^*/dt_{max}$

In order to compute the contractility index by employing Equation 3.4, we employ a sixth-order polynomial function to curve-fit the volume–time data and then calculate the volume rate (dV/dt) by differentiating it. The contractility index $d\sigma^*/dt_{max}$ is then calculated as [6]

$$\frac{d\sigma^*}{dt_{max}} = \left|\frac{d(\sigma_\theta/P)}{dt}\right|_{max} = \frac{3}{2V_m}\left|\left(\frac{dV}{dt}\right)\right|_{max} \tag{7.9}$$

where the myocardial volume V_m can be conveniently measured at the end-diastolic phase.

7.5.2 Clinical Results

All 40 patients were treated with CABG and SVR (endoventricular circular patch plasty). The age of the patients averaged 69 years (range, 52–84 years). Among them, 19 patients had severe mitral regurgitation and received additional MVS; 28 patients had CHF. The baseline patient characteristics are summarized in Table 7.4.

7.5.3 Left Ventricular Functional Index Changes Pre- and Post-Surgery (MRI Parameters)

Figure 7.7 shows typical short-axis and long-axis magnetic resonance images of patient pre- and post-SVR, and illustrates the shape, eccentricity, and sphericity indices. It is noted

TABLE 7.4

Patients' Characteristics and Clinical Data ($n = 40$)

Variables	Value
Male:female	36:4
Age (years)	69 ± 9
Body surface area (m²)	1.98 ± 0.18
Coronary artery disease	39 (98%)
Hypertension	19 (48%)
Diabetes mellitus	13 (33%)
Tobacco	23 (58%)
Congestive heart failure	28 (70%)
Peripheral arterial disease	3 (8%)
Stroke	2 (5%)
Creatinine (mg/dL)	1.17 ± 0.29
Prior cardiac surgery	19 (48%)
New York Heart Association class	
I–II	26 (65%)
III–IV	14 (35%)
Surgery	
Surgical ventricular restoration + coronary artery bypass grafting	21 (52%)
Surgical ventricular restoration + coronary artery bypass grafting + mitral valve surgery	19 (48%)

Values are mean ± SD or numbers of patients (percentages).

that the long-axis decreased more dramatically when compared with the short-axis dimension, thereby producing a more spherical LV. Figure 7.8 shows typical 3D modeling of LV from CMR images, using LV tools pre- and post-SVR.

The intraobserver and interobserver data (namely, EDV, ESV and mass) for the pre- and post-surgery groups are shown in Table 7.5. Table 7.6 summarizes the mean LV functional indexes pre- and post-SVR. It is seen that following SVR, there was a significant decrease in the dimensions of both the long- and short-axes of the LV. The long-axis dimension of the LV decreased more than the short-axis dimension, however, resulting in a more spherical ventricle post-SVR. There was a significant reduction in end-diastolic volume index (EDVI), end-systolic volume index (ESVI), LV stroke volume index (SVI), LV mass index, and peak normalized wall stress after SVR (Table 7.6). The values of LV EDVI, ESVI, LVEF, and the contractility index $d\sigma^*/dt_{max}$ pre- and post-SVR (as computed from Equation 7.9) are also shown in the scatter plots of Figure 7.9.

Table 7.6 provides the sphericity index (SI) values in end-diastole and end-systole and its diastolic–systolic change, as well as the percentage shortening of the long- and short-axes. During a cardiac cycle, LV shape becomes less spherical in systole (SI smaller) than in diastole (SI closer to "1"). The diastolic–systolic change in SI (i.e., $SI_{ED} - SI_{ES}$) is significantly augmented by the operation, despite the LV chamber becoming more spherical. The percentage shortening of long-axis is not significantly altered, but the percentage shortening of the short-axis is significantly increased by the operation. Despite the seemingly unfavorable spherical LV shape post-SVR, the LV contractile function is significantly improved, as indicated by the increased value of $d\sigma^*/dt_{max}$.

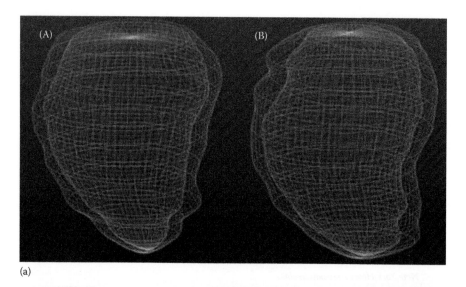

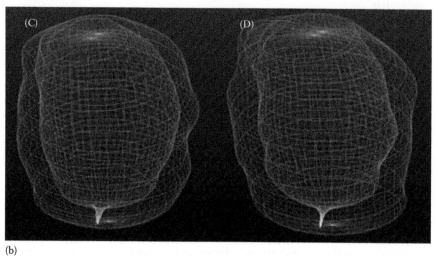

FIGURE 7.8

3D reconstructions during end-diastole (panels A and C) and end-systole (panels B and D) phases: (a) pre-SVR ED and ES (panels A and B) and (b) post-SVR ED and ES (panels C and D) using LV tools. It is created from the endocardial and epicardial contours, which were drawn for calculations of ventricular volumes and function from the multiple short-axis cines (Figure 7.7). (Based on Zhong, L. et al., *Am. J. Cardiol.*, 103(5), 674, 2009.)

The scatter plots of Figure 7.9 graphically illustrate pre- and post-SVR values of ventricular end-diastolic volume, end-systolic volume, LVEF, and contractility index $d\sigma^*/dt_{max}$. From Tables 7.5 and 7.6, we can note a significant reduction in end-diastolic volume (318 ± 63 mL vs. 206 ± 59 mL, $p < 0.01$), end-systolic volume (228 ± 58 mL vs. 133 ± 61 mL, $p < 0.01$), LV mass (204 ± 49 g vs. 187 ± 53 g, $p < 0.01$), and peak normalized wall stress (PNWS) (4.64 ± 0.98 vs. 3.72 ± 0.87, $p < 0.01$). Increased sphericity index SI (0.57 ± 0.094 vs. 0.67 ± 0.13, $p < 0.01$) and increased shape factor S (0.44 ± 0.085 vs.

TABLE 7.5

Reproducibility Data in Patients Pre- and Post-SVR

	Pre-SVR			Post-SVR		
	End-Diastolic Volume (mL)	End-Systolic Volume (mL)	LV Mass (g)	End-Diastolic Volume (mL)	End-Systolic Volume (mL)	LV Mass (g)
Intraobserver						
Mean	318 ± 63	228 ± 58	204 ± 49	206 ± 59	133 ± 61	187 ± 53
Mean difference	1.1 ± 8.60	−1.4 ± 8.38	−5.1 ± 7.96	0.3 ± 6.94	−1.5 ± 3.20	0.6 ± 8.51
Correlation coefficient	0.99	0.99	0.99	0.99	0.99	0.99
t-test *p*	N.S.	N.S.	N.S.	N.S.	N.S.	N.S.
% Variability	1.50 ± 1.99	2.13 ± 2.45	3.74 ± 3.71	2.42 ± 2.32	1.79 ± 1.77	4.09 ± 3.02
Interobserver						
Mean	318 ± 65	231 ± 61	206 ± 52	207 ± 60	135 ± 62	189 ± 51
Mean difference	0.3 ± 10	7.9 ± 10	7.6 ± 14	2.0 ± 8.9	5.5 ± 10	3.1 ± 9.8
Correlation coefficient	0.99	0.99	0.97	0.99	0.99	0.98
t-test *p*	N.S.	N.S.	N.S.	N.S.	N.S.	N.S.
% Variability	2.73 ± 1.58	4.11 ± 2.93	5.90 ± 3.13	3.44 ± 2.94	5.87 ± 6.23	4.81 ± 2.49

Data are mean ± SD.
N.S., not significant.

TABLE 7.6

Patients' Data Pre- and Post-SVR

Variables	Pre-SVR (*n* = 40)	Post-SVR (*n* = 40)
Cardiac index (L/min/m²)	2.84 ± 0.74	2.59 ± 0.74
Mean arterial pressure (mmHg)	85 ± 14	84 ± 8
Systolic blood pressure (mmHg)	115 ± 20	113 ± 10
Diastolic blood pressure (mmHg)	71 ± 12	70 ± 8
End-diastolic volume index (mL/m²)	156 ± 39	110 ± 33[a]
End-systolic volume index (mL/m²)	117 ± 39	77 ± 31[a]
Stroke volume index (mL/m²)	39 ± 9	33 ± 8[a]
Left ventricular ejection fraction (%)	26 ± 7	31 ± 10[a]
LV mass index (g/m²)	112 ± 25	101 ± 23[a]
End-diastolic long axis, BA_{ED} (cm)	10.89 ± 1.16	8.31 ± 1.00[a]
End-diastolic short axis, AP_{ED} (cm)	7.00 ± 0.80	6.64 ± 0.78[a]
End-systolic long axis, BA_{ES} (cm)	10.37 ± 1.20	7.87 ± 1.05[a]
End-systolic short axis, AP_{ES} (cm)	5.86 ± 0.98	5.23 ± 1.06[a]
End-diastolic sphericity index, SI_{ED}	0.65 ± 0.087	0.81 ± 0.11[a]
End-systolic sphericity index, SI_{ES}	0.57 ± 0.094	0.67 ± 0.13[a]
Difference between end-diastolic and end-systolic sphericity index, $SI_{ED} - SI_{ES}$	0.077 ± 0.043	0.14 ± 0.059[a]
Long-axis shortening (%)	4.8 ± 3.6	5.4 ± 4.4
Short-axis shortening (%)	16.4 ± 6.8	22 ± 9.7[a]
dV/dt_{max} (mL/s)	364 ± 83	401 ± 81[a]
Pressure normalized wall stress	4.30 ± 0.95	3.31 ± 0.75[a]
Stroke work (mmHg·L)	6.61 ± 1.96	5.46 ± 1.64[a]
$d\sigma^*/dt_{max}$ (s⁻¹)	2.69 ± 0.74	3.23 ± 0.73[a]

Values are mean ± SD.
[a] $p < 0.05$.

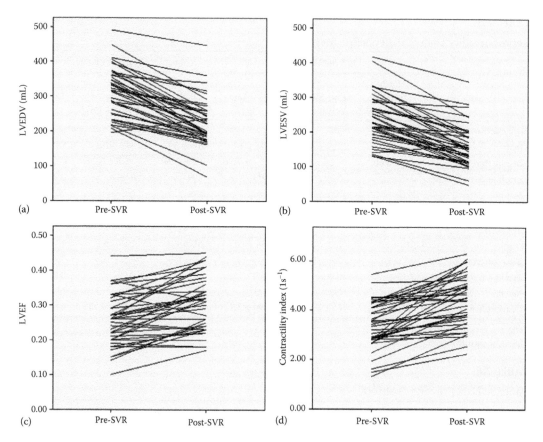

FIGURE 7.9
Changes in (a) end-diastolic volume (EDV), (b) end-systolic volume (ESV), (c) LVEF, and (d) contractility index $d\sigma^*/dt_{max}$ after SVR. (Adapted from Zhong, L. et al., *Am. J. Cardiol.*, 103(5), 674, 2009.)

0.54 ± 0.089, $p < 0.01$) during end-systole indicates that the LV became more spherical after SVR.

The primary effect of SVR may be viewed as (1) a decrease in myocardial oxygen consumption by reduction of LV peak normalized wall stress, resulting in improved functioning of LV, and (2) augmentation of value of the contractility index $d\sigma^*/dt_{max}$ (2.69 ± 0.74 s^{-1} vs. 3.23 ± 0.73 s^{-1}, $p < 0.01$) as seen in Table 7.6. This improvement may be attributed to (1) increased maximal flow dV/dt_{max} with reduced LV mass, and (2) improved regional contraction and contractility of the remote myocardium. The improvement in remote myocardial performance is likely due to reduced myocardial stress, along with effective and complete revascularization. This is because the SVR procedure reduces the volume by more dramatically reducing the long-axis dimension compared with the short-axis dimension and producing a more spherical ventricle.

Based on Table 7.6, increased LV contractile function $d\sigma^*/dt_{max}$ can be associated with increased maximal flow dV/dt_{max} and reduced LV mass, as well as with increased maximal change rate of shape factor dS/dt_{max} ($r = 0.414$, $p < 0.001$). We can also note good correlation between $d\sigma^*/dt_{max}$ and LVEF ($r = 0.69$, $p < 0.001$, pre-SVR; $r = 0.77$, $p < 0.001$, post-SVR) in Figure 7.10.

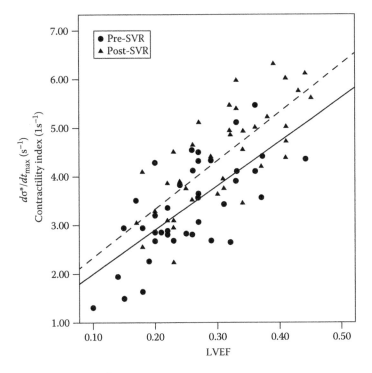

FIGURE 7.10
Association between $d\sigma^*/dt_{max}$ and left ventricular (LV) ejection fraction (EF) pre- and post-SVR. (Solid line: $d\sigma^*/dt_{max} = 9.045 \times EF + 1.091$, $r = 0.69$, $p < 0.001$ for pre-SVR; dash line: $d\sigma^*/dt_{max} = 9.969 \times EF + 1.337$, $r = 0.77$, $p < 0.001$ for post-SVR). (Adapted from Zhong, L. et al., *Am. J. Cardiol.*, 103(5), 674–679, 2009.)

7.6 Conclusion

The hearts of MI patients undergo substantial remodeling and loss of contractility and can progress to HF. Echocardiographic texture analysis enables determination of the percentage volume of the infarcted segments in the ventricular volume.

The ventricular remodeling is defined in terms of reduced alteration in curvedness index (%ΔC) from end-diastole to end-systole. The cardiac contractility is assessed in terms of the value of the index $d\sigma^*/dt_{max}$.

With the help of these three indices of percentage volume of MI segments, curvedness index and contractility index, we can track and assess LV progression to HF, and its recovery following CABG, SVR, or other treatments.

References

1. MV Kamath, RC Way, DN Ghista, TM Srinivasan, C Wu, S Smeenk, C Manning, J Cannon. Detection of myocardial scars in neonatal infants form computerised echocardiographic texture analysis, *Eng Med*, 15(3):137–141, 1986.

2. Y Su, L Zhong, CW Lim, D Ghista, T Chua, RS Tan. A geometrical approach for evaluating left ventricular remodeling in myocardial infarct patients, *Comput Methods Programs Biomed*, 108(2):500–510, 2012.
3. L Zhong, S Sola, RS Tan, DN Ghista, V Kurra, JL Navia, GS Kassab. Effects of surgical ventricular restoration on left ventricular contractility assessed by a novel contractility index in patients with ischemic cardiomyopathy, *Am J Cardiol*, 103(5):674–679, 2009.
4. DD Streeter Jr, WT Hanna. Engineering mechanics for successive states in canine left ventricular myocardium. I. Cavity and wall geometry, *Circ Res*, 33:639–655, 1973.
5. DN Ghista. *Applied Biomedical Engineering Mechanics*, CRC Press, Boca Raton, FL, 2009.
6. L Zhong, RS Tan, DN Ghista, EYK Ng, LP Chua, GS Kassab. Validation of a novel noninvasive cardiac index of left ventricular contractility in patients, *Am J Physiol Heart Circ Physiol*, 292(6):H2764–H2772, 2007.

8

Vector Cardiogram Theory and Clinical Application

Dhanjoo N. Ghista and Thurairaj Nagenthiran

CONTENTS

8.1 Introduction

In this chapter, we present the theory, development, and clinical application of vector cardiogram: How the three-lead ECG voltages are derived from the projection of the equivalent-dipole heart electrical-activity vector (HAV) on the sides of the Einthoven's triangle, and the development of the heart-depolarization vector-locus cardiogram (HDVLC) from the ECG leads and its clinical diagnostic application.

We start out with a conducting cardiac tissue cylinder, which is depolarized by an action potential $V_i(x)$. We put down the expression for the extracellular current or the transmembrane current dI_o, leaking out through the membrane into the external medium, in terms of the membrane conductivity. We then provide the equation for the electrical potential at a point $dV_o(r)$ due to the current source dI_o. The total potential at point 0 due to a continuous leakage of current along the length of the dipole within the cylindrical cardiac tissue can then be expressed in terms of the magnitude of the electrical activity vector.

In the Einthoven's triangle electrocardiographic model, the cardiac source is a 2D dipole represented by the equivalent-dipole HAV located at the circumcenter O. We then demonstrate how the three-lead ECG voltages are derived from the projection of the equivalent-dipole HAV on the sides of the Einthoven's triangle. We can determine the magnitude and direction of the HAV $\overrightarrow{OP}$, in terms of its x and y components P_x and P_y. The HAV $\overrightarrow{OP}$ is then plotted on a plane representing the frontal plane of the torso, as depicted in Figure 8.4. The line drawn by the tip of the HAV $\overrightarrow{OP}$ (derived from Leads I and II), as it traces the path of the depolarization electrical vector during the progression of QRS complex, constitutes the front-plane HPVLC, which is actually a loop with initial and terminal points at the origin (equivalent to the isoelectric baseline).

We then demonstrate the reconstruction of the equivalent HAV for the QRS complex from limb lead voltages of a sample ECG recording and plot the progression of the cardiac vector during the QRS complex. A realistic visualization of the progression of the equivalent-dipole HAV during the QRS complex is demonstrated by staging the heart-depolarization vector locus cardiogram (HP-VCG) of the QRS complex from the onset of the QRS until the end of the depolarization stage, in the form of a loop. We have constructed VCGs for a normal subject, and three patients with ventricular hypertrophy, bundle branch block, and inferior myocardial infarction.

Then in order to distinguish VCG shapes of diseased and normal subjects, we have introduced two VCG diagnostic parameters, namely, VCG loop area and loop sling length. Figure 8.8 provides the HDVC parametric space with loop area and loop sling length as coordinates, for 35 subjects representing healthy control and abnormal electrocardiological states. It can be seen that each diagnostic class has its own zone in the parametric space. The subtle changes in the ECG are reflected more distinctly in the VCG loop and in the VCG parametric space. Hence, VCG can even help to diagnose cardiac disease at an early stage.

We can also characterize VCG shapes by means of an analytical function. By studying the HPVLC for various electrocardiological disorders, it is possible to determine the ranges of the analytical function's parameters for normal and disordered electrocardiological states, for diagnostic purpose.*

8.2 Developing the Expression for the Electrical Activity Vector

8.2.1 Depolarized Cardiac Tissue and the Electrical Potential at an External Point due to the Current within It

According to the centric dipole assumption, the electrical activity of the heart (as sensed on the torso) can be represented by a single lumped dipole moment located at the center of the torso [4]. In an in vivo cardiac tissue depolarized by the action potential $V_i(x)$, the depolarization wave front (caused by the action potential) can be represented by an equivalent dipole in the direction of the electrical wave propagation.

---

* This chapter is based on lecture notes Theory of ECG, Ghista DN [1], which were converted Heart depolarization vector cardiogram and its clinical diagnostic applications, Nagenthiran T, Ghista DN, Prasad VR, *Journal of Mechanics in Medicine and Biology* [2], and Frontal plane vectorcardiograms: Theory and graphics visualization of cardiac health status, Ghista DN, Acharya UR, Nagenthiran T., *Journal of Medical Systems* [3].

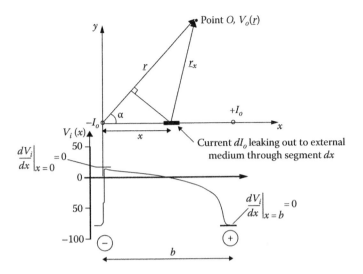

FIGURE 8.1
Illustration of a cardiac tissue depolarized by the action potential $V_i(x)$, wherein the depolarization wave front (caused by the action potential) is represented by an equivalent dipole in the direction of the electrical wave propagation. The dipole consists of a sink $-I_o$ at origin and a source I_o at radius vector x, shown with respect to action potential. Also illustrated is a potential point at radius vector r and polar angle. (Based on Nagenthiran, T. et al., *J. Mech. Med. Biol.*, 12(5), 1240024, 2012.)

The dipole consists of two monopoles of opposite sign but equal strength I_o (often termed as source and sink) separated by a small length b, which is depolarized by the action potential.

The quantity p is the *dipole moment* or dipole magnitude. Figure 8.1 illustrates the action *potential $V_i(x)$* and the associated dipole, whose negative pole is located at the origin and the positive pole is located along the x-axis at a distance b from it. The dipole moment p is the vector whose direction is defined from the negative point source to the positive, along the x-axis.

8.2.2 Potential at a Point Exterior to the Depolarized Cardiac Tissue

This derivation is based on our earlier papers on Frontal plane vector cardiogram [3] and Heart-depolarization vector cardiogram [2].

The current $I_i(x, t)$ flowing within this tissue cylinder is given (by Ohm's law) as

$$I_i(x,t) = \frac{\Delta V_i}{R} = \frac{\partial V_i}{\partial x} \cdot \frac{\partial x}{R} \tag{8.1}$$

Putting $R = \partial x / \pi a^2 \sigma_{ci}$ (based on Ohm's law), we get

$$I_i(x,t) = \sigma_{ci} \pi a^2 \frac{\partial V_i}{\partial x} \tag{8.2}$$

where σ_{ci} is the conductivity of the intracellular medium = 2 S m^{-1}.

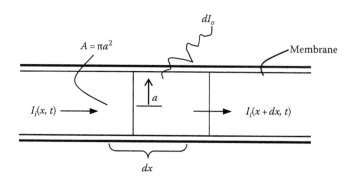

FIGURE 8.2
Segment of the cardiac tissue cylinder into which the depolarization wave front has advanced during depolarization, showing the transmembrane leakage current given by Equation 8.3. (Based on Ghista, D.N. et al., *J. Med. Syst.*, 34(4), 445, 2010.)

Then, the expression for the extracellular current or the transmembrane current dI_o (leaking out through the membrane into the external medium) is given (as depicted in Figure 8.2) by

$$dI_o = I_i(x,t) - I_i(x + dx, t)$$

$$= \frac{\partial I_i(x,t)}{\partial x} \cdot dx \qquad (8.3)$$

$$= \pi a^2 \sigma_{ci} \frac{\partial^2 V_i}{\partial x^2} dx$$

Using the definition of electrical potential at a point O (due to a small current source dI_o), the potential at point $O(r)$ due to this small leakage current dI_o is given by

$$dV_o(\underline{r}) = \frac{dI_o}{4\pi\sigma_{co}r_x} \qquad (8.4)$$

where σ_{co} is the myocardial conductivity $= 0.2$ S m^{-1}.
   Combining Equations 8.3 and 8.4, we get

$$dV_o(\underline{r}) = \frac{\pi a^2 \sigma_{ci}}{4\pi\sigma_{co}r_x} \frac{\partial^2 V_i}{\partial x^2} dx \qquad (8.5)$$

The total potential at point O due to a continuous leakage of current along the length (b) of the dipole (or the extent of the action potential) within the cylindrical cardiac tissue (from the negative point source to the positive) is obtained by integrating the contribution of all the elements of the current within the dipole. We thus obtain the expression for the total potential at point O due to a continuous leakage of current along the length of the dipole from the negative point source to the positive [2,3], as

$$V_o(\underline{r}) = \frac{P \cos \alpha}{4\pi\sigma_{co}r^2} = \frac{\underline{p} \cdot \underline{r}}{4\pi\sigma_{co}r^3} \qquad (8.6)$$

wherein we define the magnitude (P) of the electrical activity vector ($\underline{p}$) as $P = \pi a^2 \sigma_{ci} \Delta V$ and $\Delta V = V(0) - V(b)$.

Now, let us consider two points $A(\underline{r_1})$ and $B(\underline{r_2})$ in the external myocardial medium far from the conducting tissue fiber, such that $|\underline{r_1}| = |\underline{r_2}| = \underline{r}$. Then, we have

$$V_o(A) = V_o(\underline{r_1}) = \frac{\underline{p} \cdot \underline{r_1}}{4\pi\sigma_{co}r^3} \tag{8.7}$$

$$V_o(B) = V_o(\underline{r_2}) = \frac{\underline{p} \cdot \underline{r_2}}{4\pi\sigma_{co}r^3} \tag{8.8}$$

Therefore, the potential difference between points A and B is given by

$$V_o(\underline{r_1}) - V_o(\underline{r_2}) = \frac{\underline{p} \cdot (\underline{r_2} - \underline{r_1})}{4\pi\sigma_{co}r^3}$$

$$= \frac{\underline{p} \cdot (\underline{r_2} - \underline{r_1})}{4\pi\sigma_{co}r^3}$$

$$= \frac{P(\underline{r_2} - \underline{r_1})}{4\pi\sigma_{co}r^3} \tag{8.9}$$

This is the expression for the potential difference between two external points A and B due to the electrical activity vector $\underline{p}$ of magnitude $P(= \pi a^2 \sigma_{ci} \Delta V_i)$.

8.3 Modified Einthoven's Triangle

8.3.1 Expressing the Three Bipolar Lead ECG Voltages in Terms of the Heart Electrical-Activity Vector

We will now demonstrate how the three-lead ECG voltages are derived from the projection of the equivalent-dipole HAV on the sides of the Einthoven's triangle [2,3].

In the Einthoven's electrocardiographic model, the cardiac bioelectrical source is a 2D equivalent-dipole HAV, located at the centroid O of the modified Einthoven's triangle (MET) in the frontal plane, as shown in Figure 8.3a. The MET is not an equilateral triangle but is defined by taking the actual physical dimensional angles between the bipolar leads. The magnitude and direction of this HAV vector $(\overrightarrow{OP})$ will vary from instant to instant during a cardiac cycle.

$$r_A = r_B = r_C = r = 36 \text{ cm}$$
$$\sigma_{ci} = 2\,\text{S m}^{-1}; \quad \sigma_{co} = 0.2\,\text{S m}^{-1}$$

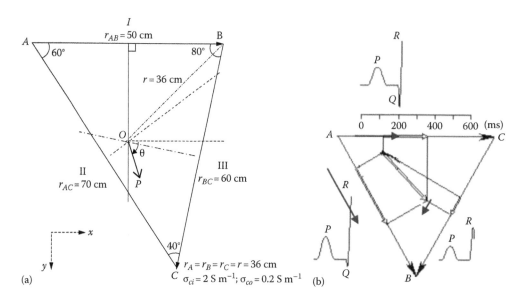

FIGURE 8.3

(a) Modified Einthoven's triangle, in which the vertices A, B, C are the three bipolar leads and the HAV $\overrightarrow{OP}$ is located at its centroid. A typical sample set of dimensions of the Einthoven's triangle is provided in the figure. (Based on Nagenthiran, T. et al., *J. Mech. Med. Biol.*, 12(5), 1240024, 201.) (b) Projections of the heart vector onto the leads, with corresponding limb lead ECG voltages. (Based on Ghista, D.N. et al., *J. Med. Syst.*, 34(4), 445, 2010.)

We now employ Equation 8.9 to develop the expressions for the potential differences between the vertices (A and B, B and C, C and A) of the Einthoven's triangle. The equation of potential difference between two points on the torso, in terms of the equivalent-dipole HAV $\overrightarrow{OP}$, is as follows:

$$V(\underline{r_2}) - V(\underline{r_1}) = \frac{\overrightarrow{OP} \cdot R}{4\pi\sigma_{co} r^3} \tag{8.10}$$

where $R = \underline{r_2} - \underline{r_1}$.

The potential differences $A - B$, $A - C$, and $B - C$ are considered to be the scalar components of the HAV (along AB, AC, and BC), as shown in Figure 8.3a. The three bipolar lead voltages are expressed as the projections of the heart vector ($\overrightarrow{OP}$) onto each side of the Einthoven's triangle [2,3]. Using Equation 8.10, we can put down

$$\text{Lead I} = V_I = V_B - V_A = \frac{Pr_{AB}\cos\theta}{D} = \frac{P_x r_{AB}}{D} \tag{8.11}$$

wherein (1) P is the magnitude of the cardiac vector $\overrightarrow{OP}$, (2) P_x is the magnitude of the component of $\overrightarrow{OP}$ vector along the x-axis (or along AB), (3) r_{AB} is the length of side AB of the MET, (4) D equals to $4\pi\sigma_{co}r^3$, with the myocardial conductivity (σ_{co}) assumed to be 0.2 S m^{-1}, and (5) $P(= \pi a^2 \sigma_{ci} \Delta V_i)$, with the intracellular medium conductivity $\sigma_{ci} = 2$ Sm^{-1}.

$$\text{Lead II} = V_{II} = V_C - V_A = \frac{Pr_{AC}\cos(\theta - 60°)}{D}$$

$$= \frac{(P_x \cos 60° + P_y \sin 60°)r_{AC}}{D} \tag{8.12}$$

wherein (1) P_y is the magnitude of the y-axis component of $\overrightarrow{OP}$ vector, (2) r_{AC} is the length of the side AC of the MET, and (3) θ, measured clockwise by convention from the horizontal axis, defines the instantaneous electrical axis of the heart.

$$\text{Lead III} = V_{III} = V_C - V_B = \frac{P r_{BC} \cos(100° - \theta)}{D}$$

$$= \frac{(P_x \cos 100° + P_y \sin 100°) r_{BC}}{D} \tag{8.13}$$

where

  P is the magnitude of the cardiac vector $\overrightarrow{OP}$

  θ, measured clockwise by convention from the horizontal axis, is defined as the *instantaneous electrical axis* of the heart

  $D = 4\pi\sigma_{co}r^3$

So, the three bipolar lead ECG voltages, as depicted in Figure 8.3a and b theoretically represent the three projections of the heart vector onto each side of the Einthoven's triangle. Conversely, since the three-lead voltages can be monitored, they can be employed to reconstruct the HAV, from which we can then generate the vector cardiogram, as shown in the next section.

8.3.2 Reconstruction of HAV (From the Limb Leads) and Heart-Depolarization VCG Generation

A simplified approach is used for the inverse reconstruction of the HAV $\overrightarrow{OP}$ from any two of the bipolar leads. Using Lead I and Lead II and Equations 8.11 through 8.13, we can determine the magnitude and direction of the HAV $\overrightarrow{OP}$, in terms of its x and y components P_x and P_y given by

$$P_x = \frac{V_I D}{r_{AB}}$$

$$P_y = \frac{((V_{II}D/r_{AC}) - P_x \cos 60°)}{\sin 60°}$$

$$\theta = \tan^{-1}\left(\frac{P_y}{P_x}\right) \tag{8.14}$$

Now, by using values of Lead I and II voltages, obtained from an ECG sample for Leads I, II, and III provided in Figure 8.4 for the QRS complex (and tabulated in Table 8.1), we can determine P_x and P_y, and hence the magnitude and direction of the HAV $\overrightarrow{OP}$.

8.3.3 Construction of the Heart Depolarization Vector Locus Cardiogram

The HAV $\overrightarrow{OP}$ is now plotted on a plane representing the frontal plane of the torso, as depicted in Figure 8.5. The curve drawn by the tip of the HAV $\overrightarrow{OP}$ (derived from Leads I and II), as it traces the path of the depolarization electrical vector, during the progression of QRS complex, is the front-plane HPVLC. Thus, the HPVLC is actually a loop, with initial and terminal points at the origin (equivalent to the isoelectric baseline).

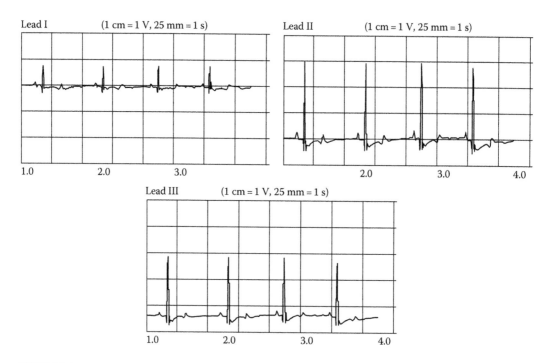

FIGURE 8.4

Sample ECG recording used for sampling of Leads I, II, and III voltages during QRS complex. (Adapted from Nagenthiran, T. et al., *J. Mech. Med. Biol.*, 12(5), 1240024, 2012.)

TABLE 8.1

Readings at Intervals of 6 ms during the Progression of the QRS Complex

Point	V_I (mV)	V_{II} (mV)	V_{III} (mV)	p_x	p_y	P (mV)	θ (°)
1	0	0.01	0.01	0.00E+00	−4.83E−05	4.83E−05	−89.99
2	−0.2	−0.45	−0.25	−4.69E−05	−6.57E−05	8.07E−05	−125.48
3	0.8	3.0	2.20	1.88E−04	1.18E−04	2.22E−04	32.16
4	−0.1	−0.25	−0.15	−2.34E−05	−7.73E−06	2.47E−05	−161.72
5	−0.1	−0.3	−0.2	−2.34E−05	−1.55E−05	2.81E−05	−146.56

8.4 Progression of a Typical Vector Locus Cardiogram during a QRS Complex

A realistic progression of the equivalent-dipole HAV during the QRS complex can be visualized by staging the HPVLC of the QRS complex from the onset of the QRS until the end of the depolarization stage.

Figure 8.6a is depicting the HPVLC during ventricular activation, when electrical impulses are first conducted down the left and right bundle branches on either side of the septum. This causes the septum to depolarize from left-to-right as depicted by the HAV.

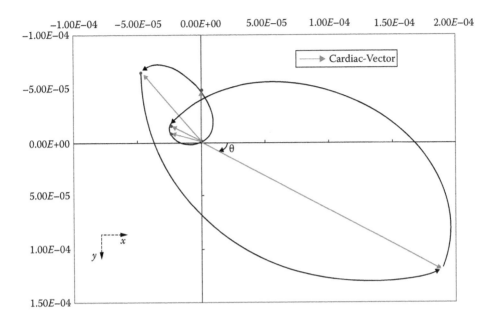

FIGURE 8.5
Heart-depolarization vector locus cardiogram (HPVLC) for a QRS complex. The plot was done by using five separate readings at interval of 6 ms (in Table 8.1) during the progression of the QRS complex.

This vector is heading away from the positive electrode and therefore will record a small negative deflection (Q wave of the QRS complex).

As the electrical wave propagation proceeds along the Purkinjie fibers to the inner walls of the ventricles, ventricular depolarization starts first from the left side of the interventricular septum. The resultant dipole from this septal activation points to the right, as can be seen from the left orientation of the path of the depolarization vector in Figure 8.6b.

Depolarization then propagates through the walls of the ventricles. Because the left ventricle wall is thicker, activation of the left ventricular free wall continues even after depolarization of a large part of the right ventricle has depolarized. As seen in Figure 8.6c, the resultant depolarization vector reaches its maximum and points toward the right in this phase, due to non-compensating right depolarization.

Figure 8.6d shows that the depolarization front continues propagation along the left ventricular wall toward the back. Finally, the ventricular wall surface area decreases continuously and (as shown in Figure 8.6e) the magnitude of the resultant vector decreases until the entire ventricular muscle is depolarized.

By characterizing this HAV tip-locus (HAV-TL) curve by an analytical function of a known curve (such as a limacon), we can determine the parameters (e.g., p_1 and p_2 for a limacon) of the curve. By studying the HAV-TL for various electrocardiological disorders, we can determine the ranges of the HAV-TL parameters for normal and disordered electrocardiological states. This can facilitate the assessment of intra-myocardial depolarization activity, in terms of the values of the two parameters, plotted as points on the (p_1, p_2) plane. On this plane, we can designate the zones of normal and diseased states for diagnostic usage.

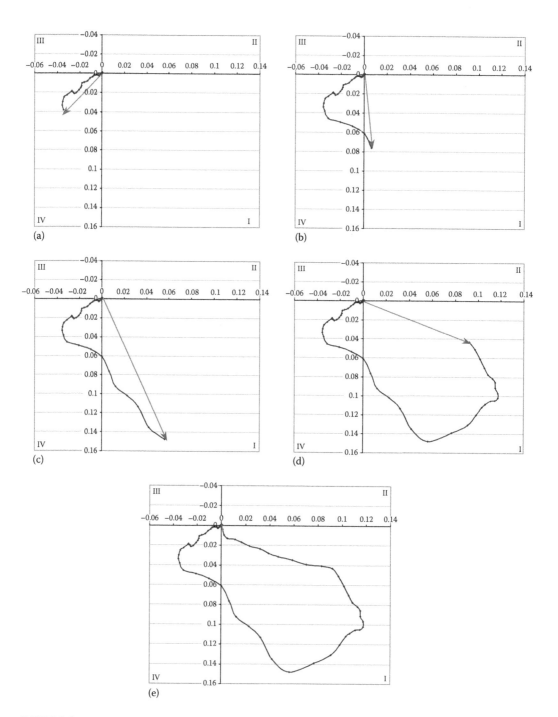

FIGURE 8.6

Illustration of the progression of the heart depolarisation vector tip, for a normal subject, during a QRS complex. (a) During ventricular activation, (b) during septal activation, (c) during right ventricle depolarization, (d) during left ventricle depolarization, and (e) entire ventricular muscle depolarized.

8.5 Heart-Depolarization Vector Cardiograms for Distinguishing Cardiac Disorders

8.5.1 Constructing VCGs for Different Cardiac Disorders

We now construct VCGs for different cardiac disorders. For a VCG construction, we (1) reconstruct the HAV at each instant from the ECG recordings (such as shown in Figure 8.4), (2) plot the heart-depolarization vector cardiogram (HDVC), and (3) associate its shape with cardiac disorders, as depicted in the following [2,3].

So for this purpose, ECG recordings from the PTB* Arrhythmia database have been used for the reconstruction of the HAV and the plotting of the HDVC. The sampling frequency is 1000 Hz with resolution 0.5 µV bit^{-1}, and 10 s of each ECG recording was downloaded. The Lead I and II voltages were normalized to the isoelectric baseline (0 V).

In Figure 8.7, plots of the HDVC on the frontal plane are provided, for a healthy control subject in Figure 8.7a and one for each abnormal electrocardiological state in Figure 8.7b through d.

The start of the vector cardiogram is assumed to be the first departure of either Lead I or II voltages from the isoelectric baseline. The end of vector cardiogram is assumed to be the return of Lead I or II voltages to the isoelectric baseline after S wave, whichever is later. Since the *T wave* can be negative for disordered electrocardiological states and the *ST segment* can be depressed in ischemia, the return to isoelectric baseline for vector cardiogram of diseased states could be after ST segment. This is especially so for hypertrophy.

The left-hand side of the figures of Figure 8.7a through d shows the ECG voltages (normalized with respect to the bioelectric baseline) at Leads I and II. The right-hand side of these figures shows the VCG loops. Herein, we have used the Cartesian coordinate system to explain the display system.

Figure 8.7a shows the HDVC for a *normal* subject. In this plot, the loop is pointing more downward and is prominent in the first quadrant with a small portion in the fourth quadrant.

In the case of *ventricular hypertrophy* in Figure 8.7b, the loop of the vector cardiogram is pointing upward and is distributed in the first and the second quadrant.

Figure 8.7c shows the VCG for the *bundle branch block* disease. The loop of the VCG is spread in the first and second quadrants, and is pointing downward. There is a small closed loop present in the third quadrant.

The VCG graph of the *inferior myocardial infarction* is shown in Figure 8.7d. The loop of the plot is almost equally distributed in the first and second quadrants, with a small area in the fourth quadrant.

For diagnostic purposes, it is helpful to characterize these VCG graphs in the form of shape functions and their parameters and, then, characterize the cardiac disorders in terms of these parameters.

---

* Physikalisch-Technische Bundesanstalt (PTB), the National Metrology Institute of Germany.

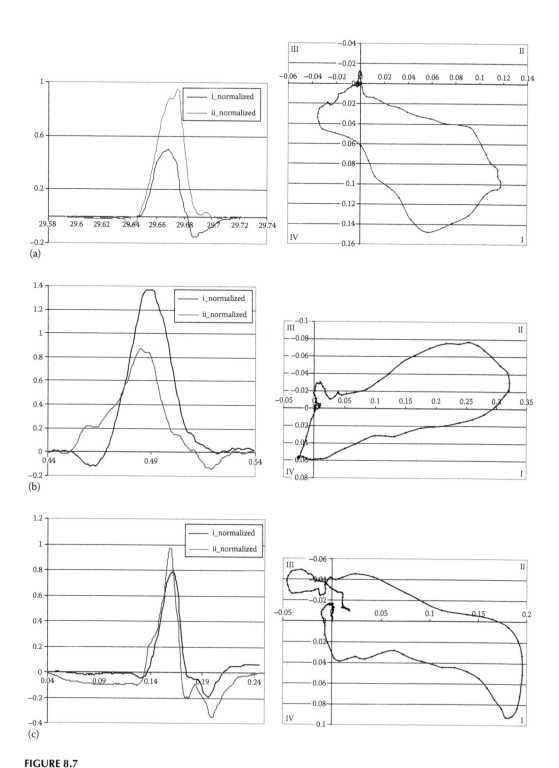

FIGURE 8.7
Typical Leads I and II ECG signals and resulting VCG plots for: (a) normal subject (patient 105). Typical Leads I and II ECG signals and resulting VCG plots for: (b) ventricular hypertrophy subject (patient 159), (c) bundle branch block subject (patient 202).

(Continued)

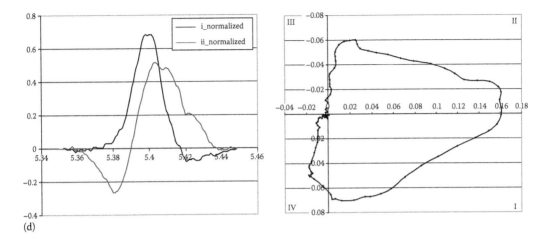

(d)

FIGURE 8.7 (Continued)
Typical Leads I and II ECG signals and resulting VCG plots for: (d) inferior myocardial infarction subject (patient 11).

8.5.2 Frontal Plane Vector Cardiogram Parameters

We now introduce two VCG diagnostic parameters, namely, VCG loop area and loop sling length. These two parameters are explained as follows.

8.5.2.1 Frontal Vector Cardiogram QRS Loop Area

The area of the vector cardiogram loop is of great clinical significance, and is more convenient to employ for cardiac disease diagnosis compared to 1D ECG signals [4]. Let us assume two vectors $\vec{A}$ and $\vec{B}$. The result of their cross-product $\vec{A} \times \vec{B}$ is a vector perpendicular to both $\vec{A}$ and $\vec{B}$ which is $\vec{C}$. The absolute value of $\vec{C}$ is two times the area spanned by the vectors $\vec{A}$ and $\vec{B}$. Calculating the area for the whole loop means calculating each separate area between vectors pointing from point 1 (at the origin) to point $(i + 1)$ and $(i + 2)$, where $i = 1, ..., N - 2$ for a loop containing N points [4].

Thus, the QRS loop area is given by

$$\sum_{i=2}^{N-2} \frac{1}{2} \left(|(\tilde{a}_i - \tilde{a}_1) \times (\tilde{a}_{i+1} - \tilde{a}_1)| \right) \tag{8.15}$$

where $\tilde{a}_i$ is the position vector of point i.

8.5.2.2 Frontal Vector Cardiogram QRS Loop Sling Length

The length of the loop, which we call the sling length, is calculated by adding the distances between consecutive points together. As mentioned earlier, the loop sling length could provide correlated information about the length of the QRS complex. The distance between two points is given as

$$D = \sqrt{(X_i - X_{i+1})^2 + (Y_i - Y_{i+1})^2} \tag{8.16}$$

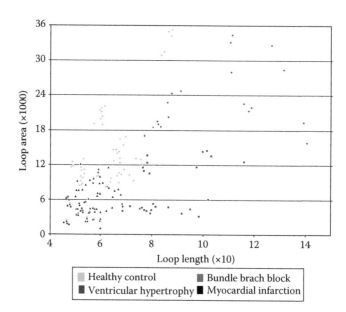

FIGURE 8.8
HDVC parametric space with zones for diagnostic classes.

8.5.2.3 HDVC Parametric Space

Figure 8.8 provides the HDVC parametric space covered by the loop area and loop sling length parameters, for a total of 35 subjects representing healthy control and abnormal electrocardiological states. It can be seen that each diagnostic class has its own zone in the parametric space. To verify the results obtained in Figure 8.8, we need to study the correlation between the ECG features for abnormal states and the parametric space ranges occupied by data from each diagnostic class.

It can be seen from Figure 8.8 that the HDVCs from the diagnostic class of *bundle branch block* have long loop length but relatively small loop area. This is in agreement with the expected long QRS duration (>120 ms) but small R wave for this abnormal class. HDVCs from subjects with *ventricular hypertrophy* occupy the parametric space with long loop length and large loop area. This is in correlation to the large R wave (>15 mm) expected of such diagnostic class. Similarly, HDVC loop area and loop length are small for the *myocardial infarction* cases, due to the loss of R waves.

8.6 Conclusion

Herein, we have presented the theory, construction method, and clinical application of the HDVLC. The HDVCG provides a visual graphics display of various cardiac disorders. The orientation and the magnitude of the loop indicate the type of heart disease. The subtle changes in the ECG are reflected more distinctly in the VCG loop and in the VCG parametric space. Hence, HDVCG helps to identify the disease at an early stage.

VCG has been found to be more reliable than the electrocardiogram, for the diagnosis of atrial enlargement and right ventricular hypertrophy [5]. It is more sensitive than the electrocardiogram in the detection of myocardial infarction, especially if the infarction is inferior or if it occurs in the presence of left bundle branch block. It is also helpful in the diagnosis of ventricular pre-excitation and in the localization of the bypass tract. Some repolarization abnormalities are more clearly demonstrated by the vector display.

In this chapter, we have provided studies of the usefulness of vector cardiography in the diagnosis of heart diseases. The method of reconstruction of the equivalent heart vector for the QRS complex from limb lead voltages of a sample ECG is provided. We have illustrated a typical progression of the equivalent-dipole HAV during the QRS complex, by staging the HPVLC from the onset of the QRS until the end of the depolarization stage. Thereby, a visual display platform of VCG, for the study of subtle changes in the QRS complex using bipolar lead voltages of ECG, is developed.

Hence, the VCG parametric space derived from the frontal plane VCG can help to define classification zones for different ECG abnormalities. This VCG visual display technique makes it easier to identify cardiac abnormalities. The orientation and shape of these loops are unique for each disease. The technique is simple to operate and does not involve extensive computations. This method can also be employed to test the efficacy of drugs, treatment, and therapy.

Different patterns of HDVC for cardiac states such as normal, bundle branch block, ventricular hypertrophy, and myocardial infarction are considered in this chapter. Especially, the QRS loop vector (based on the MET) is studied for both normal and abnormal cases. Significant changes in morphology, contour, and spatial orientation of QRS vectors can be seen in the VCG loops. The VCG is a useful adjunct to electrocardiography in the diagnosis of congenital heart disease. For diagnosis of many cardiac bioelectrical abnormalities and disease conditions, it even proves to be a superior technique, since it provides more illustrative graphical displays of the electrical events in the VCG, thereby making this technique very valuable in the diagnosis of various forms of congenital and acquired heart diseases.

References

1. Ghista DN. Theory of ECG, NTU M6521 Cardiovascular Engineering Lecture Series, July–October 2003.
2. Nagenthiran T, Ghista DN, Prasad VR. Heart depolarization vector cardiogram and its clinical diagnostic applications. *J Mech Med Biol* 12(5), 1240024, 2012.
3. Ghista DN, Acharya UR, Nagenthiran T. Frontal plane vectorcardiograms: Theory and graphics visualization of cardiac health status. *J Med Syst* 34(4), 445–458, 2010.
4. Malmivuo J, Plonsey R. *Bioelectromagnetism: Principles and Applications of Bioelectric and Biomagnetic Fields*. Oxford University Press, New York, 1995, pp. 119–130, Chapter 6.
5. Chou TC. When is the vectorcardiogram superior to the scalar electrocardiogram? *J Am Coll Cardiol* 8, 791–799, 1986.

Section II

ECG Signal Analysis, Left Ventricular Pumping (Intra-Ventricular, Aortic and Coronary Flow) Characteristics, Coronary Bypass Surgery Design, and Their Implications in Clinical Cardiology and Cardiac Surgery

9

ECG Waveform and Heart Rate Variability Signal Analysis to Detect Cardiac Arrhythmias

Dhanjoo N. Ghista, Vinitha Sree Subbhuraam, G. Swapna, U. Rajendra Acharya

CONTENTS

9.1 Introduction

Today electrocardiogram is the most commonly used noninvasive technology for monitoring the heart electrical activity, for evaluation of the heart condition of patients with cardiac complaints and to evaluate cardiac arrhythmias, ischemic heart disease, and myocardial infarction. The origin of the electrocardiogram dates back to 1811, when Dr. Augustus Waller, a British physiologist of St Mary's Hospital Medical School in London, published the first human electrocardiogram using a capillary electrometer with electrodes placed on the chest and back of a human; he demonstrated that electrical activity preceded ventricular contraction. Then, many years later, Dr. Willem Einthoven, a Dutch physiologist, further refined the capillary electrometer and was able to demonstrate five deflections, which he named as ABCDE as illustrated in Figure 9.1.

To adjust for inertia in the capillary system, Einthoven implemented a mathematical correction, which resulted in the curves that we are familiar with today; he named these deflections as PQRST. Einthoven coined the term *electrocardiogram* to describe the cardiac electrical activity wave forms at the Dutch Medical Meeting of 1893. He went on to develop (in 1901) a new string galvanometer, which he used in his electrocardiograph device, illustrated in Figure 9.2.

As the string galvanometer electrocardiograph became available for clinical use, improvements were made to make it more practical. The earlier electrocardiograms used 5 electrodes, 1 on each of the 4 extremities and the mouth, with 10 leads derived from the different combinations. Einthoven reduced the number of electrodes to the three-lead system used to construct Einthoven's triangle, which is an important concept to this day and referred to in our chapter. In 1924, Einthoven was awarded the Nobel Prize in physiology and medicine for the invention of electrocardiogram. By 1930, the importance of electrocardiogram in diagnosing the cause of cardiac chest pain had become universally recognized and adopted.

So with this historical background, we embark in this chapter on ECG waveform analysis to detect cardiac arrhythmias, and thereafter conduct heart rate variability signal processing and analysis to detect cardiac arrhythmias. We first study the electrical activity of the heart and the different phases of the action potential. We then discuss the Einthoven triangle, the relationship between the Einthoven vector and each of the three frontal limb leads (leads I, II, and III), and the method of measuring ECG by using electrodes attached to the body surface and connected to an instrumentation amplifier. We then present (1) how the ECG waveform evolves and develops the PQRST complex, (2) detection of

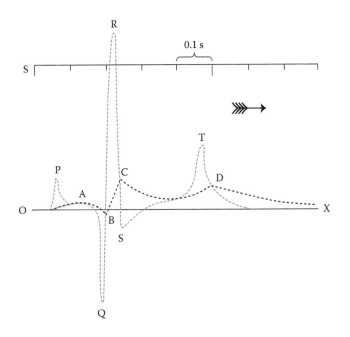

FIGURE 9.1
Two superimposed ECGs are shown. The uncorrected curve is labeled ABCD. This tracing was made with refined Lippmann capillary electrometer. The other curve was mathematically corrected by Einthoven to allow for inertia and friction in the capillary tube. (From AlGhatrif, M. and Lindsay, J., *J. Comm. Hosp. Intern. Med. Perspect.*, 2, 2012.)

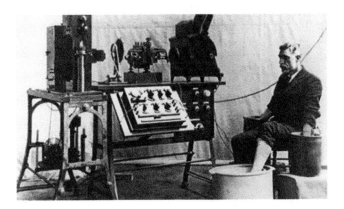

FIGURE 9.2
Old string galvanometer electrocardiograph showing the big machine with the patient rinsing his extremities in the cylindrical electrodes filled with electrolyte solution. (From AlGhatrif, M. and Lindsay, J., *J. Comm. Hosp. Intern. Med. Perspect.*, 2, 2012.)

P, QRS, and ST-segments of the ECG waveform, and (3) ECG waveform abnormalities in terms of P-wave amplitude, P–R interval, and QRS width.

We then proceed to the next part of our chapter on heart rate variability (HRV) signal, processing, and analysis methods for studying heart rate rhythms and how to detect arrhythmias from the normal sinus rhythm (NSR). We study the steps of how the HRV signal is employed for diagnosis, involving (1) continuous wavelet transform (CWT) application, resulting in a series of wavelet coefficients in the form of a scalogram signal, and (2) principal component analysis (PCA) to reduce the dimension of the data and identify the patterns expressed in terms of their differences and similarities, by performing a covariance analysis. From the covariance matrix, we calculate the eigenvectors and eigenvalues, which constitute the extracted features of signal patterns. We study the distribution of these eigenvalues over the NSR and the four arrhythmias, and find considerable overlap for some arrhythmias. Hence, we develop single Physiological Index number called the HRVID Index by combining these eigenvalues, and find that this HRVID Index can effectively separate out the different arrhythmia classes from the NSR category. We hence make a case for the adoption of this HRVID Index for arrhythmia detection.*

9.2 Electrical Activity of the Heart

The electrocardiogram (ECG) is a biosignal representing the combined activity of millions of cardiac depolarization potentials. ECG genesis is due to the electrical activity occurring in the heart. A potential difference exists in each cell. In order for the cell to constantly maintain this potential difference, positive ions are pumped out of the cell and negative ions are pumped into the cell. There is a dipole moment at any point on the cell membrane, which is caused by the difference in charge between the inner and outer cell membranes. This difference in charge will be canceled out by an identical dipole moment occurring at the opposite side of the cell. The heart contains a specialized group of muscle cells called the myocardium. When the myocardium is electrically stimulated, an action potential (AP) is created. The term AP describes the momentary change in the electrical potential across a cell membrane. Figure 9.3 shows the course of action potential occurring in a cell.

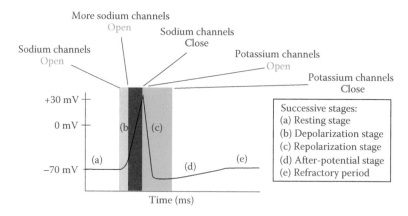

FIGURE 9.3
The course of action potential occurring in cells.

---

* This chapter was based on Swapna et al. 2012. ECG signal generation and heart rate variability signal extraction: Signal processing, features detection, and their correlation with cardiac diseases. *Journal of Mechanics in Medicine and Biology* (*Special Issue*) 12:1240012-1–1240012-26 and Vinitha Sree et al. 2012. Cardiac arrhythmia diagnosis by HRV signal processing using principal component analysis. *Journal of Mechanics in Medicine and Biology* 12:1240032-1–1240032-16 with permission from World Scientific Publishers.

9.2.1 Different Stages of Action Potential

The course of action potential across a cell membrane consists of five stages: *resting, depolarization, repolarization, after-potential,* and *refractory period.* These stages are briefly explained as follows (Swapna et al. 2012).

> *Resting stage (stage "a" in Figure 9.3):* Resting potential (RP) is due to the presence of electrical charge across the membrane of a cell. The RP of the myocardium's inner cell membrane is relatively negative. It also varies at different locations of the heart. For example, the myocardium's RP is approximately –70 mV in the sino-atrial (SA) node. The resting potential is due to the difference in the concentration of ions (electrically charged molecules) on different sides of the cell membrane. Sodium (Na^+), chloride (Cl^-), and potassium (K^+) are the ions present in the cells. The concentration of ions outside the cell is comprised of Na^+ and Cl^-, while K^+ and organic anions comprise the concentration inside the cell. To maintain a cell's resting potential, a membrane protein, known as sodium–potassium pump, pumps outside three Na^+ ions, in exchange for two K^+ ions that are pumped inside the cell. A shift from resting to depolarization stage is caused by an external electrical stimulus from the nervous system.
>
> *Depolarization (stage "b" in Figure 9.3):* The stage after resting is depolarization. It consists of two sub-stages: partial and rapid depolarization. When partial depolarization reaches the activation threshold, the voltage-gated sodium ion channels open. Then, rapid depolarization occurs leading to the rushing in of sodium ions and causing the membrane potential to change from –70 to +40 mV.
>
> *Repolarization (stage "c" in Figure 9.3):* When depolarization reaches a certain stage, the voltage-gated potassium ion channels open, allowing K^+ ions to rush out of the cell. Along with these, voltage-gated sodium ion channels will close and become refractory. This is the repolarization stage that causes the positive potential to decrease, cross zero and increase in the negative direction. This process causes the membrane to be repolarized and then hyperpolarized as shown by the "c" stage of Figure 9.3.
>
> *After-potential stage and refractory period (stages "d" and "e" in Figure 9.3):* After repolarization, the potassium channels will close and the sodium channels are reset. This is the after-potential stage followed by the refractory period where there is no occurrence of depolarization. Ions diffuse away from the area, and the polarization is maintained by the sodium–potassium transporter. The cell membrane can then repeat its cycle.

Figure 9.4 shows the different stages of action potential occurring between the membranes of the cells, as explained earlier.

The specialized action potential occurring in the heart is called cardiac action potential. The action potential is generated in the heart due to the movement of ions through the transmembrane ion channels. Due to the property of cardiac muscle automaticity, the cardiac muscles can depolarize spontaneously without external electrical stimulation from the nervous system. The property of automaticity is profoundly found in the SA node of the heart. The SA node contains cells which are the fastest in undergoing spontaneous depolarization. Hence, the SA node is known as the pacemaker of the heart (the SA node cells are called the pacemaker cells), since it sets the heart rate. Electrical activity gets

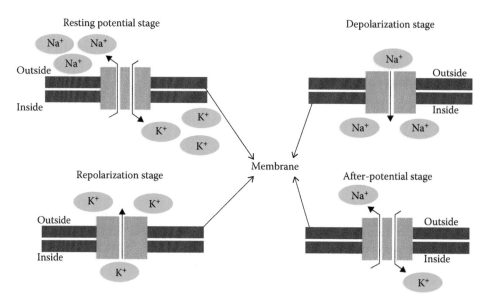

FIGURE 9.4
Different stages of action potential occurring between the membranes of the cell.

originated from the SA node and spreads to the ventricle muscle passing through different regions like atrial muscle, atrioventricular (AV) node, common bundle, bundle branches, and Purkinje fibers. The combined electrical activity is represented by the ECG waveform. Figure 9.5 shows a cross-sectional view of the heart and the respective electrical activity from various regions.

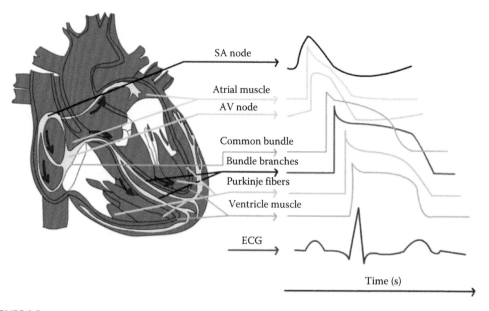

FIGURE 9.5
Cross-sectional view of the heart and the respective electric activity from its various regions.

9.2.2 Different Phases of Action Potential Generation

The course of action potential can also be explained in an alternate way in the form of various phases. The different phases of the AP generation in the myocardium are phases 0, 1, 2, 3, and 4. Depending on the type of cell involved, different behaviors are observed in each phase.

Phase 4 is the resting potential, which is the membrane potential when the cell is not subjected to electrical stimulation typically from an adjacent cell. Once the cell is stimulated, it starts a sequence of actions involving an exchange of positive and negative ions in and out of the cell, causing an action potential that propagates to the adjacent cell. The electrical stimulation is thus conducted and propagated to all the parts of the heart.

Phase 0 occurs when there is an initiation of depolarization marked by an upstroke of the AP in the SA node and Purkinje fibers. This is caused by the net entry of positive charges carried by sodium ions and the resulting potential is approximately +20 mV. The behavior of phase 0 is similar to the rapid depolarization stage explained earlier. Next is phase 1. Phase 1 occurs when a rapid repolarization occurs in the Purkinje fibers due to a rapid inactivation of the fast sodium channels. It is also due to the presence of an outward current, which is carried not only mostly by potassium ions but also by chloride ions. Phase 2 occurs when there is a potential plateau for a period at its depolarized value in the Purkinje fibers only. This is due to the near balance of several opposing currents, mainly due to the inward movement of calcium ions and outward movement of potassium ion. The outward potassium current is slowly being activated.

Phase 3 is the rapid repolarization phase of action potential due to the latter potassium current, which is being activated more fully in a time-dependent manner while the calcium channels are closed. Thus, a net positive current flows outward, resulting in negative changes to the potential of the cell membrane leading to the opening of more potassium channels, which again cause more potassium flow to the outside of the cell. The total repolarization of the cell occurs during phase 4 where it reaches the resting potential, and it remains in this phase until another electrical stimulation occurs.

Although the SA node is acting as a self-sufficient pacemaker, it is still heavily innervated by the nerves of the sympathetic and parasympathetic nervous systems. Stimulation of the SA node by the parasympathetic nervous system will decrease its pace, while stimulation by the sympathetic nervous system will increase its pace. This is because the sympathetic and parasympathetic nervous systems regulate the depolarization rate and duration of the action potential of the SA node cells. Stress, exercise, and heart disease cause sympathetic stimulation. Parasympathetic activity is the result of functioning of internal organs, trauma, allergic reactions, and the inhalation of irritants.

9.3 ECG Generation and Basic ECG Components

9.3.1 ECG Generation

Electrocardiography is the process of recording the electrical activity of the heart. It is a noninvasive and effective diagnostic tool for studying cardiac rhythm and understanding arrhythmias. Its first version known as electrocardiogram was invented by Einthoven in 1902. Einthoven also proposed and developed the model of human cardiac excitation. He modeled cardiac excitation as a vector and came up with the Einthoven triangle. Figure 9.6 shows the Einthoven triangle that was drawn using the two shoulders and the

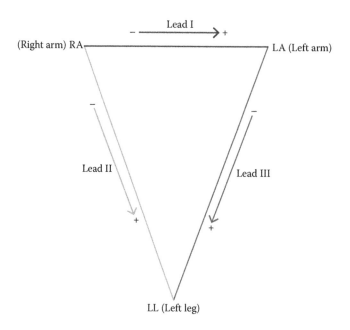

FIGURE 9.6
Einthoven triangle.

navel as vertices. It also shows the relationship between the Einthoven vector and each of the three frontal limb leads (leads I, II, and III). The three electrodes are generally colored as per the standards of the American Heart Association (AHA) and the International Electrotechnical Commission (IEC). The color code described in the following is as per AHA standard. The W (white) lead, which always has the negative polarity, is placed over the right arm (RA). The B (black) lead, which is positive for lead I and negative for lead II, is placed over left arm (LA). The R (red) is always of positive parity (positive polarity for both leads II and III connected to it) and is usually placed near the left lateral base of the chest (LL). This position is near the apex of the heart. The arrow shown parallel to lead III represents a vector. The potential difference measured between two vertices or limbs of the triangle is proportional to the projection of the vector on the side of the triangle that connects the limbs, unless the vector representing the spread of cardiac excitation is unknown.

Figure 9.7 shows the method of measuring ECG by using electrodes attached to the body surface and the way of connecting the electrodes to an instrumentation amplifier. The electrodes are connected to an approximate lead II configuration. The output ECG signal can be either positive or negative. In order to observe a positive-going output ECG signal, the points in time for the vector need to be pointing toward the electrode connected to the positive terminal of the amplifier and vice versa. Figure 9.7 also shows the body surface ECG for one heartbeat with its characteristic P wave, QRS complex, and T wave, produced by the time-varying motion of the cardiac vector.

9.3.2 Basic ECG Components—Generation and Their Associated Heart Events

The cardiac spread of excitation represented by a vector at different points in time is shown in Figure 9.8, as per measurements taken according to the configuration shown in Figure 9.7. The ECG is made up of a series of waves and lines, and it can be displayed on

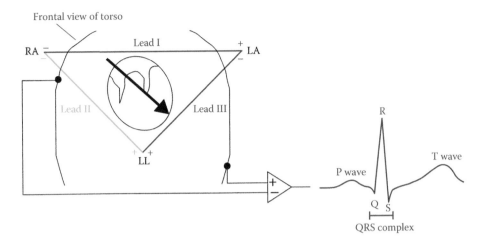

FIGURE 9.7
ECG measurement.

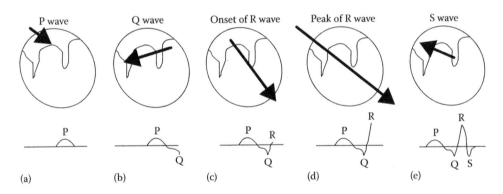

FIGURE 9.8
The cardiac spread of excitation represented by a vector at different points in time. (a) P wave, (b) Q wave, (c) onset of R wave, (d) peak of R wave, and (e) S wave.

a screen or recorded on an ECG paper. Figure 9.9 is a typical ECG waveform, with time in seconds as the *x*-axis and surface potential in millivolts as the *y*-axis. Some of the basic ECG components are P wave, Q wave, R wave, S wave, PR interval, ST-segment, and QRS complex. The interval is the time from the start of one wave to the start of another wave, while the segment is the time between waves. This implies that interval should include at least one wave, while segment does not contain any wave.

Figure 9.8 along with Figure 9.5 represent how the ECG waveform evolves, starting with an impulse generated in the SA node located in the right atrium. The action potential created in the SA node conducts to the AV node through the intermodal tracts. When the SA node depolarizes, it leads to the contraction of a cascade of myocardial tissue, resulting in the ejection of blood from the atrium to the ventricles. The process of conduction is delayed momentarily when it reaches the AV node. This delay is to ensure that ventricles are completely filled with blood. After the delay, the conduction process is continued through the His-Purkinje fibers (located at the septum of the heart) across the ventricles, resulting in the pumping of blood from ventricles to the lungs and remaining part of the body. As the

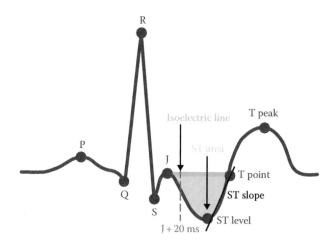

FIGURE 9.9
Various features of an ECG waveform.

action potential that originates in SA node traverses to the ventricles, the different parts of the ECG waveform like P wave, Q wave, etc., are formed.

Figure 9.8a shows the P wave that represents the slow-moving depolarization of the atria that begins at the SA node. The P wave starts with the first deviation from the baseline and ends when the wave again touches the baseline. The isoelectric line or baseline is the section where the voltage of the cardiac cells does not change. The depolarization of the ventricles is represented by the QRS complex. The start of the depolarization results in a small downward or negative deflection called Q wave. In other words, the first narrow negative deflection present in the QRS complex represents the Q wave. Figure 9.8b presents the Q wave indicating that the Purkinje system starts delivering the stimulus to the ventricular muscle after the appearance of the isoelectric region, after the P wave due to a delayed signal in the AV node. This isoelectric region is the PR segment, which occurs between the end of the P wave and the start of the QRS complex. The time taken to conduct through the AV section is reflected in the PR segment.

The R wave is due to the rapid depolarization of the ventricular muscle (Figure 9.8c). The R wave is the first positive deflection of the QRS complex above baseline. Figure 9.8d shows the peak of the R wave, which represents the point of the maximal vector in time when most of the cells are depolarized. Finally, Figure 9.8e shows the occurrence of the final phase of ventricular depolarization due to the excitation spreading toward the base of the ventricles, which gives rise to the S wave. The S wave dips below the baseline and then flattens out indicating the end of the S wave namely the J point. It is not essential for the QRS complex to have all these three waveforms of Q, R, and S.

9.4 Detection of P, QRS, and ST-Segments of the ECG Waveform

9.4.1 QRS Detection Algorithm

Pan and Tompkins (1985) developed a real-time QRS detection algorithm that can recognize QRS complexes based on analyses of amplitude, width, and slope of the ECG signal. Figure 9.10 shows the different filters involved in the analysis of the ECG signal.

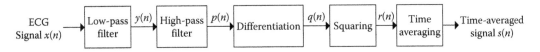

FIGURE 9.10
Flowchart depicting the various processes involved in the QRS detection.

The signal has to be passed through a bandpass filter composed of cascaded low-pass and high-pass integer filters. Differentiation, squaring, and time averaging of the ECG signal are involved in the subsequent processes.

The bandpass filter comprising of low-pass and high-pass filters was designed from a special class of digital filters that require only integer coefficients as it permits the microprocessor to perform the signal processing using only integer arithmetic. The input to the bandpass filter is $x(n)$, and $p(n)$ is its output. The filtered signal $p(n)$ is then differentiated to find the high slopes that distinguish the QRS complexes from the other waves in the ECG. Differentiation is done using linear digital filters to obtain $q(n)$. After the process of differentiation is completed, point-by-point squaring of the signal samples is required. It is a nonlinear transformation, which serves to make all the data positive before subsequent integration can take place. Higher frequencies in the signal obtained from differentiation process are also accentuated by squaring. Usually, the QRS complex is characterized by these higher frequencies.

In order to integrate the squared waveform $r(n)$, it is passed through a moving window integrator to get $s(n)$. The integrator will sum the area under the squared waveform over an interval of 150 ms, advance one sample interval, and will integrate the new 150 ms window. It is required to ensure that the window's width is not only short enough so that there is no overlapping of both QRS complex and T wave, but also long enough to include the time duration of extended abnormal QRS complexes.

Based on continuously updated estimates of peak noise and peak signal level, adaptive amplitude thresholds are then applied to both the moving integration waveform and the bandpass-filtered waveform. Finally, the detection process will determine whether the detected event is a QRS complex or not after preliminary detection by adaptive thresholds. As each QRS complex is detected, the QRS duration is calculated using a measurement algorithm. Thus, the QRS duration and RR interval are calculated for subsequent arrhythmia analysis. The algorithm for QRS detection is described in more detail as follows.

9.4.1.1 Bandpass (Low-Pass and High-Pass) Filtering

In order to reduce noise in the ECG signal, there is a requirement for the bandpass filter to be included in the QRS detection algorithm. It helps to attenuate the baseline wander, T wave interference, 60 Hz interference, and the noise due to muscle. It comprises of the low-pass filter and high-pass filter. The low-pass filter is defined by Equation 9.1 and the high-pass filter by Equation 9.2.

$$y(n) = \frac{x(n) + 2 \times x(n-1) + x(n-2)}{4} \tag{9.1}$$

$$p(n) = y(n) - y(n-1) \tag{9.2}$$

9.4.1.2 Differentiation

In order to find the slope of the QRS complex, the signal has to undergo differentiation after bandpass filtering. This procedure is characterized by Equation 9.3. After the ECG signal has undergone bandpass filtering and differentiation, the peak-to-peak signal corresponding to the QRS complex will be further enhanced, while T and P waves will be attenuated.

$$q(n) = \frac{p(n) + 2 \times p(n-1) + p(n-2)}{4} \tag{9.3}$$

9.4.1.3 Squaring

After bandpass filtering and differentiation, the ECG signal will be squared. Squaring is a nonlinear operation that not only makes all the data points in the signal become positive but also amplifies the output of the derivative process. Thus, this process emphasizes the higher frequencies in the signal, which mainly belong to the QRS complex. Equation 9.4 presents the equation used for squaring.

$$r(n) = (q(n))^2 \tag{9.4}$$

9.4.1.4 Moving Window Integral

Due to the presence of long durations and large amplitudes in many abnormal QRS complexes, detecting the QRS through the slope of R wave alone is not a guaranteed method. Therefore, moving window integration is performed on the squared signal in order to extract more information from the signal. Equation 9.5 defines the moving-window integration process.

$$s(n) = \frac{1}{N}(r(n-(N-1)) + r(n-(N-2)) + \cdots + r(n)) \tag{9.5}$$

9.4.2 ST-Segment Detection Analysis

The segment of the ECG signal after depolarization and before repolarization represents the ST-segment. The ST-segment is between the QRS complex and the T wave (Figure 9.9). If there is a deficiency in the blood supply to the heart muscle, it will be indicated by the changes in the ST-segment. Therefore, the ability to perform measurements of the ST-segment would be crucial for diagnosing cardiovascular abnormalities. In order to detect the ST-segment, it is important to detect the QRS waveform first. To obtain the maximal value of the R wave peak, the interval corresponding to 60 ms after the QRS detection mark has to be searched. Before the R wave is observed, the first inflection point is the Q wave and is recognized by a significant change in the slope. The inflection point, as per differential calculus, is a point on a curve where the sign of the curvature changes. To calculate the slope, the three-point difference derivative method is applied. To calculate the slope of a noisy ECG signal, a low-pass digital filter has to be applied first to filter out the noise of the ECG signal.

The next part of the ECG to be located and measured is the isoelectric line. The location of the isoelectric line in the ECG waveform is performed by searching for a 30 ms interval of near-zero slope between the P and Q waves. The end of the QRS duration is determined by locating the S point, which is the first inflection point after the R wave. It is important to obtain the R-peak magnitude relative to the isoelectric line, RR intervals, and the QRS duration.

After the S point, the first inflection point is the J point. The T point that marks the onset of the T wave is observed by locating the peak of T wave, which has a maximal absolute value. This value is relative to the isoelectric line and is between J + 80 ms and R + 400 ms. By looking for a 35 ms period on the R side of the T wave, the T point can be found. The T point is one of the most difficult features to be found in ECG waveform. Hence, it will be assumed to be J + 120 ms if it is not detected.

A windowed search method is applied to measure the ST-segment after various ECG features have been identified. The two window limits are defined by two boundaries, which are at J + 20 ms and T point. The elevation, also known as point of maximal depression, in the window, is then identified. The absolute change relative to the isoelectric line can be used to express the level of the ST-segments.

Other parameters such as the ST slope, ST area, and ST index are calculated apart from the ST-segment level. The amplitude difference between the ST-segment point and T point divided by the corresponding time interval is used to define the ST slope. By summing all sample values between the T and J points after subtracting isoelectric line value from each point, the value of the ST area can be calculated. Calculating the sum of the ST-segment level and 1/10th of ST slope will give the ST index.

9.4.3 Filtered ECG Waveforms Showing the Detected Features: P Wave, R–R Peak, ST-Segment, and T Wave

Figure 9.11 shows a few waveforms of the ECG signal, after it has gone through the various filter stages of the QRS detection algorithm described in Section 9.4.1. The first waveform in Figure 9.9 depicts the unfiltered ECG input signal. The second waveform represents the output after bandpass filtering and differentiation. From this waveform, it can be observed that the T wave is absent in the ECG signal. It may be due to the high-pass filter that helps to attenuate the T wave in the ECG signal. The third waveform shows the ECG signal after it has gone through bandpass filtering, differentiation, and squaring. The fourth waveform shows the result of the moving window integration.

Figure 9.12 shows the detected components of the ECG signal. The first waveform is the low-pass filtered ECG signal. The other waveforms show the detected P wave, R–R peak, ST-segment, and the T wave. The second waveform in Figure 9.12 indicates the detected P peaks. The relationship of the P waves and QRS complexes is used in the identification of various cardiac arrhythmias. A patient with hypokalemia can be identified if there is a presence of larger amplitude of the P wave. The third waveform in Figure 9.10 shows the detected R–R peak. By locating the R point for each beat of the signal, all other characteristic points on the ECG signal can also be determined using this R point as a reference point. The fourth waveform in Figure 9.12 shows the start and end points of the ST-segments. After the determination of the width of the start and end points of the ST-segment, it is possible to determine the ST-segment region area, characteristic features of the ST-segment slope, and ST-segment deviation. The fifth waveform in Figure 9.12 indicates the detected T peaks. The time interval between the R peak and the T peak of the same beat of ECG signal is known as the RT interval. In order to obtain the RT interval in the ECG, the peak of the T wave needs to be determined. The time interval between adjacent QRS complexes is called RR interval (t_{R-R}). Heart rate (HR) in terms of beat per minute (bpm) is given by HR = $60/t_{R-R}$.

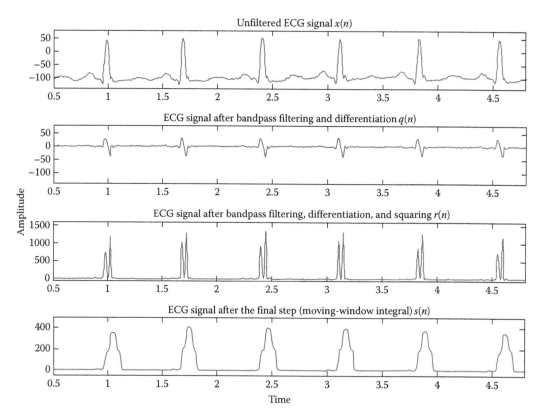

FIGURE 9.11
ECG waveform output after various stages of filtering in the QRS detector.

9.5 ECG Waveform Abnormalities in Terms of P-Wave Amplitude, P–R Interval, and QRS Width

The activity of the autonomic nervous system (ANS), which controls the rhythm of the heart, is reflected in the ECG. Research over decades has underlined the relation between ANS and cardiovascular mortality (Schwartz and Priori 1990, Levy and Schwartz 1994, Task Force 1996). Therefore, cardiac health can be assessed from ECG (Sokolow et al. 1990). The abnormalities in the ST-segment, QRS, and P wave in the ECG waveform are indicators of cardiovascular diseases. The anomalies of the heart cause anatomical differences in the structure of atria and ventricles and produce changes in its sequential activation, depolarization, and repolarization. These changes are reflected by the deviations of the ECG waveform from its normal shape and size. It may so happen that the correct sequence of P–QRS–T may not occur. Hence, cardiac rhythm analysis is an important method to diagnose cardiac abnormalities. A brief description of some of the indications of normal and abnormal heart conditions (Malmivuo and Plonsey 1995) is given in the following:

Normal heart: Normal heart produces normal P–QRS–T waveform in the ECG. In the normal ECG waveform, the QRS amplitude is about 1 mV and its duration is about 0.08–0.09 s. The P-wave amplitude is about 0.1 mV with duration of 0.1 s. T-wave

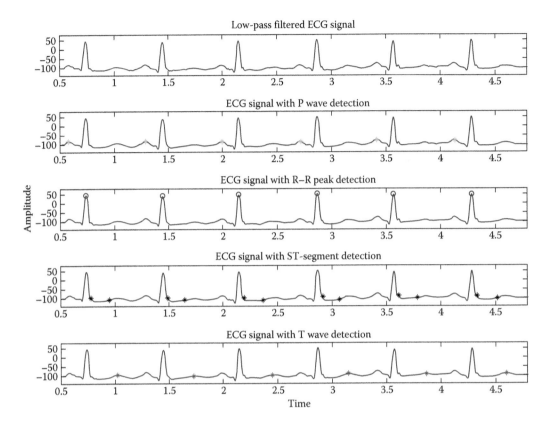

FIGURE 9.12
ECG waveforms indicating various detected features.

amplitude and duration are roughly double that of the P-wave. T-wave occurs about 0.2 s after the occurrence of QRS waveform.

Normal sinus rhythm: A healthy normal heart produces a normal sinus rhythm with a frequency between 60 and 100 min^{-1}. The name sinus comes from the fact that the sinus node is the originating point that triggers the cardiac activation. The three deflections, P–QRS–T, of the ECG waveform follow in this order and are clearly differentiable.

Sinus bradycardia: An increased vagal or parasympathetic tone may result in a sinus rhythm having a frequency less than 60 min^{-1}. This type of sinus rhythm is called sinus bradycardia. Sinus bradycardia falls under the category of supraventricular (above the ventricles) cardiac rhythm. Supraventricular rhythms originate in the atria or AV junction, and they travel to the ventricles.

Premature ventricular contraction: This arrhythmia comes under the category of ventricular arrhythmias, where the originating point of the activation is not in the AV node and/or it proceeds to the ventricles in a method quite different from the normal that results in a relatively short duration QRS complex. A premature ventricular contraction occurs abnormally early. If the originating point is in the atrium or in the AV node, it is said to be of supraventricular origin and the duration of the corresponding QRS complex is less than 0.1 s. If the originating point is in the ventricular muscle, then the QRS complex has a very abnormal form, and its duration is longer than 0.1 s.

Bundle-branch block: This condition denotes a defect in the conduction of activation in either of the bundle-branches or in either fascicle of the left bundle-branch. If there is simultaneous block in the two bundle-branches, then there is complete inhibition in the progress of activation from the atria to the ventricles resulting in third-degree (total) atrioventricular block. This is reflected as a total lack of synchronism between the P wave and the QRS complex. Bundle-branch block thus results in bizarre-shaped QRS complexes with abnormally longer durations. According to the location of the bundle where the defect lies, there is right bundle-branch block and left bundle-branch block.

Paroxysmal atrial tachycardia (PAT): In this condition, P waves occur as a result of a reentrant activation front (circus movement) in the atria, usually involving AV node. The rate of activation is very high, usually in the range of 160–220 min^{-1}. The isoelectric baseline usually lies between the T wave and the next P wave.

Atrial flutter: The arrhythmia where the heart rate is sufficiently high, so that the isoelectric interval between the end of T and beginning of P disappears, is called atrial flutter. This arrhythmia involves a reentrant atrial pathway. The frequency lies between 220 and 300 min^{-1}. Every second or every third atrial impulse (2:1 or 3:1 heart block) activates the AV-node and then the ventricles.

Atrial fibrillation: This arrhythmia produces irregular fluctuations in the baseline due to the fully irregular and chaotic activation in the atria. The ventricular rate is also rapid and irregular, while the QRS contour is usually normal. Rheumatic disease, atherosclerotic disease, hyperthyroidism, and pericarditis may cause atrial fibrillation.

In Table 9.1, the various cardiac disorders are designated in terms of the values of heart rate, P–R interval, QRS width, and P-wave amplitude measured from normal and different abnormal ECG waveforms. From this table, it can be observed that although some of the abnormalities can occur in the same part of the heart such as the atria, they can still be distinguished as different abnormalities based on these measurements. These measurements can be done by performing QRS detection and identifying the important features of the ECG. Thus, this table emphasizes the importance of the QRS detection and ST-segment analysis methods mentioned previously.

9.6 Heart Rate Variability Signal and HRV Analysis Methods for Studying Cardiac Disorders

9.6.1 Limitations of ECG Signal Analysis

From Table 9.1, it is evident that the information to be extracted from ECG signal lies in the shape and size of the P-QRS-T wave, the time intervals between its various peaks, etc. It is this subtle information that indicates the nature of disease affecting the heart. However, it is very difficult to manually monitor these subtle details visually. Also, these indicators may be present at all times or may occur at random times (Acharya et al. 2005).

TABLE 9.1

Heart Rate, P–R Interval, QRS Width, and P-Wave Amplitude of Normal and Abnormal Heart Conditions

Types	Heart rate (bpm)	P–R interval (s)	QRS width (s)	P-wave amplitude (mm)
Normal	60–90	0.12–0.21	0.06–0.08	2.0–2.5
Sinus bradycardia	40–60	0.12–0.21	0.06–0.08	2.0–2.5
Premature ventricular contraction	90–140	P wave absent	0.12–0.21	Absent
Bundle branch block	60–140	0.12–0.2	0.12>	>2.5
Atrial premature contraction	60–140	0.12–0.21	>0.2 or <0.12	<2.5
Sinus arrest	75	0.2	0.08 (missing during pause)	2.0–2.5 (missing during pause)
Sinoatrial exit block	60 (before SA block)	0.16	0.08 (missing during pause)	Periodically absent
Sick sinus syndrome	43–150	Varies with rhythm	0.10	Varies with prevailing rhythm
Premature atrial contraction	90	0.12–0.18	0.08	Premature and abnormally shaped with PACs
Atrial tachycardia	200	Not visible	0.10	Hidden in preceding T wave
Atrial tachycardia with block	140–250	Can vary but is usually constant for conducted P waves	0.06–0.08	Slightly abnormal
Multifocal atrial tachycardia	100–250 (atria and ventricle)	Varying	Abnormal	varying
Paroxysmal atrial tachycardia	140–250	Immeasurable	Abnormal	Inverted
Atrial flutter	280 (atria) 60 (ventricle)	Immeasurable	0.08	Classic sawtooth appearance
Atrial fibrillation	Indiscernible (atrial) 130 (ventricle)	Indiscernible	0.08	Absent

Thus, visual examination of ECG waveform signals for the diagnosis of diseases is highly subjective (Acharya et al. 2002). Randomness in the occurrence of symptoms necessitates the careful analysis of ECG waveform over sufficient time durations which may even extend to several hours. Furthermore, morphologies of the ECG waveform show large variations even within the same patient. These factors led to the thought of transforming the shape-related information in ECG to digital signal-related information.

Heart rate variability (HRV) signal is one such discrete signal, wherein the complete information lies in the value of each discrete data sample. HRV signals are reliable, accurate, reproducible, yet very simple to measure and process. The ECG-to-HRV conversion not only removes the subjectivity factor in analysis, but also makes the data suitable to be analyzed using computers. Kleiger et al. (1991) and Ge et al. (2002) showed that HRV measurements have good reproducibility when done under standardized conditions and are easy to perform.

9.6.2 HRV Signal and Its Use in Diagnosing Diseases

The HRV signal is obtained from the measurements of the time interval between two consecutive R waves. HRV is the variation of the heart beat period measured in time units. The instantaneous heart rate is decided by a variety of hormonal, neural, and myocardial factors (Constant et al. 1999). Like ECG, the HRV signal also represents the electrophysiological properties of the heart. HRV signals indicate the sympathetic–parasympathetic autonomic balance and serve as a warning signal about the risk for sudden cardiac death (SCD) (Acharya et al. 2006). These signals serve either as indicators of a disease already present or as predictors of impending cardiovascular diseases. It is shown that decreased heart rate variability is a strong indicator of the increased risk of cardiovascular diseases (Acharya et al. 2008). The HRV method is sensitive enough to detect cardiac autonomic impairments before traditional cardiovascular autonomic function tests like Ewing battery can do so (Schroeder et al. 2005).

The HRV is a reflection of the state of ANS. The ANS is affected by a lot of factors like blood pressure, diabetes, myocardial infarction (MI), renal problems, drugs, smoking, alcohol, age, gender, and sleep. HRV analysis can be used to analyze many situations, and it can serve as an indicator to several diseases affecting the ANS (Acharya et al. 2006). For example, acute MI is associated with an increase of sympathetic activity and decrease in parasympathetic activity (Rothschild et al. 1988). Brain damage and depression reduces the normal cyclic changes in the HR (Lowensohn et al. 1977, Acharya et al. 2003a). For diabetic patients, the parasympathetic autonomic activity is reduced much before the clinically distinguishable symptoms appear (Pfeifer et al. 1982, Singh et al. 2000). Also, HRV analysis can help in monitoring post-infarction and diabetic patients. Nocturnal heart period analysis using time–frequency parameters and wavelet decomposition can serve as an effective tool for obstructive sleep apnea syndrome diagnosis (Roche et al. 2003).

9.6.3 Techniques for HRV Analysis

HRV analysis is widely employed as a noninvasive tool for assessing the activities of the ANS. The system that generates the HR signal is not simply linear, and thus, the HR signal has significant nonlinear content. HRV is not only nonlinear but also nonstationary. The HRV signals can be analyzed using methods based on time domain, frequency domain, time–frequency domain, and also geometric and nonlinear methods. This section presents a brief summary of these techniques.

9.6.3.1 Time Domain–Based Techniques

The most important time domain measure of HRV is the value of RR interval. A number of parameters are derived from the RR interval value. Among them, there are measures of variance like SDNN (also called SDRR) and error measures like SENN. The SDNN (ms), which is an indicator of total variability, is the standard deviation of all RR intervals about mean RR for the entire recording. SENN is the standard error of the mean RR or NN interval and is calculated by measuring the standard deviation of the sampling distribution of means, based on data. These parameters reflect vagal (i.e., parasympathetic) as well as sympathetic modulations over the normal heart rate.

Measures like RMSSD and Edinburgh index analyze differences between adjacent RR intervals. The RMSSD (unit ms) is the square root of the mean of sum of the squares of the differences between adjacent normal RR intervals measured over entire 24 h ECG recording. RMSSD is an indicator of high-frequency variations in heart rate; it mainly reflects parasympathetic activity. The Edinburgh index (also called SNN50 counts) is the number of times the differences between adjacent normal RR intervals exceeds 50 ms. NN50 is calculated over the 24 h ECG recording while PNN50 (%) is the percentage of the aforementioned difference.

SDSD is the standard deviation of differences between adjacent NN intervals. The parameters RMSSD and NN50 reflect short-term HRV. They represent changes in vagal tones, and hence, these parameters are named as vagal indexes. Abnormalities of heart, like preventricular contraction (PVC) and atrial fibrillation (AF), cause higher RR variation resulting in higher values of time domain parameters SDNN, SENN, SDSD, RMSSD, and PNN50%. For heart problems like complete heart block (CHB), ischemic/dilated cardiomyopathy, etc., these parameters show smaller value, since RR signals slowly vary for these abnormalities. There are geometrically representable time domain features such as the triangular index and TINN. These measures are highly insensitive to artifacts and ectopic beats.

The disadvantage of time domain parameters is that their mean values can be easily affected by artifacts and outliers. Hence, such measures require elimination of artifacts before data analysis.

9.6.3.2 Frequency Domain–Based Techniques

The main frequency domain method is the analysis of power spectral density (PSD). It is shown that the spectral analysis of the short-term variability of HR helps in the quantitative assessment of neurogenic oscillations that decide the instantaneous heart rate (Akselrod et al. 1985, Pomeranz et al. 1985). Typical power spectrum of the heart rate signal has the following three main frequency regions (Akselrod et al. 1981).

- The high-frequency (HF) power band (HF: 0.15–0.5 Hz)
- The low-frequency (LF) power band (LF: 0.04–0.15 Hz)
- The very-low-frequency (VLF) power band (VLF: 0.0033–0.04 Hz)

The HF region analysis can give vital information about the respiratory sinus arrhythmia and cardiac vagal activity, while LF shows baroceptor control mechanisms and the combined effect of vagal and sympathetic systems. Information about the thermoregulatory, vascular mechanisms, and renin–angiotension systems can be obtained by studying the VLF power region. In other words, the high-frequency region represents the parasympathetic activity, and the low-frequency region represents the combined effect of sympathetic and parasympathetic activity. The total power indicates the sympathetic/parasympathetic balance of the system (Myers et al. 1986, Saul et al. 1988, Ryan et al. 1992).

The Fourier transform technique is not much suitable in analyzing nonstationary signals because it does not provide the exact time localization. The reliability of the determined spectral power decreases with decrease in the signal power and the signal-to-noise ratio (Acharya et al. 2006). Fast Fourier transform (FFT) is normally employed for estimating PSD. Spectral leakage effects due to windowing can be avoided by using the parametric or model-based power spectrum estimation methods. Another advantage of this method is its improved frequency resolution compared to the classical or nonparametric method. AR (autoregressive) modeling is another popular method under the frequency domain, which is better suited for biosignals like EEG and ECG than traditional Fourier domain–based methods. EEG signals have been analyzed for distinguishing alcoholic and epileptic stages from normal by AR methods (Faust et al. 2008, 2010).

9.6.3.3 Wavelet Transform–Based Techniques

To overcome the limitations of Fourier techniques in analyzing nonstationary signals, several methods have been proposed. The time–frequency techniques like short-time Fourier transform (STFT) technique can provide better time localization, but with poorer frequency resolution. Wavelet transform is the best method among time–frequency techniques suitable for nonlinear and nonstationary signals like HRV. Wavelet analysis involves comparison of the signal with a chosen (finite duration) wavelet and recording the correlation coefficient (Vetterli 1992). There are two types of wavelet analysis: continuous wavelet transform (CWT) and discrete wavelet transform (DWT) (Meyer 1992). Sampling of CWT in a dyadic grid gives DWT. The DWT coefficients are determined for discrete values of scale factor and translation factors with the increments in the dyadic scale (Vetterli 1992).

9.6.3.4 Nonlinear Methods

Nonlinear methods are more suitable to analyze biosignals like ECG and HRV that are nonlinear and nonstationary in nature (Subha et al. 2010). The nonlinear dynamical theory is based on the concept of chaos. Cohen et al. (1996) showed that chaos theory-based methods have been used for HRV signal analysis and prediction of events like ventricular tachycardia (VT).

Poincare Plot and Recurrence Plot: Poincare plot is a graphical display of the correlation between consecutive RR intervals. The plot can provide the detailed beat-to-beat information about the heart (Kamen et al. 1996). Each RR interval is plotted as a function of the previous RR interval. Analysis implies visually examining the shape of the Poincare plot, and then categorizing it into functional classes that can indicate the degree of the heart failure in a subject. Poincare plot gives information about the nature of RR interval fluctuations. Recurrence plot measures the nonstationarity of the time-series. This graphical tool determines hidden periodicities in a signal in time domain, which is not easily noticeable.

Approximate Entropy (ApEn): ApEn takes a positive number corresponding to a time series. More complex or irregular data produces a higher ApEn value. Thus ApEn measures the disorder in HR signal. Its value reduces as HR variation reduces. For cardiac impairment cases, the HR variation is small, and hence, the ApEn value is also small.

Sample Entropy (SampEn): SampEn also measures the complexity and regularity of time-series data. It is an improved measure compared to ApEn.

Fractal Dimension (FD): A fractal is a set of points that resembles the whole set, even when looked at smaller scales (Mandelbrot et al. 1983). FD is a measure of the complexity of time series. This parameter can be used in ECG and EEG analysis to identify and distinguish specific states of physiological functions (Acharya et al. 2005).

Detrended Fluctuation Analysis (DFA): DFA parameter can assess the fractal scaling properties of short-term RR interval signals (Peng et al. 1996). The fluctuation is quantified by a factor "α" which is an indicator of the roughness of the time series. Smoother time series have larger values for "α." The value of "α" falls in different ranges for different types of cardiac abnormalities.

Largest Lyapunov Exponent (LLE): LLE defines the predictability of the signal or system and the sensitivity of the system to initial conditions. The Lyapunov exponent is positive and indicates chaos. LLE searches for nearest neighbor of each point in phase-space and tracks their separation over certain time evolution.

Correlation Dimension (CD): Correlation dimension is a nonlinear measure by which biosignals like ECG can be analyzed for diagnosing possible pathologies. CD is also a popular measure of fractal dimension. The value of CD will be high for chaotic type RR signal variations, while it will be low for low or rhythmic RR signal variations.

Higher Order Spectra (HOS): Higher order spectral analysis is a powerful tool for analyzing nonlinear and nonstationary physiological signals like EEG and ECG. The HOS (also known as poly spectra) is the spectral representation of higher order statistics (i.e., moments and cumulants of third and higher order). HOS analysis can detect nonlinearity, and deviations from Gaussianity. It helps to understand the phase relationships between harmonic components of the signal, since HOS preserves the true phase character of signals. Authors have used HOS for the analysis of nonlinear EEG signals for classifying them to normal, pre-ictal (background) and epileptic categories (Chua et al. 2009a,b), sleep stages (Acharya et al. 2010), and cardiac abnormalities (Chua et al. 2008a).

Recurrence Quantification Analysis (RQA): Recurrence quantification analysis is one of the methods used for nonlinear data analysis. In a state space trajectory of a dynamical system, RQA can be used to quantify its number and duration of recurrences. A cross recurrence plot (CRP) reveals all the times at which the phase space trajectory of the first dynamical system visits approximately the same area in the phase space where the phase space trajectory of the second dynamical system is located. It can be a nonsquare CRP matrix if the data length of both the systems is different. It can be applied to all the physiological signals to study the nonlinear and nonstationary behavior (Acharya et al. 2011).

9.6.4 Importance of Automation in HRV Analysis

As mentioned earlier, the indicators of the disease may occur at random. To look for the presence of these indicators, we need to collect, store, and analyze HRV data over long durations of time, extending to several hours. Computer-based analytical tools mentioned earlier are employed to (1) process and analyze the HRV signals by means of the aforementioned methods and measures, (2) characterize the features of the signals in terms of these measures and then feed them into classifiers for grouping into categories—normal subjects and those with disorders such as cardiac disorders and diabetes, and (3) thereby carry out diagnosis. These heart rate signals and patient information can be interleaved within the images with the different error correcting codes in a noisy environment, without affecting the hidden information (Acharya et al. 2001, 2003b).

9.6.5 Summary of Studies Using ECG and HRV for Detecting Cardiac Disorders

In this section, a brief summary of some of the key studies related to HRV analysis for cardiac disorder detection is presented.

Ge et al. (2002) classified cardiac arrhythmia into six classes by using autoregressive modeling and obtained an accuracy ranging from 93.2% to 100%. Acharya et al. (2002)

found that the ranges of the correlation dimension and detrended fluctuation analysis parameters fall in distinct ranges for the different states or diseases of the heart, like normal, ectopic, sick sinus syndrome, and complete heart block. The automated classification of heart rate data was performed by using nonlinear methods of Poincare plot geometry, largest Lyapunov exponent, and spectral entropy with artificial neural network (ANN) and fuzzy classifiers (Acharya et al. 2003a). An average accuracy of 95% for four classes was reported.

Acharya et al. (2004) analyzed eight types of cardiac classes such as atrial fibrillation using different nonlinear and linear methods and found out different ranges of values for each of the used linear and nonlinear parameters with a classification accuracy of 85%. Faust et al. (2004) calculated Renyi's entropy from the input HRV signals using time–frequency analysis and spatial filling index. The HR corresponding to different cardiac arrhythmias was proposed using wavelet transform. In another study by Acharya et al. (2005), cardiac health was analyzed using fractal dimension (FD) and wavelet transformation methods. It was shown that FD showed a better performance and provided more than 90% confidence interval in classifying cardiac data. Kannathal et al. (2006) used nonlinear features, such as SD1/SD2 (low range variability/long range variability), largest Lyapunov exponent and Hurst exponent coupled with adaptive neuro-fuzzy inference system (ANFIS) classifier, to achieve classification accuracy of 94% in distinguishing 10 cardiac classes. Chua et al. (2008a) classified five classes of heart rate signals using higher order spectra (HOS) features and support vector machine (SVM) classifier with an accuracy of 85%. Chua et al. (2008b) proposed different ranges of sample and approximate entropies, recurrence plots and Poincare plots for eight cardiac classes. They also proposed unique recurrence and Poincare plots for each disease. Acharya et al. (2008) analyzed HRV signals for the study of nine cardiac classes by using fast Fourier transform and three modeling techniques: autoregressive (AR), moving average (MA), and the autoregressive moving average (ARMA). It was shown that the ARMA modeling technique performed better than the other methods with an accuracy of 83.83%. Patil et al. (2010) classified QRS complexes of ECG waveforms as normal or myocardial ischemic by using discrete wavelet transform (DWT).

In another study by Acharya et al. (2013), normalized bispectrum entropies (P1 and P2), approximate entropy (ApEn), sample entropy (SampEn), and recurrence entropy (REN) were used to detect eight cardiac conditions. A cardiac integrated index was formulated by using these features. However, this index showed overlaps among few of the conditions, and hence, a better formulation of an Integrated Index is necessary so that there is effective separation of the values for the different disease states without overlap. In the following section, another unique novel formulation of an integrated index to differentiate normal sinus rhythm and four other types of cardiac arrhythmias is presented.

9.7 Application of HRV Analysis for the Detection of Normal Sinus Rhythm and Cardiac Arrhythmias

In this section, a technique for analyzing the HRV signal in order to differentiate normal sinus rhythm and four other types of cardiac arrhythmias is presented (Vinitha Sree et al. 2012).

9.7.1 Description of the Cardiac Conditions

The following is a brief description of the cardiac conditions that are to be differentiated by the HRV analysis technique. A few of these conditions have also been described briefly in Section 9.5.

Normal Sinus Rhythm (NSR) is generated by the sinus node and travels in a normal fashion in the heart. In the typical ECG signal, P waves are first observed. After a brief pause (of less than 20 s), a QRS complex is observed, and finally a T wave. The P wave morphology and axis must be normal. The PR interval ranges between 120 and 200 ms. The NSR is characterized by a usual rate of any value between 60 and 100 bpm.

Atrial Fibrillation (AF) constitutes random activation of different parts of the atria at different times, due to multiple patterns of electrical impulses traveling randomly through the atria. In the ECG signal, AF is noted by absence of P waves and irregularity of R–R interval. These may be due to irregular conduction of impulses to the ventricles. The heart rate for patients with AF may range from 100 to 175 bpm.

In *Pre-Ventricular Contraction (PVC)*, the regularity of the underlying rhythm of the heart is interrupted, as the heartbeat comes earlier than expected and causes problems outside the sinus atrial node. In the ECG signal, the QRS complex is not only widened, but it is also not associated with the preceding P wave. Usually, the T wave is observed to be in opposite direction from the R wave. Two consecutive PVCs exist in couplets, and a compensatory pause usually follows a PVC signal.

Complete Heart Block (CHB) is a disease of the heart's electrical system, which does not enable the electric signals of the heart to pass from the upper to the lower chambers. Thereby, all the impulses generated from the sinus node in the right atrium are not conducted into the ventricles. This causes ventricles to contract and pump the blood at a slower rate. Hence, there is a reduction of the heart rate (as low as 30 bpm). In patients with CHB, there is no normal relationship between the P and the QRS waves in ECG.

Ventricular Fibrillation (VF) is a condition that causes the heart's electrical activity to become disordered, causing the heart to fibrillate very rapidly (sometimes at 350 bpm or more). VF commonly occurs in severe coronary artery disease and cardiac arrest patients. In VF, instead of pumping blood, ventricular muscles contract randomly, causing complete failure of ventricular function. It is observed that there is irregular chaotic electrical activity in the ECG. There is usually no recognizable QRS complex in patients with VF.

9.7.2 Data Acquisition and Preprocessing

The ECG data used in this study were acquired from Kasturba Medical Hospital, Manipal, India after the required Institutional Review Board approval. The ECG was captured for a 15 min duration and was then digitized at the sampling frequency of 320 samples/s. The number of data sets acquired in each class of patients is shown in Table 9.2.

TABLE 9.2

Number of Data Sets for Different Cardiac Health States

Class	NSR	AF	PVC	CHB	VF
Number of data sets	90	20	27	22	21

NSR, normal sinus rhythm; AF, atrial fibrillation; PVC, premature ventricular contraction; CHB, complete heart block; VF, ventricular fibrillation.

In order to preprocess the acquired ECG data, a low-pass filter with a cut-off frequency of 35 Hz was first employed to remove the unwanted high frequencies. A high-pass filter with cut-off frequency 0.3 Hz was then applied to suppress the baseline wander. To suppress the power-line interference noise, a band-stop filter of cut-off frequencies 50 or 60 Hz was used. Finally, a median filter was used to extract the baseline wander present in the processed ECG signal. In order to effectively remove the baseline wander, the extracted wander was subtracted from the processed ECG signal. The Tompkins algorithm (Jiapu and Tomkins 1985, Wariar and Eswaran 1991) was then used to detect the R peaks.

Between two successive QRS complexes, there exists an interval, which can be defined as the RR interval (t_{R-R}, s). The heart rate (HR) (bpm) is given by the following equation:

$$HR = \frac{60}{t_{R-R}} \tag{9.6}$$

9.7.3 HRV Analysis Technique

A generalized predictive analytics classification framework comprises of (1) data preprocessing, (2) feature extraction, (3) feature selection, (4) classifier development, and (5) classifier evaluation elements. This framework is usually employed to determine the feature subset–classifier combination (also called as the predictive model) that presents the highest classification accuracy in detecting the classes. The classification framework used for classification of normal sinus rhythm and five other types of cardiac arrhythmias is visually represented in Figure 9.13. In this technique, the extracted HRV signals were analyzed in the wavelet domain. Thus, continuous wavelet transform (CWT) was first used to

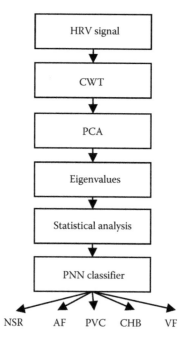

FIGURE 9.13
Proposed HRV analysis technique for classification of cardiac arrhythmias.

transform the signal into wavelet domain, and then principal component analysis (PCA) was performed on the extracted CWT coefficients in order to extract the eigenvalues. Only the first three eigenvalue features were selected and used to develop and evaluate the probabilistic neural network (PNN) classifier.

9.7.3.1 Continuous Wavelet Transform

Fourier transform uses complex exponential functions of infinite duration to represent biosignals of finite interval, thereby making it not very suited for analysis of nonstationary biosignals. Wavelet analysis, on the other hand, provides a better insight into both the timing and intensity of transient events. There are two types of wavelet analysis as described earlier—CWT and DWT. Wavelet is a small wave with finite energy and finite duration that is correlated with the signal to obtain the wavelet coefficients (Vetterlin 1992, Vetterli and Koyacevic 1995). The reference wavelet is known as the mother wavelet, and in this technique the Morlet (morl) wavelet was used to perform CWT (Figure 9.14).

The continuous wavelet transform $W_\psi(s, \tau)$ of a signal $f(x)$ is given by

$$W_\psi(s, \tau) \int_{-\infty}^{\infty} f(x) \psi_{s,\tau}(x) dx \tag{9.7}$$

The mother wavelet $\psi_{s,\tau}(x)$ is given by

$$\psi_{s,\tau}(x) = \frac{1}{\sqrt{s}} \psi\left(\frac{x-\tau}{s}\right) \tag{9.8}$$

where τ and s are called translation and scale parameters. The transformation is obtained from the mother wavelet through scaling and translation. The scale parameter corresponds to the frequency information. Scaling either expands or compresses the signal.

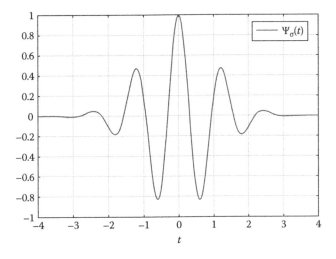

FIGURE 9.14
Morlet wavelet (morl).

Large scales (low frequency) will either dilate or expand the signal. This will provide detailed hidden information in the signal. Small scales (high frequency) will cause the signal to be compressed, and this will provide global information of the signal. The translation parameter refers to the location of the wavelet function as it is being shifted through the analyzed signal. Mathematically, continuous wavelet transform can be defined as the sum over all times of the signal $f(t)$ multiplied by shifted and scaled versions of the analyzing wavelet. The end result of the continuous wavelet transform will be a series of wavelet coefficients, which are a function of these shift and scale parameters. The resulting signal is known as scalogram.

9.7.3.2 Principal Component Analysis

Principal component analysis (PCA) is a technique that can be used to reduce multidimensional data into lesser dimensions without much loss of information of the data. It is one of the most successful techniques that have been used in data recognition and compression. PCA can reduce the dimension of the data by identifying the patterns that are expressed in terms of their differences and similarities by performing a covariance analysis. This will describe the strong correlation relationship between the observed variables in a multi-dimensional data set. Covariance (Equation 9.9) is used to measure the variation of the dimensions from the mean with respect to each other.

$$\text{cov}(X,Y) = \frac{\sum_{i=1}^{n}\left(X_i - \bar{X}\right)\left(Y_i - \bar{Y}\right)}{(n-1)} \tag{9.9}$$

where the terms Y or $\bar{X}$ refer to the mean of set Y and set X, respectively, while the total number of elements is represented by n. The process of subtracting the mean value from each of the data dimensions is performed by PCA. The mean value is the average for respective dimensions. Hence, this will cause all the y values to have y and all the x values to have $\bar{x}$. The result will be a zero mean for the data set, and the covariance matrix is calculated.

From the covariance matrix, the eigenvectors and eigenvalues, which provide the information about the patterns in the data, are calculated. The eigenvalue can be defined as a scalar of a square matrix; it is a requirement for an eigenvector to be a nonzero vector. Eigenvalues and eigenvectors usually come in pairs. Given a complex square matrix $\mathbf{A}$ and a nonzero complex column vector $\mathbf{X}$, λ is a complex number that has to satisfy $\mathbf{AX} = \lambda$ $\mathbf{X\cdot X}$ (this equation is known as the eigenvector), and λ will be known as the eigenvalue of matrix $\mathbf{A}$. The eigenvectors will appear on the diagonal lines, and they are perpendicular to each other. Therefore, this will allow the data to be expressed in terms of these perpendicular eigenvectors, instead of expressing it in terms of the x and y axes, which will show how the data sets are related along the lines. The x and y axes will not show exactly how the points are related to each other in the data. Therefore, we will be able to extract the lines that characterize the data, by calculating the eigenvectors of the covariance matrix. All eigenvectors have to be rearranged from highest to lowest eigenvalues, and the eigenvectors corresponding to the largest eigenvalues have the most significant information on the data. In this technique, the top three eigenvalues obtained after performing PCA on the CWT coefficients were used as features in the classifier.

TABLE 9.3

Results of ANOVA for the Three Eigenvalues of the Five Classes of Heart Rate Rhythms (Normal Sinus Rhythm and Four Classes of Arrhythmias)

Features (eigenvalues)	NSR	AF	CHB	PVC	VF	*p*-value
λ_1	−1090.8 ± 138	−959.15 ± 166	−457.00 ± 32.0	−1061.2 ± 173	−1644.8 ± 454	<0.0001
λ_2	−53.530 ± 36.6	−42.151 ± 33.9	−25.088 ± 1.66	−59.394 ± 28.1	−92.155 ± 28.5	<0.0001
λ_3	−40.584 ± 30.0	−28.939 ± 17.8	−11.593 ± 6.89	−6.9314 ± 31.5	−53.558 ± 42.9	<0.0001

Note: Entries in the columns (except for the last column) correspond to mean ± standard deviation.

9.7.3.3 Quantitative Analysis

The extracted features were subjected to the analysis of variance (ANOVA) test, to determine whether their means are different for the different classes of cardiac conditions. The ANOVA test, sometimes known as the *F*-test, which is closely related to the *t*-test, is a statistical method which uses *variances* to determine whether the *means* are different. The main difference between ANOVA and the *t*-test is that ANOVA measures the differences between the means of two or more groups while the *t*-test measures the differences between the means of two groups. If the ANOVA test gives high observed differences, the feature is considered to be statistically significant. The *p*-values shown in Table 9.3 (in Section 9.7.4.1) were obtained by using the ANOVA test.

9.7.3.4 Probabilistic Neural Network

PNN is a special type of neural network that learns to approximate the probability density function (pdf) of the training data. PNN is a kind of two-layer radial basis network suitable for classification problems. When an input is presented, the first layer (radial basis layer) computes distances from the input vector to the training input vectors and produces a distance vector whose elements indicate how close the input is to a training input. The second layer (competitive layer) sums these contributions for each class of inputs to produce a vector of probabilities as its net output. Then, the compete transfer function applied on the output of the second layer picks the maximum of these probabilities and assigns a class label 1 for that class and a 0 for the other classes.

9.7.4 Results

9.7.4.1 Eigenvalues for Normal Sinus Rhythm and Arrhythmia

Table 9.3 shows the range of the top three eigenvalues (λ_1, λ_2, λ_3) for the five classes of heart rate rhythms. The result of ANOVA (*p*-values) on these eigenvalues obtained from PCA for the various cardiac conditions is also listed in Table 9.3. These values are clinically significant because the *p*-values are very less (<0.0001). The heart rate will vary continuously between 60 and 80 bpm for normal sinus rhythm (NSR). Since there is higher variation in the heart rate, the eigenvalues (λ_1, λ_2, λ_3) appear to be high for NSR (Table 9.3).

For NSR, the mean values of eigenvalues (λ_1, λ_2, λ_3) are −1090.8, −53.530, and −40.584, respectively. There may be a possibility that these values are related to the rate of breathing and its harmonics, as we have to take into consideration the modulating effect on the heart rate variability due to the breathing pattern. The heart has to work harder in order to meet higher body demands. Hence, the HRV will be high. For CHB, the heart rate variation is low, due to inability of the A node to send electrical signals rhythmically to the ventricles. Compared to NSR, there is a reduced beat-to-beat variation for CHB as indicated by their low mean values of eigenvalues (457.00, –25.088, and –11.593, respectively).

In the case of ventricular fibrillation (VF), the heart fibrillates very rapidly, causing the heart rate variation to be high. Therefore, compared to NSR, the mean values of eigenvalues are higher for VF (–1644.8, –92.155, and –53.558, respectively). In the case of atrial fibrillation (AF), there is a random activation of different parts of the atria at different times. Compared to NSR, the mean values of eigenvalues are higher for AF, but lower than VF (–959.15, –42.151, and –28.939, respectively). In the case of premature ventricular contraction (PVC), there is an ectopic beat beginning from one of the ventricles. The mean values are now –1061.2, –59.39, and –6.93, respectively. The distribution of these three eigenvalues for the five classes is shown in Figure 9.15a through c.

9.7.4.2 Classification Results

The number of samples used for training and testing the PNN classifier is presented in Table 9.4. Table 9.5 shows the results of the classification efficiency of the PNN classifier obtained using the 10-fold cross validation method. The results indicate that the PCA method can be used for the detection of the unknown cardiac class with an average accuracy of about 80%, specificity of 85.6%, and sensitivity of 82%. Sensitivity is the probability that a test will produce a positive result when used on diseased population. Specificity is the probability that a test will produce a negative result when used on disease-free population. Accuracy is the ratio of the number of correctly classified samples to the total number of samples.

9.7.5 Formulation of an Integrated Index That Gives Better Separation of the Various Cardiac Rhythms

In spite of the eigenvalues having high degree of accuracy, sensitivity, and specificity, it can be seen from Figure 9.15 that the distribution of these eigenvalues exhibits considerable overlap for some arrhythmias. Hence, we cannot effectively employ these eigenvalue parameters to specifically distinguish the four arrhythmias from one another and from the normal sinus rhythm. Therefore, based on the concept of a single Physiological Index number (Ghista 2004, 2009), a new integrated index called the HRVID Index was empirically formulated using λ_1, λ_2, and λ_3. HRVID is given by the following equation.

$$\text{HRVID Index} = \left| \frac{\lambda_1 * \lambda_2 * \lambda_3}{100,000} \right| \tag{9.10}$$

Table 9.6 shows the range of HRVID Index values for different cardiac states. It is seen that this HRVID Index can effectively separate out the different arrhythmia classes from the NSR category. Also, it is now possible to clearly distinguish VF and CHB from each other as well as from AF and PVC. Then, the eigenvalue λ_3 can be used to further separate PVC and AF.

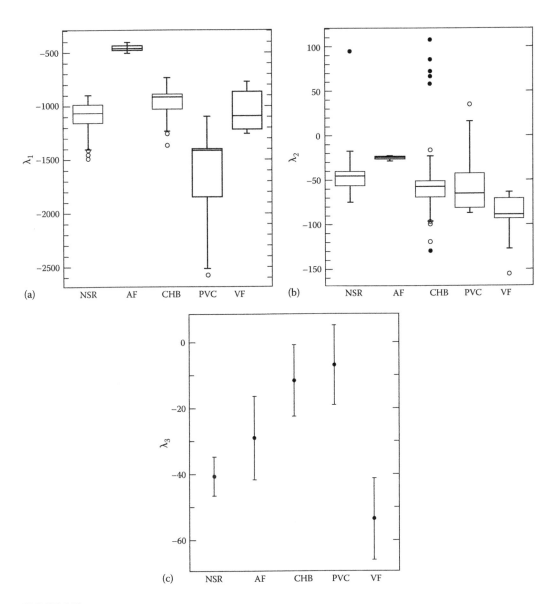

FIGURE 9.15

Distributions of eigenvalues extracted from the heart rate signals: (a) eigenvalue 1 (λ_1), (b) eigenvalue 2 (λ_2), and (c) eigenvalue 3 (λ_3).

TABLE 9.4

Number of Training and Testing Samples Used in Each Class

	NSR	AF	PVC	CHB	VF	Total
Training	81	18	25	20	19	163
Testing	9	2	2	2	2	17

TABLE 9.5

Average Values of the Accuracy, Positive Predictive Value (PPV), Sensitivity, and Specificity over the 10-Folds for the PNN Classifier

Classifier	Avg. TN	Avg. FN	Avg. TP	Avg. FP	Avg. accuracy (%)	Avg. PPV (%)	Avg. sensitivity (%)	Avg. specificity (%)
PNN	7	2	7	1	80	85	82	85.6

True Positive (TP), number of diseased patients for whom the test results were positive; True Negative (TN), number of disease-free patients for whom the test results were negative; False Positive (FP), number of disease-free patients for whom the test results were positive; False Negative (FN), number of diseased patients for whom the test results were negative.

TABLE 9.6

Range of HRVID values for NSR and four arrhythmia states: AF, CHB, PVC, VF

Index	NSR	AF	CHB	PVC	VF	*p*-value
HRVID	32.429 ± 15.9	17.340 ± 12.9	1.4787 ± 0.544	21.956 ± 17.0	102.95 ± 55.5	<0.0001

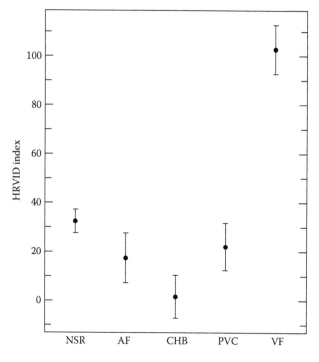

FIGURE 9.16
Variation of HRVID Index values for different cardiac states.

Figure 9.16 shows the distributions of this HRVID Index for normal and arrhythmias classes. It is evident that there is effective separation of AF, PVC, CHB, and VF from NSR. Also, there is effective separation of VF and CHB from each other as well as from AF and PVC. However, there is not significant separation between AF and PVC. So we are recommending that this HRVID Index be employed to first decide the presence of NSR or VF or CHB. However, if, based on the HRVID Index, there is evidence of presence of AF or PVC, then we should employ the value of the eigenvalue λ_3 to decide between AF and PVC. This procedure can be implemented clinically by means of a Decision Tree (or a Neural Network) and can also be incorporated into the Electronic Medical Records.

9.8 Summary

ECG signal analysis has become one of the most important methods to determine the heart condition of the patient. In this chapter, a detailed description of the electrical activity of the heart is presented with emphasis on the different stages and phases of action potential generation. This is followed by the discussion on how ECG signals and its components like the P, Q, and R waves are generated. The algorithms used to detect the various components of the ECG signal like the P wave, QRS complex, and the ST-segment are then presented. Subsequently, a description of how these components vary for the various cardiac disorders is given and explained in more detail with the inclusion of the values of heart rate, P–R interval, QRS width, and P-wave amplitude measured from normal and different abnormal ECG waveforms.

Owing to the limitations of manual analysis of the ECG signals, the most commonly used HRV-based ECG analysis methodology is then presented along with discussions on how the HRV signal is useful in diagnosing diseases, along with the various techniques used for HRV analysis. A brief summary of several studies in literature pertaining to ECG-HRV analysis is then provided. We have then presented our HRV analysis study to classify and distinguish abnormal rhythms from normal cardiac arrhythmias. The classification methodology comprises of (1) signal pre-processing, (2) feature extraction, (3) feature selection, (4) classifier development, and (5) classifier evaluation elements. The classification framework used for classification of normal sinus rhythm and cardiac arrhythmias is displayed in Figure 9.13. In this technique, the extracted HRV signals were analyzed in the wavelet domain; continuous wavelet transform (CWT) was used to transform the signal into wavelet domain. Then, principal component analysis (PCA) was performed on the extracted CWT coefficients in order to extract the eigenvalues. Only the first three eigenvalue features (λ_1, λ_2, and λ_3) were selected and used to develop and evaluate the probabilistic neural network (PNN) classifier.

In spite of these eigenvalues having high degree of accuracy, sensitivity, and specificity, it can be seen from Figure 9.15 that the distribution of these eigenvalues exhibits considerable overlap for some arrhythmias. Therefore, a new integrated index was formulated by suitably combining these eigenvalues (λ_1, λ_2, and λ_3) into a novel HRVID Index, given by Equation 9.10. Table 9.6 shows that this HRVID Index can effectively separate out the different arrhythmia classes from the normal sinus rhythm category. We are hence recommending that this HRVID Index be employed for the detection of cardiac arrhythmias.

References

Acharya UR, Anand D, Bhat S, Niranjan UC. 2001. Compact storage of medical images with patient information. *IEEE Transactions on Information Technology in Biomedicine* 5:320–323.

Acharya UR, Bhat PS, Iyengar SS, Rao A, Dua S. 2003a. Classification of heart rate data using artificial neural networks and fuzzy equivalence relation. *Journal of Pattern Recognition* 36:61–68.

Acharya UR, Bhat PS, Kannathal N, Rao A, Lim CM. 2005. Analysis of cardiac health using fractal dimension and continuous wavelet transformation. *Innovations and Technology in Biology and Medicine* 26:133–139.

Acharya UR, Bhat PS, Sathish Kumar S, Min LC. 2003b. Transmission and storage of medical images with patient information. *Computers in Biology and Medicine* 33:303–310.

Acharya UR, Chua EPC, Chua CK, Lim CM, Tamura T. 2010. Analysis and automatic identification of sleep stages using higher order spectra. *International Journal of Neural Systems* 20:509–521.

Acharya UR, Ghista DN, Faust O, Vinitha Sree S, Alvin APC, Chattopadhyay S, Lim CT. 2013. A systems approach to cardiac health diagnosis. *Journal of Medical Imaging and Health Informatics* 3:261–267.

Acharya UR, Kannathal N, Krishnan SM. 2004. Comprehensive analysis of cardiac health using heart rate signals. *Physiological Measurement* 25:1139–1151.

Acharya UR, Lim CM, Joseph P. 2002. HRV analysis using correlation dimension and detrended fluctuation analysis. *Innovations and Technology in Biology and Medicine* 23:333–339.

Acharya UR, Paul Joseph K, Kannathal N, Lim CM, Suri JS. 2006. Heart rate variability: A review. *Medical and Biological Engineering Computing* 44:1031–1051.

Acharya UR, Sankaranarayanan M, Nayak J, Xiang C, Tamura T. 2008. Automatic identification of cardiac health using modeling techniques: A comparative study. *Information Sciences* 178:4571–4582.

Acharya UR, Vinitha Sree S, Yu W, Chattopadhyay S, Alvin APC. 2011. Application of recurrence quantification analysis for the automated identification of epileptic EEG signals. *International Journal of Neural Systems* 21:199–211.

Akselrod S, Gordon D, Madwed JB, Snidman DC, Cohen RJ. 1985. Hemodynamic Regulation: Investigation by spectral analysis. *American Journal of Physiology* 249:H867–H875.

Akselrod S, Gordon D, Ubel FA, Shannon DC, Berger AC, Cohen RJ. 1981. Power Spectrum analysis of heart rate fluctuation: A quantitative probe of beat-to-beat cardiovascular control. *Science* 213:220–222.

AlGhatrif M, Lindsay J. 2012. A brief review: History to understand fundamentals of electrocardiography. *Journal of Community Hospital Internal Medicine Perspectives* 2.

Chua KC, Chandran V, Acharya UR, Lim CM. 2008a. Cardiac state diagnosis using higher order spectra of heart rate variability. *Journal of Medical Engineering and Technology* 32:145–155.

Chua KC, Chandran V, Acharya UR, Lim CM. 2008b. Computer-based analysis of cardiac state using entropies, recurrence plots and Poincare geometry. *Journal of Medical Engineering and Technology* 32:263–272.

Chua KC, Chandran V, Acharya UR, Lim CM. 2009a. Analysis of epileptic EEG signals using higher order spectra. *Journal of Medical Engineering and Technology* 33:42–50.

Chua KC, Chandran V, Acharya UR, Lim CM. 2009b. Automatic identification of epileptic encephalographic signals using higher-order spectra. *Proceedings of Institution of Mechanical Engineers, Part H: Journal of Engineering in Medicine* 223:485–495.

Cohen ME, Hudson DL, Deedwania PC. 1996. Applying continuous chaos modeling to cardiac signal analysis. *IEEE Engineering in Medicine and Biology Magazine* 15:97–102.

Constant I, Laude D, Murat I, Elghozi JL. 1999. Pulse rate variability is not a surrogate for heart rate variability. *Clinical Science* 97:391–397.

Faust O, Acharya UR, Alen A, Lim CM. 2008. Analysis of EEG signals during epileptic and alcoholic states using AR modelling techniques. *Innovations and Technology in Biology and Medicine* 29:44–52.

Faust O, Acharya UR, Krishnan SM, Lim CM. 2004. Analysis of cardiac signals using spatial filling index and time-frequency domain. *Biomedical Engineering Online* 3:30.

Faust O, Acharya UR, Lim CM, Sputh BHC. 2010. Automatic identification of epileptic and background EEG signals using frequency domain parameters. *International Journal of Neural Systems* 20:159–176.

Ge D, Srinivasan N, Krishnan SM. 2002. Cardiac arrhythmia classification using autoregressive modeling. *Biomedical Engineering Online* 1:5.

Ghista DN. 2004. Physiological systems' numbers in medical diagnosis and hospital cost effective operation. *Journal of Mechanics in Medicine and Biology* 4:401–418.

Ghista DN. 2009. Non-dimensional physiological indices for medical assessment. *Journal of Mechanics in Medicine and Biology* 9:643–669.

Jiapu P, Tompkins WJ. 1985. Real time QRS detector algorithm. *IEEE Transactions on Biomedical Engineering* 32:230–223.

Kamen PW, Krum H, Tonkin AM. 1996. Poincare plot of heart rate variability allows quantitative display of parasympathetic nervous activity. *Clinical Science* 91:201–208.

Kannathal N, Lim CM, Acharya UR, Sadasivan PK. 2006. Cardiac state diagnosis using adaptive neuro-fuzzy technique. *Medical Engineering and Physics* 28:809–815.

Kleiger RE, Bigger JT, Bosner MS, Chung MK, Cook JR, Rolnitzky LM, Steinman R, Fleiss JL. 1991. Stability over time of variables measuring heart rate variability in normal subjects. *American Journal of Cardiology* 68:626–630.

Levy MN, Schwartz PJ. 1994. *Vagal Control of the Heart: Experimental Basis and Clinical Implications.* Armonk, NY: Futura.

Lowensohn RI, Weiss M, Hon EH. 1977. Heart-rate variability in brain-damaged adults. *Lancet* 1:626–628.

Malmivuo J, Plonsey R. 1995. *Bioelectromagnetism: Principles and Applications of Bioelectric and Biomagnetic Fields*, Chapter 19. New York: Oxford University Press.

Mandelbrot BB. 1983. *The Fractal Geometry of Nature*, pp. 1–468. San Francisco, CA: WH Freeman & Co.

Meyer Y. 1992. *Wavelets and Applications.* Paris, France: Springer Verlag.

Myers GA, Martin GJ, Magid NM, Barnett PS, Schaad JW, Weiss JS, Lesch M, Singer DH. 1986. Power spectral analysis of sudden cardiac death: Comparison to other methods. *IEEE Transactions in Biomedical Engineering* 33:1149–1156.

Pan J, Tompkins WJ. 1985. A real-time QRS detection algorithm. *IEEE Transactions in Biomedical Engineering* BME-32:230–236.

Patil GM, Subba Rao K, Niranjan UC, Satyanarayan K. 2010. Evaluation of QRS complex based on DWT coefficients analysis using Daubechies wavelets for detection of myocardial ischaemia. *Journal of Mechanics in Medicine and Biology* 10:273–290.

Peng CK, Havlin S, Hausdorf JM, Mietus JE, Stanley HE, Goldberger AL. 1996. Fractal mechanisms and heart rate dynamics. *Journal of Electrocardiology* 28:59–64.

Pfeifer MA, Cook D, Brodsky J, Tice D, Reenan A, Swedine S, Halter JB, Porte D Jr. 1982. Quantitative evaluation of cardiac parasympathetic activity in normal and diabetic man. *Diabetes* 3:339–345.

Pomeranz B, Macaulay RJB, Caudill MA, Kutz I, Adam D, Kilborn KM, Barger AC, Shannon DC, Cohen RJ, Benson H. 1985. Assessment of autonomic function in humans by heart rate spectral analysis. *American Journal of Physiology* 248:H151–H153.

Roche F, Pichot V, Sforza E, Court-Fortune I, Duverney D, Costes F, Garet M, Barthe Lemy J-C. 2003. Predicting sleep apnea syndrome from heart period: A time-frequency wavelet analysis. *European Respiratory Journal* 22:937–942.

Rothschild M, Rothschild A, Pfeifer M. 1988. Temporary decrease in cardiac parasympathetic tone after acute myocardial infarction. *American Journal of Cardiology* 18:637–639.

Ryan SM, Goldberg AL, Ruthazer R, Mietus J, Lipsitz LA. 1992. Spectral analysis of heart rate dynamics in elderly persons with postprandial hypotension. *American Journal of Cardiology* 69:201–205.

Saul PL, Arai Y, Berger RD, Lilly LS, Colucci WS, Cohen RJ. 1988. Assessment of autonomic regulation in chronic congestive heart failure by heart rate spectral analysis. *American Journal of Cardiology* 61:1292–1299.

Schroeder EB, Chambless LE, Liao D, Prineas RJ, Evans GW, Rosamond WD, Heiss G. 2005. Diabetes, Glucose, Insulin, and Heart rate variability, The Atherosclerosis Risk in Communities (ARIC) study. *Diabetes Care* 28:668–674.

Schwartz PJ, Priori SG. 1990. Sympathetic nervous system and cardiac arrhythmias. In *Cardiac Electrophysiology. From Cell to Bedside*, ed. Zipes DP, pp. 330–343. Philadelphia, PA: Elsevier Saunders.

Singh JP, Larson MG, O'Donell CJ, Wilson PF, Tsuji H, Lyod-Jones DM, Levy D. 2000. Association of hyperglycemia with reduced heart rate variability: The Framingham heart study. *American Journal of Cardiology* 86:309–312.

Sokolow M, Mcllroy MB, Chiethin MD. 1990. *Clinical Cardiology*. VLANGE Medical Book, University of Michigan, Ann Arbor, MI.

Subha DP, Joseph PK, Acharya UR, Lim CM. 2010. EEG signal analysis: A survey. *Journal of Medical Systems* 34:195–212.

Swapna G, Ghista DN, Martis RJ, Alvin APC, Vinitha Sree S. 2012. ECG signal generation and heart rate variability signal extraction: Signal processing, features detection, and their correlation with cardiac diseases. *Journal of Mechanics in Medicine and Biology* (*Special Issue*) 12:1240012-1–1240012-26.

Task Force of the European Society of Cardiology and North American Society of Pacing and Electrophysiology. 1996. Heart rate variability: Standards of measurement, physiological interpretation and clinical use. *European Heart Journal* 17:354–381.

Vetterli M. 1992. Wavelet and filter banks: Theory and design. *IEEE Transactions in Signal Processing* 40:2207–2232.

Vetterli M, Kovacevic J. 1995. *Wavelets and Subband Coding*. Englewood Cliffs, NJ: Prentice-Hall.

Vinitha Sree S, Ghista DN, Ng KH. 2012. Cardiac arrhythmia diagnosis by HRV signal processing using principal component analysis. *Journal of Mechanics in Medicine and Biology* 12:1240032-1–1240032-16.

Wariar R, C Eswaran C. 1991. Integer coefficient bandpass filter for the simultaneous removal of baseline wander, 50 and 100 Hz interference from the ECG. *Medical and Biological Engineering and Computing* 29:333–336.

10

Left Ventricular Blood Pump Analysis: Intra-LV Flow Velocity and Pressure for Coronary Bypass Surgery Candidacy

Dhanjoo N. Ghista, Foad Kabinejadian, K. Subbaraj*, and Ernie Fallen

CONTENTS

10.1 Introduction

Despite significant developments in cardiac physics, there is still a need for standardized means for assessment of intrinsic left ventricular (LV) pumping function in the presence of regional myocardial ischemia. Currently employed measures of cardiac pumping function or contractility [1] include holistic parameters such as ejection fraction (ejection volume/maximum filling volume of the LV chamber), dP/dt—the rate at which LV

---

* The late Dr. Subbaraj contributed extensively to this chapter.

chamber pressure develops, and endocardial motion kinematics. None of these indices is truly intrinsic to myocardial pumping capability, whose outcome can be best represented in terms of spatial and temporal blood flow-velocity and pressure-differential distributions within the LV chamber.

Global indices such as *dP/dt* and ejection fraction are influenced by variations in preload (end-diastolic filling volume) and after-load (aortic impedance due to arterial disease or vasoconstriction), and hence, unable to reflect the intrinsic pumping ability of the left ventricle. The ejection fraction cannot convey regional variation in contractility. Segmental wall motion kinematics can identify asynergic myocardial segments but cannot indicate whether such segments will result in recirculating (or stagnant) flow zones or adverse blood pressure gradients within the LV chamber.

In order to address this problem, we have developed a method of computing intra-LV blood flow-velocity and pressure-differentials at different instants of the cardiac cycle derived from sequentially digitized cine-ventriculograms, as a prelude to development of indices for LV pumping efficiency based on these comprehensive data.

Regional variations in LV wall distensibility and contractility caused by diseased myocardial segments or intra-myocardial conduction abnormalities will influence wall motion kinematics during the filling and systolic phases of the cardiac cycle, and thereby set up variations in characteristic intra-LV flow and pressure-gradient distributions. Indeed, the intra-LV flow patterns during a cardiac cycle are governed by both biomechanical and bioelectrical properties of the myocardial wall. By employing finite element modeling, we can determine intra-LV flow-velocity and pressure-gradient distribution from sequential analog images of contrast ventriculograms. The intra-LV pressure gradients during ejection constitute a signature of regional myocardial function. On the other hand, intra-LV flow-velocity distribution can identify the presence of stagnant or recirculating flow zones, and can help delineate sites of mural thrombus formation.

We present herein the requisite analysis, technology, and methodology for the computation of flow-velocity distribution in the left ventricle as well as the results of clinical applications in a couple of patients suspected of having coronary artery disease. A 2D inviscid fluid flow finite element analysis is carried out in the antero-posterior projection plane, by assuming a quasi-steady flow in the time interval between successive frames. The flow is governed by the potential equation $\nabla^2\phi = 0$, where ∇^2 is the Laplacian operator, ϕ is the velocity potential, and $\nabla\phi$ is the velocity vector. In order to solve the earlier equation for the velocity potential (ϕ), the requisite boundary conditions are (1) the specification of ϕ over a part of the boundary and (2) the specification of the normal derivative of the velocity potential, $\partial\phi/\partial n$ (=V_n, the normal velocity of the boundary or the normal velocity of blood in contact with the boundary), over the remaining part of the boundary.

Now, from the endocardial outlines of the sequential instants, we obtain the value of wall motion velocities, which equal the blood velocities at the endocardial boundary; therefrom, the values of $\partial\phi/\partial n = V_n$ can be determined. We then compute the values of instantaneous ϕ in the interior of the LV chamber by solving $\nabla^2\phi = 0$, by using the finite element method, for the designated instantaneous V_n at the wall boundary. From the computed values of ϕ at each internal point, we can obtain the instantaneous maps of blood flow-velocity patterns.

The intra-LV pressure distribution at points within the LV chamber is then obtained from the Bernoulli equation for unsteady potential flow, given by

$$P + \frac{1}{2}\rho V^2 + \rho\frac{\partial\phi}{\partial t} + \rho gh = C(t)$$

where
P is the pressure
$1/2(\rho V^2)$ is the dynamic pressure
ρ is the density of blood
V is the velocity of blood
$\rho(\partial\phi/\partial t)$ is the effect due to acceleration
ρgh is the constant hydrostatic pressure
$C(t)$ represents the total pressure as sensed by a pressure probe facing the oncoming

The partial derivative, $\partial\phi/\partial t$, is computed from the value of ϕ at the same point at successive instants, by using the finite difference scheme.

Therefrom, the differential pressure $(p_s - p_0)$ is expressed and displayed, in nondimensional form, as

$$C_p = \frac{(p_s - p_0)}{1/2(\rho V_0^2)}$$

where C_p is the nondimensional pressure coefficient. The instantaneous graphical display of the relative pressure distribution in the LV chamber provides an indication of the effectiveness of the LV contraction in setting up the appropriate pressure distribution in the chamber so as to promote adequate emptying.

The clinical application of the finite element methodology described earlier is carried out for three subjects: Patient 1 is a case with anterior wall akinesis, Patient 2 is a case with inferior wall hypokinesis, and Patient 3 had severe ischemic heart disease with large akinetic segments in the anterior and apical wall. In the analyses and results, we have displayed the superimposed sequential diastolic and systolic endocardial frames for these patients. From these images, the instantaneous wall displacements during the four equal time intervals of diastole and systole are computed. Then from the endocardial wall velocities, the intra-LV blood flow velocities are computed by finite element analysis. The intracardiac pressure distribution at any point is then obtained from the Bernoulli equation for unsteady potential flow.

For Patient 3, we have made inferences concerning candidacy for surgery, by comparing the intra-LV velocity and pressure-differential distributions before and after administration of nitroglycerin (a vasodilating agent). Following administration of nitroglycerin, the intra-LV velocity distributions (in Figure 10.5b) demonstrate improved filling-flow and ejection-phase flow-velocity patterns (in Figure 10.5c). In Figure 10.5d, the diastole pressure-differential distributions, before and after nitroglycerin administration, are compared. We can note the substantial deleterious pressure gradient characterizing resistance-to-LV filling before nitroglycerin administration, and how this pressure gradient is distinctly reduced after nitroglycerin is given. Likewise, Figure 10.5e illustrates improvement in the pressure gradient conducive to ejection, following administration of nitroglycerin. This patient is thereby deemed to be a candidate for coronary bypass surgery.

10.2 Methodology

We will present the methodology for (1) obtaining sequential instantaneous digitized endocardial outlines of the LV chamber, and computing therefrom the instantaneous velocity distribution of the LV endocardial (or inner) wall, and (2) determining, therefrom, the intra-LV blood pressure and flow-velocity distributions, by finite element analysis of intra-LV blood flow.

10.2.1 Digitization of Instantaneous LV Chamber Outlines

During routine ventriculography, 45–60 mL of radio-opaque meglumine diatrizoate is power-injected into the LV cavity through a multiple-hole catheter. A video-angiographic sequence of x-ray images of the left ventricle in the 30° right anterior oblique position is recorded on videotape at 30 fps. The LV chamber endocardial wall motion (and segmental motion abnormalities) can be followed on video through a complete cardiac cycle, and thereby a qualitative assessment of cardiac pumping function is carried out. Conventionally, the endocardium is hand digitized at two instants of the cardiac cycle, end-diastole and end-systole. The volumes of the LV chambers are determined from these geometries by means of certain standard formulae and therefrom the stroke volumes and ejection volumes are determined.

We carry out an automated detection and digitization of the instantaneous LV endocardial boundaries, involving video digitization of each frame to 64 K picture elements, with 8 bits per element. For the purpose of digitization, since the ventricular cavity is made radio-opaque relative to the surrounding myocardium, the endocardial boundary is distinguished and demarcated as the line of maximal rate of change of picture brightness. The spatial derivative of the image brightness is calculated, using the Sobel operator. An algorithm for obtaining the endocardial outline, using the thresholding technique on the spatial derivatives was described in our pilot paper [2]. The cineangiogram processing and frame digitization is illustrated in Figure 10.1.

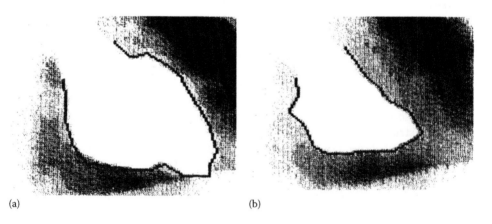

(a)   (b)

FIGURE 10.1

Typical micro-computerized cineangiogram processing and digitization of endocardial boundary of a left ventricle at (a) end-diastole and (b) end-systole.

10.2.2 Determination of Instantaneous Displacements of the Endocardial Wall

In response to blood filling during diastole as well as to LV contraction and blood ejection during systole, the LV undergoes rigid-body motion about its anchorage to the aorta, due to the momentum imparted to it by the blood entering and leaving the LV.

Additionally, in response to blood-flow-generated wall pressures during diastole, the wall undergoes elastic deformation. In systole, it is the elastic wall deformation generated by the contracting LV myocardium that gives rise to intra-LV blood flow. Hence, in both diastolic and systolic phases, for analysis of intra-LV blood flow-velocity and pressure-differential distributions, we need to remove the rigid-body displacements from the LV wall displacements.

Since the LV is essentially suspended from the aorta, one way to remove rigid-body LV displacements would be to translate and rotate each LV frame, so as to match, for all frames, the aortic valve center and the line joining it to the apex of the LV, a method conventionally used to assess regional wall motion.

Once this mode of reorientation of LV frames has effected, the instantaneous wall displacements (at time t) are obtained from the sequential endocardial outlines of the LV at times t and $t + \Delta t$, Δt being the time interval between successive frames. This is done by assuming that for each frame the endocardial points $S(i, t)$ at the intersection of an equal number of minor chords (obtained by dividing each frame's long axis, joining the midpoint of the aortic valve and the apex, into an equal number of parts and having minor chords pass through these points at right angles to the long axis), with the endocardial boundary of frame (t), traverse to points $S(i, t + \Delta t)$ at the intersection of the minor chords with the endocardial boundary of the next instant or frame ($t + \Delta t$).

Figure 10.2 illustrates the endocardial wall displacement vector, resulting from the two sequential frames:

$$\Delta S(i,t) = S(i,t+\Delta t) - S(i,t) \tag{10.1}$$

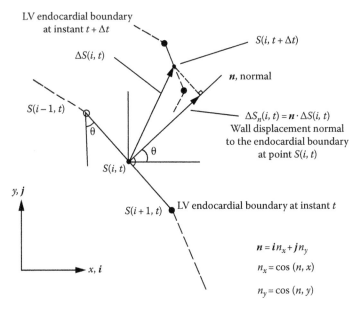

FIGURE 10.2
A typical endocardial wall displacement vector, resulting from two sequential frames.

The wall displacements along the normal n to the endocardial boundary segment of frame t, at a point S, are obtained as $\Delta S_n(i, t) = n \cdot \Delta S(i, t)$, where $n = in_x + jn_y$, with n_x and n_y being the direction cosines of the normal n so that $n_x = \cos(n, x)$ and $n_y = \cos(n, y)$ and (i, j) are unit vectors. The normal n to the endocardial boundary at a point $S(i)$ is defined as the normal to the line joining the points at $S(i - 1)$ and $S(i + 1)$.

Figure 10.3b and c illustrates the endocardial normal wall displacements during diastolic and ejection phases, associated with superimposed sequential diastolic and ejection frames (as described earlier to remove rigid-body displacements) shown in Figure 10.3a. The instantaneous endocardial normal wall velocities are then obtained as

$$V_n(i, t) = \frac{S_n(i, t)}{\Delta t} \tag{10.2}$$

10.2.3 Analysis of Intracardiac Pressure and Velocity Distributions

Intracardiac flow pressure and velocity distributions are computed from digitized LV chamber instantaneous wall velocity data. For intracardiac velocity (V) of the order of 25 cm/s, LV chamber local radius (r) of the order of 2 cm, blood viscosity (μ) of 0.0036 kg/m·s and density (ρ) of 1060 kg/m^3, the Reynolds number $(\rho r V/\mu)$ is of the order of 1500. This means that viscous effects are confined to a thin layer near the ventricular wall, and the flow in the interior of the chamber may hence be considered inviscid [3].

A 2D inviscid fluid flow finite element analysis is carried out in the antero-posterior projection plane, by assuming a quasi-steady flow in the time interval between successive frames. The flow is governed by the potential equation:

$$\nabla^2 \phi = 0 \tag{10.3}$$

where
  ∇^2 is the Laplacian operator
  ϕ is the velocity potential
  $\nabla \phi$ is the velocity vector

In order to solve the earlier equation for the velocity potential (ϕ), the requisite boundary conditions are (1) the specification of ϕ over a part of the boundary, and (2) the specification of the normal derivative of the velocity potential, $\partial \phi/\partial n$ $(=V_n$, the normal velocity of the boundary or the normal velocity of blood in contact with the boundary), over the remaining part of the boundary.

Now, from the endocardial outlines of the sequential instants, we obtain the value of wall motion velocities that equal the blood velocities at the endocardial boundary; therefrom, the values of $\partial \phi/\partial n = V_n$ can be determined. We then compute the values of instantaneous ϕ in the interior of the chamber by solving $\nabla^2 \phi = 0$, using the finite element method, for the designated instantaneous V_n at the wall boundary. From the computed values of ϕ at each internal point, we can obtain the instantaneous maps of blood flow patterns.

The governing differential equation $(\nabla^2 \phi = 0)$ is discretized to obtain the finite element analog, using the Galerkin weighted residual approach. The flow domain is divided into triangular finite elements. Within each domain, the velocity potential ϕ is approximated to vary linearly. For each triangular element, the values of ϕ are evaluated at the nodal vertices. A discrete analog for the flow domain, for the nodal values of ϕ, is obtained by assembling the finite element contributions from each domain. The velocity components

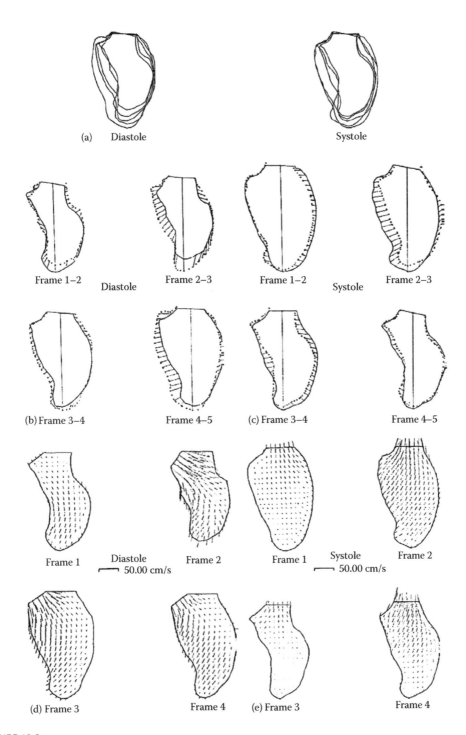

FIGURE 10.3
Patient 1: (a) superimposed sequential diastolic and systolic endocardial frames, whose aortic valve centers and the long axis are matched, (b) instantaneous endocardial wall displacement distortions during the periods of diastole, (c) instantaneous endocardial wall displacement distortions during the periods of systole, (d) instantaneous intra-LV velocity distributions during the periods of diastole, and (e) instantaneous intra-LV velocity distributions during the periods of systole.

for each triangular element are obtained by computing the derivatives of the potential; the nodal values of the velocity components are given by the average of the contributory values from the triangles joining at the node.

The intracardiac pressure distribution at any point is then obtained from the Bernoulli equation for unsteady potential flow [4], given by

$$P + \frac{1}{2}\rho V^2 + \rho \frac{\partial \phi}{\partial t} + \rho gh = C(t) \tag{10.4}$$

where
  P is the pressure
  $1/2(\rho V^2)$ is the dynamic pressure
  ρ is the density of blood
  V is the velocity of blood
  $\rho(\partial\phi/\partial t)$ is the effect due to acceleration
  ρgh is the constant hydrostatic pressure
  $C(t)$ represents the total pressure as sensed by a pressure probe facing the oncoming fluid [5]

$C(t)$ = constant, if the gravitational or hydrostatic effects are neglected. The partial derivative, $\partial\phi/\partial t$, is computed from the value of ϕ at the same point at successive instants, by using the finite difference scheme.

If we want the procedure to not utilize the catheter pressure data, we can obtain the pressure distribution relative to a reference point in the chamber, say at the center of the aortic or mitral orifice. Hence the differential pressure field at a point s, in terms of the pressure p_0 at the inlet (during diastole) or outlet (during the ejection phase) of the ventricle, is given by

$$p_s - p_0 = \frac{1}{2}\rho\left(V_0^2 - V_s^2\right) + \rho\left(\left.\frac{\partial\phi}{\partial t}\right|_0 - \left.\frac{\partial\phi}{\partial t}\right|_s\right) \tag{10.5}$$

where V_0 and V_s, are, respectively, the velocity of blood flow at the center of the orifice (i.e., at the aortic or mitral orifice during systolic or diastolic phase) and at a point s inside the LV chamber. The differential pressure $(p_s - p_0)$ is expressed and displayed, in nondimensional form, as

$$C_p = \frac{(p_s - p_0)}{1/2(\rho V_0^2)} \tag{10.6}$$

where C_p is the nondimensional pressure coefficient.

This instantaneous graphical display of the relative pressure distribution in the LV chamber can provide an indication of the effectiveness of the LV contraction in setting up the appropriate pressure distribution in the chamber so as to promote adequate emptying.

10.2.4 Finite Element Formulation of Intra-LV Blood Flow

The governing differential equation (10.3)

$$\frac{\partial^2\phi}{\partial x^2} + \frac{\partial^2\phi}{\partial y^2} = 0 \tag{10.7}$$

for a 2D planar flow domain, is transformed to a finite element equation form [6], by making use of the Galerkin weighted residual procedure, that is, by taking a scalar product of

Equation 10.7 with arbitrary weighting function W_k, which must be zero if approximated ϕ satisfies Equation 10.7 throughout the flow domain, that is,

$$\int_A \left(\frac{\partial^2 \phi}{\partial x^2} + \frac{\partial^2 \phi}{\partial y^2} \right) W_k \, dA = 0 \tag{10.8}$$

Equation 10.8 represents the desired averaged residual within the domain A. By applying Green's theorem to the second order derivatives, we obtain*

$$\int_A \left(\frac{\partial \phi}{\partial x} \frac{\partial W_k}{\partial x} + \frac{\partial \phi}{\partial y} \frac{\partial W_k}{\partial y} \right) dA = \int_l W_k \upsilon_n \, dl \tag{10.9}$$

where υ_n represents the normal velocity at the boundary

$$\upsilon_n = n_x \frac{\partial \phi}{\partial x} + n_y \frac{\partial \phi}{\partial y} \tag{10.10}$$

n_x and n_y are the directional cosines of the outward normal n to the boundary l.

Upon summing up the contributions from the elements, as per the finite element procedure, we obtain

$$\sum_e \left[\int_{A^e} \left(\frac{\partial \phi}{\partial x} \frac{\partial W_k}{\partial x} + \frac{\partial \phi}{\partial y} \frac{\partial W_k}{\partial y} \right) dA - \int_{l^e} W_k \upsilon_n \, dl \right] = 0 \tag{10.11}$$

Within each element, the unknown function, ϕ, is approximated as

$$\phi = \sum_{i=1}^m N_i \phi_i; \quad \phi = \phi(x, y), \ N_i = N_i(x, y) \tag{10.12}$$

where

m is the number of nodes associated with the element
N_i is the element shape function corresponding to node i
ϕ_i is the value of ϕ at node i

---

* Green's theorem in the form required here is obtained by taking the usual form

$$\int_A \left(\frac{\partial U}{\partial x} + \frac{\partial V}{\partial y} \right) dx \, dy = \int_l (U n_x + V n_y) dl$$

and substituting

$$U = W_k \frac{\partial \phi}{\partial x} \quad \text{and} \quad V = W_k \frac{\partial \phi}{\partial y}$$

In the Galerkin procedure, the number of weighting functions must equal the number of unknown nodal values, and they are conveniently chosen such that $W_i = N_i$, where W_i is the weighting function corresponding to node i.

Substituting Equation 10.12 in Equation 10.11, and assembling the element contributions, results in a matrix system of algebraic equations

$$[K]\{\phi\} = \{F\} \tag{10.13}$$

in which typical element components of the matrix are

$$k_{ij}^e = \int_{A^e} \left(\frac{\partial N_i}{\partial x} \frac{\partial N_j}{\partial x} + \frac{\partial N_i}{\partial y} \frac{\partial N_j}{\partial y} \right) dx dy \tag{10.14}$$

and

$$f_{ij}^e = \int_{l^e} \upsilon_n N_i dl \tag{10.15}$$

where l^e refers to elements with external boundary on which the normal velocity υ_n is specified.

The matrix system of Equation 10.13 can be solved for ϕ at nodal points in the flow domain, by specifying ϕ at those points on the boundary where υ_n is not specified. Also by specifying ϕ to be constant along the open boundaries, the flow can be constrained to be normal to the open boundary. This constraint also allows the solution to obtain a flow balance. The value of this constant ϕ is arbitrary, because only derivatives of the shape functions N_i are used in the computational process (Equation 10.14). In the present analysis, $\phi = 0$ is specified along the open boundary.

The matrix system $[K]$ in Equation 10.13 is symmetric and banded. Equation 10.13 is solved for ϕ by using a Gaussian elimination method, which transforms the matrix system $[K]$ into an equivalent triangular system whose solution can be obtained by back substitution [7].

10.3 Clinical Applications

The clinical application of finite element methodology described earlier is now presented for three subjects. The digitized video-angiographic images during all phases of the cardiac cycle are shown for each of the three patients (before and after administration of nitroglycerin). Patient 1 is a case with anterior wall akinesis, Patient 2 is a case with inferior wall hypokinesis, and Patient 3 had severe ischemic heart disease with large akinetic segments in the anterior and apical wall.

The wall velocities presented here are referred to a stationary aortic valve orifice, as the LV is assumed to be suspended from the aorta, while its apex is relatively free to move. In response to blood filling during diastole as well as to LV contraction and blood ejection during systole, the LV undergoes rigid-body motion about its anchorage to the aorta, due to the momentum imparted to it by the blood entering and leaving the LV. In addition, in response to blood-flow-generated wall pressures during diastole, the wall undergoes elastic deformation. In systole, it is the elastic wall motion generated by the contracting LV myocardium that gives rise to intra-LV blood flow during ejection.

Hence, in both diastolic and systolic phases, for analysis of intra-LV blood flow-velocity and pressure-differential distributions, the rigid-body displacements must be first removed from the LV wall displacements; since the LV is essentially suspended from the aorta, rigid-body LV displacements can be effectively removed by matching the aortic valve center and the line joining it to the apex of the LV for all frames. Figures 10.3a, 10.4a, and 10.5a display the superimposed sequential diastolic and systolic endocardial frames for Patients 1–3, respectively. From these images, the instantaneous wall displacements during the four equal time intervals of diastole and systole are computed, and shown in Figures 10.3b, c, 10.4b, c, and 10.5b, c. From the endocardial wall velocities, the intra-LV blood flow velocities are computed by finite element analysis, and shown in Figures 10.3d, e, 10.4d, e, and 10.5d, e.

10.3.1 Intra-LV Flow during Diastolic Filling

How well and how easily the LV fills is depicted by the instantaneous intra-LV flow distribution and the inter-frame variations in flow distribution that are governed by the segmental stiffness of the LV, and are manifestations of resistance-to-filling. In general, the flow is highest during the first half of the diastole (20–30 cm/s) in all patients, and the relative flow during all phases of diastole is at a maximum in the inflow segment of the LV, just below the mitral valve. The results, depicting high velocities during mid-filling phase, suggest that the early filling phase could possibly be due to the actively relaxing LV wall setting up a pressure gradient, conducive to filling, instead of the concept of LV wall motion responding passively to blood flow. Subsequently, during late-filling phases, the increasing stiffness of the LV wall (due to increasing LV volume) develops the intra-LV pressure gradient that provides increased resistance to LV filling in the form of reduced flow.

10.3.2 Intra-LV Flow during Systolic Ejection

During systolic contraction, the overall direction of the velocity vector shifts toward the aortic valve. In the two ventricles with asynergy (Patients 1 and 2), the maximum velocity occurs during the first half of systole (Figures 10.3e and 10.4e). During the systolic phase of maximum velocity, the nonischemic or contralateral segments in the two patients with asynergy (Patients 1 and 2), appear to contribute more to the magnitude of the velocity vector during the phase of maximum velocity flow (Figures 10.3e and 10.4e). Here, the maximum velocity is occurring in the upper half of the ventricular cavity just below the aortic valve (Figures 10.3e and 10.4e) and is of the order of 40–50 cm/s. In both the asynergic ventricles (Patients 1 and 2), the direction of flow velocity is from the contralateral wall throughout systole (Figures 10.3e and 10.4e), the only exception being an attempt by the anterior akinetic segment in the case of Patient 1 to increase the flow during the first phase of systole.

Finally, when the primary direction of flow is from the anterior wall there is a counterclockwise blood flow. Alternatively, there is a clockwise blood flow when the major direction is from the posterior wall.

The ideal situation is for the wall contraction to be so graded that adequate flow is generated in the apical region and a near-uniform flow is maintained throughout the

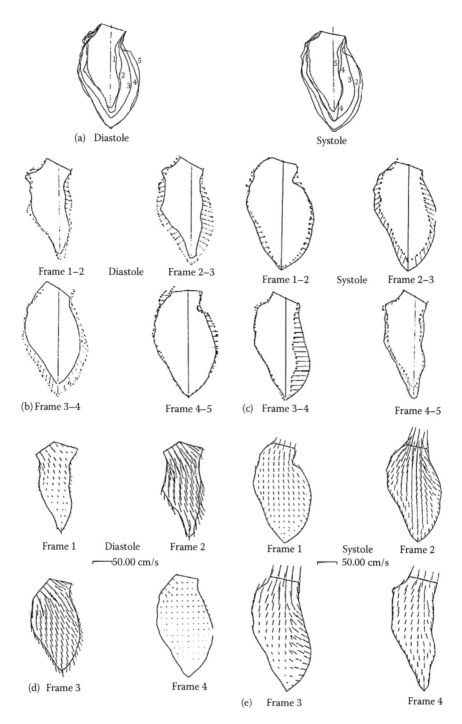

FIGURE 10.4

Patient 2: (a) superimposed sequential diastolic and systolic endocardial frames, whose aortic valve centers and the long axis are matched, (b) instantaneous endocardial wall displacement distortions during the periods of diastole, (c) instantaneous endocardial wall displacement distortions during the periods of systole, (d) instantaneous intra-LV velocity distributions during the periods of diastole, and (e) instantaneous intra-LV velocity distributions during the periods of systole.

LV chamber. From Equation 10.8, the factors contributing to an adequate intra-LV flow and cardiac output, with a smooth washout, are strong LV wall contraction and uniformly accelerating wall motion. If following administration of nitroglycerin, the LV wall can contract more uniformly and thereby set up a more favorable intra-LV velocity field, instead of a pattern of compensatory regional hypercontractility (and associated high wall tension and oxygen demand) to make up for a region of hypocontractility, then such a patient would be a good candidate for coronary bypass surgery.

10.3.3 Assessment of Ventricular Dysfunction in a Candidate for Surgery (Patient 3)

Figure 10.5a displays the superimposed sequential diastolic and systolic endocardial frames. Figure 10.5b and c provides displays of intra-LV flow distributions during filling

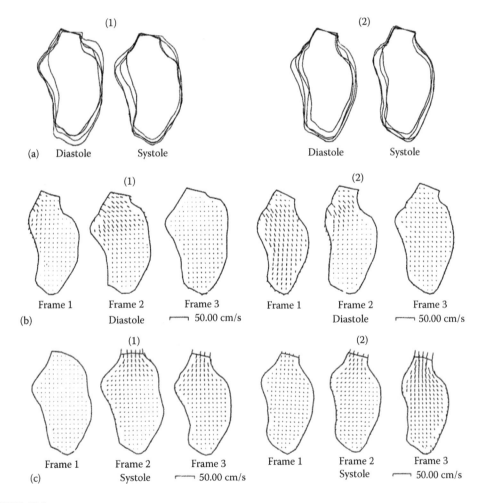

FIGURE 10.5

Patient 3: (a) superimposed sequential diastolic and systolic endocardial frames (whose aortic valve centers and the long axis are matched) before (a1) and after (b2) administration of nitroglycerin, (b) instantaneous intra-LV distributions of velocity during diastole, before (b1) and after (b2) administration of nitroglycerin, (c) instantaneous intra-LV distributions of velocity during ejection phase, before (c1) and after (c2) administration of nitroglycerin. *(Continued)*

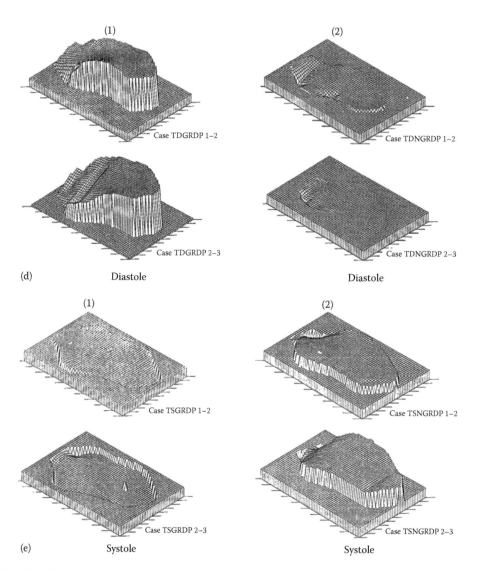

(1)

Case TDGRDP 1–2

(2)

Case TDNGRDP 1–2

Case TDGRDP 2–3

Case TDNGRDP 2–3

(d)   Diastole   Diastole

(1)

Case TSGRDP 1–2

(2)

Case TSNGRDP 1–2

Case TSGRDP 2–3

Case TSNGRDP 2–3

(e)   Systole   Systole

FIGURE 10.5 (*Continued*)
Patient 3: (d) Instantaneous intra-LV distributions of pressure-differentials during diastole, before (d1) and after (d2) administration of nitroglycerin, and (e) instantaneous intra-LV distributions of pressure-differentials during ejection phase, before (e1) and after (e2) administration of nitroglycerin.

and ejection stages of Patient 3 with anterior and apical wall akinesis, before and after administration of nitroglycerin. Following administration of nitroglycerin, the intra-LV velocity distributions in Figure 10.5b demonstrate slightly improved filling-flow compared to the pre-nitroglycerin state, and a slightly improved ejection-phase flow and contractility can be observed compared to the pre-nitroglycerin state in Figure 10.5c. This patient is a candidate for coronary bypass surgery.

For this patient, it is more interesting to make inferences concerning candidacy for surgery, by comparing the intra-LV pressure-differential distributions before and after administration of nitroglycerin. From a computational viewpoint, the intra-LV flow is determined from the LV wall motion boundary condition to the potential flow Equation 10.3, and the intra-LV pressure gradient can in turn be computed from the flow by employing Equation 10.4. However, we could interpret the phenomenon as if the LV wall stiffness were providing the resistance to wall motion for filling during diastole, and the contracting LV is facilitating emptying of the LV during systole, thereby setting up the requisite intra-LV pressure-gradient and velocity distributions.

In Figure 10.5d, the diastole pressure-differential distributions, before and after nitroglycerin administration, are compared. Note the substantial deleterious pressure gradient characterizing resistance-to-LV filling before nitroglycerin administration; this pressure gradient is distinctly reduced after nitroglycerin is given. Similarly, Figure 10.5e illustrates improvement in the pressure gradient conducive to ejection, following administration of nitroglycerin. Thereby, this patient is deemed to be a candidate for coronary bypass surgery.

10.4 Discussion

10.4.1 Limitations

We make the assumption that the LV in the 30° RAO view displays the necessary endocardial segments and reveals the ventricle along its longest axis. While single plane quantitative ventriculography is an accepted method, it is somewhat limited especially in ischemic heart disease, by failing to reveal segments in other planes. However in this context, we are working toward conducting the intra-LV flow analysis in a number of planes containing the long axis of the LV.

We have the potential to analyze more than five frames during each of diastole and systole phases, but decided to restrict ourselves to this number of frames, in order to lessen the computational effort, time, and expense. At the same time, we felt that we had sufficient frames to obtain results that would be of diagnostic value to the cardiologist; although we could increase the number of frames, we feel that five frames is a reasonable compromise.

Our choice of superimposing sequential frames along an axis from mid-aortic valve to apex is designed to remove rigid-body motion of the LV (although it tends to fix the apical segments and possibly underestimate the regional wall motion), and accounts only for elastic motion of the wall interacting with the hydrodynamic forces of intra-LV flood flow. Since it is not possible to delineate valve-leaflet motion in angiograms, the flow patterns presented here do not include the effects of valve-leaflet motion. Other technical limitations include the necessity for operator intervention with respect to endocardial border detection (although this is indeed semi-automated), problems with magnification and X-ray distortion seen in both cine and video images, and the blood-flow analysis being confined to 30° RAO plane. While it is important to bear these limitations in mind, it should be appreciated that this method provides comprehensive information concerning the magnitude and nature of intraventricular flows that are very sensitive to segmental myocardial disorders. The resulting information can help provide an insight not only into the etiology of intramural thrombus formation but also it is a step toward the intrinsic assessment of LV function and dysfunction.

10.4.2 Clinical Applications

An important prognostic indicator for patients with coronary artery disease is the degree of LV dysfunction following myocardial infarction. Although global indices such as ejection fraction are useful as a rough guide to the separation of high-risk from low-risk patients, these indices can be misleading, since coronary artery disease is a segmental disorder, and most quantitative studies on LV function appear to be focused on quantification of regional wall motion. It is now recognized that qualitative or subjective assessment of contrast ventriculograms are fraught with large inter-observer variability. Numerical values for sequences of endocardial wall motion is useful, but it is basically nonstandardized at the present time; moreover, it yields no information on the manner in which the endocardial wall imparts energy or force to the intracavitary blood volume.

Finite element analysis of intraventricular flow distribution provides a wealth of dynamic information, which can be proven to be very useful in clinical decision making. For instance, the distribution and sequence of flow within the LV cavity during both diastole and systole may reveal stagnant zones of recirculation due to impaired regional function or intercavitary thrombus formation. The magnitude and direction of the velocity vectors within the cavity can also provide some useful information on the efficiency of contraction.

Hypokinesis of a wall segment may be due either to scar tissue or to an area of reversible ischemia. It is possible, with the use of interventions such as nitroglycerin, that finite element modeling could help identify (by means of flow distributions) those segments of reversible ischemia that would benefit by revascularization, as well as areas of scar formation more amenable to aneurysmectomy.

References

1. E. Braunwald, J. Ross, and E.H. Sonnenblick, *Mechanism of Contraction of the Normal and Failing Heart*, Little Brown, Boston, MA (1976).
2. R.C. McFadden, G.R. Barnes, D.N. Ghista, E.L. Fallen, and T.M. Srinivasan, Microcomputer analysis of left ventricular video-angiograms, *Proceedings of the Canadian Medical and Biological Engineering Conference*, Ottawa, Ontario, Canada (1984).
3. C.Y. Wang and E.H. Sonnenblick, Dynamic pressure distribution inside a spherical ventricle, *J. Biomech.*, 12, 9–12 (1979).
4. A.G. Hansen, *Fluid Mechanics*, Wiley, New York (1967), p. 349.
5. L.M. Milne-Thompson, *Theoretical Hydrodynamics*, 4th edn., MacMillan, New York (1965).
6. O.C. Zienkiewicz, *The Finite Element Method*, McGraw-Hill, London, UK (1977), pp. 423–449.
7. J.E. Akin, *Application and Implementation of Finite Element Methods*, Academic Press, London, UK (1982).

11

Cardiac Perfusion Analysis and Computation of Intra-Myocardial Blood Flow Velocity and Pressure Patterns

Dhanjoo N. Ghista, Eddie Y.K. Ng, Ru San Tan, Jian-Jun Shu, and Reginald Jegathese

CONTENTS

11.1 Introduction

Myocardial perfusion is the most important designation and determinant of cardiac function, as it affects cardiac contractility, ejection fraction, and blood supply to all the organs and to the coronary tree. Hence, mapping and quantification of myocardial perfusion is very important. This chapter is divided into two parts. Section 11.2 is about the quantification of cardiac myocardial perfusion and function by single photon emission computed tomography (SPECT) imaging, in terms of intra-myocardial radionuclide tracer maps. Section 11.3 provides further substantiation of myocardial perfusion by computing intra-myocardial pressure and velocity distribution patterns.

In Section 11.2, we begin with myocardial ischemia physiology, ischemia cause and diagnosis, and coronary autoregulation. With exercise stress, tissue accumulation of metabolites occurs, which relaxes the arteriolar wall smooth muscle cell contraction. Arterioles further dilate (representing coronary hyperemia) by varying amounts depending on the basal coronary tone. The coronary blood flow (CBF) in nonstenosed arteries expands more than in stenosed arteries, because arterioles supplied by the stenosed arteries are already semi-dilated even before exercise begins. Hence, the coronary flow reserve (CFR), defined as the ratio of stress to rest CBF, is lower in stenosed arteries compared to normal arteries.

To assess CBF and CFR, we carry out radionuclide myocardial perfusion imaging (MPI) by SPECT acquisition technique. The MPI is performed with intravenously injected technetium-99m-based agents. These tracers are trapped in the myocardium in proportion to the regional CBF. SPECT enables 3D image reconstruction and good separation of the different heart chambers in space. The acquisition, computer processing, and display of scintigraphic (radionuclide imaging) data by high-speed computing constitute fundamental steps in the process of nuclear imaging. SPECT allows evaluation of perfusion patterns in reconstructed thin slices of the myocardium. Comparison of stress and rest images helps in differentiating ischemia from infarct scar. A perfusion abnormality present in the stress study that is resolved in the rest study represents ischemia, whereas a perfusion abnormality on both the stress and rest studies represents a scar.

Figure 11.5 displays myocardial perfusion SPECT imaging. Therein, the maximal tracer uptake (which implies high CFR) is depicted in bright orange, and areas of perfusion defect are in graduated darker hues of blue-green. Large area of stress perfusion defects can be seen at the apex, lateral, and inferior walls that is largely reversible on the rest images. This patient exhibits severe coronary ischemia corresponding to multiple epicardial coronary arterial territories. Figure 11.7 depicts myocardial perfusion SPECT in a patient with a large anterior myocardial infarct. The regional tracer uptake is normalized with respect to the maximum tracer activity detected count in the myocardium, and then displayed according to deciles of percentage maximal counts by using a stepped color scale (right). We can note the large area of stress perfusion defect at the inferior, septal, distal anterior, and apical walls that is nonreversible at rest. Also, the tracer activity in these areas is less than 50%–60% of maximum counts, implying that they are nonviable and are unlikely to improve with revascularization of the diseased coronary arteries.

We then discuss automated SPECT quantization of myocardial perfusion and the available software algorithms for it. Most quantitative analyses display the tomographic slices in a polar map format. The individual patient's polar map perfusion can then be compared with a parametric reference polar map derived from disease-free normal patients, with low likelihood of coronary artery disease (CAD) and visually normal images, as depicted in Figures 11.8 and 11.9. The criteria for abnormality are derived from the mean and standard deviation of the count uptake in each region of the left ventricle (LV). Figure 11.8 displays polar map quantification. Therein, the tracer activity at the LV apex is depicted in the center. Count activities in the short-axis slices are displayed around the center, as successive flat annular rings of increasing radii as the slices progress toward the base of the LV. It can be noted that the subject exhibits a large perfusion defect in the left anterior descending artery (LAD) territory that largely spares the left circumflex (LCX) and right coronary artery (RCA) territories.

Left ventricular ejection fraction (LVEF) assessment from gated perfusion SPECT measurements (of technetium-99m tracer) is highly reproducible. Gated SPECT acquisition can be performed at rest following either stress or rest radionuclide injections. In the case of stress radionuclide injections, there is potential for stress-induced ischemia to persist (known as myocardial stunning), causing abnormal wall motion and a reduction in measured LVEF. The presence of post-stress regional wall motion abnormalities not present at rest is a specific indicator of severe coronary stenosis. Figure 11.10 displays quantitative wall motion assessment of gated perfusion SPECT using AutoQuant (QGS) program. From transmural radionuclide count profiles, the endocardial and epicardial surfaces are determined, from which LV cavity and myocardial volumes are estimated and the ejection fraction is calculated. Also, regional wall motion (endocardial surface displacement) and wall thickening are evaluated. Post-stress gated SPECT in this patient shows normal wall motion in all segments. We can conclude that gated SPECT LVEF measurements are generally accurate and reliable, even in the presence of large defects.

Section 11.3 primarily deals with perfusion analysis of the myocardium. In order to gain further quantitative insight into LV intra-myocardial flow, we have developed a biomechanics model of intra-myocardial blood flow through a porous myocardium medium, using a modified form of Darcy's law in which the blood velocity is dependent on intra-myocardial pressure gradient (∇p), myocardial permeability (k) as well as myocardial stress-dependent hydrostatic pressure (H).

The governing equations required to compute intra-myocardial pressure and velocity distributions involve equations for the incompressible and viscous fluid (blood), incompressible and elastic solid (myocardium), and fluid–solid interaction. Specifically, these equations are (1) continuity equation for the fluid, (2) momentum equations for both the fluid and solid mediums, (3) constitutive equations for both solid and fluid mediums, and (4) Darcy's law. With some appropriate assumptions (such as small interconnected pores), we can express the blood velocity in terms of the pressure head gradient, myocardial tissue permeability, blood viscosity, and density. The pressure head ϕ is a function of the fluid pressure and potential gradient. Darcy's law is expressed in terms of the hydraulic conductivity C as a function of myocardial permeability and blood viscosity. Finally, we can express the blood velocity V in terms of C and spatial derivative of pressure, as given by Equation 11.28. We then provide a flow chart (Table 11.5) of this poroelastic fluid-structure analysis, for computing the streamlines, pressure, and velocity distributions.

We then display the computed results of pressure and velocity variations in annular myocardial segments, based on specified inlet and outlet pressures in Table 11.4. Figure 11.13a indicates the specified inlet and outlet pressures, for which Figure 11.13b displays the computed intra-myocardial pressure distribution and Figure 11.14 displays the intra-myocardium velocity distribution. Likewise, Figure 11.15a indicates another format of specified inlet and outlet pressures, for which Figure 11.15b displays the computed intra-myocardial pressure distribution and Figure 11.16 displays the intra-myocardium velocity distribution.

This chapter hence provides the methods for (1) determining myocardial perfusion by SPECT imaging and detecting ischemia regions, based on myocardial radionuclide tracer maps, and (2) quantifying myocardial perfusion in terms of pressure and velocity distributions in the myocardial segments.*

11.2 Quantification of Cardiac Perfusion and Function Using Nuclear Cardiac Imaging

11.2.1 Physiology of Myocardial Ischemia

11.2.1.1 Definition

The coronary arteries transport oxygen- and nutrient-rich blood to the myocardium (heart muscle) to sustain the heart's normal contractile pumping function. The pumping heart in turn generates pressure and flow within the coronary circulation to supply blood and oxygen to the heart. In CAD, atherosclerotic fatty deposits in the coronary artery wall narrow the lumen (opening) of the arteries, compromising blood flow and oxygen delivery to the heart. Myocardial ischemia is said to occur when CBF or perfusion is insufficient for myocardial metabolic needs. This can occur when there is a reduction in blood flow due to a severe obstruction of the coronary arteries, or when increased metabolic demands are not met by an increased supply of oxygen, such as during physical exercise.

During exercise, the workload of the heart increases, so as to increase cardiac output to meet the increased requirements of the skeletal muscle. This increased workload requires an increase in coronary blood supply, which is met by vasodilation of the arteriolar bed. However, in patients with CAD, this normal increase in CBF with exercise may be limited due to narrowing (stenosis) of one or more coronary arteries. Thus in a patient with a coronary stenosis, ischemia may arise when myocardial metabolic requirements and oxygen demand increase but supply is limited by coronary disease, such as when the heart is stressed during exercise. Hence, a decrease in myocardial perfusion and/or an increase in myocardial metabolism impose an imbalance in supply-demand that results in ischemia (Figure 11.1).

11.2.1.2 Ischemic Cascade

The onset and manifestations of myocardial ischemia usually occur in a stepwise sequence, which has been termed the ischemic cascade. The initial abnormality is that of insufficient CBF, either a reduction in CBF or an increase in metabolic demand that is not matched by an increase in blood supply. There is heterogeneity of CBF with lower blood flow in ischemic territories (supplied by diseased coronary arteries) compared to nonischemic

* This chapter is based on Quantification of cardiac perfusion and function using nuclear cardiac imaging, RS Tan, L Zhong, T Chua, and DN Ghista, and Left ventricular pumping-perfusion analysis: Myocardial properties, intra-LV velocity and pressure, detection of myocardial ischemic and infarcted segments, perfusion depiction by SPECT imaging, computation of blood flow pressure and velocity patterns within myocardial regions, E Y-K Ng, DN Ghista, J-J Shu, RC Jegathese, and M Sankaranarayanan in *Cardiac Perfusion and Pumping*, DN Ghista and E Y-K Ng, eds., World Scientific, 2006.

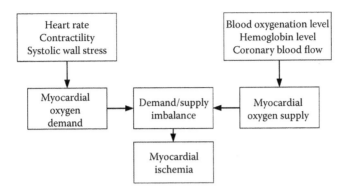

FIGURE 11.1
Factors influencing myocardial ischemia.

territories and also from the subendocardium to the subepicardium. Impairment of myocardial myofiber-active relaxation and contraction ensue, resulting in diastolic (relaxation) and systolic (contraction) dysfunction, respectively. Depending on the extent of myocardial involvement and adequacy of compensatory hyperfunction of nonischemic myocardium, global myocardial function, LVEF, and stroke volume deteriorate variably. Ischemic changes on surface electrocardiograms (ECG) appear late, often heralding the onset of anginal symptoms. The evaluation of ischemia relies on the detection and measurement of these event parameters. Using various imaging and diagnostic technologies, alterations in coronary perfusion, myocardial contractile function, and ECG may be identified and quantified (Figure 11.2).

11.2.1.3 Coronary Autoregulation

Coronary arteries arborize into a network of fine arterioles. The walls of these arterioles contain smooth muscle cells that contract in the basal state, contributing to coronary tone and resistance. When a proximal epicardial coronary artery develops stenosis, the corresponding distal arterioles dilate in response, thus lowering coronary resistance and effectively maintaining unchanged CBF. With exercise stress, tissue accumulation of metabolites occurs, which relaxes arteriolar wall smooth muscle cell contraction. Arterioles further dilate (coronary hyperemia) by varying amounts depending on the basal coronary tone. CBF in nonstenosed arteries expands more than in stenosed arteries, because arterioles supplied by the stenosed arteries are already semi-dilated even before exercise begins. Hence, the CFR, defined as the ratio of stress to rest CBF, is lower in stenosed arteries compared to normal arteries (Figure 11.3).

11.2.2 General Principles of Myocardial Perfusion Imaging

11.2.2.1 Myocardial Perfusion Tracer Agents

Blood flow to the myocardium may be tracked by using parenterally administered compounds, such as radioisotope-labeled tracers, echocardiographic microbubbles, magnetic resonance relativity, and x-ray contrast agents. Besides CBF, other factors determine myocardial blood flow tracer uptake characteristics, including the relative distribution of the tracer between intravascular (within blood vessels) and extravascular compartments, the degree of trapping within versus redistribution outside

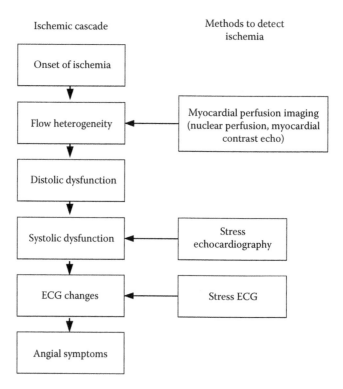

FIGURE 11.2
Diagnosis of ischemia by detection of abnormalities associated with the ischemic cascade of events.

myocardial cells, and the radionuclide half-life in the case of radiopharmaceuticals. The latter two factors determine persistence of the tracer in the myocardium. If persistent, MPI may be performed at any convenient time after the tracer has been administered. For blood flow tracers that transit briefly and rapidly clear from the myocardium, MPI must be performed during their initial passage through the myocardium and is technically more challenging.

11.2.2.2 Assessing Coronary Flow and CFR

It is possible to quantify absolute CBF (expressed as mL/min/g of myocardial tissue) in human beings using pure intravascular flow agents, such as radiolabeled ^{15}O-water, ^{13}N-ammonia, or rubidium-82, all positron emission tomography (PET) tracer agents. However, its expense, the limited availability of PET facilities, and expertise impede widespread application of the technology.

More commonly, the relative CFR of areas of myocardium supplied by normal versus stenosed coronary arteries are assessed by performing MPI at rest and under conditions of exercise, pharmacologically induced cardioexcitatory, or vasodilatory stress. While CBF in all myocardial territories may be equal at rest (yielding homogeneous tracer uptake in all myocardial regions), attenuated amplification of regional CBF during stress implies presence of physiologically significant coronary stenosis in the corresponding proximal epicardial arterial territory (Figure 11.3). Alternatively, MPI during acute ischemic episodes, for example, during anginal chest pain at the coronary care unit or emergency department, may similarly uncover heterogeneity of myocardial tracer uptake.

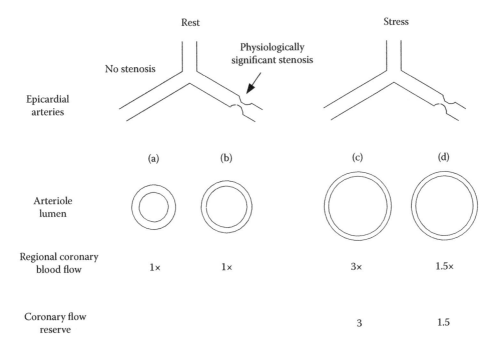

FIGURE 11.3
CFRs in normal and stenotic coronary arteries. In normal arteries, arteriolar wall contraction maintains coronary tone at rest (a). With proximal epicardial coronary artery stenosis, the corresponding distal arterioles dilate, lowering resistance and maintaining normal CBF (b). With exercise stress, arterioles dilate (coronary hyperemia). The quanta of increase, thence CFR, are greater in normal (c) versus stenotic (d) arteries because of the former's greater basal coronary tone. With pharmacologic vasodilatory stress, there is maximal arteriolar dilation and even greater CBF enhancement.

11.2.2.3 MPI Techniques

Various MPI techniques are employed to visualize the distribution and concentration of perfusion tracers within the heart. These techniques exploit the heterogeneity of blood flow between myocardial regions that are perfused by normal coronary arteries and regions that are supplied by coronary vessels with physiologically significant coronary artery stenoses. Table 11.1 lists these techniques, their strengths, and limitations. Of these, nuclear MPI is arguably the most established and commonly used technique.

11.2.3 Nuclear MPI

Nuclear cardiology studies use small doses of radioactive material to assess myocardial blood flow, evaluate the pumping function of the heart, as well as visualize the size and location of a heart attack.

11.2.3.1 Nuclear Myocardial Perfusion Tracer Agents

MPI is performed with intravenously injected radionuclides, thallium-201- or technetium-99m–based agents (sestamibi, tetrofosmin, and teboroxime compounds). These tracers are trapped in the myocardium in proportion to the regional CBF. Further, intact cell membrane and mitochondrial function are obligatory for radioactive

TABLE 11.1

Comparison of MPI Techniques

Technique	Tracer	Parameter	Quantitative analysis	Spatial resolution (mm)	Renal risk	Ionizing radiation	Limitations
PET	$^{15}O-H_2O$, $^{13}N-NH_3$, Rb-82	CBF, CRF	Yes	5–6	–	++	High cost, limited availability
SPECT	Th-201, Tc-99m agent	CRF	Yes	10–12	–	++	Attenuation, long scan protocols
MRI	Gadolinium	CBF, CRF	Yes	2–3	+[a]	–	Pacemakers, ICD contraindicated
MCE	Microbubble	CBF, CRF	Yes	1–2	–	–	Little consensus on echo technique
Angiography	X-ray contrast	Myocardial blush grade	No	0.1	+++	++	Invasive method, qualitative test
CT scan	X-ray contrast	CRF	No	0.5	+++	+++	Early development

CBF, coronary blood flow; CRF, coronary flow reserve; CT, computed tomography; ICD, implantable cardioverter-defibrillator; MCE, myocardial contrast echocardiography; MRI, magnetic resonance imaging; PET, positron emission tomography; SPECT, single photon emission computed tomography.

[a] Rare cases of a serious generalized skin condition, nephrogenic, fibrosing dermopathy, have been reported in subjects with impaired kidney function.

thallium-201- or technetium-99m–based tracers, respectively, to enter myocardial cells. Hence, myocardial uptake of these tracers reflects both myocardial perfusion and myocardial viability.

Thallium-201 was one of the earliest tracers to be used for MPI, with an excellent tissue extraction fraction.[1] The rate of tracer uptake by the myocardium is almost linearly correlated to CBF, except at very high levels of CBF, when it starts to plateau. Thallium-201 has however, some limitations. First, its relatively long half-life (73 h) exposes the patient to prolonged radioactivity, limiting the dose that can be administered. Second, its main photopeak is suboptimal for gamma camera imaging (see the following). These disadvantages adversely impacted the technical quality of the images, providing incentive for the development of the newer technetium-99m–based tracers. The tissue extraction fractions of the commonly used technetium-99m–based tracers (sestamibi and tetrofosmin) are less than that of thallium-201. In spite of this, the latter's image quality is superior due to a more favorable photon energy (140 keV) as well as the higher amounts of radioactive technetium-99m that can be administered due to its shorter half-life (6 h) and the persistence of the tracer in the myocardium. Unlike thallium-201, which slowly redistributes from perfused into nonperfused myocardial tissue, technetium-99m (sestamibi and tetrofosmin) persists in the perfused myocardial tissue. This enables MPI to be conveniently performed long after initial injection of the tracer.[2] It also allows for repeat scanning without concern that the tracer has washed out or redistributed from its initial pattern of uptake, if there is a technical problem such as patient motion that requires a repeat scan.

11.2.3.2 Stress Agents and Scan Protocols

Graded exercise stress is performed either on a treadmill or a bicycle ergometer, using various standardized protocols. The ubiquitous symptom-limited Bruce treadmill exercise protocol consists of consecutive 3 min exercise stages at successively faster speeds and steeper gradients. Exercise stress induces coronary hyperemia, resulting in heterogeneous increase in regional CBF in nonstenosed arteries (with high basal coronary tone) versus stenosed arteries (with lower basal coronary tone) due to their different CFR.

For patients who are unable to exercise adequately, the physiologic effects of exercise may be simulated by infusion of drugs. The adrenergic drug dobutamine, administered at a dose of 5 µg/kg/min with increment every 3 min to 40 µg/kg/min, increases heart rate and myocardial contractility, thereby growing myocardial oxygen demand that leads to coronary hyperemia.

Other pharmacologic agents may also directly induce coronary hyperemia. Intravenous adenosine or dipyridamole, administered at a dose of 140 µg/kg/min, maximally dilates coronary arterioles, augmenting flow heterogeneity in myocardial territories supplied by normal versus stenosed epicardial arteries. This is known as vasodilator stress imaging and is the most commonly applied radionuclide pharmacologic stress technique.

All stress procedures are performed with continuous monitoring of patients' vital signs (symptoms, blood pressure, and pulse rate) and ECG. Radionuclide tracers are administered during maximal exercise, pharmacologic cardioexcitatory, or vasodilatory stress. As the radionuclide tracers persist in the myocardium for some time, MPI can be delayed allowing sufficient time for patient to be transferred to the scanner after the stress. Technetium-99m–based agents provide more counts than thallium-201 and offer the possibility of imaging of the tracer as it passes through the heart after rapid bolus infusion of tracer. This is known as first-pass imaging and allows additional information to be obtained such as an estimation of LV function during exercise. To take advantage of this possibility, a gamma camera capable of rapid counts, such as a multi-crystal gamma camera, is recommended.

First-pass imaging during rapid bolus infusion of radioactive tracer is less commonly performed, as it requires the patient to be in the scanner during the stress procedure (which limits the choice of exercise stress possibilities).

Different scan protocols may be employed. Separate day acquisitions for stress and rest scans allow sufficient time for the radioactive tracer to be washed out between scans through radioactive decay and bodily excretion. For technetium-99m–based agents with short radioactive half-life, the same day stress-rest or rest-stress acquisition is feasible, with the two radionuclide boluses administered a few hours apart. As thallium-201 redistributes from nonischemic into ischemic tissues, a second scan may be performed a few hours (or even 24 h) after tracer administration to assess rest (redistribution) perfusion. In addition, a dual-tracer protocol combining rest thallium-201 followed shortly by stress technetium-99m (sestamibi) injections may be employed. This exploits the distinct photopeaks associated with each tracer to enable rest and stress perfusion images to be separately acquired at one sitting.[3]

11.2.3.3 Image Acquisition and Processing

Radionuclides administered into patients course through the blood circulation and enter perfused viable myocardial cells, from where they emit gamma radiation, a form of electromagnetic energy. The gamma rays are detected using scintillation counters mounted onto photomultipliers. Gamma particles interact with matter within the scintillator (usually made of sodium iodide crystal) to produce photoelectrons with characteristic energy quanta, photopeaks, specific to the radionuclide. These generate light flashes that are in turn converted to electric pulses by a system of photomultiplier tubes. The electric pulses, with voltages proportional to the energy of the original electrons, are sorted and analyzed by computers to form 2D spatial images of the scintillation count densities, which reflect the distribution and relative concentration of radioactive tracer present in the heart.

Imaging the heart from fixed standard external positions yields simple projection perfusion images (planar imaging). This has now been superseded by SPECT acquisition technique. In SPECT, multiple projection images at equally spaced angular displacement intervals are acquired of the chest by one or more gantry-mounted scintillation detectors, positioned near the chest wall, that rotate around the patient's body axis as the patient lies supine on the SPECT table. 3D image reconstruction using filtered back-projection[4] enables good separation of different heart chambers in space, which surmounts the problem of structure overlap inherent in planar imaging (Figure 11.4). Further, SPECT offers improved perfusion defect detection (because of enhanced contrast resolution), localization, and sizing compared to planar imaging.[5]

In general, myocardial perfusion SPECT acquisition takes from 10 to 30 min, depending on the number of detectors and the type and dose of the radiopharmaceutical. ECG gating can be performed using electrodes and a gating device. This yields temporally resolved SPECT data sets (usually eight per heart cycle) that when lined up sequentially and displayed as a cine loop enables visualization and quantification of cardiac contractile function.

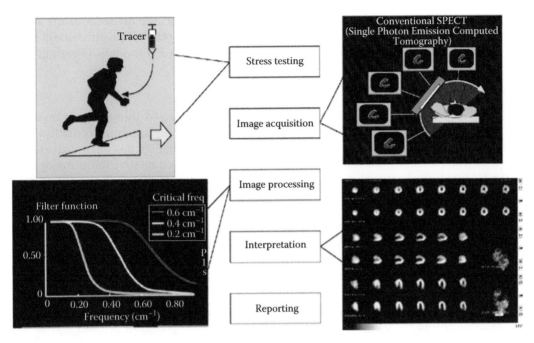

FIGURE 11.4
Stress myocardial perfusion SPECT.

11.2.4 Interpretation of Myocardial Perfusion SPECT

The acquisition, computer processing, and display of scintigraphic (radionuclide imaging) data by high-speed computers constitute a fundamental step in the process of nuclear imaging. Quantitative analysis of the digitized information reduces the subjectivity of visual assessment and augments the reproducibility of evaluation and interpretation of perfusion SPECT data.[6]

11.2.4.1 Inspection of Raw Projection Data

The rotating raw projection images are first reviewed to ensure that they have been acquired over the appropriate acquisition arc and are devoid of artifacts such as excessive motion between projections. Motion artifacts may result from either excessive patient movement within the scanner or a post-exercise gradual shift in the position of the diaphragm from a lower (more inflated lung) to a higher position ("upward creep") when the patient is lying supine during the course of image acquisition. As technetium-99m tracers, sestamibi and tetrofosmin, are excreted through the intestines, there may occasionally be areas of increased tracer uptake in gut tissue near the inferior surface of the heart. These potentially cause error during image reconstruction and must be eliminated either by digital image post-processing or repeat image acquisition. In addition, abnormal extracardiac loci of high radionuclide tracer uptake may rarely be found in the lungs or other organs within the imaging field. These warrant further investigation to determine their nature and exclude malignant lesions.

One common problem encountered in ECG-gated SPECT is inaccurate gating due to arrhythmia or poor ECG signal. This may manifest as a "flashing" appearance.

Rejected beats and low counts in some projections result in line artifacts in the back-projected reconstructed volume. Where there is concern that gated acquisition could have introduced error into perfusion data, the acquisition is repeated without ECG gating.

11.2.4.2 Visual Assessment of SPECT Myocardial Perfusion

SPECT allows evaluation of perfusion patterns in reconstructed thin slices of myocardium. While the 3D SPECT perfusion image data set may be freely reformatted and manipulated at will, a uniform approach to SPECT image display has been universally adopted. The reconstructed tomographic images are reoriented relative to the major axes of the LV yielding short-axis, vertical long-axis, and horizontal long-axis slices. Imaging slices from different acquisitions (i.e., stress-rest, stress-redistribution) are displayed in an interleaved fashion, and aligned to ensure that each slice of the stress MPI correctly matches its corresponding rest slice. Comparison of stress and rest images help in differentiating ischemia from infarct scar. A perfusion abnormality present in the stress study that is resolved in the rest study represents ischemia, whereas a perfusion abnormality on both the stress and rest studies represents scar (Figure 11.5).

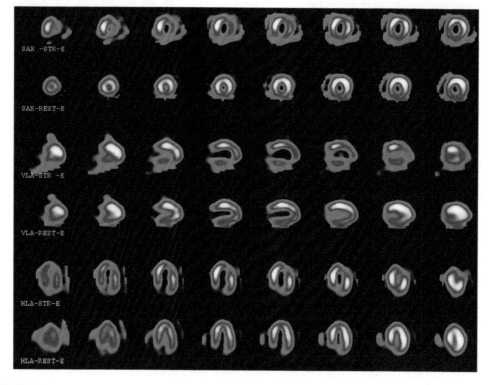

FIGURE 11.5

Myocardial perfusion SPECT. Alternating rows of stress and rest images are aligned. Contiguous thin slices of myocardium are displayed, from left to right: apical to basal short-axis slices (top 2 rows), septal to lateral vertical long-axis slices (middle 2 rows), inferior to superior horizontal long-axis slices (bottom 2 rows). Maximal tracer uptake (which implies high CFR) is depicted in bright orange and areas of perfusion defect are in graduated darker hues of blue-green. Note the large area of stress perfusion defect at the apex, lateral, and inferior walls that is largely reversible on the rest images. This patient exhibits severe coronary ischemia that corresponds to multiple epicardial coronary arterial territories.

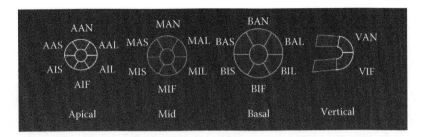

FIGURE 11.6
The 20-segment model of the LV. The entire LV is represented by three short-axis slices (apical, mid, and basal) that are each subdivided into six segments (clockwise when viewed from the apex: anterior, anterolateral, inferolateral, inferior, inferoseptal, and anteroseptal), as well as two apical segments (anteroapical, inferoapical) visualized in the mid-vertical long-axis imaging slice. Each segment constitutes approximately 5% of the LV volume. The extent of perfusion defect can be estimated by counting the number of segments involved.

An alternative explanation for a persistent perfusion defect is an attenuation artifact. This is caused by the nonuniform decrease in gamma radiation as the rays traverse soft tissue of varying thicknesses before hitting the scintillation detector surface. These attenuation artifacts typically produce nonreversible perfusion defects present both on the stress and rest studies and are associated with characteristic locations (e.g., the basal inferior wall in men, anterior wall in women). The absence of wall motion abnormality on gated SPECT helps to distinguish these nonreversible defects from scarring due to prior myocardial infarction and damage. Special hardware and software may be used to correct for soft tissue attenuation.

The LV may be divided into 17 or 20 segments for semiquantitative analysis. Our laboratory uses the latter system (Figure 11.6). Each segment is scored according to a five-point scheme: 0, normal; 1, slight reduction of tracer uptake; 2, moderate reduction of tracer uptake; 3, severe reduction of tracer uptake; and 4, absence of tracer uptake. Post-processing of SPECT images to yield a stepped color display facilitates visual assessment of regional relative CFR (Figure 11.7). This systemic approach to SPECT myocardial perfusion interpretation is conceivably more reproducible than simple qualitative evaluation.

11.2.4.3 Quantitative Assessment of SPECT Myocardial Perfusion

The quantitative approach is generally recognized as a desirable tool to standardize analysis and improve the reproducibility of the nuclear cardiac assessment. When quantitative methods are used, the reported sensitivities and specificities are 90% and 70% for thallium-201 SPECT imaging,[6–13] versus 83% and 82% for technetium-99m SPECT images analyzed using one commonly used commercial automated software (AutoQuant, Cedars-Sinai).[14,15] The apparent decline in specificity may be due partially to the effect of referral bias[16] increasing over time. Once a diagnostic test becomes widely accepted, patients with abnormal test results are more likely to be referred for angiography than patients with normal results. Although this is appropriate clinically, it has a profound effect on test specificity since patients with normal coronary arteries are unlikely to undergo angiography unless they have false-positive test results.

Various software algorithms are employed to isolate and automatically segment the LV for analysis (Table 11.2).[14,15,17–21] Nevertheless, all quantitative output for myocardial perfusion should be checked visually for accuracy of the program in defining the myocardial borders. It may be necessary to adjust the gain settings for patients with severe perfusion

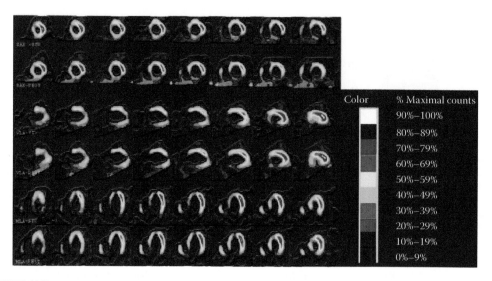

Color	% Maximal counts
	90%–100%
	80%–89%
	70%–79%
	60%–69%
	50%–59%
	40%–49%
	30%–39%
	20%–29%
	10%–19%
	0%–9%

FIGURE 11.7

Myocardial perfusion SPECT in a patient with a large anterior myocardial infarct. The regional tracer uptake is normalized with respect to the maximum tracer activity detected count in the myocardium, and then displayed according to deciles of percentage maximal counts using a stepped color scale (right). Note the large area of stress perfusion defect at the inferior, septal, distal anterior, and apical walls that is non-reversible at rest. In addition, the tracer activity in these areas is less than 50%–60% of maximum counts, implying that they are nonviable and are unlikely to improve with revascularization of the diseased coronary arteries.

TABLE 11.2

Available Software for Automated SPECT Quantization Of Myocardial Perfusion

Name	Software function and components
CEqual[17]	Automated sampling of LV volume (40 points per circumferential profile) to yield 2D polar maps, which are compared to normal database of patients with normal perfusion, low likelihood of CAD, and visually normal images. Criteria for abnormality are derived from the mean and standard deviation of the count uptake in each LV region. The patient's stress profiles are normalized to the normal database, by dividing the heart is divided into 10 regions and scaling the most normal patient sector (highest average counts) to the corresponding sector of the normal database.
CardioMatch[18]	Automated registration of 3D stress and rest images, comparison with normal database to generate measurements of perfusion defect size and extent. Database is stratified by gender, age, weight, and heart size.
Emory Toolbox[18]	CEqual software, databases for different protocols, automated calculation of transient ischemic dilation ratio, gated SPECT display, 3D display of perfusion with coronary artery tree overlay (PerSPECTive), expert systems analysis of results (PERFEX).
3D-MSPECT[19]	Automated processing and comprehensive quantitative analysis of perfusion and function, 3D SPECT, gated SPECT, and attenuation-corrected SPECT with normal databases.
Yale-CQ[20,21]	Automated sampling of LV circumferential count profiles using an automatic algorithm to localize the center and define the edges of short-axis SPECT slices.
AutoQuant[14,15]	Uniformly distributed 3D sampling of LV employing an ellipsoid model. Counts are averaged across the entire myocardial thickness. Integrated program for simultaneous assessment of perfusion (QPS) and function (QGS, using gated SPECT). Automated perfusion quantification, calculation of LVEF, volumes, lung–heart ratio, transient ischemic dilation ratio, regional wall thickening, wall motion. Standard normal databases, plus optional user-defined database generation.

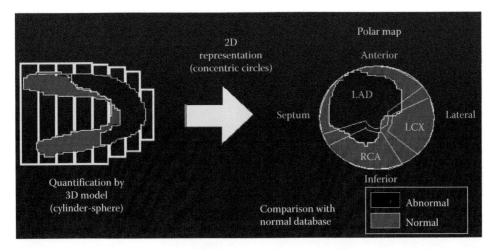

FIGURE 11.8
Polar map quantification. Tracer activity at the LV apex is depicted in the center. Count activities in the short-axis slices are displayed around the center as successive flat annular rings of increasing radii as the slices progress toward the base of the LV. In this diagram, the subject exhibits a large perfusion defect in the left anterior descending artery (LAD) territory that largely spares the left circumflex (LCX) and right coronary artery (RCA) territories.

defects to do this. The potential for failure of automated edge-detection programs exists, particularly in patients with extra-cardiac activity close to the heart or with large and severe defects such as those observed in LV aneurysms.

Most quantitative analyses display the tomographic slices in a polar map format. This provides a comprehensive representation of the extent, severity, and reversibility of regions of perfusion abnormality expressed as percentages of the entire LV, on a single compact 2D image. The individual patient's polar map perfusion can then be compared with a parametric reference polar map derived from disease-free normal patients, with low likelihood of CAD, and visually normal images (Figures 11.8 and 11.9). The criteria for abnormality are typically derived from the mean and standard deviation of the count uptake in each region of the LV. It is important to note that normal databases are usually specific to the scan protocol, gender, and tracer (thallium-201, technetium-99m sestamibi or tetrofosmin, the dual isotope) used. Acquisition and image processing parameters (filters) need also be specified.

11.2.4.4 Quantitative Assessment of Myocardial Viability from Perfusion SPECT

The likelihood of functional recovery subsequent to successful revascularization has been shown to be proportional to the amount of tracer uptake within each myocardial region. A cut off value of 50%–60% of maximal counts appears to best identify LV segments that will recover functionally following coronary revascularization.[22,23] Normal myocardial perfusion tracer uptake at rest or redistribution implies the presence of myocardial viability. Sublingual nitrate (which dilates the coronary vasculature, hence improving coronary flow) administered prior to rest tracer injection augments the detection of viable myocardium.[24] If a region has severely reduced or no uptake of radioactivity in these settings, then it is considered to be nonviable (Figure 11.7). Areas with moderate reduction of counts are usually partially viable, and patients in this group have a variable response in terms of recovery of myocardial contractile functional improvement after operation.

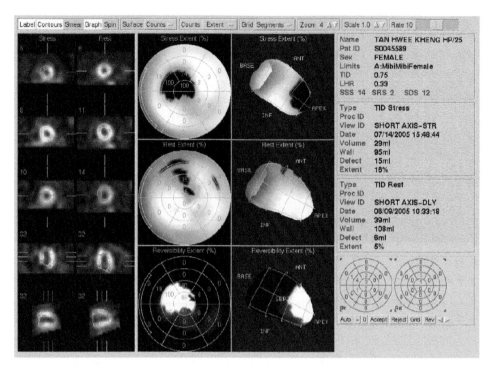

FIGURE 11.9

Quantitative myocardial perfusion assessment using AutoQuant (QPS) program. Algorithm-derived myocardial borders and segmentation are superimposed on reconstructed myocardial tomographic slices, facilitating visual check of the accuracy of myocardial border definition (left column). Stress and rest perfusion polar maps, as well as 3D displays, show a moderate-sized partially reversible defect at the apex, distal anterior, and anteroseptal walls (middle two columns). Calculated numerical data on perfusion defect size and severity are also depicted (right column). Automated quantitative regional perfusion scores at stress and rest (bottom right corner) yield sum stress score (SSS) 14, sum rest score (SRS) 2, and sum difference score (SDS) 12, implying significant ischemia (top right corner). The quantitative algorithm compares acquired perfusion data sets with normal databases that are gender, radionuclide, and protocol dependent.

Dichotomous classification of perfusion defects on thallium-201 imaging into reversible or nonreversible using qualitative assessment fails to detect many visually nonreversible defects that exhibit evidence of viability on PET imaging (considered the gold standard for viability assessment) or functional recovery after revascularization. However, when defects are quantitated, correlation between thallium-201 and PET imaging[25] improves substantially to about 80%; and agreement between thallium-201 and technetium-99m sestamibi imaging improves to 96%.[26] Thus, quantification of defect severity is highly recommended for the assessment of myocardial viability.

11.2.4.5 Assessment of LV Function from Gated Perfusion SPECT

LVEF assessment from gated perfusion SPECT (especially of technetium-99m tracer) can be achieved at very little additional cost. In general, gated perfusion SPECT measurements of LVEF are highly reproducible and correlate well with other imaging modalities.[19,27–34] However, in patients with small LV volumes (end-diastolic volume < 70 mL), the LV cavity may appear obliterated (especially at end-systole) due to the limited resolution of gamma camera systems.[35] This results in overestimation of LVEF.[36,37]

TABLE 11.3

Techniques for Automated Gated SPECT LV Function Assessment

Technique	Software function and components
Quantitative gated SPECT[29]	Automatic isolation and segmentation of the LV using an ellipsoid model. Extracted transmural count profiles are fitted to Gaussian curves and epicardial and endocardial surfaces calculated based on curve spread (Figure 11.10). Global and regional LV functional parameters are automatically determined.
St Luke's Roosevelt Hospital method[30]	Automatic determination of mid-myocardial borders by radial sampling and defined thresholds, using operator-selected bi-planar vertical and horizontal long-axis images. The endocardial surface is calculated by inward threshold searching and LV determined by Simpson's method. Computer count enhancement in severely hypoperfused myocardium assist in visualization of segmental wall motion.
Image inversion[31]	Digital inversion of long-axis images yields increased signal within the LV cavity and absent myocardial signal. A region-of-interest placed around the LV cavity is used to automatically generate time resolved regions-of-interest for each gating frame. LVEF is calculated from end-diastolic and -systolic counts.
Partial volume effect-based methods[32]	Besides tracer activity, object size also determine count levels (especially when object is less than twice the FWHM resolution of the image) through partial volume effects. LV wall thickening per se will cause changes in count recovery and wall brightness. Quantifying these count-based changes allows assessment of regional wall thickening and LVEF (assuming an ellipsoid LV with constant myocardial volume). This method makes no geometric assumptions and is not dependent on edge detection.

Gated SPECT acquisition may be performed at rest following either stress or rest radionuclide injections. In the former, there is potential for stress-induced ischemia to persist (myocardial stunning) causing abnormal wall motion and a reduction in measured LVEF. Indeed, the presence of post-stress regional wall motion abnormalities not present at rest is a specific indicator of severe coronary stenosis.[38]

As with the assessment of SPECT perfusion, a systematic approach to the assessment of ventricular function from the gated SPECT is recommended. This includes segmental wall motion, segmental wall thickening, and LVEF calculation. Segmental wall motion analysis may be visually assessed using a semiquantitative score: 0, normal; 1, mild hypokinesia; 2, moderate hypokinesia; 3, severe hypokinesia; 4, akinesia; and 5, dyskinesia. Similarly, segmental wall thickening evaluation is valuated using a 4-point score: 0, normal; 1, mild reduction; 2, moderate reduction; and 3, no detectable thickening. Assessment of regional wall motion by gated perfusion SPECT has been shown to correlate well with echocardiography and other noninvasive imaging modalities.[39-44] It adds value to perfusion imaging by increasing confidence in the interpretation of images, especially in differentiating attenuation artifact from infarct.[45-47]

Many automated and semiautomated computer programs have been developed that allow the measurement of LVEF using a variety of techniques (Table 11.3).[29-32] One advantage of quantification is that it may improve the reproducibility and objectivity of assessment (Figure 11.10). Heterogeneity of regional function in the normal heart has been demonstrated, necessitating region-specific normal limits.[48]

11.2.4.6 Accuracy of SPECT-Assessed LVEF in the Presence of Severe Perfusion Defect

Concerns have been raised about the accuracy of automated edge detection programs in the presence of severe or large perfusion defects, where the computer programs may

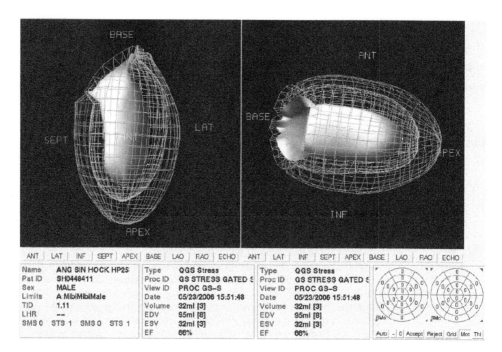

FIGURE 11.10

Quantitative wall motion assessment of gated perfusion SPECT using AutoQuant (QGS) program. The LV mid-myocardial surface is fitted to an ellipsoid using an iterative process. Transmural radionuclide count profiles with peaks at the mid-myocardial surface are fitted to asymmetric Gaussian curves whose standard deviations define the epicardial and endocardial surfaces. Calculating these surfaces for each gating interval, LV cavity and myocardial volumes can be estimated, and ejection fraction calculated. Note that these curve-fit volumes are in fact relative volumes and do not reflect authentic ventricular volumes. Nevertheless, the LVEF obtained is robust. Regional wall motion (endocardial surface displacement) and thickening are evaluated using modified centerline method, and count-based methods, respectively. Post-stress gated SPECT in this patient shows normal wall motion in all segments with sum motion score (SMS) of 0, and normal LVEF 66%.

have difficulty detecting the myocardial wall due to severe reduction in tracer uptake.[49] To investigate this, we prospectively measured LVEF using Quantitative Gated SPECT software (QGS, Cedars-Sinai) from rest-injected gated technetium-99m perfusion SPECT in a group of CAD patients, a majority of whom had prior myocardial infarction and compared the results to equilibrium radionuclide angiocardiography (ERNA) and echocardiography.

Gated SPECT LVEF has correlated well with ERNA (correlation coefficient: 0.94), even in subgroups of subjects with severe defects (>20%), prior infarction and large infarction, in whom the capability of an automated approach would be most severely tested. Further, we have demonstrated good agreement between gated SPECT and echocardiographic assessment of regional function. We can conclude that gated SPECT LVEF measurements are generally accurate and reliable, even in the presence of large defects.[50]

11.2.5 Clinical Applications of Quantitative Myocardial Perfusion SPECT

In general, quantification has previously not had a major impact on the diagnostic accuracy of perfusion SPECT, although the advent of more sophisticated computer programs is changing this. Indeed, interpretation of studies using polar map quantification alone without visual assessment of the tomographic slices is not advisable. Nevertheless, quantification provides a means of describing the extent and severity of perfusion abnormalities, and may call attention to subtle decreases in tracer uptake below the normal limits that might otherwise go unnoticed on visual inspection. In contrast, quantification has been an important factor in the success of gated perfusion SPECT because of its ability to provide reliable reproducible LVEF measurements.

Beyond the simple detection of CAD, nuclear cardiology has enormous value as a tool for risk-stratification and selection of patients for medical management or interventional therapy because of the large database of studies demonstrating its ability to prognosticate. Semiquantitative scoring systems of visually interpreted images, in particular, have been shown to be an effective method. The development of automated programs for obtaining semiquantitative perfusion scores may improve their reproducibility and reduce variability in interpretation between different laboratories. Berman et al. showed that the automatic scoring program (AutoQuant/QPS) has equivalent prognostic accuracy compared to expert visual assessment. Stress defects > 10% and reversibility > 5% of LV are associated with worse outcome.[51] Similarly, in patients undergoing risk stratification following myocardial infarction, stress perfusion defects and defect reversibility quantified by polar map programs appear to be correlated with prognosis.[52]

In addition to the widely accepted value of LVEF, volume measurements by gated SPECT have been shown to have prognostic value in a large study involving dual isotope rest thallium stress sestamibi gated SPECT. Sharir et al. showed that LVEF < 45%, end-diastolic volume > 120 mL, and end-systolic volume > 70 mL were associated with adverse prognosis.[53] The advent of quantitative gated SPECT has made automated measurement of volumes routinely feasible and highly reproducible. The ability of gated SPECT to provide additional information on LV function contributes further to the prognostic power of nuclear cardiology.

11.3 Computation of Intra-Myocardial Blood Flow Velocity and Pressure Patterns

11.3.1 Myocardial Perfusion

11.3.1.1 Perfusion Based on SPECT Imaging

MPI is a noninvasive method for assessing the regional myocardial flow, by means of radioactive tracers (thallium-201, technicium-99) injected intravenously. Ischemic areas, pertaining to little blood flow, do not take up these tracers. These tracers get trapped in the myocardium in proportion to the regional blood flow. This trapping allows external imaging, using gamma cameras to assess myocardial perfusion.

Myocardial perfusion provides added information about the hemodynamic viability of myocardial segments. Assessment of myocardial perfusion is performed using SPECT or PET. However, even though SPECT imaging is widely used, this method suffers from attenuation artifacts and also exposes the patient to radiation.

SPECT allows evaluation of perfusion patterns in thin slices of myocardium. Comparative studies of stress-to-rest images helps in differentiating ischemia from scar. A perfusion

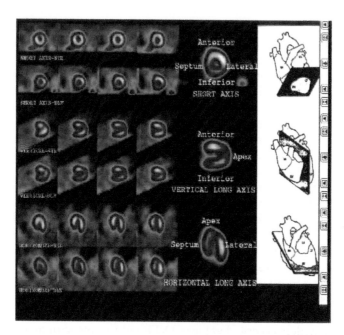

FIGURE 11.11
Perfusion pattern images of a 35-year-old man with a low probability of coronary artery disease.

abnormality present on both the stress and rest studies represents scar, while a perfusion abnormality that is present in stress study alone represents ischemia. The images shown in the following (in Figure 11.11) were obtained during exercise in a 35-year-old man, with a low probability of coronary disease.

Figure 11.11 describes a SPECT-computed 3D perfusion profile of the heart, containing serial slices of the LV in the short axis (beginning at the apex and ending at the base), vertical long axis (beginning at the septum and ending at the lateral wall), and horizontal long axes (beginning at the inferior wall and ending at the anterior wall). For each tomographic plane, the stress images are shown at the top followed by the rest images.

Figure 11.12 describes perfusion images obtained by SPECT of a 52-year-old patient, who suffers from 85% stenosis of the RCA. The stress images are the upper set of each pair of horizontal row of images, and the rest images are the corresponding lower set of each pair. The images reveal that the stress images are abnormal, while the rest images are normal. The stress images show severely reduced tracer uptake in the inferior wall of the heart, indicating the presence of a significant stenosis in the RCA. At rest, the tracer uptake is normal. This implies that there is a large potentially reversible perfusion defect of the inferior wall.

11.3.1.2 Computational Perfusion Analysis

In order to gain further insight into the intra-myocardial flow in the LV section, we have developed a biomechanics model of intra-myocardial blood flow through a porous myocardium medium, using a modified form of Darcy's law in which blood velocity is dependent on intra-myocardial pressure gradient (∇p), myocardial permeability (k) as well as myocardial stress-dependent hydrostatic pressure (H).

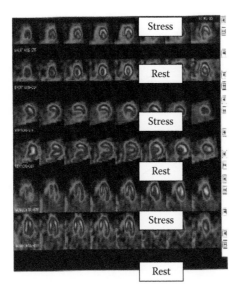

FIGURE 11.12
Perfusion images of a 52-year-old patient suffering from 85% stenosis of the right coronary artery. The abnormal stress images are shown.

The equation governing blood flow through the porous but stressed myocardium is Darcy Darcy's law,[54] for a porous media given by

$$V = -\frac{k}{\mu}(\nabla p - H)$$ (11.1)

where
V is the velocity of blood flow
k is the permeability of the tissue
μ is the dynamic viscosity of blood
p is the pressure
H is the hydrostatic pressure

The hydrostatic pressure is calculated by

$$H = \frac{1}{3}(\sigma_r + \sigma_\theta + \sigma_\phi)$$ (11.2)

and for a thick-walled spherical shell, we have[54,55]:

$$\sigma_\theta = \sigma_\phi = \frac{p(a^3/b^3 + a^3/2r^3)}{1 - a^3/b^3} \quad \text{and} \quad \sigma_r = \frac{p(a^3/b^3 - a^3/r^3)}{1 - a^3/b^3}$$ (11.3)

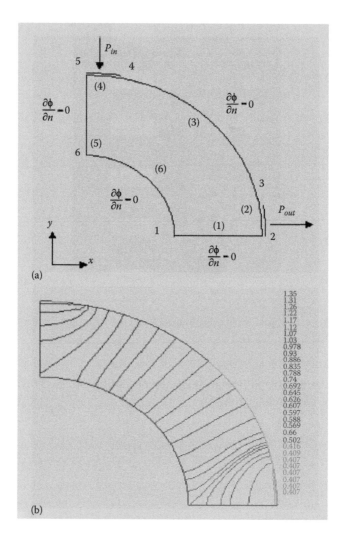

FIGURE 11.13
LV annular myocardial wall model (with inlet, P_{in} = 100 mmHg, and outlet, P_{out} = 30 mmHg, at a distance) (a), depicting pressure variation (kPa) inside the segment (b).

The intra-myocardial pressure is calculated analytically by solving the Laplace equation $\nabla^2 p = 0$, subject to input and output pressure conditions depicted in Figures 11.13 and 11.14. Thereafter, we determine the intra-myocardial blood flow velocity, using Equation 11.1.

In order to analyze this myocardial perfusion model, we first solve the Laplace equation $\nabla^2 p = 0$, to obtain the p variation in the LV myocardial sector. We then determine the H distribution for the LV, using Equation 11.2, corresponding to its geometry and the computed p distribution. Thereafter, we employ Equation 11.1 to compute the V distribution. The pressure and velocity distribution for specific cases in the sector of the LV are shown in Figures 11.13 and 11.14.

Now, if we wish to also simulate the SPECT data, we would need to vary the permeability parameter k according to the digitized SPECT images. Then for the patient, we would also need to know the inlet and outlet pressures for the sector. These data are difficult to obtain. On the other hand, if we primarily want to study and compare the perfusion

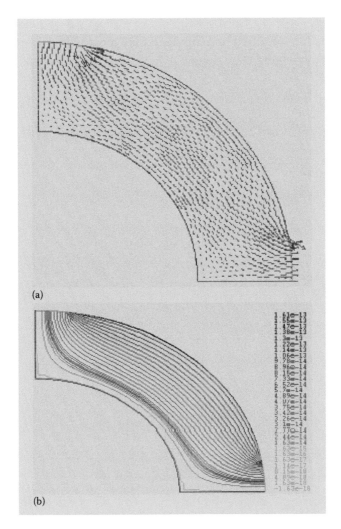

FIGURE 11.14
LV annular myocardial wall segment model having flow configuration and conditions as in Figure 11.13 (a) velocity (maximum vector of 0.9 m/s), (b) streamlines, 0 for the case of Figure 11.13a.

flow patterns in the LV myocardial sectors (to understand how intra-myocardial stress also affects intra-myocardial perfusion), then we can adopt (1) P_{in} (inlet pressure at the sector) to be equal to the mean LV pressure and (2) P_{out} (the exit pressure at the sector) to be equal to the right atrial pressure. Thereby, we can employ catheterized LV pressures along with SPECT data to obtain the detailed V distribution profiles in the various sectors.

On the other hand, if we intend to noninvasively evaluate the intra-myocardial flow distributions, we can adopt P_{in} (= mean ausculatory pressure) and P_{out} (= zero), LV filling pressure = 10 mmHg. The steps to elucidate the SPECT data with complimentary intra-myocardial perfusion profiles entail (1) determining P_{in} (= mean ausculatory pressure); (2) from LV geometry for the sector, to solve $\nabla^2 p = 0$, to obtain p distribution in the sector corresponding to P_{in}; (3) compute H variation corresponding to the LV filling pressure; (4) solve Equation 11.1 to obtain the velocity distribution.

11.3.1.2.1 *Theory and Governing Equations*

The governing equations required to compute intra-myocardial pressure and velocity distributions are given as follows[55,56]:

Continuity equation:

$$\nabla \cdot (\phi_s \vec{u}_s + \phi_f \vec{u}_f) = 0 \tag{11.4}$$

$$\phi_s + \phi_f = 1 \tag{11.5}$$

Momentum equations:

$$\nabla \cdot \sigma_s + \vec{b}_s = 0 \tag{11.6}$$

$$\nabla \cdot \sigma_f + \vec{b}_f = 0 \tag{11.7}$$

Constitutive equations:

$$\sigma_s = -\phi_s p\mathbf{I} + \tilde{\sigma}_s \tag{11.8}$$

$$\sigma_f = -\phi_f p\mathbf{I} \tag{11.9}$$

Effective solid stress:

$$\tilde{\sigma}_s = B_s tr(\mathbf{T}_s)\mathbf{I} + 2\mu_s \mathbf{e}_s \tag{11.10}$$

Darcy's law:

$$\vec{b}_s - \vec{b}_f = \frac{\mu_f}{\kappa}(\phi_f \vec{u}_f - \phi_s \vec{u}_s) \tag{11.11}$$

where
  subscripts s and f refer to the incompressible, elastic solid phase and incompressible, viscous fluid (blood) phases, respectively
  ∇ is the gradient operator
  ϕ is the volumetric concentration
  $\vec{u}$ is the velocity vector of solid
  σ is the partial stress
  $\vec{b}$ is the diffusive body force vector
  p is the hydrostatic pressure
  $\mathbf{I}$ is the identity tensor
  $\tilde{\sigma}_s$ is the effective solid stress tensor
  B_s is the elastic bulk modulus
  $tr(\cdot)$ is the trace operator that yields first invariant of its tensorial argument
  $\mathbf{T}_s$ is the solid strain tensor
  μ_s is the elastic shear modulus
  $\mathbf{e}_s = \mathbf{T}_s - (1/3)tr(\mathbf{T}_s)\mathbf{I}$ is the deviatoric component of solid strain tensor
  μ_f is the fluid dynamic viscosity
  κ is the permeability

In our situation, we assume that $\phi_f \gg \phi_s$ (i.e., $\phi_f \to 1$, $\phi_s \to 0$). Equations 11.3 through 11.11 may be rewritten as

Continuity equation:

$$\nabla \cdot \vec{u}_f = 0 \tag{11.12}$$

Momentum equations:

$$\nabla \cdot \sigma_s + \vec{b}_s = 0 \tag{11.13}$$

$$\nabla \cdot \sigma_f + \vec{b}_f = 0 \tag{11.14}$$

Constitutive equations:

$$\sigma_s = \tilde{\sigma}_s \tag{11.15}$$

$$\sigma_f = -p\mathbf{I} \tag{11.16}$$

Effective solid stress:

$$\tilde{\sigma}_s = B_s \mathrm{tr}(\mathbf{T}_s)\mathbf{I} + 2\mu_s e_s \tag{11.17}$$

Darcy's law:

$$\vec{u}_f = \frac{\kappa}{\mu_f}(\vec{b}_s - \vec{b}_f) \tag{11.18}$$

Inserting Equations 11.13 through 11.16 into Equation 11.18, Darcy's law becomes

$$\vec{u}_f = -\frac{\kappa}{\mu_f}(\nabla p - \vec{b}_s) \tag{11.19}$$

or

$$\vec{u}_f = -\frac{\kappa}{\mu_f}(\nabla p + \nabla \cdot \tilde{\sigma}_s) \tag{11.20}$$

In Equation 11.19, since the body force $\vec{b}_s$ is a field force ($\nabla \times \vec{b}_s = 0$ in Equation 11.13), $\vec{b}_s$ can be rewritten as $\vec{b}_s = \rho_f \nabla \Omega$, where ρ_f is the fluid density and W is the potential.

In Equation 11.20, if we can put $H = -\nabla \cdot \tilde{\sigma}$ for the ideal myocardium perfusion modeling case with a thick-walled spherical shell, Equations 11.1 through 11.3 are recovered.

The set of equations given earlier enable us to analyze the behavior of (1) the incompressible, elastic solid phase and (2) the incompressible, viscous fluid phase. For the analysis,[57] the bulk blood velocity is given by Darcy's law, under the assumption that the pores are small and interconnected.

$$V = -\frac{\kappa}{\mu}(\nabla p - \rho \nabla \Omega) \tag{11.21}$$

where Ω-potential for body forces b_i;

$$b_i = \rho \frac{\partial \Omega}{\partial x_i} \tag{11.22}$$

Rewriting V gives,

$$V = -\frac{\kappa}{\mu} \rho g \left[\nabla \left(\frac{p}{\rho g} \right) - \frac{1}{g} \nabla \Omega \right] = -\frac{\kappa \rho g}{\mu} \nabla \phi \tag{11.23}$$

The pressure-head is given as

$$\phi = \frac{p}{\rho g} - \frac{\Omega}{g} \tag{11.24}$$

Darcy's law is generally expressed in terms of hydraulic conductivity

$$C = \frac{\kappa \rho g}{\mu} \tag{11.25}$$

which gives (from Equations 11.13 through 11.15)

$$V_i = -C \frac{\partial \phi}{\partial x_i} \tag{11.26}$$

For an incompressible blood, $\nabla \cdot V = 0$, and the pressure-head ϕ satisfies

$$\nabla \cdot (C \nabla \phi) = 0 \tag{11.27}$$

For an anisotropic medium,

$$V_i = -C_{ij} \frac{\partial \phi}{\partial x_j} \tag{11.28}$$

For this analysis, the last estimated value for V_i gives the velocity. Table 11.4 summarizes the parameters used for the perfusion analysis of the myocardial tissue.[57]

Figure 11.13a shows the annular model and numbering of boundary conditions (BCs) with inlet and outlet at a distance. Figure 11.13b shows the computed pressure distribution.

TABLE 11.4

Parameters Used for Analysis of Myocardium Tissue

Parameter description	Value
Density (ρ)	1000 kg/m³
Acceleration due to gravity (g)	9.81 m/s²
Dynamic viscosity (μ)	0.00015 N s/m
Permeability (k)	1×10^{-15} m²
LV wall thickness (t)	10 mm
Mean inlet pressure (P_{in})	100.0 mmHg (13.3 kPa)
Mean outlet pressure (P_{out})	30.0 mmHg (3.9 kPa)
Mean LV chamber pressure (P_1)	10.0 mmHg (1.3 kPa)

Source: Ghista, D.N. et al., Augmented myocardial perfusion by coronary bypass surgical procedure: Emphasising flow and shear stress analysis at proximal and distal anastomotic sites providing the basis of better graft patency rates, in: Ghista, D.N. and Ng, E.Y.-K., eds., *Cardiac Perfusion and Pumping*, World Scientific, 2006.

A typical flowchart of computing the streamlines, pressure, and velocity distributions is highlighted in Figure 11.15. Figure 11.14 depicts the velocity distribution and streamline pattern. In general, the axial flow is dominant in the periphery, but the normal flow is significant in the location near inlet and outlet due to the pressure variation effect at entry/exit. The pressure is uniform in the middle range, but nonuniform near inlet and outlet,

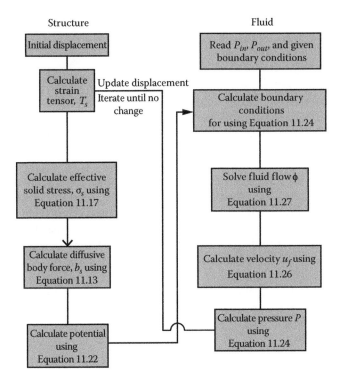

FIGURE 11.15
A typical flowchart of poroelastic fluid–structure analysis.

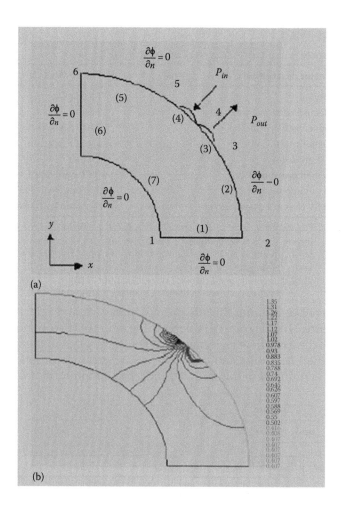

FIGURE 11.16
LV annular myocardial model (with inlet, P_{in} = 100 mmHg, and outlet, P_{out} = 30 mmHg, adjacent to each other) (a), depicting pressure variation (kPa) inside the segment (b).

which is consistent with the velocity vector plots. A typical flow chart of computing the streamlines, pressure, and velocity distributions is highlighted in Figure 11.15.

The geometry and numbering of BCs for case with inlet adjacent to the outlet are included in Figure 11.16a. Figure 11.16b shows the pressure distribution. Figure 11.17a shows the associated velocity distribution, and Figure 11.17b gives the velocity streamline plot. The pressure is uniform far away from the entry/exit region, but nonuniform near inlet and outlet, which is consistent with the velocity vector plots.

This intra-myocardial analysis and the results in Figures 11.13, 11.14, 11.16, and 11.17 can provide some insight into how perfusion occurs in the different segments of the myocardium.

11.3.2 Myocardial Reperfusion Using Coronary Bypass Surgery

It is obvious from the previous illustrations in Section 11.2.3 that there is very less amount of blood flow in some ischemic and infarcted areas of the myocardium, which suggests the severity of stenosis present in the corresponding regional coronary vessels.

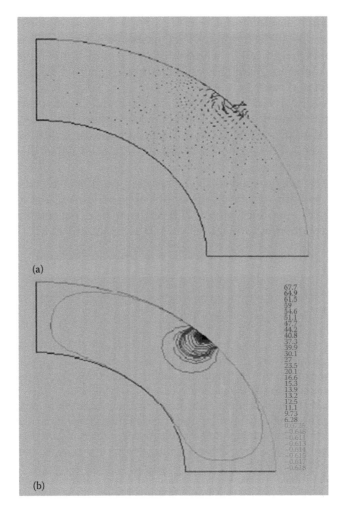

FIGURE 11.17
LV annular myocardial model having flow configuration and conditions as in Figure 11.16, (a) velocity pattern (with maximum vector of 0.88 m/s) and (b) streamlines, for the case of Figure 11.16a.

To overcome this defect, CABG surgery can be performed. The aim of CABG is thus to increase blood flow to malperfused myocardium that results in maximal perfusion through the bypass conduits. The details of this topic can be found in Sections 12.2 and 12.4 of Reference[58].

11.4 Conclusion

In Section 11.2, we have elaborated myocardial perfusion methodology for SPECT imaging and detecting ischemia regions, based on myocardial radionuclide maps. One of the major advantages that nuclear cardiology has over other imaging modalities is the ease by which nuclear cardiac data can be quantified and analyzed. In principle, quantification especially when coupled with automation of computer processing offers the potential to reduce or eliminate the subjectivity of visual assessment and to increase the reproducibility of evaluation. Quantification is also required to allow for comparison of perfusion data with a normal database thereby assisting in the detection of disease and the objective assessment of extent and severity.

In patients with CAD, the presence and extent of inducible myocardial ischemia, the extent of myocardial infarction, and LV function are among the most powerful predictors of subsequent cardiac events. These powerful prognostic indicators are provided by nuclear cardiac studies and their value is greatly enhanced when they are provided in objective, quantitative terms.

In Section 11.3, we have displayed LV myocardial perfusion results based on SPECT imaging, for patients with coronary arterial disease, in Figures 11.11 and 11.12, we have then substantiated and quantified myocardial perfusion in terms of intra-myocardial pressure and velocity distributions, in Figures 11.13, 11.14, 11.16, and 11.17.

References

1. H. F. Weich, H. W. Strauss, and B. Pitt, The extraction of thallium-201 by the myocardium, *Circulation* **56** (1977) 188–191.
2. P. Kailasnath and A. J. Sinusas, Technetium-99 m-labeled myocardial perfusion agents: Are they better than thallium-201? *Cardiology Review* **9** (2001) 160–172.
3. D. S. Berman, H. Kiat, J. D. Friedman et al., Separate acquisition rest thallium-201/stress technetium-99 m sestamibi dual-isotope myocardial perfusion single-photon emission computed tomography: A clinical validation study, *Journal of American College of Cardiology* **22** (1993) 1455–1464.
4. R. A. Brooks, and G. D. Chiro, Theory of image reconstruction in computed tomography, *Radiology* **117** (1975) 561–572.
5. D. J. Fintel, J. M. Links, J. A. Brinker, T. L. Frank, M. Parker, and L. C. Becker, Improved diagnostic performance of exercise thallium-201 single photon emission computed tomography over planar imaging in the diagnosis of coronary artery disease: A receiver operating characteristic analysis, *Journal of American College of Cardiology* **13** (1989) 600–612.
6. N. Tamaki, Y. Yonekura, T. Mukai, S. Kodama, K. Kadota, H. Kambara C. Kawai, and K. Torizuka, Stress thallium-201 transaxial emission tomography: Quantitative versus qualitative analysis for evaluation of coronary artery disease, *Journal of American College of Cardiology* **4** (1984) 1213–1221.
7. E. V. Garcia, K. Van Train, J. Maddahi et al., Quantification of rotational thallium-201 myocardial tomography, *Journal of Nuclear Medicine* **26** (1985) 17–26.
8. J. Maddahi, K. Van Train, F. Prigent, E. V. Garcia, J. Friedman, E. Ostrezega, and D. Berman, Quantitative single photon emission computed tomography for detection and localization of coronary artery disease: Optimization and prospective validation of a new technique, *Journal of American College of Cardiology* **14** (1989) 1689–1699.
9. K. F. Van Train, J. Maddahi, D. S. Berman et al., Quantitative analysis of tomographic stress thallium-201 myocardial scintigrams: A multicenter trial, *Journal of Nuclear Medicine* **31** (1990) 1168–1179.
10. E. DePasquale, A. Nody, G. DePuey et al., Quantitative rotational thallium-201 tomography for identifying and localizing coronary artery disease, *Circulation* **72** (1988) 316–327.
11. J. J. Mahmarian, T. M. Boyce, R. K. Goldberg, M. K. Cocanougher, R. Roberts, and M. S. Verani, Quantitative exercise thallium-201 single photon emission computed tomography for the enhanced diagnosis of ischemic heart disease, *Journal of American College of Cardiology* **15** (1990) 318–329.

12. S. Borges-Neto, J. J. Mahmarian, A. Jain et al., Quantitative thallium-201 single-photon emission computed tomography after oral dipyridamole for assessing the presence, anatomic location and severity of coronary artery disease, *Journal of American College of Cardiology* **11** (1988) 962.

13. A. S. Iskandrian, J. Heo, B. Kong et al., Effect of exercise level on the ability of thallium-201 tomographic imaging in detecting coronary artery disease: Analysis of 461 patients, *Journal of American College of Cardiology* **14** (1989) 1477.

14. G. Germano, P. B. Kavanagh, P. B. Waechter, J. S. Areeda, J. Gerlach, S. Van Kriekinge, T. Sharir, H. C. Lewin, and D. S. Berman, A new algorithm for the quantitation of myocardial perfusion SPECT. I. Technical principles and reproducibility, *Journal of Nuclear Medicine* **41** (2000) 720–727.

15. T. Sharir, G. Germano, P. B. Waechter, P. B. Kavanagh, J. S. Areeda, J. Gerlach, X. Kang, H. C. Lewin, and D. S. Berman, A new algorithm for the quantitation of myocardial perfusion SPECT. II. Validation and diagnostic yield, *Journal of Nuclear Medicine* **41** (2000) 720–727.

16. A. Rozanski, G. A. Diamond, D. S. Berman et al., The declining specificity of exercise radionuclide ventriculography, *New England Journal of Medicine* **309** (1983) 518.

17. K. F. Van Train, J. Areeda, E. V. Garcia et al., Quantitative same-day rest-stress technetium-99 m sestamibi SPECT: Definition and validation of stress normal limits and criteria for abnormality, *Journals of Nuclear Medicine* **34** (1993) 1494–1502.

18. P. J. Slomka, G. A. Hurwitz, J. Stephenson et al., Automated alignment and sizing of myocardial stress and rest scans to three-dimensional normal templates using an image registration algorithm, *Journal of Nuclear Medicine* **36** (1995) 1115–1122.

19. T. L. Faber, S. D. Cooke, R. D. Folks, J. Vansant, K. J. Nichols, and E. G. DePuey, Left ventricular function and perfusion from gated SPECT perfusion images: An integrated method, *Journal of Nuclear Medicine* **40** (1999) 650–659.

20. Y. H. Liu, A. J. Sinusas, P. DeMan, B. L. Zaret, and F. J. Wackers, Quantification of SPECT myocardial perfusion images: Methodology and validation of the Yale-CQ method, *Journal of Nuclear Cardiology* **6** (1999) 190–204.

21. S. Kirac, F. J. Wackers, and Y. H. Liu, Validation of the Yale circumferential quantification method using ^{201}Tl and ^{99}mTc: A phantom study, *Journal of Nuclear Medicine* **41**(8) (2000) 1436–1441.

22. J. E. Udelson, P. S. Coleman, J. Metherall et al., Predicting recovery of severe regional ventricular dysfunction: Comparison of resting scintigraphy with ^{201}Tl and ^{99}mTc-sestamibi, *Circulation* **89** (1994) 2552–2561.

23. G. J. Kauffman, T. S. Boyne, D. D. Watson, W. H. Smith, and G. A. Beller, Comparison of rest thallium-201 imaging and rest technetium-99m sestamibi imaging for assessment of myocardial viability in patients with coronary artery disease and severe left ventricular dysfunction, *Journal of American College of Cardiology* **27** (1996) 1592–1597.

24. R. Sciagra, G. Bisi, G. M. Santoro et al., Comparison of baseline technetium-99m sestamibi with rest-redistribution thallium-201 tomography in detecting viable hibernating myocardium and predicting post-revascularization recovery, *Journal of American College of Cardiology* **30** (1997) 384–391.

25. R. O. Bonow, V. Dilsizian, A. Cuocolo, and S. L. Bacharach, Identification of viable myocardium in patients with chronic coronary artery disease and left ventricular dysfunction. Comparison of thallium scintigraphy with reinjection and PET imaging with ^{18}fluorodeoxyglucose, *Circulation* **83** (1991) 26–37.

26. V. Dilsizian, J. A. Arrighi, J. G. Diodati et al., Myocardial viability in patients with chronic coronary artery disease. Comparison of ^{99}mTc-sestamibi with thallium reinjection and ^{18}fluorodeoxyglucose, *Circulation* **89** (1994) 578.

27. T. L. Faber, M. S. Akers, R. M. Peshock, and J. R. Corbett, Three-dimensional motion and perfusion quantification in gated single photon emission computed tomograms, *Journal of Nuclear Medicine* **32** (1991) 2311–2317.

28. E. G. DePuey, K. Nichols, and C. Dobrinsky, Left ventricular ejection fraction assessment from gated technetium-99m sestamibi SPECT, *Journal of Nuclear Medicine* **34** (1993) 1871–1876.

29. G. Germano, H. Kiat, P. B. Kavanagh et al., Automatic quantification of ejection fraction from gated sestamibi SPECT, *Journal of Nuclear Medicine* **36** (1995) 2138–2147.

30. K. Nichols, E. G. DePuey, and A. Rozanski, Automation of gated tomographic left ventricular ejection fraction, *Journal of Nuclear of Cardiology* **3** (1996) 475–482.

31. K. A. Williams and L. A. Taillon, Left ventricular function in patients with coronary artery disease assessed by gated tomographic myocardial perfusion images. Comparison with assessment by contrast ventriculography and first-pass radionuclide angiography, *Journal of American College of Cardiology* **27**(1) (1996) 173–181.

32. W. H. Smith, R. J. Kaster, D. A. Calnon, D. Segalla, G. A. Beller, and D. D. Watson, Quantitative gated single photon emission computed tomography imaging: A counts-based method for display and measurement of regional and global ventricular systolic function, *Journal of Nuclear Cardiology* **4** (1997) 451–463.

33. D. A. Calnon, R. J. Kastner, W. H. Smith, D. L. Segalla, G. A. Beller, and D. D. Watson, Validation of a new counts-based gated SPECT method for quantifying left ventricular systolic function: Comparison with equilibrium radionuclide angiography, *Journal of Nuclear Cardiology* **4** (1997) 464–471.

34. M. Y. Shen, Y. H. Liu, A. J. Sinusas, R. Fetterman, W. Bruni, O. E. Drozhinin, B. L. Zaret, and F. J. Wackers, Quantification of regional myocardial wall thickening on electrocardiogram-gated SPECT imaging, *Journal of Nuclear Cardiology* **6**(6) (1999) 583–595.

35. E. Vallejo, D. P. Dione, W. L. Bruni, R. T. Constable, P. P. Borek, J. P. Soares, J. G. Carr, S. G. Condos, F. J. Wackers, and A. J. Sinusas, Reproducibility and accuracy of gated SPECT for determination of left ventricular volumes and ejection fraction: Experimental validation using MRI, *Journal of Nuclear Medicine* **41** (2000) 874–882.

36. K. Nakajima, T. Higuchi, J. Taki, M. Kawano, and N. Tonami, Accuracy of ventricular volume and ejection fraction measurement by gated myocardial SPECT: Comparison of 4 software programs, *Journal of Nuclear Medicine* **42** (2001) 1571–1578.

37. P. V. Ford, S. N. Chatziioannou, W. H. Moore, and R. D. Dhekne, Overestimation of the LVEF by quantitative gated SPECT in simulated left ventricles, *Journal of Nuclear Medicine* **42** (2001) 454–459.

38. T. Sharir, C. Bacher-Stier, S. Dhar, H. C. Lewin, R. Miranda, J. D. Friedman, G. Germano, and D. S. Berman, Identification of severe and extensive coronary artery disease by postexercise regional wall motion abnormalities in Tc-99m sestamibi gated SPECT, *American Journal of Cardiology* **86** (2000) 1171–1175.

39. T. Chua, H. Kiat, G. Germano, M. Maurer, K. Van Train, J. Friedman, and D. Berman, Gated technetium-99m sestamibi for simultaneous assessment of stress myocardial perfusion, postexercise regional ventricular function and myocardial viability. Correlation with echocardiography and rest thallium-201 scintigraphy, *Journal of American College of Cardiology* **23** (1994) 1107–1114.

40. C. Anagnostopoulos, M. G. Gunning, D. J. Pennell, R. Laney, H. Proukakis, and S. R. Underwood, Regional myocardial motion and thickening assessed at rest by ECG-gated Tc-99m-MIBI emission tomography and by magnetic resonance imaging, *European Journal of Nuclear Medicine* **23** (1996) 909–1016.

41. M. G. Gunning, C. Anagnostopoulos, G. Davies, S. M. Forbat, P. J. Ell, and S. R. Underwood, Gated technetium-99m tetrofosmin SPECT and cine MRI to assess left ventricular contraction, *Journal of Nuclear Medicine* **38** (1997) 438–442.

42. J. C. Stollfuss, F. Haas, I. Matsunari, J. Neverve, S. Nekolla, J. Schneider, U. Schricke, S. Ziegler, and M. Schwaiger, Regional myocardial wall thickening and global ejection fraction in patients with low angiographic left ventricular ejection fraction assessed by visual and quantitative resting ECG-gated ^{99m}Tc-tetrofosmin single-photon emission tomography and magnetic resonance imaging, *European Journal of Nuclear Medicine* **25**(5) (1998) 522–530.

43. K. Nichols, E. G. DePuey, A. Rozanski, H. Salensky, and M. I. Friedman, Image enhancement of severely hypoperfused myocardia for computation of tomographic ejection fraction, *Journal of Nuclear Medicine* **38**(9) (1997) 1411–1417.

44. K. Nichols, E. G. DePuey, N. Krasnow, D. Lefkowitz, and A. Rozanski, Reliability of enhanced gated SPECT in assessing wall motion of severely hypoperfused myocardium: An echocardiograpic validation, *Journal of Nuclear Cardiology* 5 (1998) 387–394.
45. E. G. DePuey and A. Rozanski, Using technetium-99 m sestamibi SPECT to characterize fixed perfusion defects as infarct or artifact, *Journal of Nuclear Medicine* 36 (1995) 952–955.
46. R. Taillefer, E. G. DePuey, J. E. Udelson, G. A. Beller, Y. Latour, and F. Reeves, Comparative diagnostic accuracy of Tl-201 and Tc-99 m sestamibi SPECT imaging (perfusion and ECG-gated SPECT) in detecting coronary artery disease in women, *Journal of American College of Cardiology* 29 (1997) 69–77.
47. P. E. Smanio, D. D. Watson, D. L. Segalla, E. L. Vinson, W. H. Smith, and G. A. Beller, Value of gating of technetium-99 m sestamibi single photon emission computed tomographic imaging, *Journal of American College of Cardiology* 30 (1997) 1687–1692.
48. T. Sharir, D. S. Berman, P. B. Waehter, J. Areeda, P. B. Kavanaugh, J. Gerlach, X. Kang, and G. Germano, Quantitative analysis of regional motion and thickening by gated myocardial perfusion SPECT: Normal heterogeneity and criteria for abnormality, *Journal of Nuclear Medicine* 42 (2001) 1630–1638.
49. A. Manrique, M. Faraggi, P. Vera, D. Vilain, R. Lebtahi, A. Cribier, and D. Guludec, ^{201}Tl and ^{99m}Tc-MIBI gated SPECT in patients with large perfusion defects and left ventricular dysfunction: Comparison with equilibrium radionuclide angiography, *Journal of Nuclear Medicine* 40 (1999) 805–809.
50. T. Chua, C. Y. Lee, H. T. Tan, B. C. Tai, Z. P. Ding, and Y. L. Lim, Accuracy of automated assessment of left ventricular function using gated perfusion SPECT in the presence of perfusion defects and left ventricular dysfunction: Correlation with equilibrium radionuclide ventriculography and echocardiography, *Journal of Nuclear Cardiology* 7 (2000) 301–311.
51. D. S. Berman, X. Kang, K. F. Van Train et al., Comparative prognostic value of automatic quantitative analysis *vs* semiquantitative visual analysis of exercise myocardial perfusion SPECT, *Journal of American College of Cardiology* 32 (1998) 1987–1995.
52. H. A. Dakik, N. S. Kleinman, J. A. Farmer, Z. X. Wendt, C. M. Pratt, M. S. Verani, and J. J. Mahmarian, Intensive medical therapy versus coronary angioplasty for suppression of myocardial ischemia in survivors of acute myocardial infarction: A prospective, randomized pilot study, *Circulation* 10 (1998) 2017–2023.
53. T. Sharir, G. Germano, X. Kang, H. C. Lewin, R. Miranda, I. Cohen, R. D. Agafitei, J. D. Friedman, and D. S. Berman, Prediction of myocardial infarction versus cardiac death by gated myocardial perfusion SPECT: Risk stratification by the amount of stress-induced ischemia and the post-stress ejection fraction, *Journal of Nuclear Medicine* 42 (2001) 831–837.
54. C. R. Jegathese, E. Y.-K. Ng, and D. N. Ghista, Analysis of left ventricular myocardial properties, *Journal of Mechanics in Medicine and Biology* 4 (2004) 173–185.
55. E. Y.-K. Ng, D. N. Ghista, and C. R. Jegathese, Numerical approach to fluid-structure analysis of soft biological tissue, *Selected Paper from ICMMB-13, Journal of Mechanics in Medicine and Biology* 5 (2005) 11–28.
56. E. Y.-K. Ng, C. R. Jegathese, and D. N. Ghista, Perfusion studies of steady flow in poroelastic myocardium tissue, *International Journal of Computer Methods in Biomechanics and Biomedical Engineering* 8 (2005) 349–358.
57. D. N. Ghista, S. Meena, L. P. Chua, and Y. S. Tan, Augmented myocardial perfusion by coronary bypass surgical procedure: Emphasising flow and shear stress analysis at proximal and distal anastomotic sites providing the basis of better graft patency rates, Chapter 12, in: *Cardiac Perfusion and Pumping*, D.N. Ghista and E.Y.-K. Ng, World Scientific, 2006.
58. D.N. Ghista and F. Kabinejadian, Coronary artery bypass grafting anastomoses' hemodynamics and designs: A biomedical engineering review, *Biomedical Engineering Online*, 2013.

12

Arterial Pulse Wave Propagation Analysis: Determination of Pulse Wave Velocity and Arterial Properties

Dhanjoo N. Ghista and Foad Kabinejadian

CONTENTS

12.1 Introduction

In the circulatory system, the pulse wave travels along with the energy exchanged between the flowing blood and the elastic vessel walls. In the aorta, the pressure increases with left ventricular ejection, and blood flows through it, as it dilates and relaxes (or contracts). In situations associated with arterial stiffening (i.e., arteriosclerosis), the speed of the pulse wave increases [1], because the energy of the blood pressure pulse cannot be stored in a stiffer arterial wall. Hence, the state of the vessel can be described by the pulse wave velocity (PWV) [2], and PWV can be utilized as an index of arterial distensibility [3].

Arterial PWV describes how fast a blood pressure pulse travels from one point to another in an artery. The time difference between these two locations is known as the pulse transit time (PTT). PWV, by definition, is the distance traveled (Δx) by the wave divided by the time (Δt) for the wave to travel that distance: PWV = $\Delta x/\Delta t$. For accurate measurement of PWV (with minimal interference of the incident pressure wave by the reflected pressure wave), PWV can be measured between two sites a known distance apart, using the pressure "foot" of the waveform to calculate the transit time. In the aorta, PWV is typically measured between the carotid and femoral arteries [4]. Typically, the pulse wave is detected by pressure transducers or arterial tonometry. These methods are highly reliable but have the disadvantages of requiring specific devices and software for recording good pulse waves. These disadvantages are overcome if we take the carotid-femoral PWV measurement by ultrasound, making the assumption that real pulse wave corresponds to the flow wave of spectral Doppler.

Based on the formula of PWV $= c = (Eh/2a\rho)^{1/2}$, which we derive in this chapter, PWV is proportional to the square root of (1) the incremental elastic modulus (E) of the arterial wall, and (2) the ratio of wall thickness (h) to vessel radius (a) and blood density (ρ). Hence, PWV is a measure of arterial stiffness and an indicator for arteriosclerosis.

Arteriosclerosis, coming from the Greek for "hardening of the arteries," refers to several diseases in which the arterial wall thickens and loses its elasticity. Arteriosclerosis may be present in any artery of the body, but the disease is most concerning when it attacks the coronary arteries and threatens to cause a heart attack. The most common type of arteriosclerosis, atherosclerosis, is caused by plaque (made up of fat, cholesterol, calcium, and other substances found in the blood) building up in the vessel, resulting in arterial wall thickening and narrowing of the arterial lumen [1,5].

Arterial stiffness is now recognized as a major driver of cardiovascular disease. An increase in arterial stiffness elevates central systolic and pulse pressure, as well as left ventricular afterload and decreases coronary artery perfusion pressure. These effects increase the risk of stroke, heart failure, and myocardial infarction [6,7]. In recent years, a number of papers have been published on the diagnosis of cardiovascular diseases and mortality risk prediction using PWV [8–12].

PWV is a well-established technique for measuring the arterial stiffness parameters (because PWV is a function of the arterial wall elastic modulus), at the carotid and femoral artery sites as well as in the aorta, where it is convenient to monitor the arterial cross-sectional changes as the pulse wave propagates past an arterial cross section [13–17].

There are two types of arterial stiffness properties, in terms of (1) the arterial wall stress–strain relationship or the elastic modulus (E) as a function of arterial wall stress (σ) and (2) arterial impedance z, the ratio of the amplitudes of the pressure and flow-rate pulses, representing the incremental pressure pulse response to the incremental flow-rate pulse. This chapter presents (1) the mathematical derivation of the PWV and (2) the analytical basis for determining arterial elasticity parameters from PWV.

A pressure or flow waveform consists of forward and backward (or reflected) waves. In the aorta, the forward pressure and flow waveform comes from the heart, and the reflected wave comes from various locations in the arterial system (such as from bifurcations). The pulsatile pressure and flow can thus be viewed as the sum of forward and reflected pulse wave fronts. The relationship between blood pressure and wave reflections has long been investigated, both theoretically and experimentally [13,18–22]. Traditionally, reflection is believed to increase pressure (depending on its phase relative to the forward propagating wave) and may cause hypertension. Hence, investigators have suggested that reducing reflection should be a clinical goal for the reducing systolic hypertension [23,24]. However, based on Berger and his colleagues' work, depending on the phase difference between the forward propagating and reflected waves, reflection can even decrease stroke work and mean arterial pressure [25–27]. In this chapter, we have also provided the concept of impedance and pressure wave reflection coefficient. Based on that, we have analyzed what occurs at an arterial bifurcation. We have shown that the reflected wave can be either in phase or out of phase with the incident wave, and hence either enhance or decrease the afterload on the left ventricle. Finally, we present noninvasive methods of measurement of PWV.*

12.2 Analysis for Pulse Wave Propagation Velocity Expression

In this section, we present the analysis for expressing the PWV in terms of the arterial elastic properties and its geometrical dimensions. We will then present the manner in which the derived expression for PWV can be employed in conjunction with in vivo measurements (of PWV and arterial diameters) to obtain the values of the arterial elasticity parameters.

Figure 12.1 illustrates the arterial pressure profile, the arterial wall displacement, and the intra-arterial flow-velocity profile due to the propagating pressure (and volume) pulse wave.

Let us consider an infinitely long, isolated, circular, cylindrical, elastic vessel containing blood, as an incompressible invicid liquid. When this tube is disturbed at one place by a presure pulse entering it, the disturbance will be propagated as a wave along the tube at a finite speed. The derivation of PWV will involve (1) governing equations of fluid flow, (2) governing equations of the arterial wall motion, (3) macthing of fluid velocity at the wall with the wall motion, and (4) integrated fluid–solid interaction equation and its solution.

Figure 12.2 illustrates a segment of the artery of radius a and length dx, affected by the pressure pulse and resulting in wall displacement η. The average velocity of the fluid at the entrance is denoted by $\bar{u}$ and at the exit is $\bar{u} + d\bar{u}$.

In general, in response to the pressure pulse wave, we have fluid velocity $u = f(x, r, t)$. For *average velocity $\bar{u}$*, we put down

$$\bar{u}(x, t) = \left(\frac{1}{A}\right) \int_0^{a+\eta} u(x, r, t) 2\pi r dr \tag{12.1}$$

The *conservation-of-mass equation* (referring to Figure 12.2), is given by

$$-\bar{u} \cdot \pi a^2 + \pi a^2 \left(\bar{u} + \frac{\partial \bar{u}}{\partial x} dx\right) + (2\pi a \cdot dx) u_w = 0$$

$$\therefore u_w = -\frac{a}{2} \frac{\partial \bar{u}}{\partial x} \tag{12.2}$$

Note that at $t = 0$, $\Delta p = 0$, $\bar{u} = 0$, because the wave has not arrived at site x. When the pressure pulse (Δp) wave enters the arterial segment, the average velocity $\bar{u}$ also propagates as a wave in conjunction with the pressure pulse (Δp) wave.

---

* This work is based on Arterial Wave Propagation and Reflection at a Bifurcation Site, DN Ghista, L Zhong, E Y-K Ng, and RS Tan, in *Advances in Cardiac Signal Processing*, Springer, 2007, UR Acharya, JS Suri, JAE Spaan, and SM Krishnan, eds., with permission from Springer.

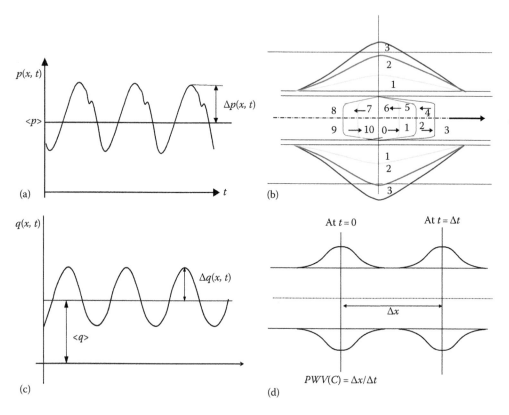

FIGURE 12.1
(a) Schematics of arterial pressure profile; (b) schematics of arterial wall displacement and flow-velocity profiles at a site during the passage of the pulse wave; (c) schematics of arterial flow profile; and (d) traveling pressure profile at two sites Δx apart, at times $t = 0$ and Δt.

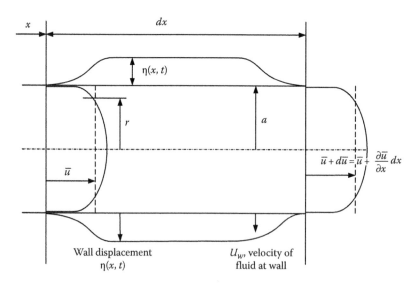

FIGURE 12.2
Flow velocity within an arterial element (of length dx).

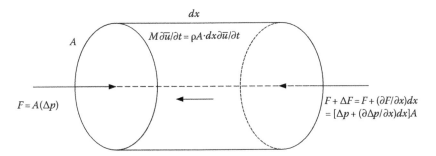

FIGURE 12.3
Forces acting on a fluid element of length dx.

Let us now put down the *momentum equations* (refer Figure 12.3):

$$\text{(a)} \quad \Delta F + M\frac{\partial \overline{u}}{\partial t} = \left(\frac{\partial F}{\partial x}\right)dx + \rho A dx \frac{\partial \overline{u}}{\partial t} = 0$$

$$\therefore \frac{-\partial F}{\partial x} + m\frac{\partial \overline{u}}{\partial t} = 0$$

where m is the fluid-element mass per unit length $= M/dx = \rho A$.
Since $\partial F/\partial x = A(\partial \Delta p/\partial x)$

$$\therefore A\frac{\partial \Delta p}{\partial x} + \rho A\frac{\partial \overline{u}}{\partial t} = 0$$

and

$$\frac{\partial \Delta p}{\partial x} = -\rho\frac{\partial \overline{u}}{\partial t} \tag{12.3}$$

that is, the pressure gradient = inertia force per unit volume.

$$\text{(b)} \quad \frac{\partial \Delta p}{\partial r} = 0$$

We now put down the *arterial wall motion equation*:
From Figure 12.4, the equilibrium equation of forces acting on the arterial wall element
is

$$\Delta p(2a \cdot dx) - 2 \cdot \Delta\sigma(h \cdot dx) - \rho_w 2\pi a \cdot h dx \ddot{\eta} = 0$$

where η is the wall displacement.
If we take reasonable values of $a = 1$ cm, $h = 3$ mm, $\eta = 2$ mm, and $\ddot{\eta} = 2$ nm/s^2.

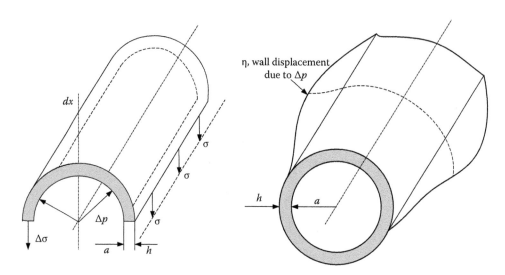

FIGURE 12.4
Schematics of wall displacement and forces acting on a wall element.

Thus, it is seen that the inertia force term ($\rho_w 2\pi a h dx \ddot{\eta}$) can be neglected, and hence we get*

$$\therefore \Delta\sigma = \frac{\Delta p \cdot a}{h} \tag{12.4}$$

Now, we take up the *arterial stress–strain σ–ε relation,* based on Figure 12.5:

$$\Delta\sigma = E\left[\frac{(2\pi(a+\eta) - 2\pi a)}{2\pi a}\right] = \frac{E\eta}{a} \tag{12.5}$$

where E is the incremental modulus of elasticity of the arterial wall.

_____

* Strictly speaking we should have

$$\therefore \Delta\sigma = \frac{\Delta p a'}{h'}$$

where the deformed internal radius $a' = a + \eta$ and the deformed wall thickness $h' = h - \Delta h$. Then, by the virtue of the incompressibility condition

$$2\pi a h = 2\pi(a+\eta)h' = 2\pi(a+\eta)(h - \Delta h) \quad \text{we get } \eta h = a(\Delta h) \text{ or } \Delta h = \frac{\eta h}{a}$$

so, we have

$$\Delta\sigma = \Delta p\left(\frac{a'}{h'}\right) = \frac{\Delta p(a+\eta)}{(h - \Delta h)} = \frac{\Delta p(a+\eta)}{(h - (\eta h/a))}$$

$$= \frac{\Delta p(a+\eta)a}{h(a-\eta)} \cong \frac{\Delta p a}{h} \quad (\because \eta \ll a)$$

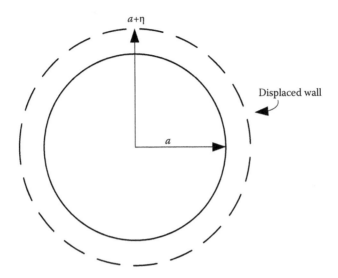

FIGURE 12.5
Arterial wall displacement.

Now let us put down the *equation of η response to Δp*.
So, by combining Equations 12.4 and 12.5, we get

$$\eta = \left(\frac{a^2}{hE} \right) \Delta p$$

$$\text{i.e., } \eta(x, t) = \left(\frac{a^2}{hE} \right) \Delta p(x, t)$$

or

$$\frac{\eta}{a} = \left(\frac{a}{hE} \right) \Delta p \qquad (12.6)$$

We now put down the *kinematics-matching relations* between the arterial wall velocity and the fluid velocity at the wall.

At the wall, the wall velocity $\dot{\eta}$ must equal the fluid velocity at the wall (u_w):

$$u_w(x, t) = \dot{\eta}(x, t) \qquad (12.7)$$

Integration of fluid and arterial wall motion equations:
From Equations 12.2, 12.6, and 12.7, we get

$$u_w = \frac{-a}{2} \frac{\partial \bar{u}}{\partial x} = \left(\frac{a^2}{hE} \right) \frac{\partial \Delta p}{\partial t} \qquad (12.8)$$

$$\therefore -\frac{\partial \bar{u}}{\partial x} = \left(\frac{2a}{hE} \right) \cdot \frac{\partial \Delta p}{\partial t} \qquad (12.9)$$

Also, from Equation 12.3

$$-\frac{1}{\rho}\left(\frac{\partial \Delta p}{\partial x}\right) = \frac{\partial \bar{u}}{\partial t} \tag{12.10}$$

By differentiating Equations 12.9 and 12.10 (with respect to t and x), as ∂ (12.9)/∂t − ∂ (12.10)/∂x, we obtain

$$\frac{\partial^2 \Delta p}{\partial x^2} = \left[\frac{1}{(Eh/2a\rho)}\right]\frac{\partial^2 \Delta p}{\partial t^2} \tag{12.11}$$

and

$$\frac{\partial^2 \bar{u}}{\partial x^2} = \left[\frac{1}{(Eh/2a\rho)}\right]\frac{\partial^2 \bar{u}}{\partial t^2} \tag{12.12}$$

Hence, the pressure-pulse wave velocity (PWV, c) expression is given by

$$c = \left(\frac{Eh}{2a\rho}\right)^{1/2} \tag{12.13}$$

In other words, Δp and $\bar{u}$ are propagating as waves. From Equations 12.6 and 12.13, we can also put down

$$c = \left(\frac{Eh}{2a\rho}\right)^{1/2} = \left(\frac{\Delta pa}{2\eta\rho}\right)^{1/2} \tag{12.14}$$

In other words, the PWV ($=c$) is (1) proportional to arterial elasticity (E) and (h/a) or (2) directly proportional to the magnitude of the pressure pulse (Δp) and inversely proportional to (η/a).

For example, in a normal adult, whose $E = 4.0 \times 10^5$ N/m^2, $h = 1.5$ mm, $a = 1.15$ cm, we get $c = 4.96$ m/s. In an atherosclerotic patient whose $E = 4.0 \times 10^5$ N/m^2, $h = 1.5$ mm, $a = 0.81$ cm (due to 50% artery occlusion), we get $c = 5.91$ m/s. For an arteriosclerotic patient whose $E = 8.0 \times 10^5$ N/m^2 (due to stiffer aortic artery), $h = 1.5$ mm, $a = 1.15$ cm, we get $c = 7.02$ m/s.

The schematics of PWV (as a function of the arterial elastic modulus) in a normal subject, atherosclerotic subject, and arteriosclerotic subject are shown in Figure 12.6. Herein, representative values of aortic diameter and wall thickness are assumed based on the echocardiography in clinical practice [28].

Based on this figure, we can develop Table 12.1. From this Table 12.1, we can see that the value of c increases from 3.5–6 m/s in normal subjects to 4.3–7.5 m/s in atherosclerotic subjects, and to 5–8.5 m/s in arteriosclerotic subjects. Correspondingly, Eh/a increases from 27–75 kPa in normal subjects to 39–119 kPa in atherosclerotic subjects, and to 54–150 kPa in arteriosclerotic subjects. The mean values of Eh/a increases from 51 kPa in normal subjects

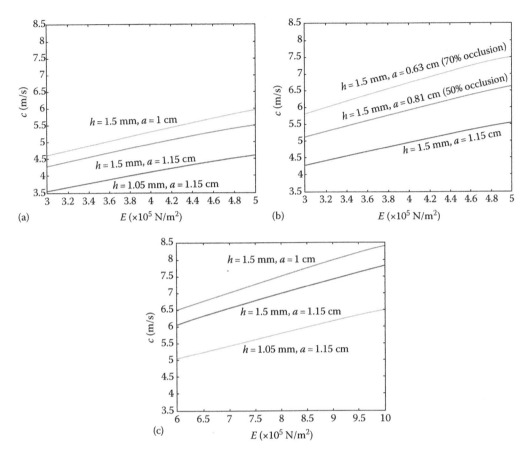

FIGURE 12.6
Schematics of pulse wave velocity in (a) normal subject, (b) atherosclerotic subject, and (c) arteriosclerotic subject.

TABLE 12.1

Data Extracted from Figure 12.6

	c (m/s)	E ($\times 10^5$ Pa)	h (mm)	a (cm)	Eh/a (kPa)
Normal subjects	3.5	3	1.05	1.15	27.39
	6	5	1.5	1	75.00
Atherosclerotic subjects	4.3	3	1.5	1.15	39.13
	7.5	5	1.5	0.63	119.05
Arteriosclerotic subjects	5	6	1.05	1.15	54.78
	8.5	10	1.5	1	150.00

to 79 kPa in atherosclerotic subjects, and to 102 kPa in arteriosclerotic subjects; this consti-tutes a distinct difference in Eh/a values of normal subjects, atherosclerotic subjects, and arteriosclerotic subjects. Hence, we can use E^* ($=Eh/a$) as an appropriate arterial stiffness parameter. The reason for our adopting E^* instead of E as an arterial stiffness parameter is because it can be obtained directly from noninvasive measurement of PWV without hav-ing to determine the arterial radius a and wall thickness h.

12.3 Depiction of Pressure Pulse Wave Propagation

$$\Delta p(x, t) = A\sin\left[\frac{2\pi(x - ct)}{\lambda}\right] + B\sin\left[\frac{2\pi(x + ct)}{\lambda}\right] \tag{12.15}$$

The first term represents a right-propagating wave and the second term represents a left-propagating wave. If we substitute Equation 12.15 in Equation 12.11, we can see that Equation 12.15 satisfies it.

Referring to Figure 12.7, if for a right-propagating pulse wave, we have

$$f(x - ct) = A\sin\frac{2\pi(x - ct)}{\lambda}$$

Then, $f(x - ct) = A\sin 2\pi x/\lambda$ at $t = T/2$, when the UVW segment of the wave has emerged into the arterial segment, and $f(x - ct) = A\sin 2\pi(x - ct_1)/\lambda$, after an additional time t_1, obtained by shifting the UVW segment by ct_1 units to the right (i.e., $f(x - ct)$ represents a wave traveling at speed c from $t = 0$ to t_1). In other words, the wave segment UVW has moved to the right by $x_1 = ct_1$ (i.e., in time $t = x_1/c = t_1$ (because $c = x_1/t_1$)).

Now, in Figure 12.8a, the UVW wave has traveled distance λ in time ct, that is, $t = T = \lambda/c$ (where T is the time required by wave to travel λ). In Figure 12.8b, at $t = 5T/4$, the wave has traveled further to the right by an amount $= \lambda/4$; note that at $x = \lambda$, $\Delta p = -A$.

Then, in Figure 12.9, (1) at $x = 0$ and $t = T = \lambda/c$, the entered wave $UVWXY = A\sin(2\pi ct/\lambda)$ is depicted in Figure 12.9a and (2) at $x = \lambda$ and after $t = 2T = 2\lambda/C$, this wave $UVWXY$ is displayed in Figure 12.9b.

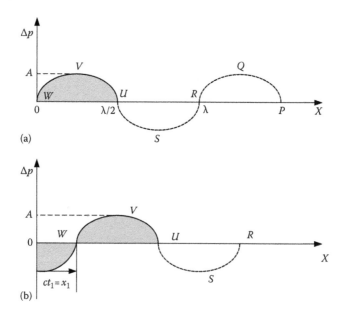

(a)

(b)

FIGURE 12.7

(a) Location of pulse wave UVW $f(x - ct) = A\sin(2\pi x/\lambda)$, at $t = 0$, at its entry into the arterial segment. The Δp wave segment UVW (from $x = 0$ to $\lambda/2$) has entered the arterial segment, while the Δp wave segment RSU is the tail end of the diastolic portion of the previous wave PQRSU (shown dotted). (b) The wave segment UVW has traveled by $x_1 (=ct_1)$ distance to the right in time t_1. $f(x - ct) = A\sin[2\pi(x - ct_1)x/\lambda]$ at $t = t_1$.

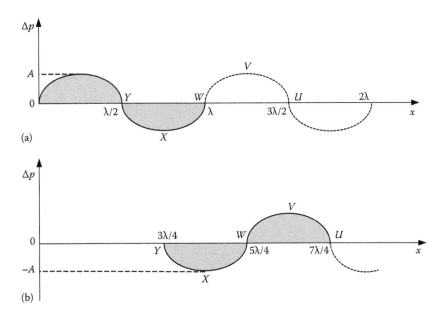

FIGURE 12.8
Locations of *UVWXY* pulse wave at $t = T$ and $5T/4$: (a) location of pulse wave $UVWXY f(x - ct) = A\sin(2\pi(x - ct)/\lambda)$, at $t = T = \lambda/c$, from the time of its entry into the arterial segment. (b) Location of pulse wave $UVWXY f(x - ct)$ at $t = 5T/4$ from the time of its entry into the arterial segment.

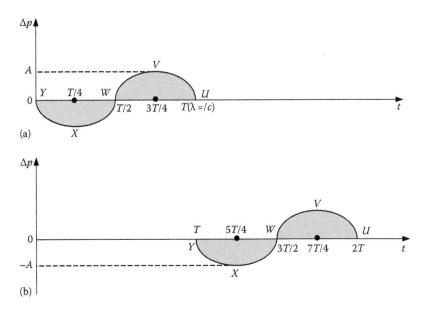

FIGURE 12.9
The wave $UVWXY = A\sin 2\pi(x - ct)$ displayed on the time scale at $x = 0$ and $x = \lambda$: (a) at $x = 0$ and $t = T$ (b) at $x = \lambda$ and $t = 2T = 2\lambda/c$.

12.4 Determination of Arterial Elasticity Parameters

In Figure 12.10, let $\langle P \rangle$ be the mean pressure before the arrival of the pulse wave. Then, the pulse wave Δp arrives at the site.

Based on Figure 12.11, we have the relationship

$$\sigma = \frac{\langle P \rangle a}{h} \quad \text{or} \quad \frac{h}{a} = \frac{\langle P \rangle}{\sigma} \tag{12.16}$$

where
$\langle P \rangle$ is the mean arterial pressure
σ is the arterial wall stress

The arterial wall elasticity E_t (as depicted by Figure 12.12) can be expressed as

$$E_t = E_0 + E_1 e^{b\sigma} \tag{12.17}$$

where
E_0 is the residual elastic modulus
E and b are the constitutive parameters

By comparing the E and σ forms of our derived arterial modulus and stress expressions (Equations 12.16 and 12.17), we note that if the values of the deformed arterial dimensions and the corresponding pressures are known, both the arterial modulus E and stress σ can be calculated. The experimental in vitro arterial data of Simon et al. [29] provides the values of pressure, dimensions a and h, and pulse velocity C, as shown in Table 12.2, corresponding to three different instants. Using these values, we compute, by means of Equation 12.16 and 12.17, the arterial modulus E and stress σ, and hence the E versus σ curve in Figure 12.13. By fitting Equation 12.17 to this curve, we obtain the values of the constitutive parameters (E_0, E, and b), as shown in Table 12.2.

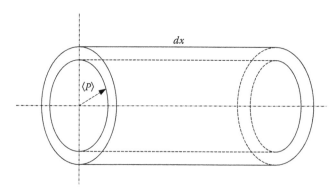

FIGURE 12.10
The arterial tube prior to arrival of the pressure pulse.

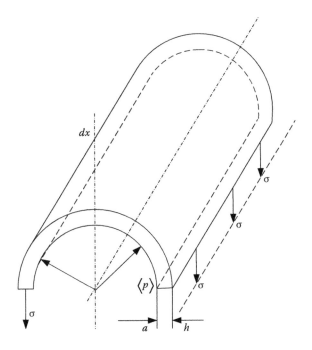

FIGURE 12.11
Relation between wall stress and internal pressure.

12.5 Determination of Arterial Impedance (Arteriosclerosis Parameter) from PWV and Arterial Cross-Sectional Area

The arterial pulse waveform is derived from the complex interaction of the left ventricular stroke volume, the physical properties of the arterial tree, and the characteristics of the fluid in the system [30]. The principal components of blood pressure, as well as of flow rate (q) and velocity (u), comprise both a steady component (mean arterial pressure and flow rate) and a pulsatile component (pulse pressure and flow rate), schematically in Figure 12.14 [31].

$$p = \langle p \rangle + \Delta p$$
$$q = \langle q \rangle + \Delta q$$

(12.18)

The pulsatile component of pressure is determined by the pattern of left ventricular ejection, the stroke volume, and the compliance characteristics of the arterial circulation [32].

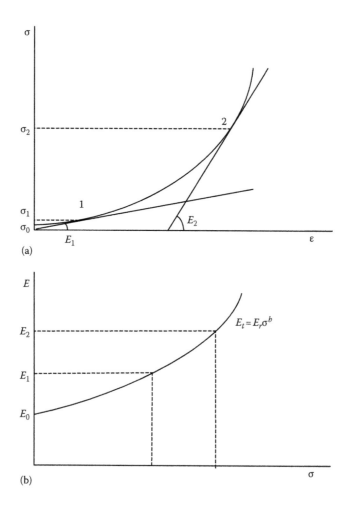

(a)

(b)

FIGURE 12.12
(a) Schematics of arterial stress–strain curve, depicting the incremental elastic modulus $E = E_1$ and E_2 corresponding to σ_1 and σ_2. (b) Schematics of E–σ property of an artery corresponding to Figure 12.12a.

TABLE 12.2

Calculating Elastic Modulus (E) Parameters

	C (m/s)	Diastolic pressure (mmHg)	a (cm)	h (cm)	σ ($\times 10^5$ Pa)	E ($\times 10^5$ Pa)	B	E_0	E_1
1	1.899	50	4.29	0.43	0.66	0.73	1.003×10^{-4}	5.63×10^4	22.96
2	2.364	56	4.37	0.41	0.79	1.20			
3	3.745	63	4.45	0.40	0.93	3.15			

Note: From the experimental data of Simon et al. [29].

Arterial compliance is defined as the change in area or volume of an artery or arterial bed for a given change in pressure [29]. The pulse pressure for a given ventricular ejection and heart rate will depend on arterial compliance, as well as the timing and magnitude of peripheral pulse wave reflection.

Impedance, a term borrowed from electrical engineering theory, describes the opposition to flow presented by a system. The impedance load of the arterial tree can be quantified by

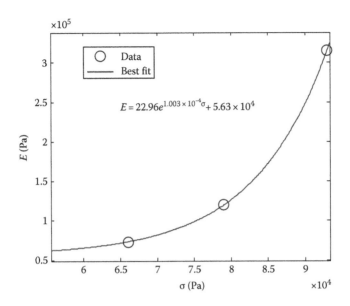

FIGURE 12.13
The computed curve of arterial modulus (E) versus arterial wall stress (σ), as obtained by Equations 12.16 and 12.17 from the experimental data of Simon et al. [29].

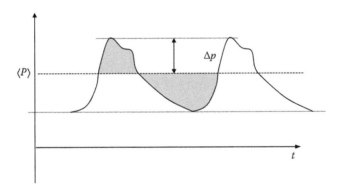

FIGURE 12.14
Pressure pulse versus time.

analyzing pulse pressure–flow relationships produced through the effects of disease on the structural and functional components of the arterial system [33,34]. Input impedance relates simultaneously recorded pressure and flow waveforms under specific mathematical conditions.

12.5.1 Peripheral Resistance

We define

$$\langle q \rangle = \frac{\langle p \rangle}{R} \tag{12.19}$$

where $R = (8\mu L/\pi a^4) = TPR$.

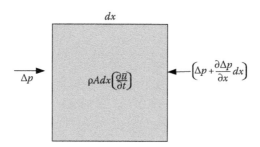

FIGURE 12.15
Force equilibrium of a fluid element; $\bar{u}$, average velocity across the cross section.

With atherosclerosis, the arterial radius (a) decreases and resistance (R) increases markedly. Hence for a given $\langle q \rangle$, $\langle p \rangle$ is increased a lot.

12.5.2 Arterial Impedance

(a) We define

$$\Delta q = \frac{\Delta p}{z_0} \tag{12.20}$$

where z_0(impedance) $= \rho c / A = \rho / A \sqrt{(Eh/2a\rho)}$.

For a given Δq, Δp is high if z_0 (impedance) is high. In other words, the impedance (z_0) is a direct measure of arterial hardening or stiffness. We will now derive Equation 12.20.

For force equilibrium (as shown in Figure 12.15),

$$-A \frac{\partial \Delta p}{\partial x} dx - \rho A dx \frac{\partial \bar{u}}{\partial t} = 0 \tag{12.21}$$

$$A\rho \frac{\partial \bar{u}}{\partial t} = -A \frac{\partial \Delta p}{\partial x} \tag{12.22}$$

Now, $\Delta q(x,t) = A\bar{u}(x,t)$

$$\therefore \rho \frac{\partial \Delta q}{\partial t} = -A \frac{\partial \Delta p}{\partial x} \tag{12.23}$$

Now, let

$$\Delta p = f_1(x - ct) \quad \left(\text{since } \frac{\partial^2 \Delta p}{\partial x^2} = \frac{1}{(Eh/2a\rho)} \frac{\partial^2 \Delta p}{\partial t^2} = \frac{1}{c^2} \frac{\partial^2 \Delta p}{\partial t^2} \right) \tag{12.24}$$

$$\Delta q = \phi_1(x - ct) \quad \left(\text{since } \frac{\partial^2 \Delta q}{\partial x^2} = \frac{1}{c^2} \frac{\partial^2 \Delta q}{\partial t^2} \right) \tag{12.25}$$

For instance, we can have $\Delta p = \Delta p_1 \sin(2\pi/\lambda)(x-ct)$ and $\Delta q = \Delta q_1 \sin(2\pi/\lambda)(x-ct)$.
Substituting Equations 12.24 and 12.25 into Equation 12.23, we get

$$-\rho c \phi_1'(x-ct) = -A f_1'(x-ct) \tag{12.26}$$

Upon integrating, we get

$$\rho c \phi_1 = A f_1 \tag{12.27}$$

Hence, for right-propagating waves $f(x-ct)$ and $\phi(x-ct)$, the impedance is given by

$$\therefore z_{01} = \frac{\Delta \vec{p}}{\Delta \vec{q}} = \frac{\rho c}{A} = \frac{\rho}{A}\left(\frac{Eh}{2a\rho}\right)^{1/2} = \frac{4\rho}{\pi}\left(\frac{Eh}{2a^5\rho}\right)^{1/2} \tag{12.28}$$

Now, for a left-propagating wave $\Delta p_2 = f_2(x+ct)$ and $\Delta q_2 = \phi_2(x+ct)$, we have $-\rho c \phi_2 = +A f_2$.
Hence, for a left-traveling wave,

$$z_{02}\left(=-\frac{\rho c}{A}\right) = -\frac{f_2}{\phi_2} = -\frac{\Delta \overleftarrow{p}_2}{\Delta \overleftarrow{q}_2} \tag{12.29}$$

(b) *Implication*: If the arterial stiffness E is high (as in arteriosclerosis), then (as per Equations 12.20 and 12.28), both z_0 and Δp will be high. Based on Equations 12.19 and 12.28, (1) if a person smokes or has atherosclerosis, $\langle p \rangle$ will be elevated; (2) if a person has hardened artery (arteriosclerosis), Δp will be elevated. Note that R (in Equation 12.19) is primarily affected by high μ and low a. On the other hand, z_0 is affected by high E as well as low a and high h.
Reiterating, for a right-propagating wave, in Equations 12.24 and 12.25.
Let

$$\Delta p = f_1 = \Delta p_1 \sin\frac{2\pi}{\lambda}(x-ct)$$

$$\Delta q = \phi_1 = \Delta q_1 \sin\frac{2\pi}{\lambda}(x-ct)$$

Then, from Equation 12.27

$$\rho c \Delta q_1 \sin\frac{2\pi}{\lambda}(x-ct) = A\Delta p_1 \sin\frac{2\pi}{\lambda}(x-ct) \tag{12.30}$$

and hence

$$z_{01} = \frac{\rho c}{A} = \frac{\Delta p_1}{\Delta q_1} \tag{12.31}$$

For a left-propagating wave,

$$\Delta p = f_2 = \Delta p_2 \sin \frac{2\pi}{\lambda}(x+ct)$$

$$\Delta q = \phi_2 = \Delta q_2 \sin \frac{2\pi}{\lambda}(x+ct)$$

Since from Equation 12.23,

$$\rho \frac{\partial \Delta q}{\partial t} = -A \frac{\partial \Delta p}{\partial x}$$

We have corresponding to Equation 12.27:

$$\frac{2\pi\rho c}{\lambda} \Delta q_2 \sin \frac{2\pi}{\lambda}(x+ct) = -\frac{A 2\pi}{\lambda} \Delta q_2 \sin \frac{2\pi}{\lambda}(x+ct) \tag{12.32}$$

$$\therefore \rho c \Delta q_2 = -A \Delta p_2 \tag{12.33}$$

$$\therefore z_{02} = \frac{\rho c}{A} = -\frac{\Delta p_2}{\Delta q_2} \tag{12.34}$$

(c) What about the constant of integration in Equation 12.27? In general, we can put down

$$\rho c [\phi(x-ct) + \phi(0)] = A[f(x-ct) + f(0)] \tag{12.35}$$

If $f(x-ct) = \Delta p_1 \sin \frac{2\pi}{\lambda}(x-ct)$ and $\phi(x-ct) = \Delta q_1 \sin \frac{2\pi}{\lambda}(x-ct)$

then, $f(0) = 0$, and also $\phi(0) = 0$ $\tag{12.36}$

If $f(x-ct) = \Delta p_1 \cos \frac{2\pi}{\lambda}(x-ct)$ and $\phi(x-ct) = \Delta q_1 \cos \frac{2\pi}{\lambda}(x-ct)$

then $f(0) = \Delta p_1$ and $\phi(0) = \Delta q_1$ $\tag{12.37}$

Hence, we have

$$\rho c [\phi(x-ct) + \Delta q_1] = A[f(x-ct) + \Delta p_1]$$

or

$$\rho c \left[\Delta q_1 \cos \frac{2\pi}{\lambda}(x-ct) + \Delta q_1 \right] = A \left[\Delta p_1 \cos \frac{2\pi}{\lambda}(x-ct) + \Delta p_1 \right] \tag{12.38}$$

i.e., $\rho c \Delta q + \rho c \Delta q_1 = A \Delta p + A \Delta p_1$

$$\therefore \rho c \Delta q = A \Delta p; \quad \text{for } z_0 = \frac{\Delta p}{\Delta q} = \frac{\rho c}{A}$$

$$\therefore \rho c \Delta q_1 = A \Delta p_1; \quad \text{for } z_0 = \frac{\Delta p_1}{\Delta q_1} = \frac{\rho c}{A} \tag{12.39}$$

i.e., $\rho c \phi(0) = A f(0)$

So, either, $\phi(0) = f(0) = 0$, based on Equation 12.36 $\tag{12.40}$

or

$\rho c \phi(0) = A f(0)$, based on Equation 12.39, for which

$$z_0 = \frac{f(0)}{\phi(0)} = \frac{\rho c}{A} \tag{12.41}$$

(d) Hence, the arterial pressure characteristics in normal, atherosclerosis, and arterio-sclerosis states will be as follows in Figure 12.16.

Summarizing, we have $\langle p \rangle = R\langle q \rangle$, given by Equation 12.19, where R is the arteriolar bed resistance, and $\Delta p = Z_0 \Delta q$, given by Equation 12.20, where Z_0 is the arterial impedance.

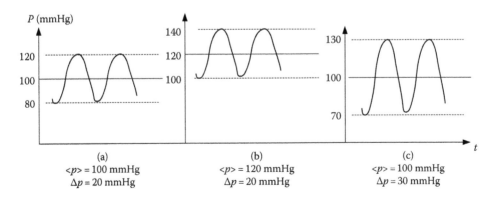

FIGURE 12.16
Schematics of pressure waveform under different situations: (a) normal, (b) atherosclerosis, and (c) arteriosclerosis.

So in a hypertensive person, we can (1) reduce $\langle p \rangle$ by reducing R, that is, by reducing blood viscosity (μ) with the help of appropriate medications, and reduce (2) Δp by reducing Z_0 (or increasing compliance), that is, by reducing the arterial wall modulus E with lifestyle changes and therapies.

12.5.3 Hypertension due to Elevated Blood Viscosity and Arterial Stiffness

Blood viscosity, referred to earlier, is a measure of the resistance of blood to flow. It can also be described as the thickness and stickiness of blood. The primary determinants of blood viscosity are hematocrit, red blood cell deformity, red blood cell aggregation, and plasma viscosity. Plasma viscosity is determined by water content and macromolecular components, so these factors that affect blood viscosity are the plasma protein concentration and types of proteins in the plasma. Nevertheless, hematocrit has the strongest impact on whole blood viscosity.

Elevation of plasma viscosity correlates to the progression of coronary and peripheral vascular diseases. Many conventional cardiovascular risk factors and outcomes have been independently correlated with whole blood viscosity. Hypertension, total cholesterol, LDL cholesterol, triglycerides, chylomicrons, VLDL cholesterol, diabetes, and metabolic syndrome have all been positively linked to whole blood viscosity.

Blood viscosity–reducing drugs are medicines that improve blood flow by making the blood less viscous (sticky). Blood viscosity–reducing drugs are available only with a physician's prescription and come in extended release tablet form. Examples of blood viscosity–reducing drugs are pentoxifylline (Trental) and oxypentifylline.

Arterial stiffness (or modulus or elastance), mentioned earlier, is associated with increased risk of cardiovascular events, dementia, and death. Increased elastance or decreased compliance of the central vasculature alters arterial pressure and flow dynamics and impacts cardiac performance and coronary perfusion. Vascular stiffening develops

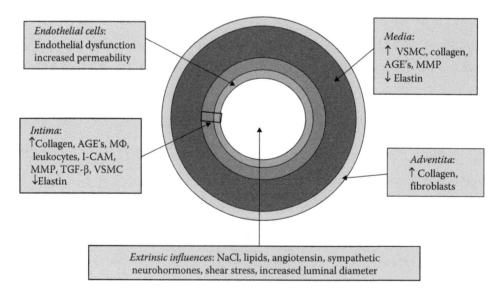

FIGURE 12.17
Summary of the multiple causes and locations of arterial stiffness. (From Zieman, S. et al., *Arterioscl. Thromb. Vasc. Biol.*, 25, 932, 2005.)

from a complex interaction between stable and dynamic changes involving structural and cellular elements of the vessel wall, as shown in Figure 12.17 [35].

Stiffened arteries require a greater amount of force to cause them to expand and take up the blood ejected from the heart. This increased force requirement is provided by the heart, which begins to contract harder to accommodate the artery. Over time, this increased load placed on the heart causes left ventricular hypertrophy and eventually left ventricular failure. Causing further damage is the increased time required for systole and the reduction of diastole. This reduction in both time and pressure during diastole decreases the amount of perfusion for cardiac tissue. Thus the heart, which is becoming hypertrophic (and with therefore a greater oxygen demand) is starved of oxygen and nutrition, adding to cardiac damage.

There are a number of strategies to reduce vascular stiffening. These involve lifestyle issues, such as reducing body weight, exercise, lowering salt intake, and moderate alcohol consumption. Other strategies are pharmacological in nature, focusing on nitric oxide-dependent pathways and antioxidants.

12.6 Pulse Wave Reflection at Arterial Bifurcation

12.6.1 Analysis

Based on Figure 12.18, we have

$$\Delta p = \Delta p' = \Delta p'_1 = \Delta p'_2 \tag{12.42}$$

$$\Delta q' = \Delta q'_1 + \Delta q'_2 = \frac{\Delta p'}{z'_{01}} + \frac{\Delta p'}{z'_{02}} = \Delta p' \left(\frac{1}{z'_{01}} + \frac{1}{z'_{02}} \right)$$

$$= \frac{2\Delta p'}{z'_0} \quad (\text{if } z'_{01} = z'_{02}) \tag{12.43}$$

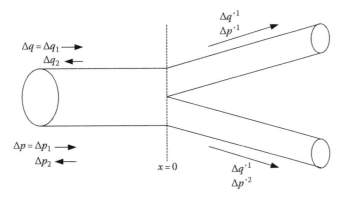

FIGURE 12.18
Schematics of pressure and flow pulses at an arterial bifurcation.

Also,

$$\Delta p = \Delta p_1 + \Delta p_2 = \Delta p' = \Delta p'_1 = \Delta p'_2 \tag{12.44}$$

and

$$\Delta q = \Delta q_1 + \Delta q_2 = \Delta q' = \Delta q'_1 + \Delta q'_2 \tag{12.45}$$

Hence, from Equation 12.45,

$$\frac{\Delta p_1}{z_0} - \frac{\Delta p_2}{z_0} = \frac{\Delta p'}{z'_0} + \frac{\Delta p'}{z'_0} = \frac{2\Delta p'}{z'_0} \tag{12.46}$$

Then, from Equations 12.46 and 12.44,

$$\frac{z'_0}{z_0} \Delta p_1 - \frac{z'_0}{z_0} \Delta p_2 = 2\Delta p' = 2\Delta p_1 + 2\Delta p_2$$

or

$$\Delta p_1 \left(\frac{z'_0}{z_0} - 2 \right) = \Delta p_2 \left(\frac{z'_0}{z_0} + 2 \right) \tag{12.47}$$

Let λ be defined as

$$\frac{z_0}{z'_0} = \left(\frac{E}{E'} \times \frac{h}{h'} \right)^{0.5} \times \left(\frac{a}{a'} \right)^{2.5} \tag{12.48}$$

Then, we have

$$\frac{\Delta p_2}{\Delta p_1} = \frac{z'_0 - 2z_0}{z'_0 + 2z_0} = \frac{1 - 2\lambda}{1 + 2\lambda} \tag{12.49}$$

Let R_f (reflection coefficient) be defined as

$$R_f = \frac{\Delta p_2}{\Delta p_1} = \frac{1 - 2\lambda}{1 + 2\lambda} \tag{12.50}$$

12.6.2 Applications

(a) So, for no reflection (as ideally expected in nature), $\Delta p_2 = 0$ and $R_f = 0$

$$\text{i.e., } \lambda = \frac{z_0}{z'_0} = 0.5 \tag{12.51}$$

$$\text{i.e.,} \left(\frac{E}{E'} \times \frac{h}{h'} \right)^{0.5} \times \left(\frac{a'}{a} \right)^{2.5} = 0.5 \tag{12.52}$$

$$\text{Suppose } a' = 0.75a \tag{12.53}$$

Then, if we can assume conservation of mass between the parent vessel and its bifurcations, we will have

$$2\pi a h = 2(2\pi a' h') \tag{12.54}$$

Hence, from Equations 12.53 and 12.54,

$$\frac{h}{h'} = 2\frac{a'}{a} = 2 \times (0.75) = 1.5 \tag{12.55}$$

$$\therefore \frac{E}{E'} = \frac{0.25}{(a'/a)^5 \times (h/h')} \tag{12.56}$$

Now since from Equations 12.53 and 12.55, $(a'/a)^5 = 0.237$ and $h/h' = 1.5$, then

$$\frac{E}{E'} = 0.703 \tag{12.57}$$

Hence, we have
For $R_f = 0$, $\Delta p_2 = 0$ or no reflection, and $\lambda = 0.5$

$$\text{i.e., } \lambda = 0.5 \text{ means } \Delta p_2 = 0 \text{ and } R_f = 0 \text{ (i.e., no reflection)} \tag{12.58}$$

(b) For

$$\lambda < 0.5, \ \Delta p_2 = R_f \Delta p_1, \text{ and } 0 < R_f < 1 \tag{12.59}$$

In this case, there is reflection with no phase change, that is, an incident expansion wave at a site will be superimposed by a reflected expansion wave (of less magnitude) at that site.
  Let us represent Equation 12.59 by

$$A_2 \sin(x + ct) = R_f A_1 \sin(x - ct); \quad 0 < R_f < 1$$

and adopt $R_f = 0.3$, so that

$$A_2 \sin(x + ct) = 0.3 A_1 \sin(x - ct)$$

This means that the reflected pulse wave amplitude will add to the amplitude of the incident wave.

(c) For $\lambda > 0.5$, $\Delta p_2 = -R_f \Delta q_2$; that is, $R_f < 0$

Let $R_f = -0.2$, then,

$$A_2 \sin(x + ct) = -\frac{1}{5} A_1 \sin(x - ct) = \frac{1}{5} A_1 \sin[(x - ct) - \pi],$$

$$\text{i.e., } A_2 = \frac{A_1}{5}$$

This means that the reflected pulse wave will be 180° out of phase with the incident way and contribute to decreasing the amplitude of the combined incident and reflected wave. This aspect has some important clinical inference. It would be interesting to verify that for normal persons, $E/E' = 0.3$ and these persons will be intrinsically normotensive persons, for whom $\lambda < 0.5$ (and say $R_f = 0.3$), will be intrinsically hypertensive. On the other hand, person, for whom $\lambda > 0.5$ (and say $R_f = 0.2$), will have intrinsically low blood pressure.

12.7 Noninvasive Determination of PWV and Arterial Stiffness

There are several methods of pulse wave measurements based on different principles and depending on the type of the pulse wave measured.

In clinical practice PWV is commonly determined by arterial tonometry, using noninvasive pressure sensors applied over carotid and femoral arteries either simultaneously or sequentially (using the electrocardiogram [ECG] as a timing reference for gating separate recordings to a fixed point in the cardiac cycle, usually the R wave of the ECG) to determine the time delay or "transit time" between the upstroke of carotid and femoral pulse waveforms.

The important point is the reference point on the waveforms. Foot-to-foot methodology is usually used, as it avoids the confounding influence of wave reflection [36]; that is, time is calculated from the foot of the pressure wave at the first point to the foot of the pressure wave as it arrives at the next point (Figure 12.19).

However, difficulties are encountered in judging accurately where the foot of the wave is [38]. For example, is it at the point of minimal diastolic pressure, or is it at the point at which the first derivative of pressure is at a maximum? Different algorithms for identification of the foot of the wave are used (including intersecting tangents, maximum upstroke of the second derivative, and 10% of the pulse pressure), as shown in Figure 12.20, among which the intersecting tangent method (looking at the point yielded by the intersection of a line tangent to the initial systolic upstroke of the pressure tracing and a horizontal line through the minimal point) is shown to be the most reliable [39,40]. This algorithm identifies the foot of the waveform as the point at which a tangent to the steepest part of the upstroke of the pressure waveform intersects with diastolic pressure.

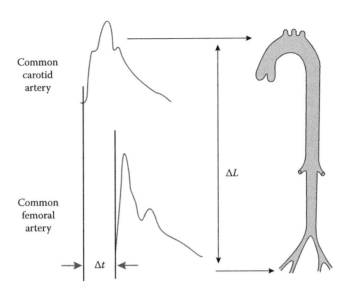

FIGURE 12.19
Principle of arterial stiffness measurement by pulse wave velocity with the foot-to-foot method. (Adapted from Safar M.E., Antihypertensive efficacy and destiffening strategy, *Medicographia*, 32, 234, 2010.)

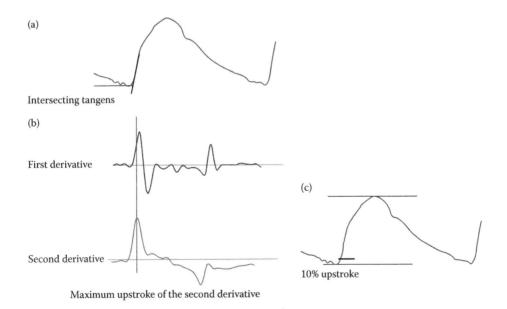

FIGURE 12.20
Different algorithms for identifying the foot of the wave. (a) Intersecting tangents; (b) maximum upstroke of the second derivative; and (c) percentage of the full amplitude of the cycle. (Adapted from Boutouyrie, P. et al., *Artery Res.*, 3, 3, 2009.)

The second derivative method and intersecting tangent method have been shown to be the most reproducible [41].

For noninvasive assessment of carotid–femoral PWV, estimation of pulse wave travel distance is critical. The simplest way to measure the distance (i.e., pathway) is to measure transcutaneously using a tape meter or a caliper. If the measurement is made between the two measurement sites, it leads to a systematic overestimation of PWV by an amount close to 30% [39]. However, it is possible to correct this. Best agreement with invasive measurements has been found for the method of subtracting carotid–suprasternal notch distance from suprasternal notch–femoral distance [42].

Various devices are commercially available and largely used worldwide. The SphygmoCor® system (ArtCor, Sydney, Australia) that has been used in large clinical trials and population survey uses a large band piezoelectric probe and allows the arterial pulse recording in succession (carotid then femoral), both signals being synchronized with the same time basis (ECG R wave) that impose to accurately check that the heart rates are quite similar at the moment of each recording to avoid any disturbance due to PWV relationship to heart rate [39].

Also, customized methods have been used in a number of clinical and population studies [43–45]. PWV can be assessed from measurement of local pressure (using applanation tonometry or piezo-electric sensors), flow velocity (Doppler ultrasound), diameter distension (ultrasound wall-tracking algorithms), or photoplethysmography (i.e., measuring local changes in blood volume). However, the problems with such techniques include the inaccessibility of the central arteries, necessitating compromise by using the nearest superficial arteries. There are also difficulties and inaccuracy in estimating the actual arterial distance between recording sites using only surface measurements [36,46].

Since magnetic resonance imaging (MRI) offers scanning sequences that allow for measurement of PWV [47–50], an alternative method of measuring PWV has been described that uses a MRI technique [51]. The major advantage of this technique is that the path length can be quantified with great accuracy, and it allows measurements to be made from inaccessible arteries; however, it is expensive, time-consuming, can only be applied to relatively large arteries at the present time, and the temporal resolution with which signals (e.g., aortic flow) can be registered is still relatively low compared with other techniques [36,52].

12.7.1 Normal and Reference Values of Pulse Wave Velocity and Arterial Stiffness

A recent study has established reference and normal values for PWV based on a sizeable European population, by gathering data from 16,867 subjects and patients from 13 different centres across 8 European countries and standardizing the results of different methods of PWV measurement [53].

Figure 12.21a demonstrates the reference values for PWV according to age and blood pressure (BP) categories. Corresponding E^* ($=Eh/a$) values are calculated (based on $\rho = 1050$ kg/m^3) and presented in Figure 12.21b. As shown in this figure, both PWV and arterial stiffness are increased with age and blood pressure. These range of values for ages < 40 years agree with those obtained earlier from Figure 12.6 and Table 12.1. Thereby we are now confirming that we can noninvasively depict arterial stiffness in terms of the parameter E^* ($=Eh/a$), which can (1) be noninvasively determined from PWV and (2) also enable us to characterize enhanced arterial stiffness in arteriosclerosis and atherosclerosis in clinical practice.

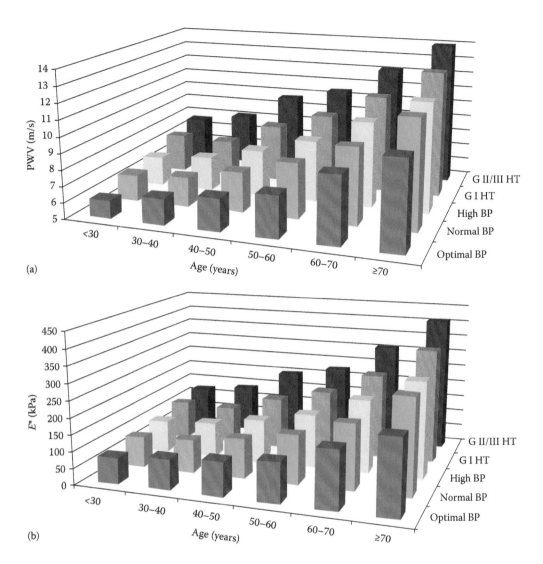

FIGURE 12.21
(a) Reference values for PWV: mean values according to age and blood pressure (BP) categories (HT: hypertension). (Adapted from Boutouyrie, P. and Vermeersch S.J., *Eur. Heart J.*, 31, 2338, 2010.) (b) E^* $(=Eh/a)$ values corresponding to the PWV measurements (calculated based on $\rho = 1050$ kg/m^3).

References

1. Ross R, Atherosclerosis an inflammatory disease, *New England Journal of Medicine*, 340, 1999, 115–126.
2. Nichols WW, O'Rourke MF, *McDonald's Blood Flow in Arteries: Theoretical, Experimental and Clinical Principles*, 4th edn., Amold, London, UK, 1998.
3. Asmar R, Benetos A, Topouchian J, Laurent P, Pannier B, Brisac AM, Target R, Levy BI, Assessment of arterial distensibility by automatic pulse wave velocity measurement, *Hypertension*, 26, 1995, 485–490.

4. Kelly RP, Hayward CS, Ganis J, Daley JM, Avolio AP, O'Rourke, MF, Noninvasive registration of the arterial pulse waveform using high fidelity applanation tonometry, *Journal of Vascular Medicine and Biology*, 1, 1989, 142–149.

5. Ghista DN, Kabinejadian F, Coronary artery bypass grafting hemodynamics and anastomosis design: A biomedical engineering review, *BioMedical Engineering Online*, 12(129), 2013.

6. Fang J, Madhavan S, Cohen H, Measures of blood pressure and myocardial infarction in treated hypertensive patients, *Journal of Hypertension*, 13, 1995, 413–419.

7. Weber T, Auer J, O'Rourke MF, Kvas E, Lassnig E, Berent R, Eber B, Arterial stiffness, wave reflections and the risk of coronary artery disease, *Circulation*, 109, 2004, 184–189.

8. Blacher J, Asmar R, Djane S, London GM, Safar ME, Aortic pulse wave as a marker of cardiovascular risk in hypertensive patients, *Hypertension*, 33, 1999, 1111–1117.

9. Laurent S, Boutouyrie P, Asmar R, Gautier L, Guize L, Ducimetiere P, Benetos A, Aortic stiffness is an independent predictor of all-cause and cardiovascular mortality in hypertensive patients, *Hypertension*, 37, 2001, 1236–1245.

10. Van Popele NM, Grobbee DE, Bots ML, Asmar R, Topouchian J, Reneman RS, Hoeks APG, van der KDAM, Hofman A, Witteman JCM, Association between arterial stiffness and atherosclerosis, *Stroke*, 32, 2001, 454–457.

11. Safar ME, London GM, Asmar R, Frohlich ED, Recent advances on large arteries in hypertension, *Hypertension*, 32, 1998, 156–161.

12. Madhavan S, Ooi WL, Cohen H, Relation of pulse pressure and blood pressure reduction to the incidence of myocardial infarction, *Hypertension*, 23, 1994, 395–401.

13. Westerhof N, Sipkema P, Van Den Bos GC, Elzinga G, Forward and backward waves in the arterial system, *Cardiovascular Research*, 6(6), 1972, 648–656.

14. Liu Z, Brin KP, Yin FC, Estimation of total arterial compliance: An improved method and evaluation of current methods, *American Journal of Physiology*, 251(3), 1986, H588–H600.

15. Laskey WK, Parker HG, Ferrari VA, Gussmaul WG, Noordergraaf A, Estimation of total systemic arterial compliance in humans, *Journal of Applied Physiology*, 69, 1990, 112–119.

16. Stergiopulos N, Meister JJ, Westerhof N, Simple and accurate way for estimating total and segmental arterial compliance: The pulse pressure method, *Annals of Biomedical Engineering*, 22, 1994, 392–397.

17. Stergiopulos N, Segers P, Westerhof N, Use of pulse pressure method for estimating total arterial compliance in vivo, *American Journal of Physiology Heart Circulation Physiology*, 276, 1999, H424–H428.

18. Noordergraaf A, *Circulatory System Dynamics*, Academic Press, New York, 1978, pp. 105–151.

19. Wemple PR, Mockros LF, Pressure and flow in the systemic arterial system, *Journal of Biomechanics*, 5, 1972, 629–641.

20. O'Rourke MF, Vascular impedance in studies of arterial and cardiac function, *Physiological Reviews*, 62, 1982, 570–623.

21. Papageorgiou GL, Jones NB, Wave reflection and hydraulic impedance in the healthy arterial system: A controversial subject, *Medical and Biological Engineering and Computing*, 26, 1988, 237–242.

22. Quick CM, Berger DS, Noordergraaf A, Construction and destructive addition of forward and reflected arterial pulse waves, *American Journal of Physiology: Heart and Circulatory Physiology*, 280(4), 2001, H1519–H1527.

23. O'Rourke M, Arterial stiffness, systolic blood pressure, and logical treatment of arterial hypertension, *Hypertension*, 15, 1990, 339–347.

24. Westerhof N, O'Rourke MF, Haemodynamic basis for the development of left ventricular failure in systolic hypertension and for its logical therapy, *Journal of Hypertension*, 13, 1995, 943–952.

25. Berger DS, Li JK, Noordergraaf A, Arterial wave propagation phenomena, ventricular work, and power dissipation, *Annals of Biomedical Engineering*, 23, 1995, 804–811.

26. Berger DS, Li JK, Noordergraaf A, Differential effects of wave reflections and peripheral resistance on aortic blood pressure: A model-based study, *American Journal of Physiology: Heart and Circulatory Physiology*, 266, 1994, H1626–H1642.

27. Berger DS, Robinson KA, Shroff SG, Wave propagation in coupled left ventricle-arterial system: Implications for aortic pressure, *Hypertension*, 27, 1996, 1079–1089.

28. Chambers J, *Echocardiography in Clinical Practice*, The Parthenon Publishing Group, London, UK, 2002.

29. Simon BR, Kobayashi AS, Strandness DE, Wiederhielm CA, Large deformation analysis of the arterial cross-section, *Journal of Basic Engineering*, 93, 1971, 138–145.

30. McVeigh GE, Bank AJ, Cohn JN, Arterial compliance, in: *Cardiovascular Medicine*, Willerson JT, Cohn JN, eds., Churchill Livingstone, Philadelphia, PA, 2000, pp. 1479–1496.

31. Smulyan H, Safar ME, Systolic blood pressure revisited, *Journal of the American College of Cardiology*, 29, 1997, 1407–1413.

32. McVeigh GE, Finklestein SM, Cohn JN, Pulse contour and impedance parameters derived from arterial waveform analysis, in: *Functional Abnormal of the Aorta*, Boudoulas H, Toutouzas P, Wooley CF, eds., Futura, Armonk, NY, 1996, pp. 183–193.

33. Finkelstein SM, Collins VR, Vascular hemodynamic impedance measurement, *Progress in Cardiovascular Diseases*, 24, 1982, 401–418.

34. Nichols WW, Pepine CJ, Geiser EA, Conti CR, Vascular load defined by the aortic input impedance spectrum, *Federation Proceedings*, 39, 1980, 196–201.

35. Zieman S, Melenovsky V, Kass D, Mechanisms, Pathophysiology, and therapy of arterial stiffness, *Arteriosclerosis, Thrombosis, and Vascular Biology*, 25, 2005, 932–943.

36. Mackenzie IS, Wilkinson IB, Cockcroft JR, Assessment of arterial stiffness in clinical practice, *QJM—Monthly Journal of the Association of Physicians*, 95, 2002, 67–74.

37. Safar ME, Antihypertensive efficacy and destiffening strategy, *Medicographia*, 32, 2010, 234–240.

38. Davies JI, Struthers AD, Pulse wave analysis and pulse wave velocity: A critical review of their strengths and weaknesses, *Journal of Hypertension*, 21, 2003, 463–472.

39. Boutouyrie P, Briet M, Collin C, Vermeersch S, Pannier B, Assessment of pulse wave velocity, *Artery Research*, 3, 2009, 3–8.

40. Millasseau SC, Stewart AD, Patel SJ, Redwood SR, Chowienczyk PJ, Evaluation of carotide-femoral pulse wave velocity: Influence of timing algorithm and heart rate, *Hypertension*, 45(2), 2005, 222–226.

41. Chiu YC, Arand PW, Shroff SG, Feldman T, Carroll JD, Determination of pulse wave velocities with computerized algorithms, *American Heart Journal*, 121, 1991, 1460–1470.

42. Weber T, Ammer M, Rammer M, Adji A, O'Rourke MF, Wassertheurere S, Rosenkranze S, Ebera B, Noninvasive determination of carotid-femoral pulse wave velocity depends critically on assessment of travel distance: A comparison with invasive measurement, *Journal of Hypertension*, 27, 2009, 1624–1630.

43. Sutton-Tyrrell K, Najjar SS, Boudreau RM, Venkitachalam L, Kupelian V, Simonsick EM et al., Elevated aortic pulse wave velocity, a marker of arterial stiffness, predicts cardiovascular events in well-functioning older adults, *Circulation*, 111(25), 2005, 3384–3390.

44. Waldstein SR, Rice SC, Thayer JF, Najjar SS, Scuteri A, Zonderman AB, Pulse pressure and pulse wave velocity are related to cognitive decline in the Baltimore Longitudinal Study of Aging, *Hypertension*, 51(1), 2008, 99–104.

45. Najjar SS, Scuteri A, Shetty V, Wright JG, Muller DC, Fleg JL et al., Pulse wave velocity is an independent predictor of the longitudinal increase in systolic blood pressure and of incident hypertension in the Baltimore Longitudinal Study of Aging, *Journal of the American College of Cardiology*, 51(14), 2008, 1377–1383.

46. Asmar R, *Arterial Stiffness and Pulse Wave Velocity. Clinical Applications*, Elsevier, Amsterdam, the Netherlands, 1999, pp. 37–55.

47. Segers P, De Backer JF, Devos D, Rabben SI, Gillebert TC, Van Bortel L, De Sutter J, De Paepe A, Verdonck PR, Aortic reflection coefficients and their association with global indices of wave reflection in healthy controls and patients with Marfan disease, *American Journal of Physiology: Heart and Circulatory Physiology*, 290, 2006, H2385–H2392.

48. Fielden SW, Fornwalt BK, Jerosch-Herold M, Eisner RL, Stillman AE, Oshinski JN, A new method for the determination of aortic pulse wave velocity using cross-correlation on 2D PCMR velocity data, *Journal of Magnetic Resonance Imaging*, 27, 2008, 1382–1387.

49. Yu HY, Peng HH, Wang JL, Wen CY, Tseng WYI, Quantification of the pulse wave velocity of the descending aorta using axial velocity profiles from phase-contrast magnetic resonance imaging, *Magnetic Resonance in Medicine*, 56, 2006, 876–883.

50. Parczyk M, Herold V, Klug G, Bauer WR, Rommel E, Jakob PM, Regional in vivo transit time measurements of aortic pulse wave velocity in mice with high-field CMR at 17.6 Tesla, *Journal of Cardiovascular Magnetic Resonance*, 12(72), 2010.

51. Mohiaddin RH, Age-related changes of human aortic flow wave velocity measured non-invasively by magnetic resonance imaging, *Journal of Applied Physiology*, 74, 1993, 492–497.

52. Segers P, Kips J, Trachet B, Swillens A, Vermeersch S, Mahieub D, Rietzschelc E, De Buyzerec M, Van Bortelb L, Limitations and pitfalls of non-invasive measurement of arterial pressure wave reflections and pulse wave velocity, *Artery Research*, 3, 2009, 79–88.

53. Boutouyrie P, Vermeersch SJ, Determinants of pulse wave velocity in healthy people and in the presence of cardiovascular risk factors: Establishing normal and reference values, *European Heart Journal*, 31, 2010, 2338–2350.

13

Simulation of Blood Flow in Idealized and Patient-Specific Coronary Arteries with Curvatures, Stenoses, Dilatations, and Side-Branches

Kelvin K.L. Wong, Dhanjoo N. Ghista, Jianhuang Wu, and Guiying Liu

CONTENTS

13.1 Introduction

13.1.1 Literature Survey: Modeling and Simulation of Coronary Arterial Hemodynamics, Vessel Wall Mechanics, and Atherosclerotic Plaque Formation

It is well established that hemodynamics and vessel wall mechanics play important roles in the initiation, development, and rupture of plaques [1,2]. Plaque progression may cause redistribution of the stresses within the vessel wall. When the stresses within the diseased arterial wall exceed their strength limit, rupture can occur. A clogged fluid domain creates significant flow resistance, large pressure drop, and wall motion patterns [3,4]. There is a complex question regarding the precise relationship between hemodynamic mechanical factors and atherosclerotic changes in the arterial wall. Studies on stenosis and plaque structure [3,5,6] have demonstrated the importance of a two-way fluid–structure interaction (FSI) analysis in stenosis arteries. It is important to understand how the flow features and the stress field change with the development of stenosis.

In addition, the acute onset of coronary heart disease causes a sharp decline in coronary blood supply with associated clinical manifestations such as myocardial infarcts. Therefore, this motivates us to study the stress over the arterial surface and within the arterial walls. In order to achieve a higher realism in our simulation, FSI is used to study the effects of solid structural deformation due to flow field changes, which can better reveal the relationship between arterial hemodynamics and atherosclerotic plaques. Numerical simulation is the ideal method of studying blood flow in diseased arteries, when in vivo or in vitro experimentation is not feasible; then, numerical simulation provides an alternative way to obtain detailed flow patterns. It is currently recognized by most scholars [5,7] the simulation of blood flow within blood vessels by using the FSI simulation methods closer to the physiological state.

Numerical simulation is now widely employed in the hemodynamic analyses of aorta, and the carotid and coronary arteries under physiological and pathological conditions [8–10]. Numerous studies have shown that the values of wall shear stress (WSS) are higher at the outer wall than at the inner wall of curved coronary artery [11]. It is found, through numerical simulation, that the local low WSS often appears in plaque-prone areas [12,13]. A local high WSS area induces the growth and rupture of the plaque by producing endothelial injury and disruption [14,15]. For the blood vessel with more complex curvature and stenosis, the WSS value and the pressure drop ΔP (between the proximal inlet and distal outlet) are much larger, which increases the severity of atherosclerosis [16]. Works on the wall pressure distribution and associated atherosclerosis [17] report that local low wall pressure is strongly correlated to atherosclerosis. Giannoglou et al. [18] have obtained the result that low wall pressure occurs at regions, which are anatomic sites prone to atherosclerotic plaques development, and that the locations of low wall pressure regions are consistent with those of low WSS; hence, they concluded that low wall pressure could be another Evaluation Index for predicting plaque-prone sites.

Further, coronary arteries display localized atherosclerotic plaques throughout their length. Based on imaging studies of intravascular ultrasound [19] and multidetector CT angiography [20], it is observed that atherosclerotic plaques develop more frequently on the myocardial side of the vessel wall and on the proximal part that is predisposed to eccentric intimal thickening in autopsy and histological studies [12,21].

It can be noted from the literature that atherosclerotic plaques are located at low WSS and wall pressure regions and are closely associated with the localized stress concentrations. These researches have led to the hypothesis that different flow patterns may determine the relative deposition and orientation of localized coronary artery disease, along with the relationship between regions of atheromas and anatomical features of coronary artery. However, it is unclear from the literature as to the precise quantitative trends of wall stress with progression of stenosis severity in the blood vessels. The aim of this work is to (1) develop an arterial stenosis models, which incorporate FSI and realistic boundary conditions, and (2) use this models to investigate the WSS, wall pressure, and von Mises stress associated with the development of atheromas in both idealized and realistic patient-specific arteries.

Atherosclerosis is the main disease of the large and medium arteries (e.g., carotid, aorta, and other proximal arteries) and tends to be localized in regions of curvature and branching in arteries. Right coronary arteries (RCAs) display localized atherosclerotic plaques throughout their length. These atherosclerotic plaques develop more frequently on the myocardial side of the vessel wall and on the proximal part, which is shown to be predisposed to eccentric intimal thickening in autopsy and histological studies [12,21–23], and imaging studies [19,20] of intravascular ultrasound and multidetector CT angiography.

Using numerical simulation, researchers have confirmed that there are more complex hemodynamic changes in S-shaped curved arteries, in terms of the large changes of pressure and WSS [24]. It has been found that atherosclerotic plaques and wall thickenings in left and right coronary arteries are localized almost exclusively on (1) the outer wall of one or both daughter vessels at major bifurcations and T-junctions, and (2) along the inner wall of curved segments, where WSS is low [11,13,25]. It has been demonstrated that WSS is clearly different in the case of small bifurcation angle in comparison to the large bifurcation angle, due to the complex hemodynamic flow effect of the bifurcation angle variation [26,27].

Further it has been discovered that high WSS also induce plaque growth and rupture; moreover, high WSS can induce plaque growth at bifurcations by producing endothelial injury and disruption [15,28,29]. Also, large WSS gradients can induce morphological and functional changes in the endothelium in regions of disturbed flow and promote the occurrence of plaque [14,30].

In addition to these atherosclerotic factors, the stress development within the arterial wall has a direct effect on the induced pressure in the flow field. Works on the wall pressure distribution and associated atherosclerosis report that low wall pressure gradient (WPG) is strongly correlated to atherosclerosis [17,18]. Thus, the locations of low and high WPG at high curvature and branch points are consistent with that of low and high WSS; hence, low and high WPG could be another "Evaluation Index" for predicting plaque-prone sites.

In conclusion, it is widely available in the literature that plaques locate at less intensified WSS and WPG regions and are closely associated with the local WSSs. These researches have led to the hypothesis that disturbed flow patterns are associated with the deposition and orientation of localized coronary artery disease; further, there appears to be a strong relationship between regions of atheromas and anatomical features of RCAs. However, it is unclear from literature as to the precise quantitative trends of WSS and WPG on different curvatures and angulations; no one has quantitatively analyzed the relationship between these hemodynamic parameters and the geometry variations in RCAs with side-branches and hemodynamics. As regards whether (1) low or high WSS are sites of atherosclerotic plaques, (2) low or high WPG are sites of atherosclerotic plaques, (3) low or high WSS gradients and WPG contribute to the development of plaque, we will determine the locations of low and high WSS and WPG regions, and thereby state the possible locations of plaques.

Computational models are adept at simulating flow in blood vessels with complicated geometries [25,31], such as the ones shown in Figure 13.1. There is a strong interest in minimally invasive operational techniques that predict the resistance to flow, caused by the impingement of atherosclerotic lesions into the lumen and the subsequent extra shear stresses on the wall [3]. Stenosed and curved arteries have been suggested as the physiological biomedical engineering model of this situation. The generation of hemodynamic parametric data, such as WSS and WPG, by this model can be more helpful in enabling cardiologists to strategize ideal medical treatment after diagnosis.

Clinically, surgeons and physicians define the degree of atherosclerosis by measuring the percentage of reduction of the vessel lumen due to accumulation of atherosclerotic plaque [32–34]. However, simply measuring the plaque height is not sufficient for clinical decision-making, as it is not the sole parameter affecting arterial flow resistance; the proportion of the diseased segment of the atherosclerotic artery and the degree of bending are also important parameters of consideration. We are providing the anatomical examination of geometrical parameters, such as arterial curvature

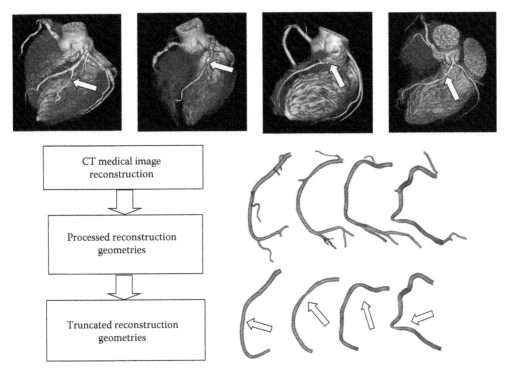

FIGURE 13.1
3D CT visualization of arteries in patient with suspected coronary disease. The arteries can be seen as a combination of various curved segments with stenoses at unspecific locations. The stenoses are observed to occur at the inner bend of the arteries as highlighted by the arrows.

α and plaque height d, that pertain to an atherosclerotic artery with an irregular curvilinear bend and their effect on the resistance to blood flow, by using and computing a series of different fluid mechanical parameters.

The adjustment of normal flow due to the growth of plaque affects the blood flow in the artery, and plaque vulnerability results in the coronary arterial disease. Vascular surgery, which is based on techniques such as balloon angioplasty [35–37], grafting coronary artery bypass [38], stenting [39] or endarterectomy [40], aims to improve blood circulation in the segment of the heart associated with the stenosed coronary artery. The localization of the diseased arterial segment and knowledge of the blood flow properties in the inspected vessel is a prerequisite in treatment planning [41]. As such, geometrical parameters (such as the number and degree of occlusions) and the abnormal deformation of artery due to the stenosis and dilatations, material properties (such as the elasticity of the arterial wall), as well as hemodynamic parameters (such as WSS, WPG, and pressure drop across the network of oxygen supplying arteries) can allow physicians to gain more insight into the coronary arterial disease and plaque growth progression.

The arterial flow parameters have been introduced and discussed thoroughly by Pincombe and Mazumdar [42–44] who have analyzed flow through atherosclerotic arteries in detail, whereby the dependent flow variables of interest are the flow resistance ratio and the WSS ratio. The former measures change in blood flow flux through the abnormal arterial segment and is effectively the ratio of flow pressure drop (FPD) of the diseased artery to that of the normal healthy one, while the latter is a measure of the shear forces along the arterial wall. An accurate measure of reduced blood flow caused by the stenosed arteries is important for assessing the degree of atherosclerosis for patients, and also indirectly assesses how oxygen-starved the tissues supplied by the artery have become.

13.1.2 Chapter Overview

In this chapter, we present simulations of blood flow in idealized and patient-specific coronary arteries with curvatures, stenoses, dilatations, and side-branches. The chapter is divided into four sections.

In Section 13.2, we present analysis of transient blood flow in a curved coronary artery with progressive amounts of stenosis and determine the variation of WSS and WPG with the degree of stenosis. Herein, computational modeling of atherosclerotic arteries has been performed, by taking into consideration the structural modifications of stenosis variations. A two-way FSI analysis is carried out between the blood vessel wall and the blood in elastic arteries with eccentric stenotic plaques, by employing ANSYS Mechanical and CFX modules. The boundary conditions of time-varying velocity and pressure waves are applied at the inlet and outlet of the artery. This information provides insight into the formation of plaque and its vulnerability.

In Section 13.3, we present analysis of blood flow in coronary arteries with varying degrees of curvature and stenosis and determine the WSS and WPG profiles in idealized artery models and realistic arteries. Our results show that increasing values of WSS, *WPG*, and *FPD* are associated with the increasing narrowing of the lumen and degree of curvature. This flow response to arterial variability framework can be used to supplement the angiographic assessment of occlusion due to lesion development in curvilinear atherosclerotic coronary arteries. The WSS and WPG plots of four patient-specific right coronary arteries (RCAs) are then carried out, to illustrate the effectiveness of our parametric study in examination of flow through idealized curved and stenosed vessels. It is observed that the WSS is maximal in the stenotic region and its maximum value increases with the curvature of the artery. The wall pressure demonstrates a similar effect, whereby it is maximum for the most curved artery. All of these results have close agreement and trends with the results obtained for the idealized arteries.

In Section 13.4, we present analysis of blood flow in straight coronary arteries with varying degrees of stenosis and dilatations. Herein, we are concerned with pulsatile flow through partially occluded arteries, to determine the hemodynamic parameters of WSS and WPG contributory to enhanced flow resistance and myocardial ischemic regions that impair cardiac contractility and cause increased work load on the heart. This investigation is undertaken by working on a set of simulations of blood flow in a straight artery containing stenotic and dilatational deformities. The results indicate that both WSS and WPG properties are shown to demonstrate significant increments at segments where the artery is more stenosed. The opposite occurs for dilatations but at much lower magnitudes. For the narrowest sections, the WSS and WPG values are significantly enhanced.

In Section 13.5, we study blood flow in right coronary arteries with varying degrees of curvature and side-branch bifurcation angles. Therein, we have employed CFD to computationally analyze the WSS and WPG variations in idealized and realistic RCA models, to (1) determine the distribution map of WSS and WPG in RCAs, by taking into account their curvatures and bifurcations; and (2) evaluate the variations of average WSS (defined as $\overline{WSS}$) on the vessel wall and pressure drop (ΔP) across the arterial inlet and outlet. Our study results have (1) confirmed that low WSS regions are located at the inner wall of the arterial curve and opposite to the flow divider and (2) depicted increased values of $\overline{WSS}$ and ΔP with higher values of curvature angle α and branch bifurcation angle γ. We can then postulate that in RCAs, the atherosclerotic plaques are more prone to be located at the relatively low WSS and WPG sites of the curved arterial trunk and its branch for arbitrary degrees of curvature.

Throughout this chapter, we have clearly presented the governing equations of modeling blood flow through idealized and realistic arteries of varying curvature amounts, stenosis and dilatation amounts, and bifurcations. The blood flow is governed by the incompressible Navier–Stokes equation and Continuity equation; for the solid segment of the artery, the elastic mechanics equation of motion are employed; the coupling of the fluid and solid domains is carried out by means of the compatibility equations of stress and displacement. The two-way FSI analysis between the blood vessel wall (and its constitutive properties) and the blood has thus been carried out. The flow simulation is based on the physiologically realistic boundary conditions of pulsatile blood flow velocity and pressure boundary conditions at inlet and outlet of the artery, acquired with an electrocardiography-gated intravascular ultrasound Doppler and pressure probe. We have provided the details of the computational methods to solve the governing blood flow FSI simulation analysis; the solid domain is constructed in the ANSYS solver, while the fluid domain is modeled in the CFX solver. Then, we have presented the results of the hemodynamic parameters, and their bearing on the formation of atherosclerotic plaques. This chapter can provide the basis for analyzing patient-specific coronary arteries and determining the risk of atherosclerotic plaque formation in these arteries.

13.2 Blood Flow in a Curved Coronary Artery with Progressive Amounts of Stenosis: Analysis of Wall Shear and Wall Pressure Gradients

In this section, we analyze transient blood flow through idealized models of elastic atherosclerotic arteries with eccentric stenotic plaques, by means of computational fluid dynamics. The two-way FSI analysis between the blood vessel wall and the blood is carried out in ANSYS mechanical and computational fluid dynamics (CFD) modules, by using the finite element method. The simulation is based on the boundary conditions of pulsatile blood flow velocity and pressure boundary conditions at inlet and outlet of the artery. The hemodynamic analysis computation of average wall shear stress ($\overline{AWSS}$) over the arterial surface, pressure drop (ΔP) between inlet and outlet of the artery, and von Mises stress at the throat of the stenosis are carried out, for varying degrees of lumen stenosis. The results show that increasing values of $\overline{WSS}$, ΔP, and von Mises stress are in positive correlation with the increasing narrowing of the lumen. Our FSI framework also examines the influence of the variability in curvilinear arterial wall geometry on the blood flow characteristics. This study can be used to provide the biomedical engineering basis of the angiographic assessment of occlusion due to lesion development in curvilinear atherosclerotic coronary arteries.

We study transient blood flow through idealized elastic atherosclerotic coronary arteries, based on medical imaging and computational fluid dynamics. In order to establish an accurate and reliable blood flow response in coronary arteries with varying stenosis due to plaque formation, we have carried out a detailed hemodynamic parametric analysis of an idealized model of a realistic arterial geometry, by incorporating the two-way FSI framework. In order to achieve realism in this simulation, we have employed physiologically realistic pulsatile blood flow velocity and pressure boundary conditions at the inlet and outlet of the artery.

13.2.1 Blood Flow Modeling

We are determining the fluid mechanics properties in high curvature coronary arterial sites of occurrence of atherosclerotic plaques. We have developed a model of blood flow through a highly curved artery, based on the degree of lumen stenosis. The model is simulated by assuming that the stenosis on the curved portion is eccentric. Figure 13.2 shows the general geometrical form of the model developed in our study. In the sketch of the longitudinal section of the curved artery in Figure 13.2, the angle a of the arc for the curved part is supposed to be 90°; D_s, D_l and D_w are the diameter of the vessel at the throat of the plaque, the length, and the height of plaque on the inner wall based on the curve, respectively (Table 13.1).

Physiologically, a plaque grows longitudinally and laterally, with a greater degree of lumen stenosis. In Figure 13.3, L_2 is the length of the plaque measured from the outer wall of the fluid domain of length of 35.3 mm; L_1 (10 mm) and L_3 (40 mm) are the lengths of the straight tube segments prior to and immediately after the bend. The vessel wall thickness H_s = 0.8 mm at the unobstructed parts. In all the cases, the unobstructed diameter D_f is

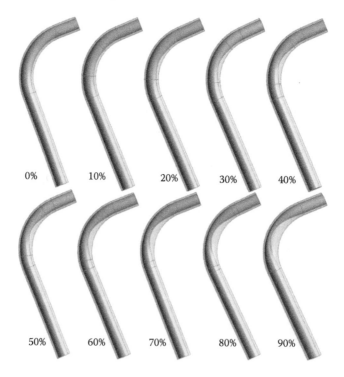

FIGURE 13.2

The coronary arteries with and without eccentric stenosis arranged from 10% to 90% based on area stenosis percentage. The colored parts are blood, while the transparent parts are the vessel wall and plaques. The stenosis site is in the most curved segment of the artery.

TABLE 13.1

Height (D_w) and Length (D_l) of the Plaques on the Inner Wall of a Curved Coronary Artery

S (%)	0	10	20	30	40	50	60	70	80	90
D_l (mm)	0	5.50	8.24	10.99	13.74	16.49	19.24	21.98	24.73	27.48
D_w (mm)	0	0.23	0.47	0.74	1.01	1.32	1.65	2.04	2.79	3.08

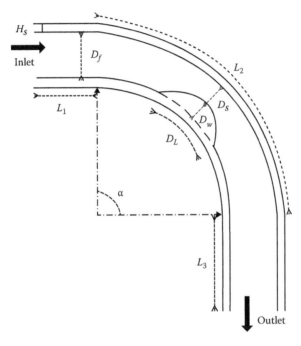

FIGURE 13.3
The longitudinal section of a curved plaqued coronary artery model. The inlet L_1 (10 mm) and outlet L_3 (40 mm) are extended parts to minimize the influence of boundary conditions.

4.5 mm; the degree of stenosis ($S\%$) is determined by the percentage of cross-sectional area occluded at the throat of the stenosis.

13.2.1.1 Numerical Analysis Details of FSI Simulation

A hexahedral finite element mesh is generated by using CFX-mesh software. The grid independence analysis is performed for: coarse, medium, and fine grid numbering about 132,000 elements, 347,000 elements, and 786,000 elements, respectively. FSI simulation is carried out with ANSYS Mechanical and CFX modules. The fluid flow is considered to be 3D, transient, isothermal, and incompressible. The arterial wall is modeled as a nonlinear isotropic and hyperelastic incompressible homogeneous material.

It has long been recognized that a high percentage of cardiovascular disease is associated with a hardening of the vessel wall or arteriosclerosis [45]. Increased stiffness of the vessel wall has gained acceptance as a fundamental risk factor for cardiovascular and many other diseases [46]. We have used a constant Young's modulus of 5 MPa and Poisson coefficient of 0.499 for the hardened incompressible arterial wall. The no slip wall boundary condition is also adopted.

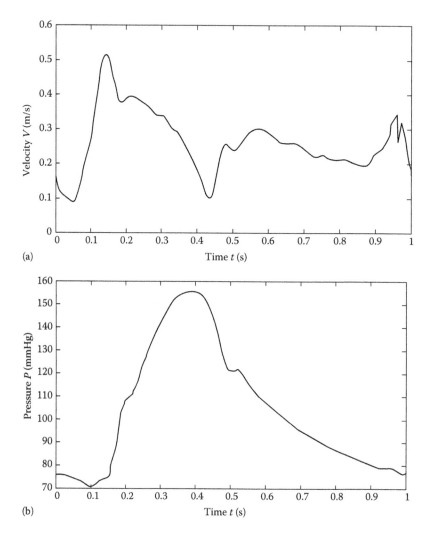

FIGURE 13.4
Physiological waveforms of velocity and pressure of inlets and outlets. The waveforms present the velocity variation (a) and pressure variation (b) in one cardiac cycle. The velocity waveform is in m/s and the pressure waveform is in mmHg.

Then, as regards the inflow–outflow boundary conditions, the time-varying velocity wave is applied at the inlet and the time-varying pressure wave is applied at the outlet (Figure 13.4), both of which were simultaneously acquired with an electrocardiography-gated intravascular ultrasound Doppler and pressure probe (ComboWire®, Volcano Corporation) in the proximal and distal artery of a suspected patient, with confirmation of unobstructed coronary artery [47]. For FSI simulation, the proximal and distal ends of the arteries are taken to be fixed, with no axial or transaxial motion.

The blood flow is governed by the incompressible Navier–Stokes equation and Continuity equation as follows:

$$\rho \frac{\partial v}{\partial t} + \rho(v \cdot \nabla)v = -\nabla P + \rho g + \mu \nabla^2 v \tag{13.1}$$

$$\nabla \cdot v = 0 \tag{13.2}$$

where
  ρ is the blood density of 1050 kg/m³
  v is the velocity
  P is the pressure
  g is the gravity constant
  μ is the dynamic viscosity of 0.035 g/cm s

For the solid segment of the artery, the elastic mechanics equation of motion is adopted (under conditions of ignoring gravity) as shown below:

$$\rho_s \frac{d^2 u_i}{dt^2} = \sigma_{ij,j} \quad (i, j = 1, 2, 3) \tag{13.3}$$

where
  σ is the stress tensor
  u is the displacement
  ρ_s is the density of the artery material

Compatibility equations of stress (τ) and displacement (u) on the coupling of fluid (f) and solid (s) domain are as follows:

$$\tau_f \cdot n_f = \tau_s \cdot n_s \tag{13.4}$$

$$u_f = u_s \tag{13.5}$$

Equation 13.4 implies that the normal component of the stress is transferred by the fluid onto the solid at the interacting point, and Equation 13.5 indicates that the displacements of the fluid and solid domain interaction nodes are equal.

The solid domain is constructed in the ANSYS solver, while the fluid domain is modeled in the CFX solver. The coupling between the solid and fluid domains is from the "setup" of the two solvers. Once the simulation is run in the "solution" window, it first begins computing iterations for the fluid domain by initiating the CFX solver, and then progresses onto the solid domain in the ANSYS solver.

Partitioned approach is used to implement FSI capability in the commercial software. Coupling between the ANSYS and CFX solvers is performed many times, until convergence of interface variables (such as displacements and pressure) is reached. At each coupling loop, the calculation of blood flow is initiated. Then, the calculated pressure field is transferred and used as an applied force in the solid solver to calculate the deformation of the artery.

In the transient analysis, the time period T of one cardiac cycle is 1.0 s, yielding a heart rate of about 60 beats/min. All simulations are carried out for three cardiac cycles, and then the variables presented in the following are collected in the third cycle. The time step was set to be 0.01 s. In the solution setting, a high resolution for advection and second order backward Euler for transient scheme is used. The convergence criterion of each time step for the relative residuals of all the dependent variables was set as 0.0001. In solving, the convergence criterion of each time step for the relative residual could reach the value of 0.0001.

13.2.2 Flow Quantification and Analysis of Stenosed Arteries

The flow simulation in the arterial vessels is performed with FSI, under the in vivo physiological conditions during the systolic and diastolic phases. The analysis results demonstrate a strong relationship between hemodynamics and percentage stenosis. All the results are collected at peak systole, when the velocity of inlet reaches the maximum. A comparative analysis of the distribution of WSS and WPG over the blood vessel wall has been conducted for varying degrees of stenosis. Then, the $\overline{AWSS}$ and the pressure drop ΔP between the inlet and outlet of the artery are computed as shown in the following and then plotted with respect to the percentage of stenotic occlusion.

13.2.2.1 Wall Shear Stress

The WSS is the shear stress experienced by the vessel wall during the flow of blood. Through the calculation of WSS, we are further exploring the WSS difference owing to different degree of stenosis of the blood vessel. The WSS is given by

$$WSS(\tau_\omega) = -\mu \frac{\partial u_t}{\partial n} \bigg| \text{wall} \tag{13.6}$$

where
   μ is the dynamic viscosity
   u_t is the wall tangential velocity
   n is the unit vector that is vertical to the vessel wall

The average WSS ($\overline{WSS}$) over the surface of the artery is given by

$$\overline{WSS} = \frac{\iiint_D \tau_\omega(x,y,z)d_x d_y d_z}{\|D\|} \tag{13.7}$$

where
   $\tau_\omega(x, y, z)$ is the WSS in the point (x, y, z)
   $\|D\|$ is the area of the blood vessel walls
   $d_x d_y d_z$ is the integral of WSS in the curved vessel

The average WSS ($\overline{WSS}$) ratio λ_1 is defined as λ_1

$$\lambda_1 = \frac{\overline{WSS_0}}{\overline{WSS_n}} \tag{13.8}$$

where
   $\overline{WSS_0}$ is the AWSS value of the unobstructed vessel at peak systole
   $\overline{WSS_n}$ pertains to that of obstructed vessels

Figure 13.5 presents the contour plot of the WSS distribution for the stenosed arteries. We can see that the values of WSS are lower at the outer wall than at the inner wall, for all the arteries.

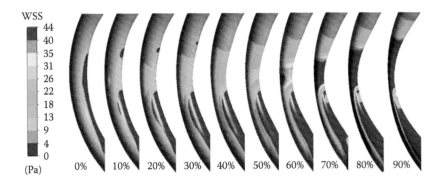

FIGURE 13.5
Detailed WSS contour plot, showing the development of wall shear stress profiles on the intima of arteries. The WSS is shown to demonstrate a larger variation with greater percentage stenosis.

TABLE 13.2

$\overline{WSS}$ Ratio (λ_1) and ΔP Ratio (λ_2) with Respect to Percentage of Occlusion

S (%)	0	10	20	30	40	50	60	70	80	90
λ_1	1.00	1.02	1.04	1.08	1.14	1.24	1.41	1.71	2.41	5.06
λ_2	1.00	1.02	1.06	1.13	1.26	1.54	2.11	3.44	7.33	30.41

Specifically, the region of WSS $\leq$ 4 Pa is generally located at the outer wall of the curved vessel, and the local high WSS ($\geq$40 Pa) emerges at the inner wall in the stenosis region when the stenosis degree is 60%. As the stenosis becomes more serious, the areas of local high WSS and $\overline{WSS}$ of the vessel become larger. With the stenosis degree of 60%, 70%, 80%, and 90%, the WSS parameter λ_1 becomes 1.41, 1.71, 2.41, and 5.06 times the normal value, respectively (Table 13.2). Therefore, the WSS value will also increase considerably for the blood vessel having more extensive stenosis. However, the relatively high WSS regions are always occurring at the inner wall.

13.2.2.2 Wall Pressure Gradient Distribution

We determine the pressure drop ΔP between the inlet and outlet of an elastic blood vessel. The reference model is the curved artery without stenosis, and its pressure drop is designated as ΔP_n. The pressure drop ratio between the stenosis model and this reference model is also known as the flow resistance ratio [4] and is calculated by means of the following equations:

$$\text{WPG} = \sqrt{\left(\frac{\partial_p}{\partial_x}\right)^2 + \left(\frac{\partial_p}{\partial_y}\right)^2 + \left(\frac{\partial_p}{\partial_z}\right)^2} \qquad (13.9)$$

$$\overline{P} = \frac{\iiint_D P(x,y,z)dxdydz}{\|D\|} \qquad (13.10)$$

$$\Delta P = \bar{P}_{inlet} - \bar{P}_{outlet} \tag{13.11}$$

$$\lambda_2 = \frac{\Delta P_0}{\Delta P_n} \tag{13.12}$$

where

P is the wall static pressure

x, y, and z are the 3D coordinates in space

$\bar{P}$ is the mean static pressure

P (x, y, and z) is the pressure at the point (x, y, and z)

$\|D\|$ is the area of the blood vessel wall

dx, dy, and dz are the infinitesimal lengths of integration of pressure over the curved surface in the x, y, and z directions

In Equation 13.12, λ_2 is the ratio of ΔP_0 and ΔP_n, the pressure drops pertaining to the atherosclerotic artery and to the normal artery, respectively.

As shown in Figure 13.6, the distribution of the pressure in the curved blood vessel wall is irregular and segmental, and the pressure at the inlet is overall larger than at the outlet. The variation of pressure drop is greater with increased amount of vessel stenosis.

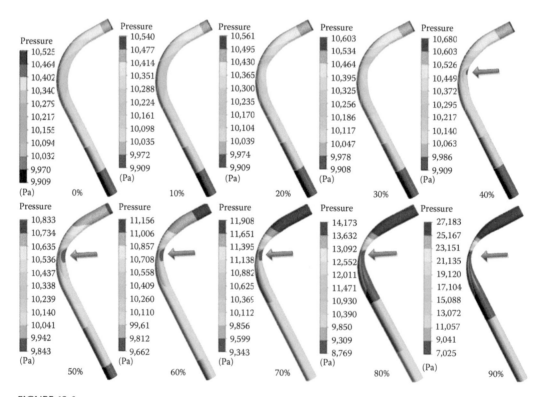

FIGURE 13.6

Detailed WPG contour plot showing the development of wall pressure gradient profiles on the intima of arteries. The arrow shows the local low pressure region occurs at the inner wall of the curved vessel.

When the strain in the stenosis segment reaches 40%, the atheromatous plaque inside the curved vessel emerges into the partial low pressure area in the narrowest region. This phenomenon becomes more obvious with increased stenosis. When the strain in the stenosis segment reaches 60%, the low pressure occurs at the inner wall of the curved vessel and is lower than in the distal part of the artery. Corresponding to the stenosis degree of 50%, 60%, 70%, 80%, and 90%, the value of the pressure drop parameter λ_2 is 1.54, 2.11, 3.44, 7.33, and 30.41 times the normal value, respectively (Table 13.2). Therefore, the wall pressure will also vary considerably for the blood vessel having more serious stenosis.

With the emergence of atheromatous plaque, the distribution of WSS also changes. In other words, the local low WSS region area along the bend moves downstream along the inner bend. As shown in Figure 13.5, with the increase of the stenosis degree, the local high WSS area spreads to the inner bend of the arterial throat, which promotes the continued development of atheromatous plaque. At the same time, the risk of the rupture of the atherosclerosis plaque also increases. When the stenosis becomes 40%, the WPG increases in the narrowest portion of the bend along the inner bend where the atheromatous plaque resides, along with a similar increase in local WSS. It is to be noted that turbulent blood flow can also accelerate the deposition of platelets in the blood on the atheromatous plaque and causing it to increase in volume and grow in the direction of blood flow. This phenomenon is consistent with the various existing studies [18,48].

13.2.2.3 von Mises Stress on the Throat Section of the Stenosis

The von Mises stress is often used for determining whether an isotropic and ductile metal will yield when subjected to a complex loading condition. This is accomplished by calculating the von Mises stress and comparing it to the material's yield stress, which constitutes the von Mises Yield Criterion. Recently, von Mises stress has been used in the numerical simulation of flow [49]. In our study, it is calculated as follows:

$$\sigma_{von\,Mises} = \frac{\sqrt{2}}{2}\sqrt{(\sigma_1 - \sigma_2)^2 + (\sigma_2 - \sigma_3)^2 + (\sigma_3 - \sigma_1)^2} \tag{13.13}$$

where σ_1, σ_2, and σ_3 are the principle stresses.

As shown in Figure 13.7, von Mises stress is nonuniformly distributed at the throat of the stenosis. It is higher on the inner wall for the unobstructed artery, while lower for the obstructed artery. The distribution of von Mises stress does not greatly vary with increased height of the plaques; it is found that the von Mises stress is highest on the intima, followed by the media and adventitia.

The principal stresses σ_1, σ_2, and σ_3 are determined in the vessel wall via force on the wall divided by unit area. The pressure data are employed to compute the principal stresses, which can then be used to generate the von Mises stress using Equation 13.13.

Quantitatively, the values of the von Mises stress are of great importance. As shown in Table 13.3, the increase in minimum and maximum of von Mises stress is positively correlated with the increased height of the plaques based on the unobstructed vessel wall. In the middle section of the unobstructed vessel wall, the maximum value of von Mises stress is 21.05 kPa. When the strain in the stenosis reaches 90%, the maximum value reaches to 43.33 kPa, which is twice that in the unobstructed vessel, and hence implies greater rupture risk in the more obstructed vessels [50,51].

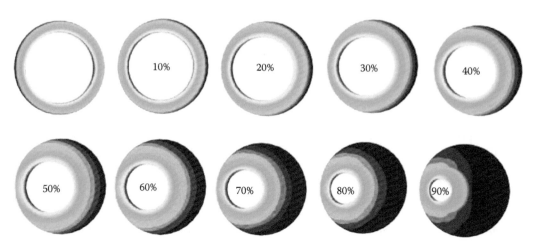

FIGURE 13.7

The contour of von Mises stress on the throat of the stenosis. The first cross section is vessel wall of the unobstructed one and the rest are of the obstructed ones.

TABLE 13.3

Minimum and Maximum of von Mises Stress at the Throat of the Stenosis

S (%)	0	10	20	30	40	50	60	70	80	90
Min (kPa)	0.34	0.53	0.99	2.02	3.14	4.97	7.46	11.06	16.25	21.70
Max (kPa)	21.05	23.37	26.74	29.02	30.97	33.15	35.13	36.32	38.64	43.33

13.2.3 Concluding Comments

The extensive flow information generated by our work can be used to gain insight into the formation of plaque and its vulnerability. Herein, computational modeling of atherosclerotic arteries has been performed, by taking into consideration the structural modifications of stenosis variations.

We can note that with the emergence of atheromatous plaque and stenosis percentage increase, the WSS distribution also changes. As the stenosis increases, the local high WSS area spreads to the inner bend of the arterial throat, which promotes the development of atheromatous plaque. When the stenosis becomes 40%, the WPG increases in the narrowest portion of the bend, with corresponding increased flow resistance along the artery. The von Mises stress also increases with the increased height of the plaques, with increased rupture risk.

13.3 Blood Flow in Coronary Arteries with Varying Degrees of Curvature and Stenosis: WSS and WPG Profiles in Idealized Artery Models and Realistic Arteries

13.3.1 Arteries with Varying Degrees of Curvatures and Stenosis

Herein, hemodynamic analysis is carried out for hemodynamic fluid parameters of AWSS over the arterial surface, WPG, and flow pressure drop (FPD) between inlet and outlet of the artery, based on the degree of lumen stenosis and curvature (based on the radius of the arterial bend curvature). We have conducted this elaborate analysis for both idealistic coronary arteries as well as patient-specific coronary arteries (arteries modeled as vessels with elastic walls). Our results show that increasing values of AWSS, WPG, and *FPD* are associated with the increasing narrowing of the lumen and degree of curvature. This flow response to arterial variability framework can be used to supplement the angiographic assessment of occlusion due to plaque lesion development in curvilinear atherosclerotic coronary arteries.

Prior to studying the realistic arteries constructed from medical images, it is necessary to reduce the complexities involved in the simulations by first (1) designing a set of idealized arteries based on a limited number of geometrical parameters, determining the correlations between their fluid mechanical properties and geometrical variations, and then (2) relating these relationships to the complex real arteries. The geometrical parameters are (as depicted in Figure 13.8 and Table 13.4) (1) the radius R (mm) from the center of arc to the arterial curve extended by angle α (radian) and (2) the percentage of occlusion S (%) that is dependent on the height of arterial throat d (mm).

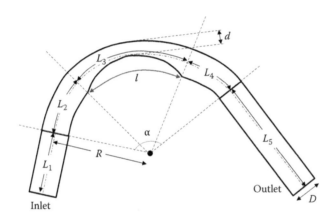

FIGURE 13.8
Model of a curved artery with a plaque in the inner wall of its curved segment: axial variation of arterial wall with lesion (or plaque) development in the sagittal plane. A single lesion segment is presented from the proximal to the distal end for the case of stenosis. The geometry of the simulated models follows the stenosis height and curvilinear configurations of the main artery (based on height d and the angle α). An aneurysm or dilatation can be constructed by negating the value of diseased wall height. The occlusion percentage $S = (D - d)/D\%$.

TABLE 13.4

Variation of Geometrical Parameters to Attain the Idealistic Arteries in Our Parametric Analysis

S (%)	0	20	40	60	80
d (mm)	4.5	4.4249	3.8857	3.2460	2.4125
α (rad)	$\dfrac{\pi}{6}$	$\dfrac{\pi}{3}$	$\dfrac{\pi}{2}$	$\dfrac{2\pi}{3}$	$\dfrac{5\pi}{6}$
R (mm)	57.32	28.66	19.11	14.33	11.465

The geometries of the idealistic models were designed based on the percentage of occlusion S (%) that is dependent on the height of arterial throat d (mm), as well as the radius R (mm) from the center of arc to the arterial curve extended by angle α (rad).

The feature of a coronary artery is mainly its bending and branching; the inner bent side of a curved segment is prone to plaque formation [12,13,21]. Figure 13.8 illustrates the model of the longitudinal section of a curved artery with a plaque in its inner wall.

Figure 13.8 presents a curved arterial segment with $\alpha \geq 30°$, the diameter of vessel lumen $D = 4.5$ mm, the thickness of vessel wall $H_s = 0.8$ mm, the straight length of inlet $L_1 = 10$ mm, the outside length of curved segments $L_2 = 7.5$ mm and $L_4 = 7.5$ mm, the straight length of outlet $L_5 = 20$ mm, d is the diameter of vessel lumen in the narrowest plane, $D–d$ is the height of plaque, $L_3 = 15$ mm is the length of the plaque. For different models, the percentage of stenosis corresponding to the area of cross section in the narrowest plane for different values of D and d is shown in Table 13.4.

Figure 13.9 illustrates the pathological variations of arteries as regards the degree of stenosis (S), based on the variation of bend angle (α), as viewed in the sagittal plane. The arterial blood flow path in the vessel is dependent on the parameters α and d, which characterize the curvature and stenosis. The data points designated along the inner surface of the artery are used to determine the hemodynamic flow properties in terms of the hemodynamic parameters.

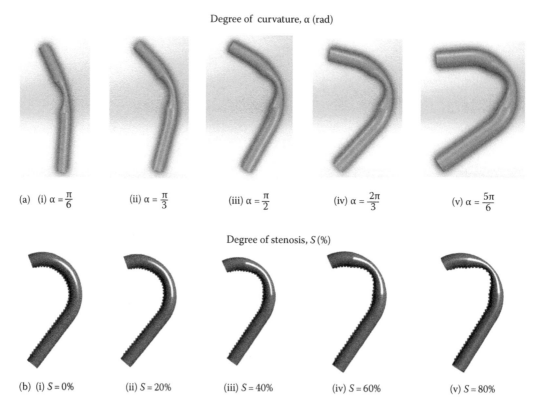

Degree of curvature, α (rad)

(a)   (i) $\alpha = \frac{\pi}{6}$ (ii) $\alpha = \frac{\pi}{3}$ (iii) $\alpha = \frac{\pi}{2}$ (iv) $\alpha = \frac{2\pi}{3}$ (v) $\alpha = \frac{5\pi}{6}$

Degree of stenosis, S (%)

(b)   (i) $S = 0\%$ (ii) $S = 20\%$ (iii) $S = 40\%$ (iv) $S = 60\%$ (v) $S = 80\%$

FIGURE 13.9
Pathological variations of the arterial wall with stenosis based on variation of bend that is viewed in the sagittal plane. The arterial variability in the vessel is dependent on (a) the bend angle α in radians and (b) the occlusion S in percentage, which control the stenosis and curvature, respectively. In this way, the variability of the arterial structuring can be controlled by only two parameters. In (b), the line of data extraction points for our flow analysis is presented by the series of points that lie along the inner wall of the arterial curve, which passes through the apex of the stenosis. For the same bend angle α, we change the degree of stenosis; for the same degree of stenosis, we change the degree of curvature. Here, we are studying the effect of these two parameters on the hemodynamic parameters.

13.3.2 CFD Analysis of Simulated Arteries

The application of medical image reconstruction for modeling blood vessels for CFD analysis has had considerable development in recent years. The typical process for performing numerical simulation of a blood vessel is based on its medical imaging, image segmentation, 3D model reconstruction, grid generation, and flow analysis [52]. The final grid is used for transient numerical simulation of blood flow, with physiological boundary conditions for making the simulation closer to physiological reality.

In this study, we want to examine how the effects of idealistic geometrical variations affect flow, under physiological flow conditions. The arterial wall is modeled as a no-slip wall. At the inlets and outlets, we have interpolated physiologically representative velocity and pressure waveforms [47]. The incompressible Navier–Stokes equations, as described by Equations 13.1 and 13.2, are used as the governing equations. We are also employing equations for the elastic vessel wall motion and compatibility equations between the wall and fluid.

Then, for the boundary conditions, the time-varying velocity is applied at the inlet cross section, while the time-varying pressure is applied at all the outlets for all the simulated arteries (as illustrated in Figure 13.10). For the solution setting, a high resolution for advection and second-order backward Euler for transient scheme is used. In our simulated artery models, in order to minimize the effects of boundary conditions, the inlets and outlets are adequately extended to (1) 10 mm for inlet and (2) 20 mm for outlet.

13.3.2.1 Examined Flow Parameters

Numerous studies show that the occurrence and development of atherosclerosis and the rupture of plaque are closely related to the hemodynamics in the vessel and the mechanical properties of the vascular wall. It is currently recognized in most works [5,7] that the

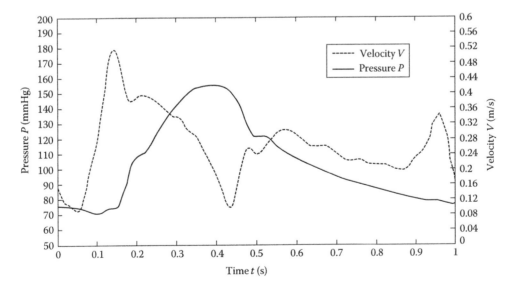

FIGURE 13.10
Physiological waveforms of velocity at inlet and pressure at outlets. The waveforms present the velocity and pressure variations in one cardiac cycle. The velocity waveform is in m/s and the pressure waveform is in mmHg.

simulation of blood flow within blood vessels is closer to the physiological state, by using the finite element FSI simulation method. It is found through numerical simulation that the local low WSS often appears in plaque-prone areas [12,13]; further, autopsy and histopathology reports provide information concerning the severity of the plaque. Local high WSS area induces the growth and rupture of the plaque [14,15]. For the blood vessel with more complex curvature and stenosis, the WSS value and the upstream and downstream flow pressure difference as indicated by the *FPD* (between the proximal inlet and distal outlet) are much larger, which increases the severity of atherosclerosis [16].

When the stenosis appears in a local blood vessel, the progression of plaque can lead to the redistribution of WSS inside the blood vessel wall. As a result of this stress change along the diseased arterial wall, plaque growth and rupture may occur. Before the rupture occurs, the stenosis can cause flow separation and oscillation, resulting in greater pressure drop and flow resistance [4,53]. All of these manifestations characterize the acute onset of coronary heart disease, resulting in a sharp decline in coronary blood supply with the associated clinical manifestations. Therefore, this correlation between the blood flow patterns and hemodynamic parameters associated with the onset of coronary heart disease motivates us to study the WSS and WPG over the arterial surface. In order to achieve a higher realism in our simulation, the fluid–structure coupling analysis (FSI) is used to study the effects of solid structural deformation due to flow field changes, which can help to better reveal the relationship of arterial hemodynamics and the atherosclerotic plaques.

We then determine the hemodynamic parameters of WSS (τ_ω), the $\overline{AWSS}$, the average WSS ratio λ_1 of $\overline{WSS}_0$ (the AWSS value in a particular artery at peak systole) and $\overline{WSS}_n$ (the AWSS in a normal straight artery), as follows.

The WSS is the shear stress experienced by the vessel wall during the flow of blood. We have given its expression earlier by Equation 13.6, but for the sake of convenience give it as

$$WSS(\tau_\omega) = -\mu \frac{\partial u_t}{\partial n} \,|\, \text{wall} \tag{13.14}$$

where
　μ is the dynamic viscosity
　u_t is the wall tangential velocity
　n is the unit vector that is vertical to the vessel wall

Through the calculation of WSS, we further explore the WSS difference owing to different degree of stenosis of the blood vessel.

The average WSS over the surface of the artery is given by Equation 13.7, and we again provide it as

$$AWSS = \overline{WSS} = \frac{\iiint_D \tau_\omega(x,y,z)d_x d_y d_z}{\|D\|} \tag{13.15}$$

where
　$\tau_\omega(x, y, z)$ is the WSS in the point (x, y, z)
　$\|D\|$ is the area of the blood vessel walls
　$d_x d_y d_z$ is the integral of WSS in the curved vessel

The expressions for WSS(τ_ω) and the average wall shear stress $\overline{WSS}$ are given earlier by Equations 13.6 and 13.7.

The average WSS ratio λ_1,

$$\lambda_1 = \frac{\overline{WSS_0}}{\overline{WSS_n}} \tag{13.16}$$

where
$\overline{WSS_0}$ is the AWSS value for a particular artery at peak systole
$\overline{WSS_n}$ pertains to that of a normal straight artery

We next determine the average pressure differences (also termed as the flow pressure drop FPD_0) between the inlet and outlet of an elastic blood vessel. The reference model is the straight artery without stenosis, and its pressure drop is designated as FPD_n. The flow pressure drop ratio between the stenosis model and this reference model is also known as the flow resistance ratio λ_2 [4] and is calculated by means of the following equations:

$$\overline{P} = \frac{\iiint_D P(x,y,z)dxdydz}{\|D\|} \tag{13.17}$$

$$FPD = \overline{P}_{inlet} - \overline{P}_{outlet} \tag{13.18}$$

$$\lambda_2 = \frac{PD_0}{PD_n} \tag{13.19}$$

where
P is the wall static pressure
$\overline{P}$ is the mean static pressure
$P(x, y, z)$ is the pressure of point (x, y, z)
$\|D\|$ is the area of the blood vessel wall

In Equation 13.17, dx, dy, and dz are the infinitesimal lengths for the integration of pressure over the curved surface in the x, y, and z directions. Equation 13.19 gives the ratio λ_2 of pressure drop PD_0 in a particular artery and PDn in a normal straight artery. It is worth noting that the FPD is also positively related to the WPG, since a higher pressure difference across the arterial segment of interest would induce a higher wall pressure. Therefore, WPG is used in our contour plots to show the effect of stenosis in generating a larger FPD.

All the results of these hemodynamic parameters are collected at peak systole, when the velocity of inlet reaches the maximum. A comparative analysis of the distribution of WSS and WPG over the blood vessel wall is conducted for varying degrees of stenosis and curvatures. Then, the AWSS and the pressure difference between the inlet and outlet of the artery are plotted with respect to the percentage of occlusion and arterial bend.

13.3.3 Flow Quantification in Curved and Stenosed Arteries

13.3.3.1 *Flow Analysis in Idealized Curved and Stenosed Arteries*

13.3.3.1.1 Parametric Analysis of WSS Distribution in Idealized Curved and Stenosed Arteries

Figure 13.11 presents the contour plots of WSS distribution for the curved and stenosed arteries. We can see that in a normal curved vessel with a low degree of stenosis, the region of WSS $\leq$ 4 Pa is generally located in the inside segment of the blood vessel. The local high WSS ($\geq$40 Pa) emerges in the stenosis region when the stenosis degree reaches 60%. As the stenosis aggravates, the regions of local high WSS and AWSS of the vessel become larger. When the stenosis degree reaches 60%, the parameter λ_1 is almost 1.5 times the normal value. Thus, it is seen that the WSS value varies considerably with the degree of stenosis.

13.3.3.1.2 Parametric Analysis of Wall Pressure Gradient Distribution

As shown in Figure 13.12, the distribution of the pressure in the curved blood vessel wall is irregular and segmental; the pressure at the inlet end is overall larger than the outlet end. The variation of the intra-vessel pressure drop is greater with increased incidence of vascular stenosis. When the strain of stenosis reaches 40%, the atheromatous plaque inside the curved vessel becomes a partial low pressure area in the narrowest region. This phenomenon becomes more obvious with increased stenosis.

13.3.3.1.3 Variational Plot and Surface Response Graphs of Wall Shear Stress and Pressure

Figure 13.13 depicts WSS and WP plots of idealistic arteries with 30°, 90°, and 150° bend, based on the line of data extraction (defined in Figure 13.9b). The magnitudes of WSS plots demonstrate a strong positive correlation with the stenotic region located at the 0.2–0.6 mm line of the data extraction; the peak magnitude at the apex of stenosis increases with the degree of curvature. A similar trend is demonstrated for WP, whereby a sudden decline in magnitude occurs at the stenosis.

The variation of *WSS* and *WP* along the inner surface of the curved arteries for 30°, 90°, and 150° bend provides insight into how the fluid mechanical properties vary with respect to the geometrical variation. The stenosis is positioned at the 0.2–0.6 mm section of the data extraction line. Figure 13.14a through c illustrates how the WSS magnitude is strongly dependent on the degree of stenosis and less dependent on the degree of curvature. The same trend is present for the *WP* plots in Figure 13.14d through f. The stenosis is responsible for restricting flow, and a higher velocity flow at its throat induces a larger *WSS* magnitude. In order to maintain the same volume flow rate, a larger pressure exists at the inlet of the artery to enable transport of the same quantity of blood. Downstream of the artery, there is the reduction in pressure when the blood passes through the stenosis. The more aggravated the stenosis, the more restrictive is the quantity of blood transport; this is confirmed by the larger pressure drop at its throat.

The flow ratios $\bar{\lambda}$ surface responses for variations of (a) AWSS and (b) flow pressure drop for an artery are presented in Figure 13.14. The response of $\bar{\lambda}$ is based on the variable grid of (h, α), that varies from [−0.5 to 0.5] and [30° to 150°]. All arterial cases are normalized with respect to that of a healthy normal straight artery whose AWSS and *FPD* are 5.221 and 327.12 Pa respectively.

These response curves present the detailed illustration of the increment of AWSS and pressure drop with the amount of stenosis degree. They demonstrate how the pressure

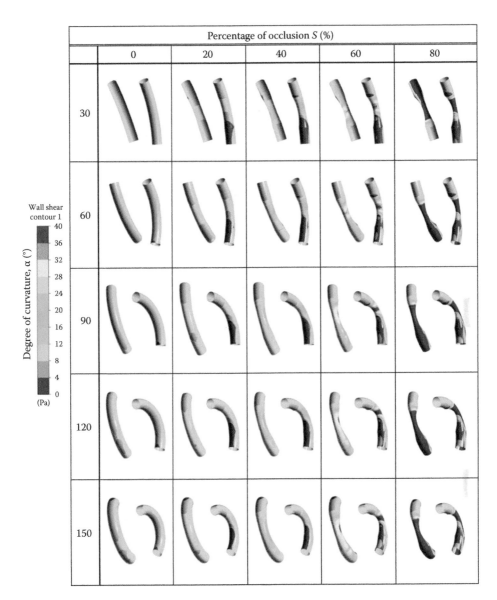

FIGURE 13.11
WSS contour plot profiles based on diseased segment height and bend variability of idealistic arteries. The percentage of occlusion and curvature vary from $S = 0\%$ to 80% and $\alpha = 30°$ to 150°. The WSS is shown to demonstrate a larger variation in more bent arteries, and particularly where the artery is stenosed at the maximum curvature portion L_3. When the occlusion percentage S and curvature angle α become maximum, the WSS value increases significantly at the narrowest section of the artery.

drop in the curved blood vessel increases with the increment of the stenosis. For the most curved artery at $\alpha = 150°$, where the stenosis area is 40%, the AWSS and pressure drop exceed 10.0328 and 614.565 Pa, respectively. Where the stenosis area is 80%, the AWSS and pressure drop increase to 30.382 and 4436.710 Pa, respectively. The same trend applies for both these parameters.

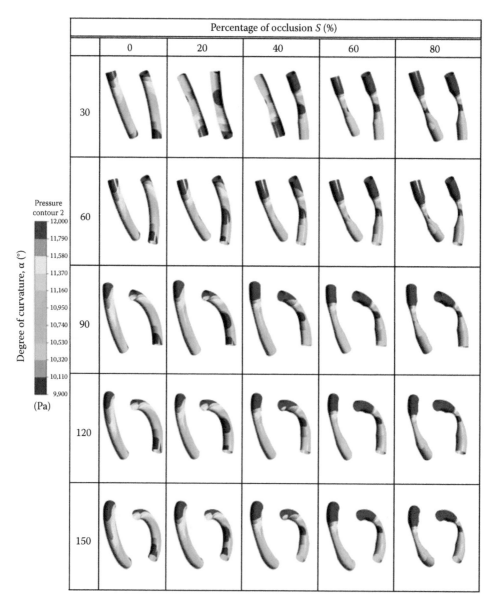

FIGURE 13.12

WPG contour plot profiles based on diseased segment height and bend variability of idealistic arteries. The percentage of occlusion and curvature vary from $S = 0\%$ to 80% and $\alpha = 30°$ to 150°. However, the *WPG* is shown to demonstrate a larger variation in the segment L_2 rather than in the segment L_3 where the stenosis occurs. This may be explained by the pressure build up at the entrance segment of each stenosis.

13.3.3.2 Patient-Specific Flow Analysis in Curved Stenosed Arteries

Now we analyze some patient-specific curved stenosed arteries and compare the results with those of the idealized arteries.

The WSS and WPG plots of four patient-specific RCAs are now presented, to illustrate the effectiveness of our parametric study in examination of flow through idealized curved and stenosed vessels. In effect, the parametric analyses may be viewed as a study based

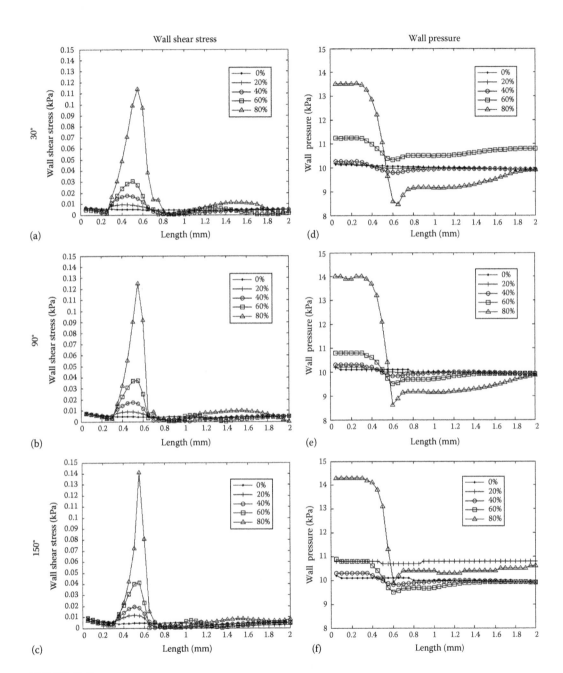

FIGURE 13.13
WSS plots (a, b, and c) and WP plots (d, e, and f) of idealistic arteries with 30°, 90°, and 150° bend based on the line of data extraction. The WSS plots demonstrate a strong positive correlation in magnitude with the stenotic region located at the 0.2–0.6 mm line of the data extraction; the peak magnitude at the apex of stenosis increases with the degree of curvature. A similar trend is demonstrated for WP, whereby a sudden decline in magnitude occurs at the stenosis.

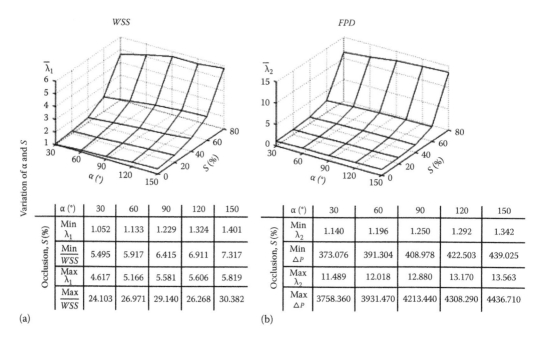

α (°)	30	60	90	120	150
Min λ_1	1.052	1.133	1.229	1.324	1.401
Min $\overline{WSS}$	5.495	5.917	6.415	6.911	7.317
Max λ_1	4.617	5.166	5.581	5.606	5.819
Max $\overline{WSS}$	24.103	26.971	29.140	26.268	30.382

Occlusion, *S* (%)

α (°)	30	60	90	120	150
Min λ_2	1.140	1.196	1.250	1.292	1.342
Min ΔP	373.076	391.304	408.978	422.503	439.025
Max λ_2	11.489	12.018	12.880	13.170	13.563
Max ΔP	3758.360	3931.470	4213.440	4308.290	4436.710

Occlusion, *S* (%)

(a) (b)

FIGURE 13.14

Flow surface response of elastic curved arteries based on average wall shear stress parameter (a) and flow pressure drop parameter (b). The surface response values pertaining to ratio λ_1 of average wall shear stress $\overline{WSS}$ and to ratio λ_2 of pressure drop *FPD* are normalized with those of the healthy artery with no wall variation that represent our standard model. Highly curved and stenosed arteries present incremental values of the λ_1 and λ_2 ratios, implying larger *WSS* and *WPG* distributions whereas gently curved and healthy arteries indicates otherwise.

on reduced complexities of overly excessive number of geometrical parameters, and using WSS and PD as exemplifications of the fluid mechanical parameters to highlight the variations in flow as a result of the geometry.

We present the patient-specific study of realistic vascular anatomies based on the framework that we have successfully established in our parametric studies. We first plot the WSS and WPG distributions of these four patient arterial samples that are reconstructed from medical images of patients diagnosed with atherosclerosis and a stenosis in the RCAs of the heart (as shown in Figure 13.15). We have selected RCAs that have increasing amounts of stenosis and curvature in the order of patients 1–4.

Now, as we know, the AWSS and PD of arteries is known to increase with complexity in geometry of the RCA vis-à-vis diseased segment and curvilinear variation, as is demonstrated by the increasing intensity of these parameters toward the stenosis in Figure 13.16a. As such, we extract these flow parameters along the inner wall of the arteries, as illustrated in Figure 13.16b. The plots of the WSS and PD variation along the line of data extraction in Figure 13.16 can be used to quantify and explain this effect even more clearly.

In Figure 13.16a, we observe that the value of patient 3 is highest in length at 0.8, and patient 1 has the lowest value at that stenotic point, so the WSS is maximal toward the stenotic region and its maximum value increases with the curvature of the artery. The wall pressure demonstrates the similar effect, whereby it is maximum for the most curved

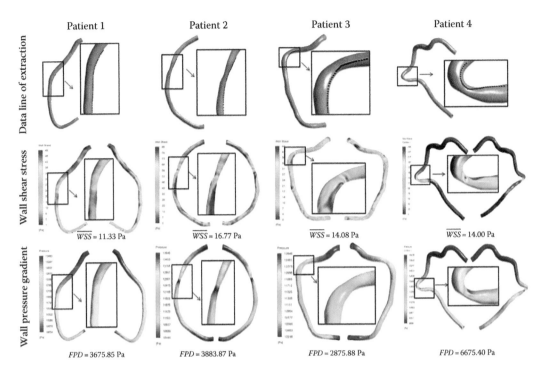

FIGURE 13.15
WSS and WPG surface plots of realistic arteries A, B, and C from two perspectives. The small squared parts are enlarged to show the detailed localized contour plots at the stenotic regions. Therein, the circular encapsulations show (1) high WSS and (2) high WPG regions at the stenosis and inner wall of the arterial curve.

artery as shown in Figure 13.16b. All of these results have close agreement and trends with the results obtained for the idealistic arteries. This goes to prove that our parametric study is robust and reliable.

13.4 Blood Flow in Straight Coronary Arteries with Varying Degrees of Stenosis and Dilatations

In the previous section, we have examined blood flow through curved and stenosed arteries. Now, we examine blood flow through straight multiply stenosed and dilated coronary arteries, using computational fluid dynamics based on a parametric framework. Our aim is to study the influence of atherosclerosis by modeling different arterial geometries and to determine the severity of this cardiovascular disease based on the degree of stenosis. Arterial hemodynamics affects atherosclerosis formation, and CFD can be employed to assist in understanding this phenomenon by providing a noninvasive method for studying the blood flow characteristics in relation to this condition. We are employing advanced CFD techniques, such as fluid structure interface (FSI) based on finite volume method. This technique represents moving boundary conditions, which replicates realistic behavior of blood flow in arteries.

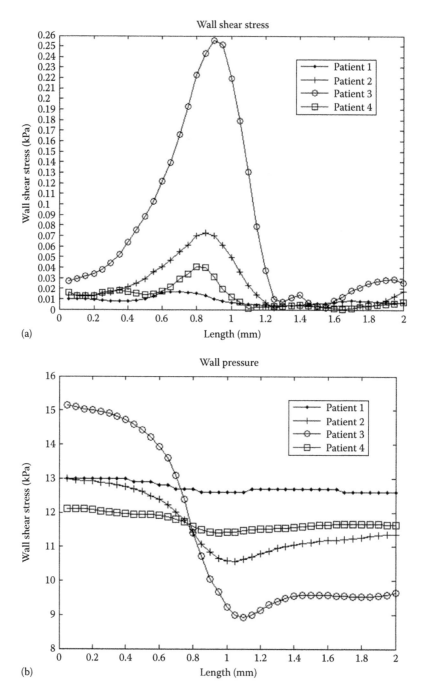

(a)

(b)

FIGURE 13.16

WSS and WP plot of realistic RCAs of arteries based on the line of data extraction. The wall shear stress plots (a) and wall pressure plots (b) of four realistic RCAs (labeled as patient 1–4) have a strong positive increasing trend with the increasing amounts of stenosis and degrees of curvature. The increasing intensity of the flow parameters toward the affected stenotic region demonstrates that the arterial geometry is responsible for influencing WSS and ultimately the aggravation of plaque in the diseased segments.

13.4.1 Motivation of CFD in Understanding Atherosclerotic Plaque Aggravation and Hemodynamic Analysis

Thickening of the artery wall has long been understood as an early process in the formation of atherosclerosis, and is one of the most widespread diseases in humans leading to the malfunction of the peripheral vascular system [33,34,54]. The gradual built up of cholesterol plaque in the artery wall and eventual rupture of the plaque can cause immediate occlusion of the artery and lead to sudden death. The causes of atherosclerosis may be high blood pressure, tobacco smoking, excessive drinking, high cholesterol, diabetes, as well as physical inactivity and obesity.

Atherosclerosis is a major clinical problem, and the disease leads patients to experience strokes and heart failures. To prevent such harm from occurring, stents are inserted into the affected regions of plaque or atheroma depositions to enhance the area of flow. The hemodynamics in stenotic elastic arteries can be properly investigated by means of CFD modeling, to investigate the regions of low WSS, WPG, and pressure drop that contribute to atherosclerotic plaque formation. Medical imaging can be used to visualize the regions of fatty deposits within arterial wall; however, this is unable to provide numerical data into the intricacies of hemodynamics. On the other hand, computational simulation models can provide an in-depth analysis on flow resistance due to shear stress on walls, which is related to flow rates and pressure drop, as illustrated by Kompatsiaris et al. [55] and Liu et al. [56]. The CFD results obtained by modeling the vessels in their affected regions can be deemed to be satisfy mathematical data standards. By combining the knowledge of clinicians and the information extracted from accurate CFD computational models, we can obtain a better understanding of the variability of flow resistance caused by stenosis.

The CFD computational results obtained by modeling the vessel in their affected regions can be used to assess disease [57,58]. As stated earlier, by combining the knowledge of clinicians based on the information extracted from medical images with the hemodynamic parametric information derived from CFD modeling, a patient-specific methodology can be developed for diagnosis of the severity of the condition of atherosclerotic arteries, in order to then determine the optimal treatment recourse. In fact, even treatment procedures can be analyzed in advance of actually carrying it out, so as to determine the optimal treatment recourse—be it coronary arterial stenting or grafting (coronary artery bypass graft [CABG]), based on the assessment of abnormal flow conditions in the stented vessel and the distal anastomosis of the CABG [7,41,59,60].

13.4.1.1 Implementation of CFD Approach and the Hemodynamic Parameters Used

This investigation involves a mathematical model representing the dynamic response of blood flow through the arteries under stenotic conditions causing the atherosclerotic plaque formation. The blood can be treated to be a generalized Newtonian fluid, and the arterial wall can be considered to be having different degrees of stenosis in its lumen, arising from various types of abnormal growth or plaque formation. The nonlinear unsteady pulsatile flow phenomenon is governed by the Navier–Stokes equations combined with the Continuity equation. In an attempt to derive physiologically significant and accurate quantities, the governing equations of motion need to be accompanied by the appropriate choice of the inlet–outlet boundary conditions, namely, physiological waveforms for velocity at the inlet and pressure at the outlet of an artery. The necessary checking for numerical stability of the computational procedure has also to be incorporated into the algorithm, for better precision of the results computed.

This investigation is concerning simulations of blood flow in a straight artery containing stenotic and dilatational deformities, to determine the hemodynamic parameters of WSS and WPG contributory to enhanced flow resistance and myocardial ischemic regions. The flow conditions, structural variation, and multiple abnormal segments all have influence on the resistance to flow. Tang et al. have explored CFD modeling to provide a noninvasive method of studying plaque rupture in carotid bifurcation arteries [14]. The main aim of harnessing computational models is to provide vascular surgeons with more flow disturbance parameters for cardiac diagnosis, based on the values of WSS and WPG.

13.4.2 Methodology

13.4.2.1 Describing the Arterial Wall Geometry and Material

The variables that influence the resistance to flow ratio are the blood viscosity, the geometry of the artery, and its wall flexibility characteristics (as given by its elastic modulus). The dimensional parameters of the typical arterial segment serve as inputs for determining the flow properties and characteristics.

The axial geometry is characterized by the nonoccluded wall height H_i for an atherosclerotic lesion of length l_i through an artery of diameter D_i. We allow for both constriction (stenosis) and dilation (aneurysm) of the lumen.

Then, the normalized diseased height is given by

$$h_i = \frac{D_i - H_i}{D_i} \quad \text{for } -0.5 \le h_i \le 0.5, \ i = 1, 2 \tag{13.20}$$

The geometrical model of a 3D artery is shown in Figure 13.17. The cylindrical domain has a total length of $L = 45$ mm, where in $L_1 = 5$ mm from the inlet segment, the first diseased segment (stenosis) has a length of $L_2 = 7.5$ mm; then after a length of $L_3 = 5$ mm the second diseased segment (dilatation) is located having the length $L_4 = 7.5$ mm and at a distance $L_5 = 5$ mm from the outlet segment. The nondiseased sections have constant diameter of $D_0 = 4.0$ mm. The variational parameters of h_1 and h_2 localized at the throats of the artery represent the heights of the diseased segments. The wall thickness $h_w = 0.2$ mm with density of $\rho = 1150$ kg/m³. The compliant vessel is modeled as an isotropic material with Poisson's ratio of $v = 0.499$ and Young's modulus $E = 5$ MPa of the solid structure [56].

13.4.2.2 CFD Modeling of Arterial Flow

The fluid flow is considered to be laminar, 3D, transient, isothermal, and incompressible. The blood fluid is modeled as an incompressible fluid, with fluid viscosity and density of $\mu = 0.035$ Pa s and $\rho = 1050$ kg/m³, and the flow is assumed to be Newtonian [61]. The arterial wall is elastic in nature and modeled as a no-slip wall. At the inlets and outlets, we have applied physiologically representative velocity and pressure waveforms that were simultaneously acquired with an electrocardiography-gated intravascular ultrasound Doppler and pressure probe [47]; the time-varying velocity is applied at the inlet cross section, while the time-varying pressure is applied at all the outlet for all the simulated models

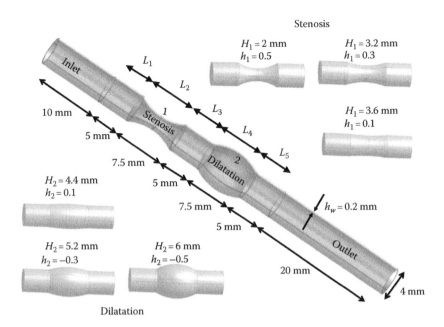

FIGURE 13.17
Geometrical model of the straight artery with stenotic and dilated segments, showing different degrees of stenotic heights and lengths of the arterial sections. The wall heights vary at different sections (L_1–L_5) of the cylindrical tube of the specific thickness representing an artery. The inlet and outlet of the tube are extended to enable the parabolic flow profile to be developed fully prior to entering the artery. The flow parameters are extracted at the beginning of L_1 and the end of L_5 surfaces, and averaged.

(as illustrated in Figure 13.18). For the solution setting, the incompressible Navier–Stokes equations are employed as the governing equations; a high resolution for advection and second-order backward Euler for transient scheme is used.

13.4.2.3 Numerical Simulation of the Structural Configurations of the Artery Model

Numerical analyses using CFD techniques have been performed on various structural configurations of the artery model in Figure 13.17. Over the past decade, with the rapid advancement of computer technology, CFD has been widely adopted to investigate the hemodynamic parameters inside various stenosed arteries as portrayed by Poiseuille [62]. Although the method requires considerably long computational time, it is well accepted as one of the more accurate approach for a detailed hemodynamic analysis. Herein, we have analyzed a sample of 36 geometrical configurations, with the diseased-to-normal wall length ratio of 1; different combinations of disease heights (h_1 and h_2), ranging from dilatation with a value of −0.5 to stenosis with a value of 0.5 [4] are generated and imported into a generic CFD package—ANSYS CFX 14.5.

Within the CFD code, the finite volume method is used to solve the detailed blood flow structure that is represented by the Navier–Stokes equations. At the inlet, we have stipulated fully developed parabolic velocity profiles corresponding to the Reynolds number, $Re = \rho VL/\upsilon$, having a range of 122–692. The imposed velocity and pressure waveforms at the inlet and outlet of the artery are shown in Figure 13.18. The details of the boundary conditions and geometrical parameters adopted are summarized in Table 13.5.

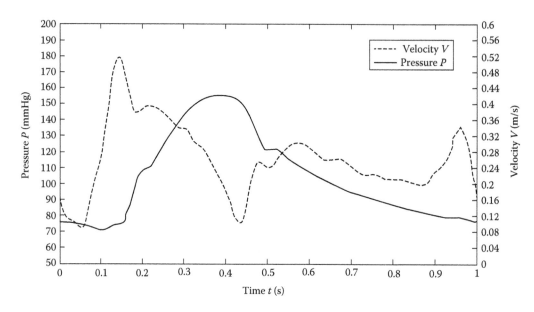

FIGURE 13.18

Physiological waveforms for velocity at the inlet and pressure at the outlet of an artery. The waveforms present the velocity (left axis) and pressure variations (right axis) at the entrance and exit of the vessel in one cardiac cycle. The velocity waveform is measured in m/s, while that of the pressure is in mmHg.

TABLE 13.5

Geometrical Parameters and Boundary Conditions Adopted in CFD Simulations

Parameter	Value
Normalized diseased height, h_1	[−0.5, −0.3, −0.1, 0.1, 0.3, 0.5]
Normalized diseased height, h_2	[−0.5, −0.3, −0.1, 0.1, 0.3, 0.5]
Normalized wall length, l_0/L	[1/6, 1/4, 1/6, 1/4]
Reynolds number, Re	122–692
Number of mesh elements	28,782

13.4.2.4 Measured Fluid Dynamics Properties

It is of interest to examine the WSS, as endothelial cells of the vessel wall tend to be aligned along the site of local WSS at the throat of the artery (as indicated by the stenosis located at Section 13.4.1 of the artery in Figure 13.17). The WSS is calculated as

$$\tau_\omega = -\mu \frac{\partial u_t}{\partial n}\bigg|\text{wall} \tag{13.21}$$

where
  μ (kg/m s) is the dynamic viscosity
  u_t (m/s) is the wall tangential velocity
  n is the unit vector perpendicular to the wall

The average wall shear stress is calculated as

$$\overline{WSS} = \frac{\iiint_D \tau_\omega(x,y,z)d_xd_yd_z}{\|D\|} \tag{13.22}$$

where
τ_w is the wall shear stress on the wall
x, y, and z are the 3D coordinates in space
D is the volume
d is the infinitisimal distance

The WPG is defined as

$$WPG = \sqrt{\left(\frac{\partial_P}{\partial_x}\right)^2 + \left(\frac{\partial_P}{\partial_y}\right)^2 + \left(\frac{\partial_P}{\partial_z}\right)^2} \tag{13.23}$$

where
P is the wall static pressure
x, y, and z are the 3D coordinates in space

The ratio λ_1 of average wall shear stress $\overline{WSS}$ pertaining to the entire wall of artery at peak systole is given by

$$\overline{\lambda_1} = \frac{\overline{WSS_1}}{\overline{WSS_2}} \tag{13.24}$$

where $\overline{WSS_1}$ and $\overline{WSS_2}$ are the average wall shear stress in the atherosclerotic artery and in the normal artery, respectively.

The flow resistance ratio [4] is defined as

$$\overline{\lambda_2} = \frac{\Delta P_1}{\Delta P_2} \tag{13.25}$$

where ΔP_1 and ΔP_2 are the pressure drops pertaining to the atherosclerotic artery and to the normal artery, respectively.

13.4.2.5 Mathematics of Fluid–Structure Interaction

In the FSI simulation, the fluid is modeled by using the Navier–Stokes equation that includes energy equation, continuity equation, and the momentum equation. These equations are then coupled with the governing equation for the solid domain. When solving the FSI, the coupling between fluid and solid solvers is governed by a set of conditions, which ensure that the dynamic and kinematic relationships of the two subdomains are properly represented.

These two conditions are employed for FSI coding, which generally adopt the partitioned approach. For following the kinematic condition, the fluid nodes on the FSI interface are updated according to their corresponding solid nodes. In the dynamic condition, the equilibrium of stress on the FSI interface is maintained, and the fluid pressure is integrated into the fluid force applied onto the solid nodes at the FSI interface. In the FSI simulation, the governing equations involved can be derived in Lagrangian, Eulerian, and Arbitrary Lagrangian–Eulerian (ALE) frame of references. These governing equations for the fluid and solid domains are given in the following.

13.4.2.5.1 Fluid Domain

The *Continuity equation* is based on the concept that the mass in the system has to be conserved. This means that the rate of change of mass within the control volume is equivalent to the mass flux crossing the surface S of volume V. After some mathematical manipulations, a general form of Continuity equation in the Eulerian frame can be written as

$$\frac{\partial P}{\partial t} + v \cdot \nabla \rho = -\rho \nabla \cdot v \tag{13.26}$$

The *Energy equation* is formulated on the physical principle that energy in the system has to be conserved. A general form of energy equation in the Eulerian frame can be written as

$$\rho \frac{\partial E}{\partial t} + \rho(v \cdot \nabla)E = \nabla \cdot (\sigma \cdot v) + v \cdot \rho b \tag{13.27}$$

The *Momentum equation* can be formulated based on the physical principle that momentum in the system has to be conserved. A general form of momentum equation in the Eulerian frame can be written as

$$\rho \frac{\partial v}{\partial t} + \rho(v \cdot \nabla)v = \nabla \cdot \sigma + \rho b \tag{13.28}$$

13.4.2.5.2 Solid Domain

The governing equation for the solid domain is formulated in the Lagrangian reference frame, as shown in the following:

$$\rho_s h_s \frac{\partial^2 d_\Gamma}{\partial t^2} + a_0 d_\Gamma - b \frac{\partial^2 d_\Gamma}{\partial x^2} = P_\Gamma \tag{13.29}$$

where
  $a_0 = (Eh_s)/r^2(1-\upsilon^2)$
  $b = K_T B h_s$. Note that K_T denotes the Timoshenko shear correction factor
  P_Γ is the structural load on the interface Γ due to the external forcing term from the fluid
  d_Γ is the displacement at the interface
  x is the position in space
  t is the position in time

When solving FSI, the fluid and solid domains are interlinked by displacement compatibility equations. The kinematic condition ensures the compatibility of displacement across FSI interface and can be written as

$$d_\Gamma^f = d_\Gamma^s$$

where
  d is displacement
  d_Γ^s and d_Γ^f are the displacements of the solid and fluid interface, respectively

The carotid artery bifurcation is one of the common sites where atherosclerotic plaque and stenosis are prone to develop. The FVI simulations have demonstrated local mechanical factors involved in the fluid vessel coupling participation in the pathogenesis of atherosclerosis.

The solid domain is constructed in the ANSYS solver, while the fluid domain is modeled in the CFX solver. The in-between coupling is from the "setup" of the two solvers. Once the simulation is run in the "solution" window, it first begins computing iterations for the solid domain by initiating the ANSYS solver, and then progresses onto the fluid domain in the CFX solver.

The combination of CFD and FEA, associated with the vessel structural analysis modules, has been developed to incorporate the dynamic interaction of blood flows with the motion of the arterial wall solid structure (to study flow-induced structural deformation), under different blood flow rates and pressure conditions.

13.4.3 Results of Quantification of Flow through Stenosed Straight Arteries

13.4.3.1 Contour Plots of WSS and WPG

Determining the local hemodynamics, temporal WSS, as well as WPG is important for understanding the mechanisms leading to various complications in cardiovascular function.

From Figures 13.19 and 13.20, it can be seen that both WSS and WPG properties are shown to demonstrate significant increments at segments where the artery is more stenosed. The opposite occurs for dilatations but at much lower magnitudes. For the narrowest sections (i.e., at the maximum h_1 and h_2), the WSS and WPG values are significant. However, for the widest sections (i.e., at the minimum h_1 and h_2), these parameter values are not changing as much as in the narrowest sections.

13.4.3.2 Surface Response Graphs of WSS and WPG

The effect of additional flow resistance can be further ascertained based on the velocity variation in an artery. For example, as the dilatation increases, the vessel cross-sectional area enlarges, and the flow velocity gradually decreases while the pressure increases; for this case, the flow resistance will be minimal. However, herein the circulating motion of the fluid induces additional energy and pressure loss to flow, causing extra flow resistance. In our current study, due to the small dilatation, the flow separations are assumed to be negligible. As such, the flow resistance will still show a decline when there is dilatation.

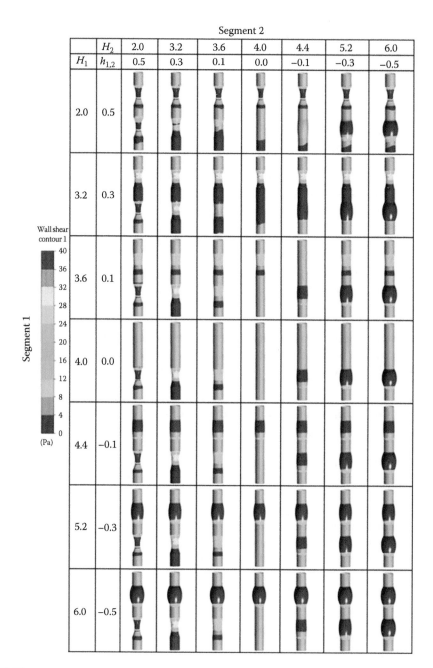

FIGURE 13.19

Detailed WSS contour plot showing the development of wall shear stress profiles for diseased segment heights h_1 and h_2. The normalized diseased wall heights vary from $h_1 = -0.5$ to $+0.5$ and $h_2 = -0.5$ to $+0.5$ at sections L_2 and L_4. The WSS is shown to demonstrate a larger variation at those sections where the artery is particularly stenosed, rather than dilated. When h_1 and h_2 become 0.5, the WSS value increases significantly at the narrowest sections. The color bar scale representing WSS values varies from 0 to 40 Pa.

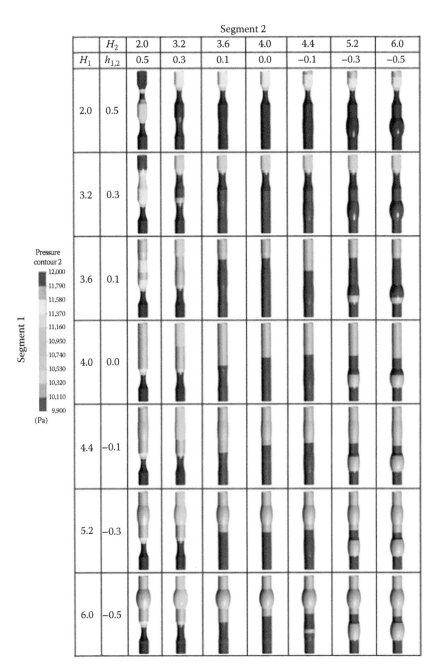

FIGURE 13.20
Detailed WPG contour plot showing the development of wall pressure gradient profiles for diseased segment heights h_1 and h_2. The normalized diseased wall heights vary from $h_1 = -0.5$ to $+0.5$ and $h_2 = -0.5$ to $+0.5$ at sections L_2 and L_4. The WPG is shown to demonstrate a larger variation at segments L_1 and L_3 rather than at segments L_2 and L_4 where the stenosis occurs. This may be explained by the pressure build up at the entrance segment of each stenosis. The color bar scale representing WPG values varies from 9,900 to 12,000 Pa.

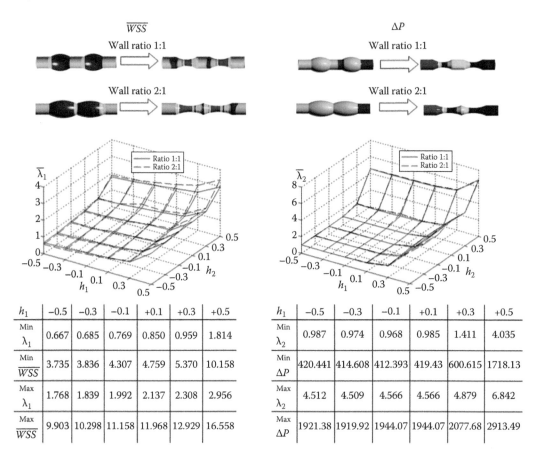

h_1	−0.5	−0.3	−0.1	+0.1	+0.3	+0.5
Min λ_1	0.667	0.685	0.769	0.850	0.959	1.814
Min $\overline{WSS}$	3.735	3.836	4.307	4.759	5.370	10.158
Max λ_1	1.768	1.839	1.992	2.137	2.308	2.956
Max $\overline{WSS}$	9.903	10.298	11.158	11.968	12.929	16.558

h_1	−0.5	−0.3	−0.1	+0.1	+0.3	+0.5
Min λ_2	0.987	0.974	0.968	0.985	1.411	4.035
Min ΔP	420.441	414.608	412.393	419.43	600.615	1718.13
Max λ_2	4.512	4.509	4.566	4.566	4.879	6.842
Max ΔP	1921.38	1919.92	1944.07	1944.07	2077.68	2913.49

FIGURE 13.21

Flow surface response of elastic arteries based on average wall shear stress and pressure drop flow parameters. The surface response values pertaining to ratio λ_1 of average wall shear stress $\overline{WSS}$ and to ratio λ_2 of pressure drop ΔP are normalized with respect to those of the healthy artery with no wall variation, which represents our standard model. Double stenosis presents incremental values of the λ_1 and λ_2 ratios, implying larger WSS and WPG distributions, whereas double dilatation indicates otherwise. For the longer diseased segments (with diseased to nondiseased segment ratio of 2:1), $\overline{WSS}$ increases in magnitude, while the change in ΔP is negligible.

As depicted in Figure 13.21, the predicted average wall shear stress $\overline{WSS}$ and pressure drop ΔP (or flow resistance ratio) surface response trends from CFD simulations are similar. In particular, for the cases with dilatation (i.e., where h_1 and h_2 are of negative value), the elastic artery has generated 3D flow response results of $\overline{WSS}$ and ΔP_{values} that are seen to decrease; however, this decline is not of the same magnitude for the two $\overline{WSS}$ and ΔP_{curves}. The minimum WSS ratio $\overline{\lambda}_1$ falls below a value of 1 to 0.667, whereas the minimum flow resistance $\overline{\lambda}_2$ is closer to 1 at 0.987. It can hence be seen that dilatations have influence on reducing WSS values with respect to the normal unstenosed artery and may also have some implications on the plaque growth. In addition, it is also observed that a longer diseased segment (based on a ratio of 2:1 for diseased to nondiseased sections) tends to increase the $\overline{WSS}$ magnitude, which can be explained by the greater narrowing resulting from a larger extension of the stenosis. However, this does not affect ΔP, since the pressure across the inlet and outlet is not dependent on the geometrical variation in-between.

On the other hand, for the stenosis cases (i.e., where h_1 and h_2 are of positive value), both the $\overline{WSS}$ and ΔP are higher in values, and their increments are much more significant. The maximum value of WSS ratio $\overline{\lambda}_1$ rises to a value of 2.956, whereas that of flow resistance ratio $\overline{\lambda}_2$ is very much higher at 6.842. The flow ratios provided by the FSI frameworks are shown in Figure 13.21, for comparison. Although both the graphs demonstrate similar trends, we can see that pressure drop ratio gives a stronger indication of variation as compared to average wall shear stress ratio.

13.4.3.3 Velocity Contour Plots of Stenosed Artery Flow

In Figure 13.22, we provide the results of the flow visualization in a stenosed artery (based on numerical simulation) in terms of the velocity contours in the X–Y plane in the idealized vessel with stenosis and dilatations. The blood flows from left to right in the figure. The flow velocity patterns in atherosclerotic arteries can assist our understanding of the flow condition within a diseased artery. For example, higher velocity flow is observed at the site of stenosis and this can cause plaque rupture. Also, sudden pressure release after the stenosis can aggravate dilatations.

13.4.4 Summary of Hemodynamic Analysis in Straight Stenosed Arteries

It can be observed in Figures 13.19 through 13.22 that double stenoses (based on $h_1 > 0$ and $h_2 > 0$) in an artery significantly influences the hemodynamic parameters of WSS and pressure drop or flow resistance, in comparison with the double dilatations case (based on $h_1 < 0$ and $h_2 < 0$). This shows that stenosis plays a more critical role in plaque growth and vulnerability in contrast to dilatation and should be the key element in cardiovascular prognosis. Through qualitative visualization coupled with the quantitative analysis of $\overline{WSS}$ and ΔP, we can gain a clearer insight into the hemodynamics of atherosclerotic arteries. The determination of these hemodynamic parameters can be helpful to cardiologists, because these parameters are directly implicated in the genesis and development of atherosclerosis.

13.5 Blood Flow in Coronary Arteries with Varying Degrees of Curvature and Side-Branch Bifurcation Angles

As presented in the previous sections, hemodynamics plays a critical role in the development and progression of plaques that are prone to sites of arterial curvatures and stenosis. The occurrence of atherosclerosis at curvatures of coronary arteries and at the bifurcation sites of their branches is of medical importance. In this section, we have employed computer simulation of coupled arterial flow hemodynamics and arterial vessel mechanics along with a hemodynamic parametric analysis, to rigorously quantify the WSS and WPG in transient idealized and image-based RCA models with side-branches, in order to explore the effects of curvature and bifurcation on blood flow characteristics and its hemodynamic variables.

Upon establishing and implementing this parametric analysis framework, we find that the relatively lower WSS and WPG regions at the curvature and branch bifurcation sites of arteries coincide with the plaque-prone points of the three investigated image-based

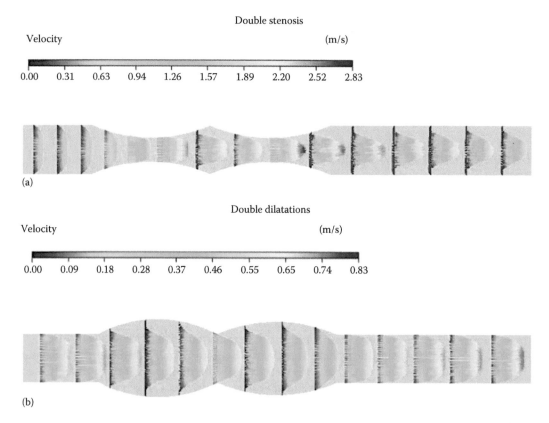

FIGURE 13.22

Flow visualization in atherosclerotic artery with stenosis and dilatations. The plots of axial velocities in a stenosed artery are presented for conditions of double stenoses (a) and double dilatations (b). The velocity distribution is taken at the center plane of a stenosed artery and can be used to compare the difference in flow due to those stenosis and dilatations. This flow visualization allows us to effectively understand the flow condition within a diseased artery, by showing the regions of high speed flow qualitatively.

arteries, to thereby confirm the correlation of the fluid mechanical properties with the arterial geometry variation in consistence with the data from existing literatures. Moreover, the average WSS and pressure drop (from inlet to outlet) are significantly increased with the more complex geometry of realistic arteries in comparison with idealized arterial models. It can hence be concluded that the geometry of curvature and angulation of the side-branches has a significant effect on the WSS and WPG in hemodynamics analysis of RCAs.

13.5.1 Introduction to Flow Characterization in Arteries of Varying Curvature and Side-Branch Bifurcations

The distribution of WSS in coronary arteries is a significant contributory factor for the onset of coronary disease. Recently, there have been some debates as to what degree of WSS or large WSS gradients is contributory to the onset of plaque formation and rupture. At the same time, various studies have gone into explaining how regions are differentiated into varying degrees of WSS and linking their implications to vessel narrowing [14,16,63,64]. It is widely available in the literature that atherosclerotic plaques are located at low WSS and WPG regions, and it is accepted that local hemodynamic forces play an important role in the formation and rupture of atherosclerotic plaques. Dynamic curvilinear arterial geometries have been demonstrated to strongly affect WSS, based on coronary artery bifurcation models [65–67]. However, a detailed quantification of the WSS increments with this arterial curvature has not been studied with sufficient analytical and computational sophistication.

The purpose of our study is hence to computationally analyze the WSS and WPG variations in idealized and realistic RCA models and focus on (1) determining the distribution map of WSS and WPG in RCAs, by taking into account their curvatures and bifurcations, and (2) evaluating the variations of average WSS (defined as $\overline{WSS}$) on the vessel wall and pressure drop (ΔP) across the arterial inlet and outlet. Despite the well-known correlation of arterial curvature with WSS and ΔP, an elaborate and concise parametric study of how the geometrical variation of the curvilinear arteries and its branches affect these physical flow properties has not been performed previously. Herein, quantitative hemodynamic analysis and the flow properties of specifically defined regions, like the inner and outer walls of the trunk, are carried out, to enable a detailed understanding of the relationship between (1) arterial trunk curvature, angle of branching, as well as curvature of the branches, and (2) the fluid mechanics of blood flow through it.

CFD is now widely employed in the hemodynamic analysis of aorta, carotid, and coronary arteries under simulated physiological and pathological conditions [7,9]. In our study, we have demonstrated earlier that there are significant differences in the magnitudes of WSS and WPG in arteries with different curvature and angulation. Herein, we are determining these hemodynamic properties in right coronary arteries sites of high curvature and branch bifurcation locations associated with occurrence of atherosclerotic plaques. As can be noted, these results reveal that curvature and branch flows have a big influence on the distributions of WSS and WPG in the coronary arterial trunk. These findings can be utilized for carrying out pre-surgical analysis of plaque-occluded arteries, in order to plan the surgical designs of CABGs, so as to minimize the adverse hemodynamic flow patterns and the values of the hemodynamic parameters in their distal anastomoses with the occluded arteries (in terms of anastomosis sites and angle of anastomosis). This can constitute an overall project of hemodynamics of coronary arteries and models of CABGs for customized optimal surgical CABG designs for maximal CABG patency.

13.5.2 Methods to Study Arteries with Varying Curvature and Side-Branch Bifurcations

This section details the procedures implemented for the hemodynamic analysis in idealized and three realistic RCA models.

The geometry of our arterial models is designed according to the anatomical details of the real RCA. The straight geometry model with angle of 60° between the trunk and side-branch in the vertical plane, as depicted in Figure 13.23, is derived as the reference model, which is then converted into idealized solid models. We have carried out simulation of different curvatures and angulations (from very small to large angulations) to perform an in-depth study of the relationship between (1) curvature and angles, and (2) the development of atherosclerosis. In this model arterial system, L_1 is the length of trunk of 30 mm, while the side-branch L_2 length is 10 mm. The inlet diameter d_1 and outlet diameter d_2 are 4.5 and 4.0 mm, respectively. The diameter d_3 of the side-branch is taken to be 2 mm.

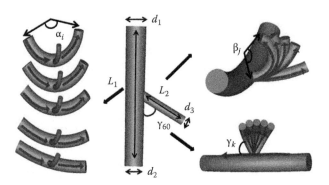

FIGURE 13.23

Geometry of the simulated models, illustrating the geometrical configurations of the main trunk and its side-branch (based on the angles α, β, and γ): variable α_i (α_{30}, α_{60}, α_{90}, α_{120}, and α_{150} from bottom to top), variable β_j (β_{30}, β_{60}, β_{90}, β_{120}, and β_{150} from right to left) and variable γ_k (γ_{60}, γ_{75}, γ_{90}, γ_{105}, and γ_{120} from left to right). Unidirectional arrows indicate the direction of blood flow. A reference model may be depicted as $\alpha_0\beta_0\gamma_{60}$.

These parametric quantifications and their subdivisions are chosen to be based on a reasonable estimation of the anatomical dimensions of the realistic RCAs image reconstruction, as illustrated in Figure 13.24. Based on this reference model, 125 other models have been generated, by changing (1) the curvature α_i of the trunk, to include 30°, 60°, 90°, 120°, and 150°, and depicted as α_{30}, α_{60}, α_{90}, α_{120}, and α_{150}; (2) the curvature β_j of the side-branch to include 30°, 60°, 90°, 120°, and 150°, and depicted as β_{30}, β_{60}, β_{90}, β_{120}, and β_{150}; (3) the angle γ_k between the trunk and side-branch to include 60°, 75°, 90°, 105°, and 120°, and depicted as γ_{60}, γ_{75}, γ_{90}, γ_{105}, and γ_{120}. All the models are denoted as $\alpha_i\beta_j\gamma_k$. Thereby, in our study, $\alpha_0\beta_0\gamma_{60}$ is treated as the standard model, which is basically a straight artery with a bifurcated straight section.

The RCA models are assumed to have rigid walls. The mesh for these idealized models consists of 3D rectangular grids and is generated by using the name of the software followed by "ANSYS Inc., Canonsburg, PA." The grid independence analysis is performed for three different levels of mesh refinement: coarse, medium, and fine grid numbering 130,000 elements, 340,000 elements, and 1,500,000 elements, respectively. Since only 2% of dissimilitude between the fine and medium mesh was observed, it was decided that the fine mesh can be used to obtain grid independent results. As such, the results are based on the computation performed with the fine mesh.

13.5.3 Data Acquisition and Reconstruction of Realistic RCA Models

Cardiac CT imaging was performed by using a 64-detector row helical scanner (Aquilion 64, Toshiba Medical Systems, Otawara, Japan), as shown in Figure 13.24a. At first, the original DICOM format images are imported into Mimics 10.01, where image segmentation is carried out by means of the thresholding function (binary), and the optimized mask model of RCA is then constructed and stored in a stereolithography (STL) file format with 100,000–200,000 number of triangular elements. Then, the optimized surface mode of RCAs is post-processed with Geomagic Studio 2012 by means of geometrical trimming and smoothing, and exported as an IGES file format model for its import into the meshing software. In Figure 13.24b, the three RCA models are depicted and labeled as A, B, and C. For our next procedure, the volume meshes and boundary layer meshes are generated in CFX, and the numerical simulation is performed.

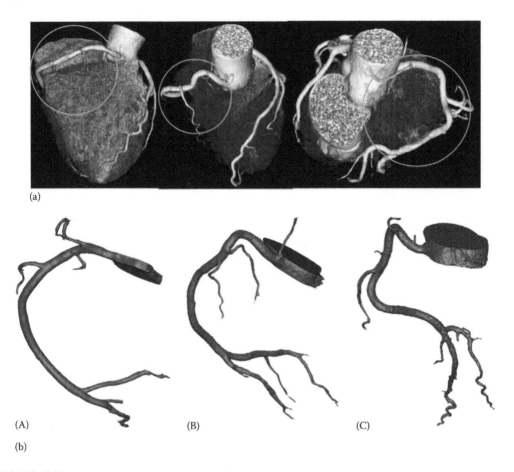

FIGURE 13.24
3D CT visualization of normal RCAs (A, B, and C) with side-branches in patients with suspected coronary disease. (a) The three RCAs (A, B, C) in the CT geometrical reconstruction are the key arteries under investigation (view of interest bounded by the circles). Note that the side-branches along the curved trunks separate at different angles. The trunk can be seen as a combination of various curved segments with side-branches at random locations. (b) The anatomical reference points for beginning to end were clearly specified when we identified and extracted the relevant arterial segments.

13.5.4 CFD Analysis of Idealized and Realistic RCAs

The application of medical image reconstruction for modeling blood vessels for CFD analysis has had considerable development in recent years. The typical process for performing numerical simulation of a blood vessel is based on its medical imaging, image segmentation, 3D model reconstruction, grid generation, and flow analysis [52]. The final grid, based on a mesh consisting of 3D tetrahedral elements, is generated in CFX-mesh software and used for transient numerical simulation of blood flow, with physiological boundary conditions close to physiological reality.

In our study, in order to minimize the effects of boundary conditions, the inlets and outlets are adequately extended to (1) 10 mm for inlet and side-branch outlets and (2) 30 mm for trunk outlet. Then, transient hemodynamic analysis is carried out by using ANSYS CFX 14.0 (ANSYS Inc., Canonsburg, PA). The fluid flow is considered to be laminar, isothermal, and incompressible. Based on the literature, the blood density is taken as 1050 kg/m^3, while the

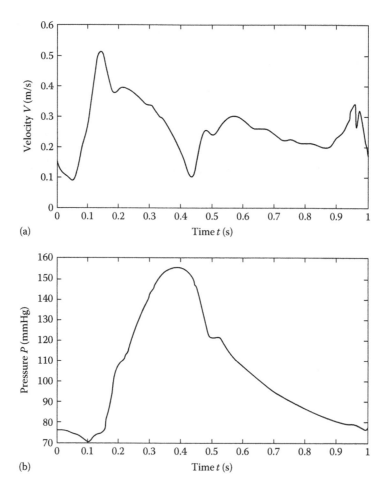

FIGURE 13.25
Physiological waveforms of (a) velocity inlets and (b) pressure outlets: the waveforms present the velocity and pressure variations for the inlets and outlets, respectively, in one cardiac cycle. The velocity waveform is in units of m/s and the pressure waveform is in units of mmHg.

blood is assumed to be a Newtonian fluid with a constant viscosity of 0.035 Pa s [61]. The arterial wall is modeled as a no-slip and rigid wall. At the inlets and outlets, we interpolate the velocity and pressure waveforms (Figure 13.25) that were simultaneously acquired with an electrocardiography-gated intravascular ultrasound Doppler and pressure probe (ComboWire®, Volcano Corporation) in the proximal and distal RCA of a patient with confirmation of unobstructed coronary artery [68]. Then as regards the boundary conditions, the time-varying velocity is applied at the inlet cross section, while the time-varying pressure is applied at all the outlets for all the idealized and realistic RCA models (illustrated in Figure 13.23 and 13.24).

For the solution setting, a high resolution for advection and second order backward Euler for transient scheme is used. The Continuity and incompressible Navier–Stokes equations are employed as

$$\rho\frac{\partial v}{\partial t} + \rho(v\cdot\nabla)v = -\nabla P + \rho g + \mu\nabla^2 v \tag{13.30}$$

$$\nabla \cdot v = 0 \tag{13.31}$$

where
  ρ is the blood density of 1050 kg/m^3
  v is the velocity
  P is the pressure
  g is the gravity constant
  μ is the dynamic viscosity of 0.035 g/cm s

For modeling solution, the temporal resolution and time step is set to be 0.01 s. A cardiac cycle length of 1 s is established and simulated over three cardiac cycles. We have ensured that transient artifacts are not present by establishing the previously defined length of the inlets and outlets. Herein, a parabolic inlet velocity profile is employed.

13.5.5 Results of Flow in Idealized RCAs through Varying Curvature and Side-Branch Bifurcations

We have selected the WSS and the WPG distribution on the artery, as well as the pressure drop (ΔP) between the inlet and outlet of the models as the simplest metrics, to illustrate the effect of curvature on the fluid mechanics of blood transport with the intention of establishing a response to geometrical parameters framework that can be clearly understood.

The idealized and realistic RCAs are studied by means of CFD analysis under the in vivo physiological conditions during the systolic phase, since the aforementioned parameters have values that are observed to be maximal during this phase. Our analysis demonstrates a strong relationship between (1) the hemodynamic characteristics and (2) the curvatures and trunk-branch angulations in all the models, and thereby confirms the rationale for performing these experiments.

13.5.5.1 WSS of Idealized RCA Models

High WSS regions (WSS $\geq$ 40 Pa) are seen to occur at the root of the side-branch adjacent to the bifurcation, while low WSS regions (WSS $\leq$ 4 Pa) are occurring at the inner and outer wall, based on the curve of the trunk and on the side-branch opposite to the bifurcation.

When the trunk displays different severities of curvature, as shown in Figure 13.26, the less intensified WSS regions are found to concentrate at the inner wall (based on curvature of the trunk) and on the side-branch opposite to the bifurcation. The WSS values are relatively higher when the curvature α of the trunk becomes larger, and the high WSS regions adjacent to the bifurcation are also found to increase. For the models with curvature α of 30° and 60°, there are small regions of low WSS on the inner and outer walls that have emerged due to the effect of the side-branch. However, as α reaches 90°, the low WSS regions are found to exclusively concentrate on the inner wall. On the other hand, Figure 13.26 demonstrates that with the branch angle γ (between the trunk and the side-branch) becoming larger, the low WSS regions reduce, while the high WSS regions increase. The $\overline{WSS}$ values become larger with a bigger angle γ between the trunk and the side-branch; it is also found that $\overline{WSS}$ increased with incremental values of α and γ. In terms of pathological implications for atherosclerosis, this has a positive effect on atherogenesis for the artery as persistently higher values of WSS has been a dominant parameter that is associated with the severity of myointimal hyperplasia and arterial occlusion.

Models		WSS contour	$\overline{\text{WSS}}$ (Pa)	Models	WSS contour	$\overline{\text{WSS}}$ (Pa)
$\alpha_i\beta_{30}\gamma_{60}$	α_{30}	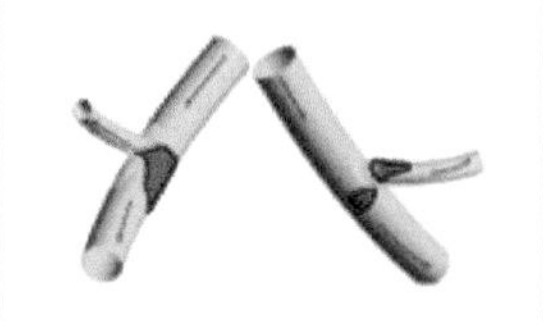	6.78	γ_{60}	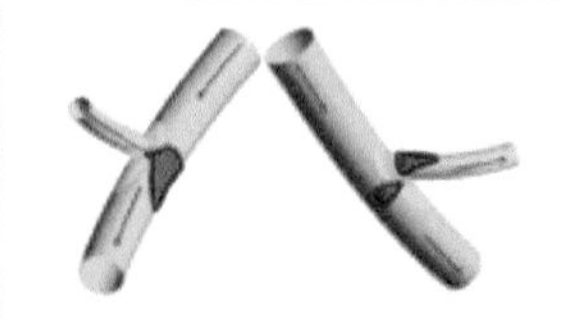	6.78
	α_{60}	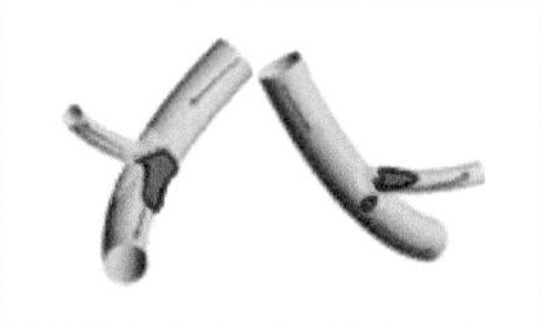	7.06	γ_{75}	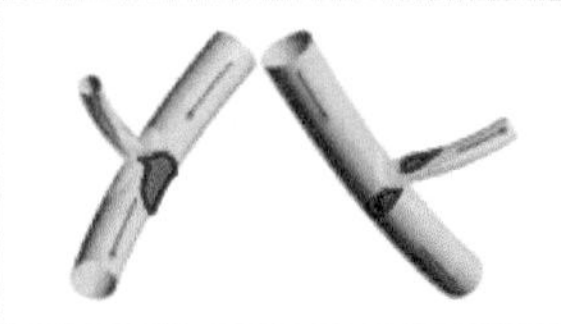	6.92
	α_{90}	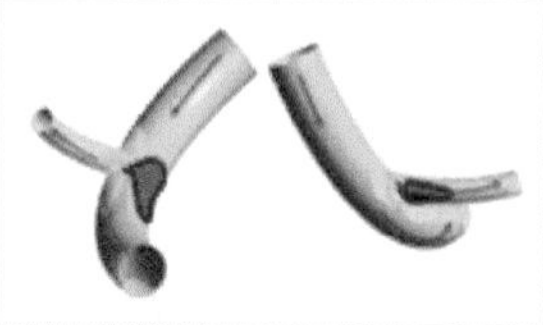	7.46	γ_{90} ($\alpha_{30}\beta_{30}\gamma_k$)	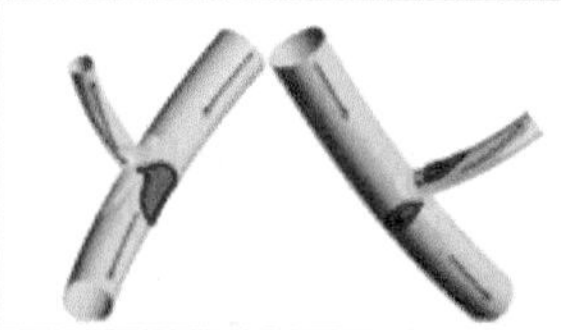	7.01
	α_{120}	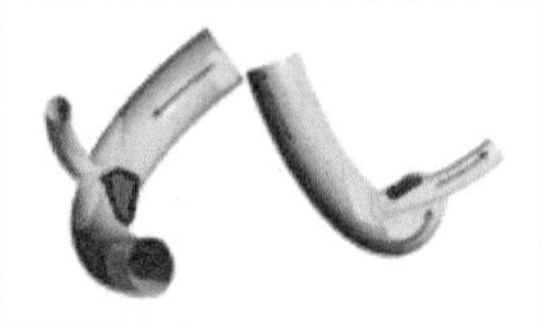	7.88	γ_{105}	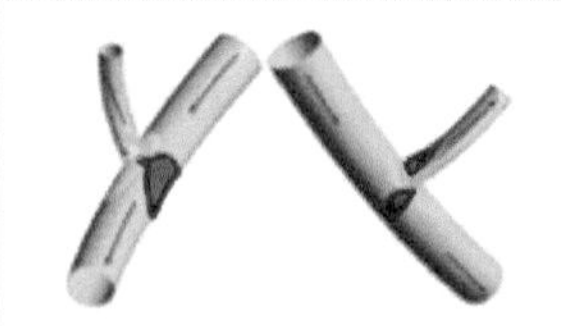	7.06
	α_{150}	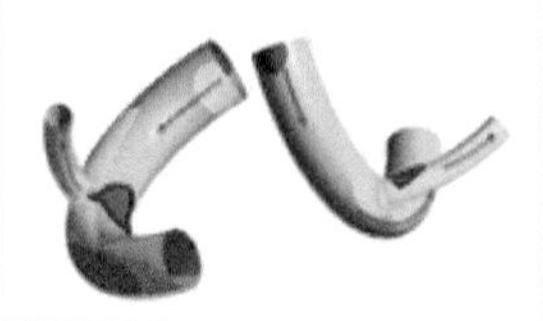	8.24	γ_{120}	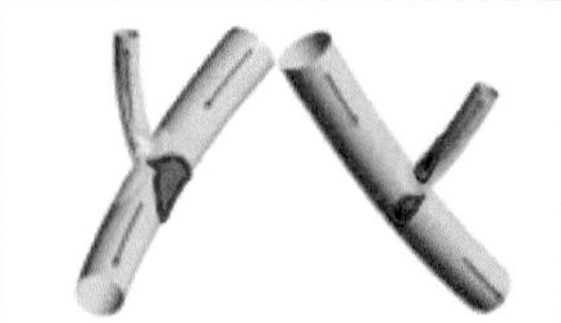	7.11

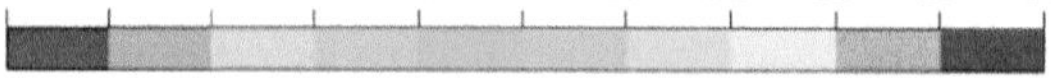

```
0    4    9   13   18   22   26   31   35   40   44
```
WSS   (Pa)

FIGURE 13.26

WSS distribution of RCAs based on the models $\alpha_i\beta_{30}\gamma_{60}$ and $\alpha_{30}\beta_{30}\gamma_k$ (with variation of the angle α and γ). The distributions of WSS are not basically the same for $\alpha_i\beta_{30}\gamma_{60}$ but same for $\alpha_{30}\beta_{30}\gamma_k$, and $\overline{\text{WSS}}$ increases with larger angles for α and γ. Note that the low WSS regions (WSS $\leq$ 0.4 Pa) are encapsulated by red boundary lines and are seen to be decreasing as γ becomes larger. On the contrary, the high WSS regions increase as shown by the more intensified colors representing high WSS values. Average WSS values are labeled on the right-hand side of every arterial simulation for the different α and γ angles.

13.5.5.2 WPG of Idealized RCA Models

The temporal WPG contours at the peak systole of the simulated RCAs are shown in Figure 13.27. Generally, the contours reveal a highly nonuniform hemodynamic environment. High WPG regions (WPG $\geq$ 10,483 Pa) co-exist with low WPG (WPG $\leq$ 9,907 Pa) values. At proximal regions, the WPG values are always higher compared to these occurring at the distal parts. The low and high WPG regions are similar to the low and high

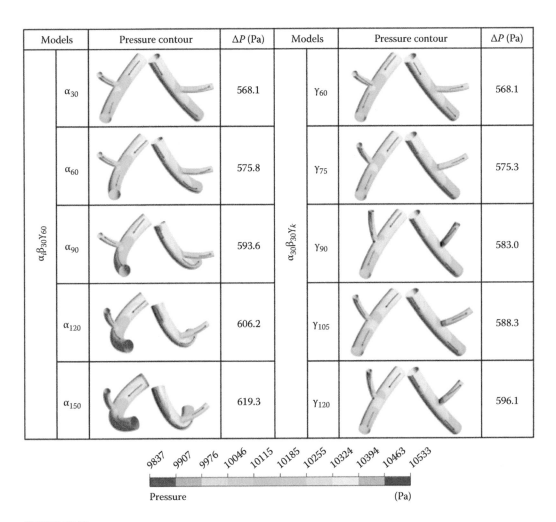

Models		Pressure contour	ΔP (Pa)	Models	Pressure contour	ΔP (Pa)
$\alpha_i\beta_{30}\gamma_{60}$	α_{30}		568.1	γ_{60}		568.1
	α_{60}		575.8	γ_{75}		575.3
	α_{90}		593.6	γ_{90}		583.0
	α_{120}		606.2	γ_{105}		588.3
	α_{150}		619.3	γ_{120}		596.1

9837　9907　9976　10046　10115　10185　10255　10324　10394　10463　10533

Pressure　　　　　　　　　　　　(Pa)

FIGURE 13.27
WPG distribution of RCAs based on models $\alpha_i\beta_{30}\gamma_{60}$ and $\alpha_{30}\beta_{30}\gamma_k$ (with variation of the angle γ). As the curvature angle α and γ increases, the WPG values at the proximal region increase and the lowest and highest WPG regions are found to be uniformly located opposite to the flow divider and at the root of the side-branch adjacent to the bifurcation. It is also noted that the low WPG regions are found to increase at the nonbifurcated areas, while the high WPG regions concentrate in the same region with larger values. It is seen that ΔP increases with bigger values of angles α and γ.

WSS regions around the bifurcation. As the branch angle γ becomes larger, the low WPG regions are found to increase, while the high WPG regions are concentrated in bifurcated regions with larger values. However, there are no localized low or high WPG regions occurring at the inner and outer walls of the trunk.

13.5.6 Flow Response Surface Plots of WSS and WPG of Idealized RCAs

In the plots, the wall shear stress values $\overline{WSS}_{\alpha_i\beta_j\gamma_k}$ are normalized against that of a standard model defined as α and β of $0°$, and γ of $60°$, which is basically a straight artery with a bifurcated section that is straight as well. This reference $\overline{WSS}_{\alpha_0\beta_0\gamma_{60}}$ value is a constant and therefore, an increase in the ratio λ_1 of $\overline{WSS}$ implies an increase in the general WSS gradient distribution.

$$\lambda_1 = \frac{\overline{WSS}_{\alpha_i\beta_j\gamma_k}}{\overline{WSS}_{\alpha_0\beta_0\gamma_{60}}} \tag{13.32}$$

In order to study the hemodynamic changes among the geometrically varying idealized models, we have plotted the surface response curve of the ratio parameter λ_1 on the whole wall at peak systole in our results.

As in the case of WSS, we have also plotted the surface response curve of the ratio parameter λ_2 of pressure drop (ΔP) between proximal inlet and distal outlet at peak systole:

$$\lambda_2 = \frac{\Delta P_{\alpha_i\beta_j\gamma_k}}{\Delta P_{\alpha_0\beta_0\gamma_{60}}} \tag{13.33}$$

The parameter λ_2 can be depicted as the flow resistance ratio, in which the pressure drop of the artery of interest is normalized against a standard reference one, which is normally perceived to lie within the range of the healthy condition [4]. This flow resistance parameter is a useful metric for evaluating the degree of vessel narrowing in clinical practice.

Figure 13.28a through c shows the surface response curves based on λ_1. We note that the more intensified curved trunk and larger bifurcation angled side-branch present bigger values of the λ_1 ratio, which implies larger WSS gradient distribution. For the highly curved model with the branch angle γ of 120°, the value of λ_1 reaches up to 1.323 with reference to the predefined standard model of α and β being 0° and γ of 60°. We see a general positive correlation of $\overline{WSS}$ with the curvature β values.

Figure 13.28d through f depicts the surface response curves of the ΔP ratio parameter λ_2. We note that the plots are relatively similar to the surface response curves of $\overline{WSS}$ ratio parameter λ_1. For the most curved model with branch angle γ of 120°, the value of λ_2 reaches up to 1.201, based on the reference model.

13.5.7 WSS and WPG in Image-Based RCA Models

A total of three realistic RCAs, with varying degrees of trunk bending with side-branches were selected for our numerical simulation study. These cases (illustrated in Figure 13.29) are labeled as artery A, B, and C. These realistic RCAs present with individual variation in the anatomy. All the reconstructed RCAs are curved with side-branches: model A appears as a C-shaped artery, model B is its S-shaped counterpart, while model C has more curves appearing at different segments along the trunk of the artery.

The analysis results of these realistic RCA models are found to be consistent with the results observed in the simulated RCA models. The low WSS regions (WSS $\leq$ 4 Pa) are seen to occur at the inner wall of the curve and opposite to the flow divider, while high WSS (WSS $\geq$ 40 Pa) are associated with angulation, showing a direct correlation between (1) the hemodynamic effects and (2) the curvature and angulation of RCAs. Figure 13.29 shows that (1) the realistic RCA shapes complex wall geometry directly affects the hemodynamic parameters WSS and WPG; (2) there are more of less intensified WSS regions opposite to the angulation and inner wall of the curve; (3) the high WSS are always located adjacent to the bifurcation; and (4) the WSS is higher at the proximal inlet, as particularly evident by contrasting the high WSS at bifurcation.

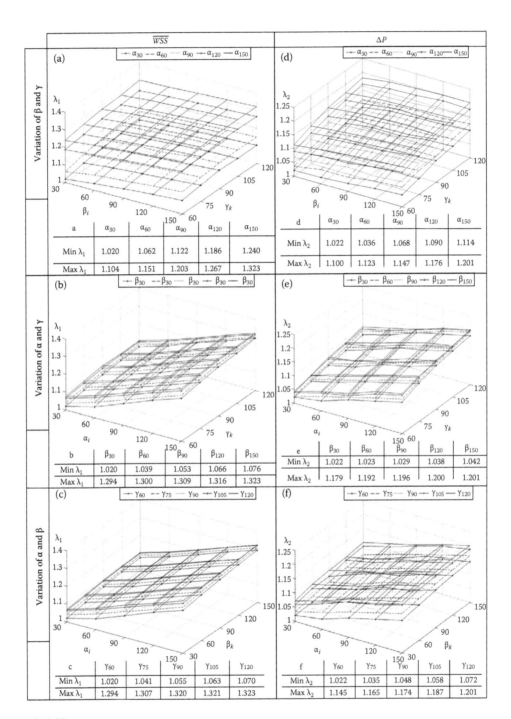

FIGURE 13.28

Surface response curves of parameter ratios λ_1 and λ_2, based on the variations of α, β, and γ. After normalization with the standard model $\alpha_0\beta_0\gamma_{60}$, the greater curved trunk and larger bifurcating side-branch are shown to present bigger values of the λ_1 and λ_2 ratios, implying larger WSS and WPG distributions. The layer-to-layer distances of the respective surfaces in the z-axis direction represent the variable α, and the plots show that the curvature of the arterial trunk plays a significant role in modifying the fluid mechanics transport of blood in the RCA.

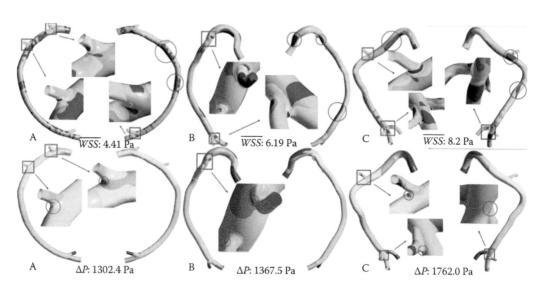

FIGURE 13.29
WSS and WPG surface plots of realistic RCAs (A, B, and C). The squared sections are enlarged to illustrate the detailed localized angulation contour. Therein, the circle boundaries show (1) low WSS regions for WSS ≤ 4 Pa opposite to the angulation and inner wall of the curve, and (2) high WSS located adjacent to the bifurcation. The $\overline{WSS}$ and ΔP of arteries increase with complexity in the geometry of the RCA.

The shape and size of quantifiable WSS regions vary with the angulation and curvature; the low WSS are distributed throughout the artery and are associated with the curvature and bifurcation. The $\overline{WSS}$ of arteries A, B, and C are 4.41, 6.19, and 8.21 Pa, with the maximum WSS value up to 67.7, 71.65, and 88.3 Pa, respectively. Obviously, there is a bigger WSS gradient for artery C. The $\overline{WSS}$ and maximum WSS of artery C are higher than that of arteries A and B, which demonstrates that the geometry plays an important role in the hemodynamics of coronary arteries. However, the localized maximum WSS regions are associated with bifurcation.

Similarly, the WPG is noticed to change in the same way as the WSS. The relatively low and high WPG regions in the three RCAs are similar to those observed in the idealized models. Generally, the wall pressure is higher at the proximal inlet than at the distal outlet at Peak systole. The ΔP of arteries A, B, and C are 1302.4, 1367.5, and 1762.0 Pa, respectively, and are 2–3 times greater than in the idealized models due to the complex geometry of realistic models. This indicates the difference between realistic RCA models and the idealized models, as the realistic models represent the patients' actual arterial geometry, while the simulated models do not incorporate the complex wall geometry such as the tortuous appearance of the vessel wall and the diameter variation along the arteries. In these RCAs, the location of the plaque in the arteries was identified to be consistent with the regions, which have relatively lower wall shear stress (WSS ≤ 4 Pa) opposite to the angulation and inner wall of the curve.

13.5.8 Discussion of Results

Our results based on idealized and realistic coronary models show that there is a direct correlation between (1) angulation and curvature, and (2) hemodynamic changes. The low and high WSS regions are observed to be affected by curvature and angulation such that the larger the curvature and angulation, the higher will be the $\overline{WSS}$ and ΔP values. The variable WSS regions are occurring at the inner wall of the curves and bifurcations, because of the irregular curves and changing locations of angulations. Furthermore, the distribution of WSS and WPG in the regions are affected by the arterial curvature and angulation in the idealized and realistic models.

Our study results based on Figures 13.26 through 13.29 have (1) confirmed that low WSS regions are located at the inner wall of the arterial curve and opposite to the flow divider and (2) depict increased values of $\overline{WSS}$ and ΔP with higher values of curvature angle α and branch bifurcation angle γ. We can then postulate that in RCAs, the atherosclerotic plaques are more prone to be located at the relatively low WSS and WPG sites of the curved arterial trunk and its branch for arbitrary degrees of curvature. In the curved segments, the low localized WSS regions are seen to occur at the inner wall of the curve, where they can be correlated with the enhanced intimal thickness and lesions progression to predict the formation of early atherosclerotic plaques. This can explain why highly curved mid-regions of RCAs develop severe narrowing of the lumen [69]. Based on the angulations, the low WSS and WPG regions are shown to appear opposite to the bifurcation, with high WSS and WPG appearing at the bifurcation sites where plaques are frequently known to occur [29,69].

It is worthwhile mentioning that the understanding of the mechanisms of plaque development mechanism is still somewhat unclear, despite intensive investigations by different schools of thoughts. A few existing studies suggest that the vessel occlusion is stimulated by low levels of WSS [54,70] and propose that (1) low and oscillating WSS increases the risk of occurrence of the disease, while (2) high WSS tends to suppress it [54]. Some researchers have believed that the disease is caused by the vessel experiencing very high WSS; an example for this is the occurrence of highly aggravated plaques at the apex of stenosis and the bifurcation point [15,71]. It is clear that these two regions experience high shear stress and stimulate the plaque progression.

With respect to the coronary arteries, many researchers have focused on the trunk of RCAs [19–21,72], but with limited studies on the side-branches in the study of location of intimal thickness and lesions in necropsy, histopathology, imaging studies, and numerical simulation. In our study, we have found that the side-branches can significantly affect the values and distribution of WSS and WPG.

Because of the simplicity of measuring intracoronary pressure, it has been concluded that combined pressure and flow velocity measurements may provide a useful tool for assessment of functional lesions on the severity of flow resistance [49,73]. In our study, we have found that the pressure drop between inlet and outlet is affected by both curvature and angulation; clearly, the correlation of the larger flow resistance, corresponding to the greater pressure drop caused by the complex geometry, cannot be neglected. Clinically, for the patients who need CABG, the CABG patency postoperatively may be influenced by the distal anastomosis sites and the angle of anastomosis. Based on our analysis, the anastomosis sites should be far away from larger curved segments and the larger angle side-branches segments. Further, the angle of anastomosis should be considered from the viewpoint of minimizing the oscillating WSS at the bifurcations.

In our study, the RCAs are assumed to have a rigid wall rather than elastic wall; therefore, the simulation does not fully reflect the realistic physiological situation as the coronary wall deforms during the cardiac cycles [74]. With elastic vascular walls and increased vascular compliance, the values of $\overline{WSS}$ and ΔP can be physiologically larger [75]. Also, for the realistic RCAs, we have ignored the diameter variation along the arteries, and WSS can further increase because of decreased diameter and tapering at distal artery [8].

The image-based models (in Figure 13.29) demonstrate that the spatial distribution of WSS and WPG varies considerably among individuals and even among branches. However, these differences cannot be explained by curvature and branch angles alone. Many other factors are at play (i.e., local cross-sectional diameter, distance from inlet, degree of developed flow, etc.), limiting the applicability of conclusions drawn from parametric models varying only the curvature or angle of branching. However, this study is performed as an exemplification of explaining how these geometrical parameters can affect the hemodynamic flow patterns and parameters with some consistency.

Likewise, from the fluid mechanics perspective, the current understanding of the role of hemodynamics in atherosclerosis is that the direction of WSS vector in addition to its magnitude is a critical determinant of the localization and progression of atherosclerosis; this requires the commonly accepted metrics of the oscillatory shear index (OSI) to be an important surface response to the arterial parameters. In fact, there also exists a variety of metrics, namely, spatial gradient of WSS, relative residence time, etc., that can be contributory to atherosclerosis formation. In our study, we have employed the two response parameters WSS and WPG as the primary metrics, to indicate the implications of varying arterial geometry, and also of the parameters λ_1 and λ_2 on plaque formation.

13.6 Discussion of Flow Quantification Used to Characterize Coronary Arterial Flow Conditions

13.6.1 Influence of Stenosis on Flow Resistance and the Threat of Ischemia

In most patients with atherosclerosis disease, there is decrease of vessel wall elasticity and high blood pressure due to the lipid deposition in the blood vessel wall, fibrosis, and partial calcification. When there is atherosclerotic stenosis in the blood vessels, the local vasculature will be stiffer, and less blood is supplied into the relevant myocardial area. In order to ensure adequate blood supply, the heart needs to work harder to overcome the increased flow resistance caused by the stenosis. When the stenosis in the artery reaches a certain limiting value, the coronary flow cannot overcome the high flow resistance. Hence, due to reduced blood flow in that coronary segment, different degrees of ischemia will appear in the stenotic areas of the blood vessel. In emergency cases, plaques may disrupt and produce overt symptoms when the stress on the vessel wall exceeds rupture limits.

For the blood vessel with stenosis, a greater pressure is required to force more blood to go through the stenosis area to the distal segment at a faster velocity. This is manifested by FSI simulation as a greater pressure drop between the entrance and exit of blood vessel. Now, as we know, Poiseuille's law demonstrates that in laminar flow through tubes, the flow resistance of blood vessel is related to the pressure drop between the inlet and outlet flow traffic as well as to the lumen radius. It is found that when the flow traffic is constant, the pressure drop is proportional to the flow resistance [76]. The research results show that greater stenosis and associated reduced lumen area leads to the larger ΔP and greater flow resistance in the blood vessels. This is also confirmed by the catheter measurement of the blood flow velocity and pressure [49,73] in the proximal and distal of blood vessels, to assess the blood flow resistance in proportion to the stenosis degree. Our study has shown that the narrower the artery, the greater is the pressure drop between the proximal and distal segments of the blood vessels.

We have employed numerical simulations of the bent stenosed artery to carry out quantitative hemodynamic analysis in terms of WSS, ΔP, and other parameters. Also, the mutual mechanical interactions between the motion of the vessel wall and fluid have been taken into account. Our utilization of the pulse wave for the physiological inlet velocity and outlet pressure of the blood makes the simulation closer to the real physiological state.

We have also made some simplifying assumptions in the fluid properties. In other words, the fluid is assumed to be a Newtonian fluid. In fact, the blood flow exhibits a non-Newtonian fluid property when the shear rate is lower than 100 s^{-1}, and a Newtonian fluid property when the shear rate is larger than 100 s^{-1} [61]. Furthermore, all blood vessels in our study are idealized as curved arteries without twist. The plaque on the bending side retains a regular shape, and is closely attached to the blood vessel wall. We have also assumed that the elastic modulus of the plaque is consistent with that of the vessel wall, and not taken into account the different elastic moduli of the plaque components such as fibrous cap, lipid pool, and calcification.

In summary, we have provided a comprehensive examination of the effect of arterial bending, curvature, and atherosclerotic plaques on (1) average wall shear stress, and (2) the pressure drop ΔP between the inlet and outlet of the blood vessels (representing the flow resistance).

13.6.2 Further Insights into Atherosclerosis Causative Mechanism

Research into the cause of atherosclerosis has been performed for decades [3,9,10]. There are various schools of thoughts on its causative mechanism. In this regard, one group believes that plaque growth is due to low wall and oscillating shear stress levels [11,19,20,45,54,77], whereas high levels of this parameter tend to suppress it [9,11,45]. In addition to the low and oscillating WSS, the intramural stress of the wall may also contribute to plaque growth at an advance stage of the disease [46].

Another group believes that vessel wall thickening occurs in the event of high shear stress (as reported by [15,71]). It is also believed that von Mises and principal stress at the apex of the plaque can be used to characterize the initialization and aggravation of its growth [49–51,78–81]. Meanwhile, the search for other indicators to better describe the causative mechanism is still on-going. We have shown in our results that the stenotic part of the arteries experiences high WSS and demonstrates to be more prone to plaque aggravation. This is consistent with the previous experimental studies.

The extensive flow information generated by our work can be used to gain insight into the formation of plaque and its vulnerability. Herein, computational modeling of atherosclerotic arteries in this research has been performed, by taking into consideration the structural modifications of stenosis variations. It has been shown that the local low WSS and wall pressure regions sites at the plaque-prone points are consistent with the data derived from literatures of anatomical and clinical researches. Likewise, there is also consistency with the literature data of the variational trends for both the magnitude and spatial distribution of WSS, wall pressure, and von Mises stress. The influence on these hemodynamic parameters due to changes in vessel geometry goes to demonstrate the hemodynamic differences among the models with anatomic diversity. Most importantly, our flow analysis hemodynamic data of WSS and pressure drop in atherosclerotic vessels is sufficient to serve as the reference data for the assessment of flow resistance through varying arterial structures and von Mises stress for predicting the plaque rupture.

In atherosclerosis, there is a decrease of vessel wall elasticity and high blood pressure due to the lipid deposition in the blood vessel wall, fibrosis, and partial calcification. In the event of stenosis of the coronary blood vessels, the local vasculature stiffens and narrows to result in less blood being supplied to the heart. In order to ensure adequate blood supply, the heart needs to work harder to overcome the increased flow resistance caused by the stenosis. When the artery stenosis reaches to a certain limitation extent, the coronary flow cannot overcome the high flow resistance; then, due to reduced blood flow in that coronary segment, different degrees of ischemia will appear in the stenotic segments of the diseased blood vessel.

Poiseuille's law demonstrates that for a laminar fluid flow through a straight and rigid cylinder, the flow resistance of blood vessel is related to the pressure difference (PD) across the inlet and outlet of the vessel and its lumen radius. For a constant flow volume, the PD is proportional to the flow resistance [76]. As such, this confirms our simulation results, whereby an aggravated stenosis and narrowing results in a larger PD, and a subsequent increase in flow resistance of blood through the diseased blood vessels. Our modeling results have proven that as narrowing becomes greater for the coronary artery, the pressure difference between the proximal and distal segments of the blood vessels also increases.

13.6.3 Elasticity of Atherosclerotic Arteries and Its Implication in Atherogenesis

Although there is no direct relationship between deformation and atherogenesis, the presence and characterization of high deformation regions at the throat of the artery has been investigated for inducing plaque rupture. Atherosclerotic plaque may be categorized into various types, such as (1) atheromatous plaque that has an artheroma or lipid pool covered with fibrous cap and (2) a nonatheromatous plaque that consists of connective issue with admixed smooth muscle cells, and the calcified plaque. We have shown that the FSI algorithm based on the dynamic equations of elastic arterial wall motion coupled with the Navier–Stokes equations for a viscous incompressible fluid captures the experimentally measured elastic properties of arterial walls in the modeled arterial length. The reduced effective model reveals several interesting features of the coupled FSI problem.

It is also of interest from the evidence of the 3D surface plots that the elastic boundary conditions seemed to have a higher resistance to that of the rigid boundary conditions. This result is because energy is taken to deform the blood vessel, and hence, there is a loss of momentum and more resistance is added due to the loss of momentum and in the direction of flow. Based on comparisons between transient and steady state flows, the transient flow conditions seem to have a higher resistance, which corresponds to a higher flow resistance ratio compared to that of steady state flow conditions. This also corresponds to the scenario in which the energy in the pulse generated by the pump (heart) begins to lose the momentum throughout the length of artery due to friction from the arterial walls.

To study the coupling between the motion of the vessel wall and pulsatile blood flow, a detailed description of the vessel wall biomechanical properties may lead to a mathematical and numerical problem whose complexity is beyond today's computational capabilities. The nonlinearity of the underlying FSI is so severe that even a simplified description of the vessel wall mechanics assuming homogeneous linearly elastic behavior leads to complicated numerical algorithms with challenging stability and convergence properties. To devise a mathematical model that can lead to producing computational solutions in a reasonable period (time frame), various simplifications need to be introduced.

13.6.4 Medical Imaging and Experimental Techniques Involved in Supporting CFD

Medical imaging modalities are able to characterize the atherosclerotic plaques in terms of their mechanical properties. Noninvasive imaging not only identifies flow-limiting vascular stenosis but can also measure the atherosclerotic plaque burden and its response to treatment, and to differentiate stable plaques from those which tend to rupture. However, the prediction of high-risk plaque rupture still requires a numerical simulation framework for quantification.

Herein, we have carried out numerical simulations of variational stenotic arteries to determine the hemodynamic parameters of WSS and ΔP. The mechanical interaction between the vessel wall and fluid is modeled by using FSI. The utilization of a pulsatile waveform for the physiological inlet velocity and outlet pressure of the blood brings the simulation closer to its real physiological state. With the application of fluid dynamics into an advanced system of coupling two fluid and structural solvers by using FSI, it is possible to determine the differences in flow behavior throughout a length of artery with variational geometrical properties. The visualization of 3D surface plots has provided a strong base to support traditional medical image diagnostic techniques and theoretical measures that lead to determination of flow resistances.

All of this work is clinically important in providing the basis and causes of flow resistance assessment causing pathological lesions and can provide a basis for surgical design and construction of coronary arterial bypass grafting.

References

1. Fry, D.L., Acute vascular endothelial changes associated with increased blood velocity gradients. *Circulation Research*, 1968. **22**(2): 165–197.
2. Fry, D.L., Certain histological and chemical responses of the vascular interface to acutely induced mechanical stress in the aorta of the dog. *Circulation Research*, 1969. **24**(1): 93–108.
3. Wong, K.K.L. et al., Modelling of blood flow resistance for an atherosclerotic artery with multiple stenoses and poststenotic dilatations. *ANZIAM Journal*, 2010. **51**: C66–C82.
4. Wong, K.K.L. et al., Theoretical modelling of micro-scale biological phenomena in human coronary arteries. *Medical and Biological Engineering and Computing*, 2006. **44**(11): 971–982.
5. Bluestein, D. et al., Influence of microcalcifications on vulnerable plaque mechanics using FSI modeling. *Journal of Biomechanics*, 2008. **41**(5): 1111–1118.
6. Tang, D. et al., Effect of a lipid pool on stress/strain distributions in stenotic arteries: 3-D fluid–structure interactions (FSI) models. *Journal of Biomechanical Engineering*, 2004. **126**: 363–370.
7. Torii, R. et al., Fluid–structure interaction analysis of a patient-specific right coronary artery with physiological velocity and pressure waveforms. *Communications in Numerical Methods in Engineering*, 2009. **25**(5): 565–580.
8. Johnston, B.M. et al., Non-Newtonian blood flow in human right coronary arteries: Transient simulations. *Journal of Biomechanics*, 2006. **39**(6): 1116–1128.
9. Vasava, P., P. Jalali, and M. Dabagh, Finite element modelling of pulsatile blood flow in idealized model of human aortic arch: Study of hypotension and hypertension. *Computational and Mathematical Methods in Medicine*, 2012. **2012**: 1–14.
10. Plank, M.J. et al., Modelling the early stages of atherosclerosis, in: A. Deutsch, L. Brusch, H. Byrne, G. de Vries, and H. Herzel (eds.), *Mathematical Modelling of Biological Systems*. Birkhäuser, Boston, MA, 2007, pp. 263–274.
11. Nosovitsky, V.A. et al., Effects of curvature and stenosis-like narrowing on wall shear stress in a coronary artery model with phasic flow. *Computers and Biomedical Research*, 1997. **30**(1): 61–82.
12. Fox, B. and W. Seed, Location of early atheroma in the human coronary arteries. *Journal of Biomechanical Engineering*, 1981. **103**(3): 208–212.
13. Asakura, T. and T. Karino, Flow patterns and spatial distribution of atherosclerotic lesions in human coronary arteries. *Circulation Research*, 1990. **66**(4): 1045–1066.

14. Tang, D. et al., Local maximal stress hypothesis and computational plaque vulnerability index for atherosclerotic plaque assessment. *Annals of Biomedical Engineering*, 2005. **33**(12): 1789–1801.
15. Wentzel, J.J. et al., Extension of increased atherosclerotic wall thickness into high shear stress regions is associated with loss of compensatory remodeling. *Circulation*, 2003. **108**(1): 17–23.
16. DePaola, N. et al., Vascular endothelium responds to fluid shear stress gradients. *Arteriosclerosis, Thrombosis, and Vascular Biology*, 1992. **12**(11): 1254–1257.
17. Giannoglou, G.D. et al., Hemodynamic factors and the important role of local low static pressure in coronary wall thickening. *International Journal of Cardiology*, 2002. **86**(1): 27–40.
18. Giannoglou, G.D. et al., Wall pressure gradient in normal left coronary artery tree. *Medical Engineering and Physics*, 2005. **27**(6): 455–464.
19. Jeremias, A. et al., Spatial orientation of atherosclerotic plaque in non-branching coronary artery segment. *Atherosclerosis*, 2000. **152**(1): 209–215.
20. Grunfeld, C. et al., Relation of coronary artery plaque location to extent of coronary artery disease studied by computed tomographic angiography. *Journal of Cardiovascular Computed Tomography*, 2010. **4**(1): 19–26.
21. Ojha, M.L. et al., Distribution of intimal and medial thickening in the human right coronary artery: A study of 17 RCAs. *Atherosclerosis*, 2001. **158**(1): 147–153.
22. Fox, B. et al., Distribution of fatty and fibrous plaques in young human coronary arteries. *Atherosclerosis*, 1982. **41**(2): 337–347.
23. McGill, H.C. et al., Effects of coronary heart disease risk factors on atherosclerosis of selected regions of the aorta and right coronary artery. *Arteriosclerosis, Thrombosis, and Vascular Biology*, 2000. **20**(3): 836–845.
24. Qiao, A. et al., Numerical study of nonlinear pulsatile flow in S-shaped curved arteries. *Medical Engineering and Physics*, 2004. **26**(7): 545–552.
25. Soulis, J.V. et al., Wall shear stress in normal left coronary artery tree. *Journal of Biomechanics*, 2006. **39**(4): 742–749.
26. Perktold, K. et al., Pulsatile non-Newtonian blood flow in three-dimensional carotid bifurcation models: A numerical study of flow phenomena under different bifurcation angles. *Journal of Biomedical Engineering*, 1991. **13**(6): 507–515.
27. Chaichana, T., Z. Sun, and J. Jewkes, Computation of hemodynamics in the left coronary artery with variable angulations. *Journal of Biomechanics*, 2011. **44**(10): 1869–1878.
28. Ross, R., The pathogenesis of atherosclerosis—An update. *New England Journal of Medicine*, 1986. **314**(8): 488–500.
29. Friedman, M. et al., Correlation between wall shear and intimal thickness at a coronary artery branch. *Atherosclerosis*, 1987. **68**(1): 27–33.
30. Kirpalani, A. et al., Velocity and WSS patterns in the human right coronary artery. *Journal of Biomechanical Engineering*, 1999. **121**(4): 370–375.
31. Perktold, K. et al., Validated computation of physiologic flow in a realistic coronary artery branch. *Journal of Biomechanics*, 1998. **31**: 217–228.
32. Worthley, S.G. et al., High resolution ex vivo magnetic resonance imaging of in situ coronary and aortic atherosclerotic plaque in a porcine model. *Atherosclerosis*, 2000. **150**(2): 321–329.
33. Worthley, S.G. et al., Serial in vivo MRI documents arterial remodeling in experimental atherosclerosis. *Circulation*, 2000. **101**(6): 586–589.
34. Worthley, S.G. et al., Coronary artery imaging in the new millennium. *Heart, Lung and Circulation*, 2002. **11**(1): 19–25.
35. Figueiredo, M.A.T. and J.M.N. Leitaeo, A nonsmoothing approach to the estimation of vessel contours in angiograms. *IEEE Transactions on Medical Imaging*, 1995. **14**(1): 162–172.
36. Sun, Y., Automated identification of vessel contours in coronary arteriograms by an adaptive tracking algorithm. *IEEE Transactions on Medical Imaging*, 1989. **8**(1): 78–88.
37. Atar, E. et al., Balloon angioplasty of popliteal and crural arteries in elderly with critical chronic limb ischemia. *European Journal of Radiology*, 2005. **53**(2): 287–292.

38. Kaul, P. et al., Coronary artery bypass grafting and concomitant excision of chest wall chondrosarcoma. *Journal of Cardiothoracic Surgery*, 2009. **4**: 7.
39. Kiemeneij, F. et al., Outpatient coronary stent implantation. *Journal of the American College of Cardiology*, 1997. **29**(2): 323–327.
40. MacGregor, F.B., J.C. Doughty, and L.D. Cooke, Vocal fold paralysis following carotid endarterectomy. *Journal of Laryngology and Otology*, 1999. **113**: 439–441.
41. Moore, J.A. et al., Numerical study of blood flow patterns in anatomically realistic and simplified end-to-side anastomoses. *Journal of Biomechanical Engineering*, 1999. **121**: 265–272.
42. Pincombe, B., A study of non-Newtonian behaviour of blood flow through stenosed arteries. PhD thesis, University of Adelaide, Adelaide, South Australia, Australia, 1998.
43. Pincombe, B. and J.N. Mazumdar, Techniques for the study of blood flow through both constrictions and post-stenotic dilatations in arteries. *Computational Methods in Biophysics, Biomaterials, Biotechnology and Medical Systems: Algorithmic Development, Mathematical Analysis and Diagnostics*, 2003. **4**: 187–246.
44. Pincombe, B. and J.N. Mazumdar, Numerical model of power law flow through an atherosclerotic artery, in: B.J. Noye, M.D. Teubner, and A. Gill (eds.), *CTAC'97*, World Scientific Press, Adelaide, Australia, 1998, pp. 563–570.
45. Simone, T. et al., Arterial stiffness is associated with cardiovascular, renal, retinal, and autonomic disease in type 1 diabetes. *Diabetes Care*, 2013. **36**(3): 715–721.
46. Simone, T. et al., Clinical application of arterial stiffness: Definitions and reference values. *American Journal of Hypertension*, 2002. **15**(5): 426–444.
47. Hadjiloizou, N. et al., Differences in cardiac microcirculatory wave patterns between the proximal left main stem and proximal RCA. *American Journal of Physiology: Heart and Circulatory Physiology*, 2008. **295**(3): H1198–H1205.
48. Bhaganagar, K., C. Veeramachaneni, and C. Moreno, Significance of plaque morphology in modifying flow characteristics in a diseased coronary artery: Numerical simulation using plaque measurements from intravascular ultrasound imaging. *Applied Mathematical Modelling*, 2012. **37**(7): 5381–5393.
49. van de Hoef, T.P. et al., Diagnostic accuracy of combined intracoronary pressure and flow velocity information during baseline conditions adenosine-free assessment of functional coronary lesion severity. *Circulation: Cardiovascular Interventions*, 2012. **5**(4): 508–514.
50. Rambhia, S.H. et al., Microcalcifications increase coronary vulnerable plaque rupture potential: A patient-based micro-CT fluid-structure interaction study. *Annals of Biomedical Engineering*, 2012. **40**(7): 1443–1454.
51. Li, Z.Y., Impact of calcification and intraluminal thrombus on the computed wall stresses of abdominal aortic aneurysm. *Journal of Vascular Surgery*, 2008. **47**(5): 928–935.
52. Steinman, D.A., Image-based CFD modeling in realistic arterial geometries. *Annals of Biomedical Engineering*, 2002. **30**(4): 483–497.
53. Li, M.X. et al., Numerical analysis of pulsatile blood flow and vessel wall mechanics in different degrees of stenoses. *Journal of Biomechanics*, 2007. **40**(16): 3715–3724.
54. Nerem, R.M., Vascular fluid mechanics, the arterial wall, and atherosclerosis. *Journal of Biomechanical Engineering*, 1992. **114**(3): 274–282.
55. Kompatsiaris, I. et al., Deformable boundary detection of stents in angiographic images. *IEEE Transactions on Medical Imaging*, 2000. **19**(6): 652–662.
56. Liu, G. et al., Numerical simulation of flow in curved coronary arteries with progressive amounts of stenosis using fluid-structure interaction modelling. *Journal of Medical Imaging and Health Informatics*, 2014. **4**: 1–7.
57. Soulis, J.V. et al., Wall shear stress in normal left coronary artery tree. *Journal of Biomechanical Engineering*, 2006. **39**(4): 742–749.
58. Prosia, M., K. Perktoldb, and H. Schimac, Effect of continuous arterial blood flow in patients with rotary cardiac assist device on the washout of a stenosis wake in the carotid bifurcation: A computer simulation study. *Journal of Biomechanics*, 2007. **40**(10): 2236–2243.

59. Chaichana, T., Z. Sun, and J. Jewkes, Hemodynamic impacts of left coronary stenosis: A patient-specific analysis. *Acta of Bioengineering and Biomechanics*, 2013. **15**(3): 107–112.
60. Chaichana, T., Z. Sun, and J. Jewkes, Hemodynamic impacts of various types of stenosis in the left coronary artery bifurcation: A patient-specific analysis. *Physica Medica*, 2013. **29**(5): 447–452.
61. Johnston, B.M. et al., Non-Newtonian blood flow in human right coronary arteries: Steady state simulations. *Journal of Biomechanics*, 2004. **37**(5): 709–720.
62. Poiseuille, J., Observations of blood flow. *Annales des Sciences Naturelles Série*, 1836. **5**: 2.
63. Schilt, S. et al., The effects of time-varying curvature on velocity profiles in a model of the coronary arteries. *Biomechanics*, 1996. **29**(4): 469–474.
64. Honda, H.M. et al., A complex flow pattern of low shear stress and flow reversal promotes monocyte binding to endothelial cells. *Atherosclerosis*, 2001. **158**(2): 385–390.
65. Weydahl, E.S. and J.J.E. Moore, Dynamic curvature strongly affects wall shear rates in a coronary artery bifurcation model. *Biomechanics*, 2001. **34**(9): 1189–1196.
66. He, X. and D.N. Ku, Pulsatile flow in the human left coronary artery bifurcation: Average conditions. *Biomechanical Engineering*, 1996. **118**(1): 74–82.
67. Pivkin, I. et al., Combined effects of pulsatile flow and dynamic curvature on wall shear stress in a coronary artery bifurcation model. *Journal of Biomechanics*, 2005. **38**(6): 1283–1290.
68. Wong, K. et al., Differences in cardiac microcirculatory wave patterns between the proximal left mainstem and proximal right coronary artery. *Medical and Biological Engineering and Computing*, 2006. **44**(11): 971–982.
69. Zarins, C.K. et al., Carotid bifurcation atherosclerosis. Quantitative correlation of plaque localization with flow velocity profiles and WSS. *Circulation Research*, 1983. **53**(4): 502–514.
70. Friedman, M.H. et al., Shear-dependent thickening of the human arterial intima. *Atherosclerosis*, 1986. **60**(2): 161–171.
71. Joshi, A.K. et al., Intimal thickness is not associated with wall shear stress patterns in the human right coronary artery. *Arteriosclerosis, Thrombosis, and Vascular Biology*, 2004. **24**(12): 2408–2413.
72. McDaniel, M.C. et al., Localization of culprit lesions in coronary arteries of patients with ST-segment elevation myocardial infarctions: Relation to bifurcations and curvatures. *American Heart Journal*, 2011. **161**(3): 508–515.
73. Sen, S. et al., Diagnostic classification of the instantaneous wave-free ratio is equivalent to fractional flow reserve and is not improved with adenosine administration. Results of CLARIFY (Classification Accuracy of Pressure-Only Ratios Against Indices Using Flow Study). *Journal of the American College of Cardiology*, 2013. **61**(13): 1409–1420.
74. Malvè, M. et al., Unsteady blood flow and mass transfer of a human left coronary artery bifurcation: FSI vs. CFD. *Journal of Physics Condensed Matter*, 2012. **39**(6): 745–751.
75. Wu, J. et al., Transient blood flow in elastic coronary arteries with varying degrees of stenosis and dilatations: CFD modelling and parametric study. *Computer Methods in Biomechanics and Biomedical Engineering*, 2014. **18**(16):1835–1845.
76. Severin, J., K. Beckert, and H. Herwig, Spatial development of disturbances in plane Poiseuille flow: A direct numerical simulation using a commercial CFD code. *International Journal of Heat and Mass Transfer*, 2001. **44**(22): 4359–4367.
77. Kleinstreuer, C. et al., Hemodynamic parameters and early intimal thickening in branching blood vessels. *Critical Reviews in Biomedical Engineering*, 2001. **29**(1): 1–64.
78. Salzar, R.S., M.J. Thubrikar, and R.T. Eppink, Pressure-induced mechanical stress in the carotid artery bifurcation: A possible correlation to atherosclerosis. *Journal of Biomechanics*, 1995. **28**(11): 1333–1340.
79. Thubrikar, M.J. and F. Robicsek, Pressure-induced arterial wall stress and atherosclerosis. *Annals of Thoracic Surgery*, 1995. **59**(6): 1594–1603.
80. Kaunas, R., S. Usami, and S. Chien, Regulation of stretch-induced JNK activation by stress fiber orientation. *Cellular Signalling*, 2006. **18**(11): 1924–1931.
81. Lee, K.W. and X.Y. Xu, Modelling of flow and wall behaviour in a mildly stenosed tube. *Medical Engineering and Physics*, 2002. **24**(9): 575–586.

14

Intra-Left Ventricular Flow Velocity Distributions, Based on Color Doppler Echo Vector Flow Mapping of Normal Subjects and Heart Failure Patients

Thu-Thao Le, Dhanjoo N. Ghista, Ru San Tan, and Sridhar Idapalapati

CONTENTS

Terminology

A	Peak flow velocity at atrial contraction phase, measured from pulsed Doppler echo
DT	Deceleration time, measured from peak to end of rapid filling phase from pulsed Doppler echo
E	Peak flow velocity at rapid filling phase, measured from pulsed Doppler echo
E'	Peak myocardial velocity, measured at the septal mitral annulus from pulsed tissue Doppler echo
PVs	Peak systolic flow velocity from pulmonary vein to LA, measured from pulsed Doppler echo
PVd	Peak diastolic flow velocity from pulmonary vein to LA, measured from pulsed Doppler echo
$\mathbf{u}_b, \mathbf{u}_v$	Basic non-vortical laminar flow and vortex flow components of Doppler velocity, respectively
$\mathbf{v}_b, \mathbf{v}_v$	Radial basic non-vortical laminar flow and radial vortex flow components, respectively

14.1 Introduction

The left ventricle (LV) is the biological pump for circulation, and the left atrium (LA) plays a major role in filling the LV in a way as to facilitate directed blood flow for ejection into the aorta by its contraction process. The LA transfers blood to LV in two steps: in the first step, the pressure gradient between LA and LV causes blood to passively flow into the LV at velocity *E*; the second step filling is caused by LA contraction, at filling velocity *A*. In a healthy heart, the *E* velocity is greater than the *A* velocity. The reduced value of the *E/A* ratio is often accepted as a clinical marker of diastolic dysfunction, in which the LV becomes so stiff as to impair proper filling, which can lead to diastolic heart failure.

Intra-cardiac flow is useful for evaluating cardiac function, as it is the end-result of cardiac myocardial abnormalities. The vortex flow during left ventricular filling is a critical determinant of directed blood flow during ejection and can offer a novel index of cardiac dysfunction. Vector flow mapping (VFM) technique has been recently developed to generate flow velocity vector fields by post-processing color Doppler echo images. In this technique, axial velocity is measured from color Doppler images, while radial velocity is computed by deconstructing the flow into a basic non-vortical laminar motion and a vortical component.

In normal subjects, after flow ejection into LV, the direction of flow is reversed toward the apex with a brief appearance of vortex at the early stage of isovolumic relaxation time. The major diastolic anterior vortex develops immediately after the onset of the early diastolic phase. This vortex continues during diastasis, persists into late LV filling phase and throughout isovolumic contraction phase and dissipates with the opening of the aortic valve and LV ejection. By using color-Doppler derived VFM, the intraventricular vortex flow can be determined for the detection of pathologically altered flow characteristics and identification of new pathophysiological mechanisms in the development of cardiac disease.

We have carried out clinical studies to determine intra-LV flow patterns for HF patients (both HFNEF and HFREF) and normal subjects. Color Doppler flow images were captured at the three-chamber view for visualization of both inflow through mitral valve and outflow into the aorta. Intra-LV flow was determined using the VFM analysis package. In this technique, color Doppler velocity (axial velocity, $\mathbf{u}$) profile was analyzed across an arc at each echo depth. The measured Doppler velocity $\mathbf{u}$ along the beam line is composed of basic non-vortical laminar flow ($\mathbf{u}_b$) and vortex flow ($\mathbf{u}_v$) components. The basic flow component $\mathbf{u}_b$ is computed as $\mathbf{u}_b = \mathbf{u} - \mathbf{u}_v$. Then the vortex flow velocity components $\mathbf{u}_v$ (along the Doppler beam) and $\mathbf{v}_v$ (perpendicular to the Doppler beam) are obtained in terms of the stream function $\psi(r, \theta)$ as $\mathbf{u}_v = (1/r)(\partial\psi/\partial\theta)$ and $\mathbf{v}_v = -(\partial\psi/\partial\theta)$. The radial basic flow component $\mathbf{v}_b$ is obtained from $\mathbf{u}_b$ as $\mathbf{v}_b = \mathbf{u}_b \tan \theta$. The flow velocity $\mathbf{U}(r, \theta)$ is then calculated as $\mathbf{U}(r, \theta) = (\mathbf{u}_b(r, \theta) + \mathbf{u}_v(r, \theta))$ $\mathbf{i}(r, \theta) + (\mathbf{v}_b(r, \theta) + \mathbf{v}_v(r, \theta))\mathbf{j}(r, \theta)$, where (1) $\mathbf{i}(r, \theta)$ and $\mathbf{j}(r, \theta)$ are the unit vectors in the axial and radial direction, respectively, at point (r, θ); (2) $\mathbf{u}_b$ and $\mathbf{u}_v$ are in the axial Doppler beam direction, while $\mathbf{v}_b$ and $\mathbf{v}_v$ are in the radial direction perpendicular to the Doppler beam.

The contractility index $d\sigma^*/dt_{max}$ is formulated as

$$\frac{d\sigma^*}{dt_{max}} = 1.5 \times \frac{dV/dt_{max}}{MV}$$

where
dV/dt_{max} is the maximal flow rate into the aorta, measured at the LVOT using VFM
MV is the myocardial volume, calculated as a quotient of LV mass (determined from M-mode images) and myocardial density (assumed to be 1.05 g/mL)

We selected two groups of subjects for our clinical study: Group 1 consists of HFNEF1 and HFNEF2 and one normal subject1; Group 2 consists of HFREF1 and HFREF2 and one normal subject2.

In diastolic flow patterns (illustrated in Figure 14.6), in the rapid filling phase, straight flow is seen to rush into the LV from the LA; circulating flow patterns are seen at the anterior and posterior walls of the LV in all subjects. In HFNEF patients there is no inflow during the diastasis phase, whereas in HFREF patients the flow continues to enter the LV with two circulating flow patterns seen at the anterior and posterior walls. The flow patterns for diastasis phase and atrial contraction phases are illustrated and are marked by circulating flow patterns, prominently at the anterior wall, until the end of atrial contraction. Markedly prolonged diastasis phase is seen in both HFNEF patients.

In systolic flow patterns (illustrated in Figure 14.8), it is seen that LV contraction produced recirculating flow patterns and directed flow toward the aortic valve. At early systole, flow is seen to be pouring out of the LV; however, recirculating flow is observed in all subjects. The flow gets ejected into the aorta rapidly at mid systole and is gradually reduced at the end of systole (frame 4). In subjects HFNEF1, HFREF1, and HFREF2, the abnormal recirculating flow patterns, formed during isovolumic contraction, are seen to remain until the end of the systolic phase. Peak flow rate out of LV is reduced in HFREF patients.

The results, as summarized in Table 14.2, show (1) substantially reduced values of contractility index for HFREF1 and HFREF2, (2) low flow rates during atrial contraction in subjects HFREF1, HFNEF2, HFREF2, and Normal2, and (3) marked reduction of peak systolic outflow rate in HFREF patients. We have been able to demonstrate the use of VFM technique to visualize blood flow patterns in HF patients and normal subjects, abnormal circulating flow patterns in filling, and irregularly directed flow patterns toward the aortic valve for HFREF patients. The VFM analysis has provided similar common flow patterns to those obtained from the combination of CFD and MRI, and contrast echo. This technique employs color Doppler echo images, which are routinely acquired in clinical settings, and thus, has great clinical potential.

14.2 Mitral Velocities, Intra-Cardiac Flow, Heart Failure, Intra-LV Flow Patterns

14.2.1 Left Ventricular and Left Atrial Dynamics

The LV is a biological pump for moving blood throughout the body. The LA is separated from the LV by the mitral valve. The LA transfers blood to LV in two steps: in the first step, the pressure gradient between LA and LV and the weight of the collected blood in LA causes blood to passively flow into the LV when the mitral valve opens. The speed at which the blood moves during this initial action is called the early or "E" filling velocity. Most filling (70%–75%) of the ventricle occurs during this phase. But some blood always remains, so toward the end of the atrial emptying cycle (diastole), the second step occurs in which the LA contracts to squeeze out that last bit ("atrial kick"). The speed of the blood filling the ventricle in this step is the "A" (for atrial) filling velocity. Mitral E velocity reflects LA–LV pressure gradient during early diastole, which is affected by LA compliance and alterations in LV relaxation. Mitral A velocity reflects active filling of LV by LA contraction setting up LA–LV pressure gradient during late diastole.

The E/A ratio is the ratio of the early (E) to late (A) LV filling velocities. Pulsed-wave (PW) Doppler echocardiography (echo) allows the measurement of velocities at the level of the sample volume as seen in Figure 14.1. In a healthy heart, the E velocity is greater than the A velocity. In certain pathologies and with aging, the left ventricular wall can become stiff, increasing the back pressure as it fills, which slows the early (E) filling velocity, thus lowering the E/A ratio. The reduced value of the E/A ratio is often accepted as a clinical marker of diastolic dysfunction, in which the LV becomes so stiff as to impair proper filling, which can lead to diastolic heart failure. The deceleration time (DT) is the time taken from the maximum E

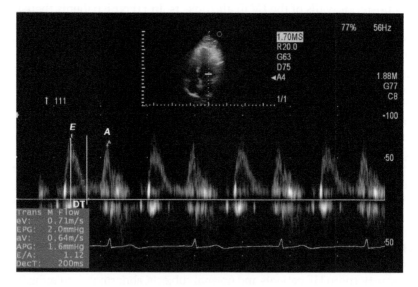

FIGURE 14.1

Mitral inflow velocities examination. Pulsed wave Doppler (PW-Doppler) allows the measurement of velocities at the level of the sample volume. Two flow velocity envelopes can be seen during diastole in persons with sinus rhythm: the E-wave, representing the early, passive filling of the left ventricle, and the A-wave, that happens late in diastole, representing the active filling, the atrial contraction.

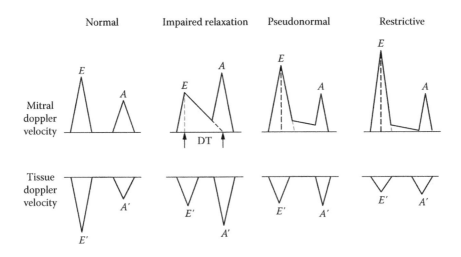

FIGURE 14.2
Changes in mitral Doppler velocity and tissue Doppler velocity with LV filling patterns: normal, impaired relaxation, pseudonormal, and restrictive.

point to baseline. DT is influenced by LV relaxation, LV diastolic pressure following mitral valve (MV) opening and LV compliance. Normally in adults it is less than 240 ms.

The velocity of early myocardial relaxation as the mitral annulus ascends during early LV filling (E'), measured by tissue Doppler imaging (TDI), correlates well with invasive hemodynamic measures of time constant of isovolumic relaxation. In healthy young subjects, septal E' is more than 10 cm/s and lateral more than 15 cm/s at rest. In patients with diastolic dysfunction related to a myocardial abnormality or disease, it is unusual that E' velocity remains normal [1] (Figure 14.2).

Based on E' velocity and E/A ratio, a number of grades of diastolic function can be determined:

1. Normal diastolic function ($E/A < 1$)
2. Impaired relaxation (E/A reversal, i.e., $E/A > 1$, DT > 240 ms, and reduced E')
3. Pseudonormal (E/A ratio appears normal, but E' is reduced)
4. Restrictive filling (E/A ratio often > 2 with a very short DT < 160 ms, reduced E')

14.2.2 Intra-Cardiac Flow Using Echocardiography

Intra-cardiac flow is useful for evaluating cardiac function as it is the end-result of cardiac myocardial abnormalities. The vortex flow that forms during left ventricular filling is a critical determinant of directed blood flow during ejection and can offer a novel index of cardiac dysfunction.

Magnetic resonance imaging (MRI) has been used for examining detailed blood flow patterns in the heart and great vessels for a range of clinical conditions [2–4]. In parallel with noninvasive imaging techniques, computational fluid dynamics (CFD) has been used for examining the global flow patterns and pressure distribution since the 1970s and 1980s [5,6]. The early models were confined to one or two dimensions with simplified geometries. With the continuing development of high-performance computing, realistic geometries, and fluid–ventricular wall interactions were subsequently incorporated into the CFD models to obtain velocity and pressure distributions in the LV, as well as stress distributions within the wall [7–9].

The integration of current state-of-the-art real-time MRI flow data and CFD enables visualization of instantaneous 3D flow field and also eliminates the need for velocity scans of the whole heart, thus enabling subject-specific intra-LV flow simulations [10,11]. However, MRI is relatively expensive and not readily available. Further, this phase contrast velocity mapping technique has limited spatio-temporal resolution, requires additional scans, and is time-consuming. It is thus not a routinely used technique in clinical settings.

Recent developments in echocardiography enable assessment of intra-cavitary blood flow patterns by tracking the patterns produced by contrast agent particles, called particle imaging velocimetry (echo-PIV) technique [12–14]. However, this technique requires injection of contrast agent, which might lead to serious side effects and has limited velocity range due to tracking algorithm.

VFM technique has been recently developed to generate flow velocity vector fields by post-processing color Doppler echo images [15]. In this technique, axial velocity is measured from color Doppler images, while radial velocity is computed by deconstructing the flow into a basic non-vortical laminar motion and a vortical component. This technique has produced reasonable accuracy when validated with numerical simulation models [16].

In normal subjects, after flow ejection into LV, the direction of flow is reversed toward the apex with a brief appearance of vortex at the early stage of isovolumic relaxation time. The major diastolic anterior vortex develops immediately after the onset of the early diastolic phase. This vortex continued during diastasis and persists into late LV filling phase. This vortex also persists throughout isovolumic contraction time and dissipates with the opening of the aortic valve and LV ejection [13].

By using echo-PIV and color-Doppler derived VFM, the intraventricular vortex flow has been successfully demonstrated and been made applicable in clinical settings, to enable comprehensive assessment of intra-cardiac structure and vortex flow for the detection of pathologically altered flow characteristics and identification of new pathophysiological mechanisms in the development of cardiac disease.

The quantitative parameters of LV vortex flow are vortex depth (VD) and vortex transversal position (VT). VD represents the vertical position of the centre of vortex relative to the LV long axis, and VT represents the transverse position relative to the posteroseptal axis, as shown in Figure 14.3. In the VD and VT configurations, we can measure the parameters of vortex length and vortex width.

14.2.3 Heart Failure with Preserved and Reduced Ejection Fractions

Heart failure (HF), a disease that causes LV dysfunction, involves high healthcare cost and has high mortality. It is one of the most common diseases in the developed world and is increasingly prevalent in developing countries, especially among the ageing population [17]. HF patients are usually stratified into two groups, based on their LV ejection fraction (EF), which is a commonly used index to assess contractile performance in clinical practice. A patient who has signs and symptoms of HF, while LVEF is normal (>50%), is characterized as HF with preserved ejection fraction (HFPEF) or HF with normal ejection fraction (HFNEF). Although the mechanisms of HFNEF are not fully understood, these patients are postulated to have diastolic dysfunction with abnormal LV relaxation during diastolic phase, slow LV filling and increased diastolic LV stiffness, while systolic function remains normal [18,19]. Thus, earlier, HFNEF was referred to as diastolic HF (DHF), while systolic HF (SHF) corresponded with HF with reduced ejection fraction (HFREF).

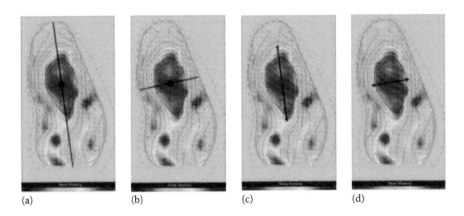

FIGURE 14.3
Description of quantitative parameters of the vortex location and shape. Vortex depth (a, black line), vortex transverse position (b, black line), vortex length (c, black arrow), and vortex width (d, black arrow). (Adapted from Hong, G.-R. et al., *J. Cardiovasc. Ultrasound*, 21(4), 155, 2013.)

However, the terms DHF and SHF have been abandoned as diastolic dysfunction has been observed in all symptomatic HF patients, regardless of EF [18].

In recent years, evidence of systolic dysfunction, to a lesser extent, has even been demonstrated in patients with HFNEF. Normal EF, apparently, does not necessarily indicate normal contractility. Regional measures of systolic function assessed by echo tissue Doppler imaging are impaired in HFNEF [20]. Other measures of myocardial contractility, assessed by mid-wall fractional shortening and particularly our wall-stress-based contractility index, $d\sigma^*/dt_{max}$ formulated as maximal rate-of-change of pressure-normalized wall stress [5] obtained from echo images, are also reduced in HFNEF, compared to healthy subjects [21,22]. However, end-systolic elastance (Ees), an intrinsic measure of contractile function, defined by the slope and intercept of the end-systolic pressure–volume relationship, is elevated in HFNEF [21]. From these findings, it is postulated that the same processes such as myocyte hypertrophy and increase in myocardial fibrosis [23] that promote diastolic stiffening also influence systolic stiffness and contribute to reduced myocardial contractility and limited systolic reserve [24].

It is still debatable whether HFNEF and HFREF exist as part of one HF spectrum with HFNEF preceding HFREF or represent two distinct syndromes of HF: HFNEF has concentric remodeling with high LV mass/volume ratio and mainly diastolic dysfunction, while HFREF has eccentric remodeling with low LV mass/volume ratio and a combination of systolic–diastolic dysfunction (HFREF) [25]. The complex mixture of systolic and diastolic dysfunction and variable degrees of LV remodeling underlying HFNEF poses challenges to diagnose and provide pharmacological treatment for HFNEF. In contrast to HFREF, research and clinical trials have not lead to a single effective treatment, and prognosis of HFNEF has remained unaltered for the past three decades [26].

14.2.4 Visualization of Intra-LV Flow Patterns as Outcomes of HFPEF and HFREF for Understanding the Pathophysiological Mechanisms in LV Remodeling Processes

LV myocardial structural remodeling processes in HFNEF and HFREF follow significantly different underlying mechanisms. In HFNEF, prominent cardiomyocyte hypertrophy is observed [27]. Cardiomyocyte diameter in HFNEF increases significantly, in contrast to minor increase in cardiomyocyte diameter in tandem with the dilated LV. Besides, although there is increased myocardial collagen deposition in both HFNEF and HFREF, the breakdown and turnover of the extracellular matrix are different [27]. This explains the different cardiomyocyte remodeling patterns: concentric hypertrophy in HFNEF and eccentric hypertrophy in HFREF. The passive force of cardiomyocytes in HFNEF is also higher than that of cardiomyocytes in HFREF, accounting for relatively more elevated LVEDP and increased myocardial stiffness in HFNEF compared to HFREF [27].

Other mechanisms underlying HFNEF include ventriculo-vascular coupling, chronotropic incompetence, LA dilatation, volume overload and pulmonary arterial hypertension, which can contribute to HF in HFNEF patients. All these concomitant structural and functional changes can affect the hemodynamics inside the LV chamber. The development of intra-LV flow patterns is the result of how (1) the LV myocardium passively responds to left atrial ejection of blood into the LV to result in diastolic filling flow patterns and pressure during diastolic filling and (2) then actively contracts to generate intra-LV flow patterns and pressure during systole to direct blood out of the LV. Therefore, the visualization of these diastolic and systolic intra-LV flow patterns can provide a wealth of dynamic information for understanding the intra-LV flow outcomes of the pathophysiological mechanisms in the LV remodeling processes.

In this regard, in Chapter 4, we have described in detail the effect of cardiomyopathy on LV remodeling process in terms of curvedness and sphericity indices. Then in Chapter 10, we have analyzed intra-LV flow and relative pressure distributions obtained by fluid–ventricular wall interactions from angiographic x-ray images of sequential LV endocardial boundaries in patients with myocardial disorders.

Herein, we apply *VFM* technique to obtain intra-LV flow patterns for patients with HFNEF, HFREF, and normal subjects, in order to characterize the LV performance outcomes of normal subjects and heart failure patients.*

14.3 Clinical Study Methodology to Determine Intra-LV Flow Patterns for HF Patients and Normal Subjects

14.3.1 Subject Recruitment

Patients who had signs and symptoms of congestive HF based on the modified Framingham criteria [29] were recruited for this study. They subsequently underwent echo scan for stratification into HFNEF (based on LVEF $\geq$ 50%) and HFREF (LVEF < 50%). Normal subjects, who had no history of heart disease or hypertension, were also recruited. For each group, two age- and sex-matched subjects were chosen. The study procedure was approved by the institutional ethical committee.

14.3.2 Echo Data Acquisition

All subjects underwent echo scans (Alpha10, Aloka). The LVEF was measured from M-mode images at the parasternal long-axis view using standard methodology. Mitral E and A

---

* This chapter is an extension of the earlier work reported by Le et al. 2012. Intra-left ventricular flow distributions in diastolic and systolic phases, based on echo velocity flow mapping of normal subjects and heart failure patients, to characterize left ventricular performance outcomes of heart failure. *Journal of Mechanics in Medicine and Biology* 12:5 with permission from World Scientific Publishers [28].

velocities DT, systolic (PVs) and diastolic (PVd) pulmonary vein velocities were measured from pulsed wave Doppler images, while the septal E' velocity was measured from pulsed tissue Doppler images. These echo measurements assess LV diastolic function.

Color Doppler flow images were captured at the three-chamber view for visualization of both inflow through mitral valve and outflow into the aorta.

14.3.3 Vector Flow Mapping Analysis

Intra-LV flow was determined using the VFM analysis package (DAS-RS1). In this technique, color Doppler velocity (axial velocity, **u**) profile was analyzed across an arc (refer Figure 14.4) at each echo depth. The Doppler velocity **u** along the beam line is composed of basic non-vortical laminar flow ($\mathbf{u}_b$) and vortex flow ($\mathbf{u}_v$) components. If the Doppler velocity profile on the arc has both negative and positive fractions, it is considered to be a combination of non-vortical and vortical laminar flows.

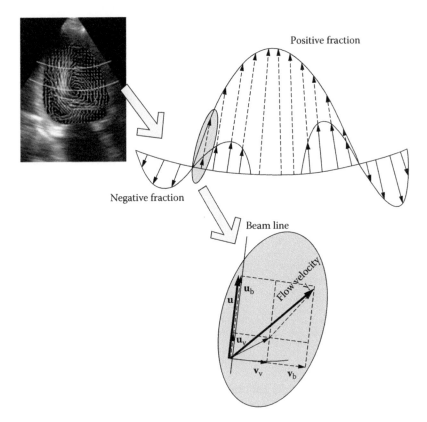

FIGURE 14.4
Velocity generated by VFM along an arc at each echo depth with a combination of single laminar flow and vortex flows (top left). Color Doppler flow data are separated into basic and vortex flow components so that vortex flow component is bilaterally symmetrical on each arc (top right); at a given pixel, color Doppler velocity **u** along the beam line is a sum of its vortex flow component $\mathbf{u}_v$ and basic flow component $\mathbf{u}_b$. The vortex flow component consists of color Doppler velocity $\mathbf{u}_v$ and radial velocity $\mathbf{v}_v$. Likewise, the basic flow component consists of color Doppler velocity $\mathbf{u}_b$ and radial velocity $\mathbf{v}_b$. Flow vector is the sum of flow vectors of basic and vortex flow components (bottom).

The vortex feature is assumed to be bilaterally symmetric, so that the negative and positive components of $\mathbf{u}_v$ perpendicular to the arc negate each other (Figure 14.4). The basic flow component $\mathbf{u}_b$ is computed as

$$\mathbf{u}_b = \mathbf{u} - \mathbf{u}_v \tag{14.1}$$

The stream function $\psi(r, \theta)$ expresses the flux of the 2D flow. The vortex flow velocity components $\mathbf{u}_v$ and $\mathbf{v}_v$ can be obtained in terms of ψ as

$$\mathbf{u}_v = \frac{1}{r}\frac{\partial \psi}{\partial \theta} \tag{14.2}$$

$$\mathbf{v}_v = -\frac{\partial \psi}{\partial \theta} \tag{14.3}$$

wherein r and θ are radial and angle coordinates expressing the location of the pixel.

From Equation 14.2, the stream function ψ can be expressed as

$$\psi(r,\theta) = \int_0^\theta \mathbf{u}_v(r,\theta)rd\theta \tag{14.4}$$

As the vortex feature is assumed to be bilateral symmetric, the flux calculated by the positive and negative components of $\mathbf{u}_v$, which intersect perpendicularly with the integration arc, negate each other.

The radial vortex flow component $\mathbf{v}_v$ can be computed from Equation 14.3.

To compute basic flow component, Ohtsuki and Tanaka [15] have proposed a flow function $F(r, \theta)$ to describe a non-vortical laminar flow within a defined plane as

$$F(r,\theta) = \int_0^\theta \mathbf{u}_b(r,\theta)rd\theta \tag{14.5}$$

To find the direction of flow vectors in the basic flow component, $F(r, \theta)$ is normalized by the total flow rate in the basic flow component across an arc, as

$$F_n(r,\theta) = \frac{\int_0^\theta \mathbf{u}_b(r,\theta)rd\theta}{\int \mathbf{u}_b(r,\theta)rd\theta} \tag{14.6}$$

The contour line connecting points that have the same value of $F_n(r, \theta)$ indicates the direction of flow vectors in the basic flow component. The radial basic flow component $\mathbf{v}_b$ can then be found as

$$\mathbf{v}_b = \mathbf{u}_b \tan\theta \tag{14.7}$$

Flow velocity $\mathbf{U}(r, \theta)$ can be calculated by

$$\mathbf{U}(r,\theta) = (\mathbf{u}_b(r,\theta) + \mathbf{u}_v(r,\theta))\mathbf{i}(r,\theta) + (\mathbf{v}_b(r,\theta) + \mathbf{v}_v(r,\theta))\mathbf{j}(r,\theta) \tag{14.8}$$

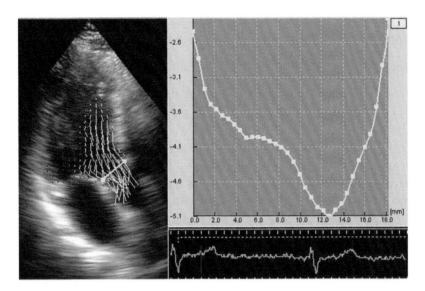

FIGURE 14.5
Measurement of maximal flow rate into the aorta using velocity flow mapping (VFM). (Left) Velocity vector distribution in the LV during systole. Arrows denote velocity vectors. Red dots indicate heads of the arrows. A line was drawn at the LVOT to determine the maximum flow rate ejected into the aorta. (Right) Flow profile through the line drawn at LVOT at a time instant.

where $\mathbf{i}(r, \theta)$ and $\mathbf{j}(r, \theta)$ are the unit vectors in the axial and radial direction, respectively, at point (r, θ). As illustrated in Figure 14.4, $\mathbf{u}_b$ and $\mathbf{u}_v$ are in the Doppler beam direction (axial), while $\mathbf{v}_b$ and $\mathbf{v}_v$ are in the direction perpendicular to the Doppler beam (radial).

The velocity vector distributions throughout the cardiac cycle are then analyzed and compared among all subjects. The LV outflow rates during systole and inflow rates during diastole were determined by computing the flow rates passing through a line drawn across the LV outflow tract (LVOT) during systole and a line across the mitral valve (MV) annulus during diastole (refer to Figure 14.5).

Figure 14.5 illustrates measurement of maximal flow rate into the aorta using VFM. The figure on the left shows the velocity vector distribution in the LV during systole; therein, the arrows denote velocity vectors, and the red dots indicate heads of the arrows; a line is drawn at the LVOT to determine the maximum flow rate ejected into the aorta. In the figure on the right, we can see the flow profile through the line drawn at LVOT at a time instant.

14.3.4 LV Contractility Index Based on LV Wall Stress

We want to define a contractility index in order to characterize HFREF (systolic heart failure) patients, who (due to myocardial disease) have depleted contractility. For this purpose, we have previously developed a LV wall-stress-based contractility index, based on the premise that in systole it is the active wall stress (produced by the actin and myosin contracting components of the myocardial structural unit) that in turn produces the intra-LV pressure, leading to the traditional contractility index dP/dt_{max}.

Our wall-stress-based contractility index, $d\sigma^*/dt_{max}$, defined as a maximal rate-of-change of pressure-normalized wall stress, has been proposed in our paper [22] as an intrinsic measure of contractile function. This index has been shown to have a good correlation with dP/dt_{max}, which is considered as a "gold standard" index for assessing myocardial contractility, and Ees, and can be determined noninvasively. We therefore apply this index to assess contractile performance of all subjects in this study.

This $d\sigma^*/dt_{max}$ index is formulated as

$$\frac{d\sigma^*}{dt_{max}} = 1.5 \times \frac{dV/dt_{max}}{MV}$$ (14.9)

where

dV/dt_{max} is maximal flow rate into the aorta, measured at the LVOT using VFM (Figure 14.5)

MV is the myocardial volume, calculated as a quotient of LV mass, determined from M-mode images using Devereaux's method, and myocardial density (assumed 1.05 g/mL)

14.4 Results of the Intra-LV VFM to Characterize the LV Performance in Heart Failure

14.4.1 Subjects' Clinical Characteristics and Echo Parameters

Clinical characteristics and echo parameters of four HF subjects and two age- and sex-matched healthy controls are shown in Table 14.1. The HFNEF1 and HFNEF2 are HF patients with normal EF. HFREF1 and HFREF2 are HF patients with reduced EF. The Normal1 and Normal2 are normal subjects with no history of cardiac problems. All HF patients were on hypertensive medication. Subject HFNEF1 had elevated systolic blood pressure while the rest were normotensive. LV hypertrophy was seen in subjects HFREF1 and HFNEF2. Dilated LA was observed in subjects HFREF1, HFREF2, and HFNEF2.

In all HF subjects, the clinical echo data have suggested abnormal filling patterns (either restrictive or pseudo-normal), with increased E/A ratio. In subjects HFREF1 and HFREF2, there was decreased DT.

All HF patients had raised E/E' ratio > 15, associated with increased filling pressure.

In general, restrictive filling pattern, with increased E/A ratio and decreased DT, were seen in patients with HFREF. Pseudo-normal filling patterns were observed in patients with HFNEF. Normal subjects had reversed E/A ratios (<1), which are common features in aging subjects.

TABLE 14.1

Subject's Clinical Characteristics and Echo Parameters

Subject	Age	Gender	LVEF (%)	E/A	E/E'	DT (ms)	PVs/PVd
HFNEF1	52	Male	64.7	2.5	19.5	210	0.90
HFREF1	53	Male	26.6	1.3	26.9	120	NA
Normal1	51	Male	60.4	0.8	5.9	184	1.27
HFNEF2	66	Female	63.3	2.7	27.7	216	0.63
HFREF2	65	Female	22.6	3.6	21.8	68	NA
Normal2	67	Female	60	0.8	6.6	168	1.61

14.4.2 Diastolic Flow Patterns

The diastolic flow patterns are shown for each of the six subjects HFNEF1, HFREF1, Normal1 (in rows 1, 2, and 3 of Figure 14.6a) and HFNEF2, HFREF2, Normal2 (in rows 1, 2, and 3 of Figure 14.6b).

After the mitral valve opens, in the rapid filling phase (frame 1), straight flow is seen to rush into the LV from the LA. Circulating flow patterns are seen at the anterior and posterior walls of the LV in all subjects, except in subject Normal2.

As inflow reduces its speed (frame 2), the circulating flow patterns are seen to become bigger. The circulating flow is seen to be more prominent at the anterior wall.

In the diastasis phase (frame 3), marked by P-wave on ECG, the flow patterns are seen to be different among the subjects. In subject HFNEF1, the flow is seen to be circulating in the LV with no inflow. In both subjects HFREF1 and HFREF2, the flow from LA is seen to be continuing to enter LV, with two circulating flow patterns seen at the anterior and posterior walls. In contrast, there is hardly any movement of blood in LV of subjects Normal1 and HFNEF2. In Normal2, continuous flow from LA to LV is seen, with a circulating flow at the anterior wall.

At atrial contraction (frame 4), after the P-wave on ECG, as LA contracts, the flow starts to again enter the LV in Normal1 and HFNEF2, after a period of no inflow into the LV. In the rest of the subjects, the flow from LA to LV is observed to have profound circulating flow patterns at the anterior wall. These circulating flow features remain until the end of atrial contraction (frame 5).

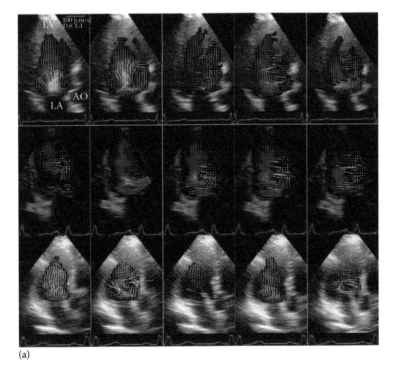

(a)

FIGURE 14.6
Diastolic flow patterns of age- and sex-matched subjects (a) HFNEF1, HFREF1, and Normal1. (*Continued*)

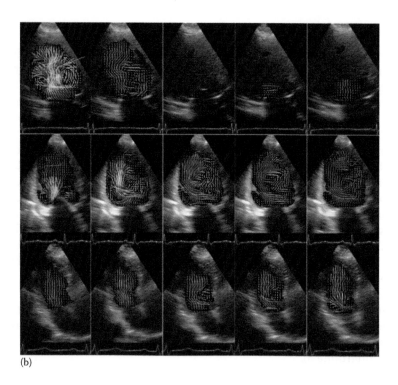

(b)

FIGURE 14.6 (*Continued*)
Diastolic flow patterns of age- and sex-matched subjects (b) HFNEF2, HFREF2, and Normal2 at (from left to right) the start of rapid filling (frame 1), late rapid filling (frame 2), diastasis (frame 3), start of atrial contraction (frame 4), and end of atrial contraction just before mitral valve closes (frame 5). Inflow toward the apex is represented in red color, outflow toward the aorta (AO) is represented in blue color.

The flow rates versus time (corrected for heart rate) of all the subjects during diastole phase, from the start of aortic valve closure to mitral valve closure, are shown in Figure 14.7.

In both HFNEF patients, prolonged diastasis phase (period of no inflow) is to be seen.

14.4.3 Systolic Flow Patterns

Systolic flow patterns are shown for each of the six subjects: HFNEF1, HFREF1, Normal1 (in rows 1, 2, and 3 of Figure 14.8a) and HFNEF2, HFREF2, Normal2 (in rows 1, 2, and 3 of Figure 14.8b).

In Figure 14.8, flow toward the aorta is illustrated in blue color, and flow toward the apex is illustrated in red color. At isovolumic contraction (frame 1), LV contraction produced recirculating flow patterns and directed flow toward the aortic valve. At early systole (frame 2), flow is seen to be pouring out of the LV; however, recirculating flow is observed in all subjects. The flow gets ejected to the aorta rapidly at mid systole (frame 3) and is gradually reduced at the end of systole (frame 4). In subjects HFNEF1, HFREF1, and HFREF2, the abnormal recirculating flow pattern, formed during isovolumic contraction, is seen to remain until the end of the systolic phase.

At isovolumic relaxation (frame 5), there is observed to be virtually no flow in the LV of HFNEF patients and normal subjects. However, some flow movement is still present in HFREF patients.

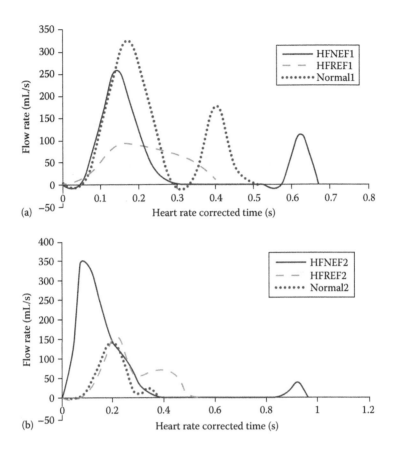

FIGURE 14.7
Flow rates from the LA into the LV versus time (corrected for heart rate) of (a) HFNEF1, HFREF1, and Normal1 and (b) HFNEF2, HFREF2, and Normal2, during diastole.

In general, persistent recirculating flow patterns are seen during the ejection phase in patients with HFREF. At isovolumic relaxation, while there is virtually no intra-LV flow in HFNEF patients and normal subjects, flow movement is still present in the LV of HFREF patients.

The instantaneous flow rates ejected into the aorta of six patients are shown in Figure 14.9. To correct for heart rate, the time intervals were divided by $\sqrt{R - R}$, based on Bazette's formula, which normalizes the heart rate to 60 beats/min.

Subject HFNEF1 is shown to have a higher peak flow rate (341.1 mL/s), compared to HFREF1 (270.5 mL/s) and Normal1 (320.8 mL/s). A steeper slope of the flow rate curve of subject HFNEF1 is seen in the graph, indicating a faster rate-of-change of flow rate, compared to HFREF1 and Normal1.

Subject HFNEF2 is shown to have a higher peak flow rate (255.4 mL/s) and faster rate-of-change of flow rate compared to HFREF2 (87.6 mL/s) and Normal2 (151.6 mL/s).

14.4.4 Contractility Index, Peak Inflow, and Outflow Rates of All Subjects

Table 14.2 lists the values of the LV myocardial volume, and the calculated values of the contractility index, peak systolic outflow rate, peak filling flow rate, peak atrial contraction flow rate, and Doppler A velocity.

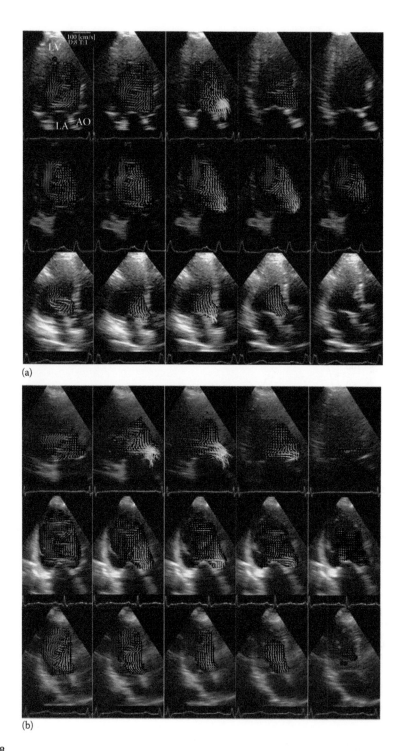

(a)

(b)

FIGURE 14.8
Systolic flow patterns of age- and sex-matched (a) HFNEF1, HFREF1, and Normal1 subjects; (b) HFNEF2, HFREF2, and Normal2 subjects at (from left to right) isovolumic contraction (frame 1), early systole (frame 2), mid systole (frame 3), end systole (frame 4) and isovolumic relaxation (frame 5). Blue indicates flow toward the aorta. Red indicates flow toward the apex. Arrow represents velocity flow vector. Red dot indicates the head of the arrow.

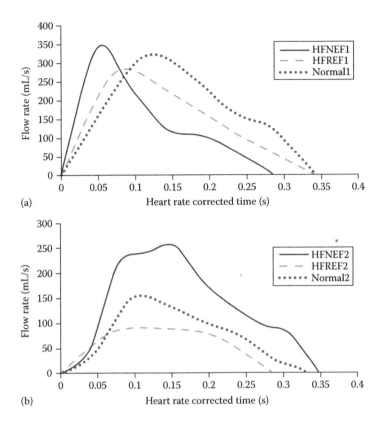

FIGURE 14.9
Flow rate from LV into the aorta versus time (corrected for heart rate) of (a) HFNEF1, HFREF1, and Normal1 and (b) HFNEF2, HFREF2, and Normal2, during systole.

As shown in Table 14.2, there is marked reduction of $d\sigma^*/dt_{max}$ in patients with HFREF; correspondingly, there is also marked reduction of peak systolic outflow rate in HFREF patients.

Despite normal values of clinical pulsed Doppler mitral *A* velocity (between 30 and 70 cm/s), low flow rates during atrial contraction are observed in subjects HFREF1, HFNEF2, HFREF2, and Normal2. The *A* velocities are 56 cm/s (HFREF1), 42.8 cm/s (HFNEF2), 34 cm/s (HFREF2), and 70 cm/s (Normal2).

TABLE 14.2

Contractility Index, Peak Outflow, and Inflow Rates of All Subjects

Subject	$d\sigma^*/dt_{max}$ (s^{-1})	Myocardial volume (mL)	Peak systolic outflow rate (mL/s)	Peak rapid filling flow rate (mL/s)	Peak atrial contraction flow rate (mL/s)	Doppler A velocity (cm/s)
HFNEF1	4.41	116	341.1	258.0	113.6	37.4
HFREF1	1.80	285	270.5	89.6	NA	56
Normal1	4.31	111	320.8	323.7	172.9	61
HFNEF2	1.31	292	255.4	344.8	40.3	42.8
HFREF2	0.62	213	87.6	158.0	73.2	34
Normal2	3.34	68	151.6	138.6	23.7	70

As seen in Table 14.2, a lower value of the contractility index $d\sigma^*/dt_{max}$ is observed in subject HFNEF2, compared to the normal subject with same age and gender, with higher peak outflow rate and increased myocardial volume. There is no difference in $d\sigma^*/dt_{max}$ between HFNEF1 and Normal1. HFREF patients are seen to have lower peak flow rate and lower $d\sigma^*/dt_{max}$ compared to HFNEF patients and normal subjects of the same age and gender.

14.5 Discussion and Conclusion

14.5.1 Intra-LV Flow Pattern Variations

Herein, the VFM analysis has provided similar common flow patterns to those obtained from combination of CFD and MRI [11] and contrast echo [13]. Even though color Doppler images have much lower temporal resolution compared to 2D echo images used for echo PIV, the current frame rates of 20–30 fps are quantifiably comparable to those obtained by phase-contrast MRI. This technique, thus, has great potential in clinical applications, as color Doppler echo is widely used in routine clinical practice.

In this study, we have demonstrated the use of VFM technique to visualize blood flow patterns in HF patients and normal subjects. Abnormal circulating flow patterns, which were observed at late systole and from late rapid filling phase to diastasis in HF patients, may suggest a stiff LV, which is resistant to expansion and contraction.

14.5.2 Contractility Index Variations

To assess the LV contractile function, the pressure-normalized wall-stress-based contractility index, $d\sigma^*/dt_{max}$, is used in this study. In systole, the wall stress, which is generated by sarcomere contraction and results in the development of pressure, can be considered as an intrinsic contractile indicator. The contractile index $d\sigma^*/dt_{max}$ is markedly reduced in HFREF patients, compared to HFNEF and normal subjects of the same age and sex. This confirms impaired contractile function in HFREF patients.

In HFNEF patients, the contractile index $d\sigma^*/dt_{max}$ is reduced in the case of HFNEF2, compared to Normal2, while for HFNEF1 it remains similar to that of the normal subject Normal1.

The contractility index $d\sigma^*/dt_{max}$ is formulated as the quotient of maximal flow rate into the aorta and myocardial volume. In both HFNEF cases, the outflow rates are higher than those of normal subjects. However, in HFNEF2, the myocardial volume is increased due to LV hypertrophy (refer to Table 14.2), probably to compensate for the increase in stroke volume. Due to this compensatory mechanism, the contractile performance assessed by pressure-normalized wall stress $d\sigma^*/dt_{max}$ is seen to be reduced.

14.5.3 Flow Rates into and out of LV

The peak flow rates out of LV are reduced in both cases of HFREF, which are associated with reduced contractile function. The peak LV outflow rates of patients with HFNEF, on the other hand, are increased compared to those of normal controls. The mechanisms underlying this observation are not quite clearly understood.

Even though diastolic dysfunction is present in both HFNEF and HFREF patients [30], different patterns of flow distribution in the diastolic phase are seen in the case of these two sets of patients. In HFREF patients, the peak inflow rates in rapid filling phase are reduced. It is noticed that during isovolumic relaxation, as both the valves were closed and LV continues to relax, the circulating flow patterns are still present. This might be due to impaired elastic recoil, influenced by reduced contractility. Intraventricular pressure, thus, may still be high in these patients during isovolumic relaxation. This may therefore affect the LV transmural pressure, and hinder LV filling.

On the other hand, HFNEF patients have prolonged diastasis phase. In HFNEF1, the circulating flow, formed at the start of rapid filling, becomes larger and has lasted throughout the diastasis phase. This may suggest high LV stiffness that is resistant to LV expansion. In HFNEF2, the LA dilation, which is evident from echo scan and is possibly resulting from increased filling pressure due to LV hypertrophy, may be the cause of delayed atrial contraction.

The discordance between normal pulsed Doppler mitral *A* velocity and low atrial contraction inflow rate into the LV might be due to the location of the velocity sample, which is placed at the tip of the mitral valve. The Doppler velocity measured at this location might be affected by the concomitant circulating flow, which is formed in the LV cavity during rapid filling phase, as shown in Figure 14.8. Therefore, Doppler *A* velocity may overestimate the actual contribution of atrial contraction to LV filling.

Thus, in future studies, both LV myocardial elastance, LV ejection force (which is an outcome measure of LV contractility) and LA ejection force (which is an outcome-based measure of LA contractility) need to be determined, in order to fully understand the mechanisms behind (1) different systolic flow patterns diastolic flow patterns and characterize systolic dysfunction, and (2) various type of diastolic flow patterns and diastolic dysfunction.

14.5.4 Intra-LV Pressure Gradients

By applying the Navier–Stokes equation, intraventricular LV pressure gradients can be calculated from the flow velocity, as performed by Subbaraj et al. [11]. This will thereby provide information on both the instantaneous intra-cavitary LV blood flow velocity field and the intra-LV pressure field, and the relationship between velocity distribution and pressure distribution. This can lend enhanced insight into the outcomes of efficiency of LV contraction and relaxation.

━━━━━

References

1. Oh JK, Park S-J, Nagueh SF: Established and novel clinical applications of diastolic function assessment by echocardiography. *Circul Cardiovasc Imag* 2011, **4**(4):444–455.
2. Buonocore MH: Visualizing blood flow patterns using streamlines, arrows, and particle paths. *Magn Reson Med* 1998, **40**(2):210–226.
3. Mohiaddin RH, Yang GZ, Kilner PJ: Visualization of flow by vector analysis of multidirectional cine MR velocity mapping. *J Comput Assist Tomogr* 1994, **18**(3):383–392.
4. Kilner PJ, Yang G-Z, Wilkes AJ, Mohiaddin RH, Firmin DN, Yacoub MH: Asymmetric redirection of flow through the heart. *Nature* 2000, **404**(6779):759–761.
5. Panerai RB, Smaill BH, Borst C, Chamberlain JH, Sayers BM: A model of left ventricular function in the denervated heart. *J Biomed Eng* 1979, **1**(3):161–171.
6. Subbaraj K, Ghista DN, Fallen EL: Intrinsic indices of the left ventricle as a blood pump in normal and infarcted left ventricles. *J Biomed Eng* 1987, **9**(3):206–215.

7. Chahboune B, Crolet JM: Numerical simulation of the blood-wall interaction in the human left ventricle. *Eur Phys J Appl Phys* 1998, **2**(03):291–297.

8. Redaelli A, Montevecchi FM: Intraventricular pressure drop and aortic blood acceleration as indices of cardiac inotropy: A comparison with the first derivative of aortic pressure based on computer fluid dynamics. *Med Eng Phys* 1998, **20**(4):231–241.

9. Watanabe H, Sugiura S, Kafuku H, Hisada T: Multiphysics simulation of left ventricular filling dynamics using fluid-structure interaction finite element method. *Biophys J* 2004, **87**(3):2074–2085.

10. Merrifield R: Patient specific modelling of left ventricular morphology and flow using magnetic resonance imaging and computational fluid dynamics. University of London, London, UK; 2003.

11. Long Q, Merrifield R, Xu XY, Kilner P, Firmin DN, Yang G-Z: Subject-specific computational simulation of left ventricular flow based on magnetic resonance imaging. *Proc Inst Mech Eng H* 2008, **222**(4):475–485.

12. Kim HB, Hertzberg JR, Shandas R: Echo PIV for flow field measurements in vivo. *Biomed Sci Instrum* 2004, **40**:357–363.

13. Hong G-R, Pedrizzetti G, Tonti G, Li P, Wei Z, Kim JK, Baweja A et al.: Characterization and quantification of vortex flow in the human left ventricle by contrast echocardiography using vector particle image velocimetry. *J Am Coll Cardiol Imag* 2008, **1**(6):705–717.

14. Hong G-R, Kim M, Pedrizzetti G, Vannan MA: Current clinical application of intracardiac flow analysis using echocardiography. *J Cardiovasc Ultrasound* 2013, **21**(4):155–162.

15. Ohtsuki S, Tanaka M: The flow velocity distribution from the Doppler information on a plane in three-dimensional flow. *J Vis* 2006, **9**(1):69–82.

16. Uejima T, Koike A, Sawada H, Aizawa T, Ohtsuki S, Tanaka M, Furukawa T, Fraser AG: A new echocardiographic method for identifying vortex flow in the left ventricle: Numerical validation. *Ultrasound Med Biol* 2010, **36**(5):772–788.

17. Cowie MR, Wood DA, Coats AJS, Thompson SG, Poole-Wilson PA, Suresh V, Sutton GC: Incidence and aetiology of heart failure; a population-based study. *Eur Heart J* 1999, **20**(6):421–428.

18. Zile MR, Brutsaert DL: New concepts in diastolic dysfunction and diastolic heart failure: Part I: Diagnosis, prognosis, and measurements of diastolic function. *Circulation* 2002, **105**(11):1387–1393.

19. Zile MR, Brutsaert DL: New concepts in diastolic dysfunction and diastolic heart failure: Part II: Causal mechanisms and treatment. *Circulation* 2002, **105**(12):1503–1508.

20. Yu CM, Lin H, Yang H, Kong SL, Zhang Q, Lee SW: Progression of systolic abnormalities in patients with "isolated" diastolic heart failure and diastolic dysfunction. *Circulation* 2002, **105**(10):1195–1201.

21. Borlaug BA, Lam CS, Roger VL, Rodeheffer RJ, Redfield MM: Contractility and ventricular systolic stiffening in hypertensive heart disease insights into the pathogenesis of heart failure with preserved ejection fraction. *J Am Coll Cardiol* 2009, **54**(5):410–418.

22. Zhong L, Poh KK, Lee LC, Le TT, Tan RS: Attenuation of stress-based ventricular contractility in patients with heart failure and normal ejection fraction. *Ann Acad Med Singapore* 2011, **40**(4):179–187.

23. Borlaug BA, Kass DA: Ventricular-vascular interaction in heart failure. *Heart Fail Clin* 2008, **4**(1):23–36.

24. Borlaug BA, Paulus WJ: Heart failure with preserved ejection fraction: Pathophysiology, diagnosis, and treatment. *Eur Heart J* 2011, **32**(6):670–679.

25. Paulus WJ, Tschope C, Sanderson JE, Rusconi C, Flachskampf FA, Rademakers FE, Marino P et al.: How to diagnose diastolic heart failure: A consensus statement on the diagnosis of heart failure with normal left ventricular ejection fraction by the Heart Failure and Echocardiography Associations of the European Society of Cardiology. *Eur Heart J* 2007, **28**(20):2539–2550.

26. Paulus WJ, van Ballegoij JJM: Treatment of heart failure with normal ejection fraction: An inconvenient truth! *J Am Coll Cardiol* 2010, **55**(6):526–537.

27. van Heerebeek L, Borbely A, Niessen HW, Bronzwaer JG, van der Velden J, Stienen GJ, Linke WA, Laarman GJ, Paulus WJ: Myocardial structure and function differ in systolic and diastolic heart failure. *Circulation* 2006, **113**(16):1966–1973.

28. Le T-T, Tan R-S, Huang F, Zhong L, Idapalapati S, Ghista D: Intra-left ventricular flow distributions in diastolic and systolic phases, based on echo velocity flow mapping of normal subjects and heart failure patients, to characterize left ventricular performance outcomes of heart failure. *J Mech Med Biol* 2012, **12**(5): 1240029.

29. Vasan RS, Larson MG, Benjamin EJ, Evans JC, Reiss CK, Levy D: Congestive heart failure in subjects with normal versus reduced left ventricular ejection fraction: Prevalence and mortality in a population-based cohort. *J Am Coll Cardiol* 1999, **33**(7):1948–1955.

30. Sanderson JE: Heart failure with a normal ejection fraction. *Heart* 2007, **93**(2):155–158.

15

Coronary Blood Flow Analysis and Coronary Bypass Graft Design

Foad Kabinejadian, Yunlong Huo, Dhanjoo N. Ghista, and Ghassan S. Kassab

CONTENTS

Acronyms

CABG   Coronary arterial bypass grafting
CAD   Coronary artery disease
CFD   Computational fluid dynamic
CT   Computed tomography
CVD   Cardiovascular disease
DAIH   Distal anastomotic intimal hyperplasia
EC   Endothelial cell
ETE   End-to-end
ETS   End-to-side
FD   Finite difference

FE   Finite element
FEM   Finite element method
HP   Hemodynamic parameter
IH   Intimal hyperplasia
IMA   Internal mammary artery
IT   Intimal thickening
LAD   Left anterior descending coronary artery
LCx   Left circumflex coronary artery
LDL   Low-density lipoprotein
LMCA   Left main coronary artery
MRI   Magnetic resonance imaging
OSI   Oscillatory shear index
PCI   Percutaneous coronary intervention
RCA   Right coronary artery
SMC   Smooth muscle cell
SQA   Sequential anastomoses
STS   Side-to-side
SVG   Saphenous vein graft
WSS   Wall shear stress
WSSG   Wall shear stress gradient

15.1 Introduction

Coronary artery disease (CAD) remains one of the primary causes of morbidity and mortality worldwide, because the coronary arteries are most vulnerable to lesions restricting blood flow (due to the heart having the highest rate of oxygen extraction from the blood, and being very sensitive to its lack). Coronary circulation is very complex due to its bifurcations and branches, which cause considerable spatial and temporal variations in the hemodynamic parameters (HPs) of wall stress, shear stress, and wall pressure gradients. Hence, coronary circulation is highly prone to atherosclerosis and consequently to myocardial ischemia, which causes decreased cardiac contractility, decreased ejection fraction, and risk of heart failure. Hence, understanding the mechanism and mechanics of atherosclerosis and its initiation and association with the complex features of coronary blood flow dynamics is very important.

Restoration of coronary flow perfusion to the myocardium is required to sustain cardiac output and prevent heart failure. In this regard, coronary arterial bypass grafting (CABG) is an effective treatment for high-risk CAD patients. Its complications and patency are known to be intertwined with the hemodynamics and vascular mechanics of bypass-grafted arterial vessels. Therefore, a hemodynamic analysis of CABG blood flow at anastomotic sites (which are prone to disturbed flow patterns and HPs) is important in order to propose anastomoses designs that can enhance CABG patency.

The blood flow in the cardiovascular system is too complex to be realistically described analytically. Experimental studies have provided valuable data, albeit being costly and time-consuming. On the other hand, computational fluid dynamics (CFD) methods have emerged as powerful tools, usually utilized in conjunction with experimental data (as boundary conditions of flow velocity and pressure at the inlet and outlet to grafted vessels) to simulate blood flow behavior and disturbances (such as flow separation, secondary flow, flow stagnation, reversed flow, and turbulence) and subsequently estimate the HPs.

Flow disturbances can locally induce abnormal biological response, such as dysfunction of endothelial cells (ECs), monocyte deposition, elevated wall permeability to macromolecules, particle migration into the vessel wall, smooth muscle cell proliferation, and microemboli formation. Since the spatial complexities of blood flow in the cardiovascular system cannot be visualized with current imaging methods, computational modeling is a necessity.

The aim of this chapter is to provide insights into the current methods of blood flow studies in coronary arteries and CABGs by means of computational fluid–solid mechanics, as well as innovative designs of CABG distal anastomotic configuration for enhancement of patency and prevention of restenosis. In Section 15.2, computational methodologies of blood flow analysis are employed to formulate and illustrate three types of coronary circulatory flows (in porcine models): pulsatile flow in the epicardial coronary tree, steady-state flow in the entire coronary arterial tree, and wave propagation in the coronary arterial tree. In Section 15.3, we have provided an overview and analysis of CABG, the preferred treatment for high-risk CAD patients. The importance and role of HPs in restenosis of CABG is analyzed. We have presented various attempts to design an optimal distal anastomotic configuration, in terms of the anastomotic angle, graft caliber (i.e., graft-to-host diameter ratio), and influence of out-of-plane graft curvature.

15.2 Coronary Circulation Analysis and Features

The blood moves through three coronary arterial trees (left anterior descending [LAD], left circumflex [LCx], and right coronary artery [RCA] trees) to the capillary network, to nourish the myocardium for preserving the pump function of the heart [1]. A coronary arterial tree is comprised of millions of arteries to arterioles with diameters of 10–5000 μm, which can be divided into epicardial, transmural, and perfusion subnetworks [2,3]. The epicardial subnetwork comprises relatively large vessels that run over the surface of the heart (epicardium), giving rise to transmural branches, which in turn penetrate the heart muscle and branch further into perfusion vessels down to the capillary network.

In contrast to transmural and perfusion vessels embedded in the myocardium [4], epicardial arteries are prone to have atherosclerosis [5]. The changes in geometry of epicardial arteries during branching can lead to significant flow disturbances (e.g., flow separation, secondary flow, stagnation point flow, reversed flow, and/or turbulence), which strongly affect various HPs, such as wall shear stress (WSS), WSS spatial gradient (WSSG), and oscillatory shear index (OSI) [5–7]. It has been found that spatial and temporal WSS and WSSG can locally induce abnormal biological response, such as dysfunction of ECs, monocyte deposition, elevated wall permeability to macromolecules, particle migration into the vessel wall, smooth muscle cell proliferation, microemboli formation, and so on [2,8,9]. In particular, the atherosclerotic-prone locations with low WSS (<4 dyn/cm²) and high OSI (>0.15) have been assumed to impair endothelial function [10–13], while the high WSSG is proposed to increase the permeability of LDL (low-density lipoprotein) at the flow reattachment [14–16].

The local flow is not amenable to direct visualization in the epicardial coronary arterial tree. With the rapid growth of computer technology, numerical simulation is an attractive methodological approach to simulate and predict what cannot be directly visualized.

The 3D CFD model has been widely used to describe the complex flow patterns in different geometries of cardiovascular system [17–21]. We have recently used the FE (finite element) method to investigate the flow patterns in the epicardial arterial tree of porcine models [6,7,22]. In addition, the CFD model has been applied to study CAD in conjunction with 3D imaging techniques (e.g., CT) [23,24].

Myocardial ischemia, a major cause of morbidity and mortality in the United States and worldwide, is transmurally heterogeneous, and the subendocardium is at a higher risk than the midwall or epicardium [25,26]. Despite its significant clinical relevance, the physical or mechanical determinants of subendocardial vulnerability remain controversial [26–31]. The reason for this is that clinical work has largely focused on the individual epicardial diseased vessels (with respect to LDL permeability and atherosclerotic plaque formation) rather than on the dynamics of the coronary blood flow system as an integrated system. The latter requires a bioengineering understanding of the complex coronary vasculature embedded in the myocardium and of the associated mechanical interactions. There are several computational approaches to blood flow analysis such as: lumped parameter (Windkessel-type) model [32–34], steady-state model in the entire coronary arterial tree [3,35,36], lumped flow model in dynamically loaded coronary microvascular vessels [37–39], Womersley-type/1D wave propagation model in entire coronary arterial tree [40,41], which are generally used to compute the distribution of blood flow in the complex coronary vasculature. Herein, we will apply these methods to formulate and illustrate three types of coronary circulatory flows (in porcine models): pulsatile flow in the epicardial coronary tree, steady-state flow in the entire coronary arterial tree, and wave propagation in the coronary arterial tree.

15.2.1 3D CFD Model in the Epicardial Coronary Tree of Porcine Model

We have used the FE method to investigate the 3D pulsatile blood flow in the epicardial coronary tree of a porcine model [7]. The governing equations are formulated for an incompressible, Newtonian fluid. The Continuity equation and Navier–Stokes equation can be written as

$$\nabla \cdot v = 0 \tag{15.1}$$

$$\rho \frac{\partial v}{\partial t} + \rho v \cdot \nabla v = -\nabla P + \nabla \cdot \mu (\nabla v + (\nabla v)^T) \tag{15.2}$$

where v, P, ρ, and μ represent the velocity vector, pressure, blood density, and viscosity, respectively. Equations 15.1 and 15.2 are solved for velocity and pressure, for appropriate boundary and initial conditions.

The solution of the governing equations is determined, subject to the following pulsatile boundary conditions:

$$v_{inlet} = v_{measured\,flow\,velocity\,at\,the\,inlet} \tag{15.3}$$

$$v_{wall} = v_{measured\,wall\,velocity} \tag{15.4}$$

$$v_{outlet} = v_{estimated\,flow\,velocity\,at\,the\,outlet} \tag{15.5}$$

Equations 15.3 through 15.5 are pulsatile inlet flow (v_{inlet}), moving wall (v_{wall}), and outlet flow (v_{outlet}) boundary conditions, respectively. The inlet flow and moving wall boundary conditions are obtained from experimental measurements. Therein, a perivascular flow probe (Transonic Systems Inc.; relative error of ±2% at full scale) was mounted on the most proximal RCA directly to determine the pulsatile inlet flow. The dynamic changes of lumen cross-sectional area of RCA were measured by using an impedance catheter, which detects the change in cross-sectional area based on electrical impedance principles. The pulsatile outlet flow boundary conditions were estimated based on scaling laws [42,43].

Because the moving wall boundary due to vessel compliance is considered, the 3D mesh moving technique is used to solve the moving fluid boundaries. The mesh is updated by solving the Laplace problem, which provides the displacement ($s = x \cdot e_1 + y \cdot e_2 + z \cdot e_3$) of each point, as follows:

$$\nabla \cdot (\nabla s) = 0 \tag{15.6}$$

After Equation 15.6 was solved, the nodal velocities (v_{node}) due to the transient changes of meshes were calculated. The convective term in Equation 15.2 was changed to $\rho(v + v_{node}) \cdot \nabla v$, based on the arbitrary Lagrangian–Eulerian frameworks.

A FORTRAN program was used to implement the FE method for the computation of pressure and flow in the epicardial coronary tree of porcine model. Before the final transient simulation, a mesh dependency was conducted, so that the relative error in two consecutive mesh refinements was <1% for the maximum velocity for steady-state flow with inlet flow velocity equal to the time-averaged velocity over a cardiac cycle. A total of almost 310,000 finite elements were required to accurately mesh the computational domains, as shown in Figure 15.1. The backward method was used for the

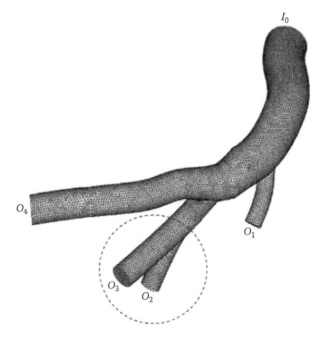

FIGURE 15.1
Finite element mesh for numerical computation of the RCA tree, where I_0 represents the inlet of RCA tree and O_1–O_4 are the outlets of RCA tree. (From Huo, Y. et al., *J. Biomech.*, 42, 594, 2009.)

time integration. A constant time step was employed, where $\Delta t = 0.005$ s with 108 total time steps per cardiac cycle. Although blood is a suspension of particles, it behaves as a Newtonian flow in tubes with diameters >1 mm [44]. The epicardial RCA vessel segments obtained from the CT images were considered to satisfy this criterion. The viscosity and density of the fluid were selected as 4.5 cP and 1.06 g/cm^3, respectively, to mimic blood flow with a hematocrit of about 45% in medium size arteries. A uniform flow velocity profile was assumed at the inlet of the RCA tree, because the RCA tree attaches to the aorta. The parabolic flow velocity profile was applied to each outlet of the RCA tree, because the inlet blunt flow velocity can quickly develop into a fully developed parabolic profile.

Based on the computed velocity and pressure of the blood flow, the Reynolds (Re) and Womersley (α) numbers are defined as follows:

$$\text{Re} = \frac{\rho V \cdot D}{\mu} \tag{15.7}$$

$$\alpha = R\sqrt{\frac{\omega\rho}{\mu}} \tag{15.8}$$

where $V = V_{min}$, V_{max}, or V_{mean}, R and D, ω, ρ, and μ represent minimum, maximum, or time-averaged velocity at the inlet of ascending aorta, radius and diameter of ascending aorta, angular frequency of beating hearts, blood mass density, and viscosity, respectively. At any point of the 3D FEM model, the stress on the wall can be represented as a nine-component tensor ($\bar{\bar{\tau}}$), which can be written as follows:

$$\bar{\bar{\tau}} = \begin{bmatrix} \tau_{11} & \tau_{12} & \tau_{13} \\ \tau_{21} & \tau_{22} & \tau_{23} \\ \tau_{31} & \tau_{32} & \tau_{33} \end{bmatrix} = 2\mu\bar{\bar{D}} = \mu \begin{bmatrix} 2\dfrac{\partial u}{\partial x} & \dfrac{\partial u}{\partial y}+\dfrac{\partial v}{\partial x} & \dfrac{\partial u}{\partial z}+\dfrac{\partial w}{\partial x} \\ \dfrac{\partial u}{\partial y}+\dfrac{\partial v}{\partial x} & 2\dfrac{\partial v}{\partial y} & \dfrac{\partial v}{\partial z}+\dfrac{\partial w}{\partial y} \\ \dfrac{\partial u}{\partial z}+\dfrac{\partial w}{\partial x} & \dfrac{\partial v}{\partial z}+\dfrac{\partial w}{\partial y} & 2\dfrac{\partial w}{\partial z} \end{bmatrix} \tag{15.9}$$

where $\bar{\bar{D}} = 0.5 \cdot [(\nabla v) + (\nabla v)^T]$ is the shear rate tensor. The stresses on the wall, its normal component and its two tangential components can be written as, respectively:

$$\vec{\tau} = \bar{\bar{\tau}} \cdot n, \quad \tau_n = n \cdot \bar{\bar{\tau}} \cdot n, \quad \tau_{t_1} = t_1 \cdot \bar{\bar{\tau}} \cdot n, \quad \text{and} \quad \tau_{t_2} = t_2 \cdot \bar{\bar{\tau}} \cdot n \tag{15.10}$$

where n, t_1, and t_2 are the unit vectors in the normal and two tangential directions, respectively. The shear component of $\vec{\tau}$ has the vector form:

$$\vec{\tau}_{shear} = \vec{\tau} - (\vec{\tau} \cdot n)n \tag{15.11}$$

Equation 15.11 is used to calculate WSS, which has the magnitude: $\left|\vec{\tau}_{shear}\right| = \sqrt{\vec{\tau}\cdot\vec{\tau}-(\vec{\tau}\cdot n)^2}$. The time-averaged WSS over a cardiac cycle (T) can be written as follows:

$$\text{time-averaged } WSS = \frac{1}{T}\int_0^T \left|\vec{\tau}_{shear}\right|\cdot dt \tag{15.12}$$

The present time-averaged OSI can be written as follows:

$$OSI = \frac{1}{2}\left(1 - \frac{\left|(1/T)\int_0^T \vec{\tau}_{shear}\right|}{(1/T)\int_0^T \left|\vec{\tau}_{shear}\right|}\right) \tag{15.13}$$

The spatial derivatives of the stress can be obtained as follows:

$$\nabla\vec{\tau} = \begin{bmatrix} \dfrac{\partial\tau_n}{\partial n} & \dfrac{\partial\tau_n}{\partial t_1} & \dfrac{\partial\tau_n}{\partial t_2} \\[2mm] \dfrac{\partial\tau_{t_1}}{\partial n} & \dfrac{\partial\tau_{t_1}}{\partial t_1} & \dfrac{\partial\tau_{t_1}}{\partial t_2} \\[2mm] \dfrac{\partial\tau_{t_2}}{\partial n} & \dfrac{\partial\tau_{t_2}}{\partial t_1} & \dfrac{\partial\tau_{t_2}}{\partial t_2} \end{bmatrix} \tag{15.14}$$

where n, t_1, and t_2 are the natural coordinates. The diagonal components $\partial\tau_{t_1}/\partial t_1$ and $\partial\tau_{t_2}/\partial t_2$ generate intracellular tension, which causes widening and shrinking of the cellular gap. However, the diagonal component $\partial\tau_n/\partial n$ can cause ECs rotation, which may also destroy the endothelial function. The WSSG is defined as follows:

$$WSSG = \left[\left(\frac{\partial\tau_n}{\partial n}\right) + \left(\frac{\partial\tau_{t_1}}{\partial t_1}\right) + \left(\frac{\partial\tau_{t_2}}{\partial t_2}\right)\right]^{1/2} \tag{15.15}$$

The time-averaged WSSG can be written as

$$\text{time-averaged } WSSG = \frac{1}{T}\int_0^T WSSG\cdot dt \tag{15.16}$$

Figure 15.2a and b show the time-averaged cross-sectional flow velocity vector profiles over a cardiac cycle along the main trunk of the RCA tree in anterior and posterior views, respectively, which has velocity values of 8.17 cm/s at the inlet and 6.05, 6.33, 6.81, and 7.29 cm/s at outlets O_1–O_4. It is seen that the blunt core velocity profile at the inlet of

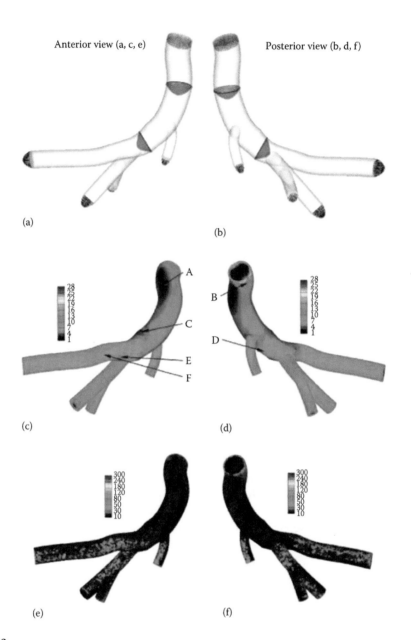

FIGURE 15.2
RCA trunk and branches: time-averaged velocity vector profiles (grid units/magnitude of velocity = 0.01) in (a) anterior view and (b) posterior view; time-averaged WSS (dyn/cm²) in (c) anterior view and (d) posterior view; time-averaged WSSG (dyn/cm³) fields over a cardiac cycle in (e) anterior view and (f) posterior view, respectively. (From Huo, Y. et al., *J. Biomech.*, 42, 594, 2009.)

RCA tree gradually develops into a parabolic velocity profile. The Reynolds number and Womersley number are about 80 and 2, respectively, at the inlet of RCA tree. Figure 15.2c through f shows the distribution of time-averaged WSS and WSSG, respectively, corresponding to Figure 15.2a and b.

Figure 15.3a through c shows the time-averaged velocity vector profile, WSS and WSSG, respectively, for diameter ratio of 0.5. Consequently, Figures 15.4a and b and 15.5a and b

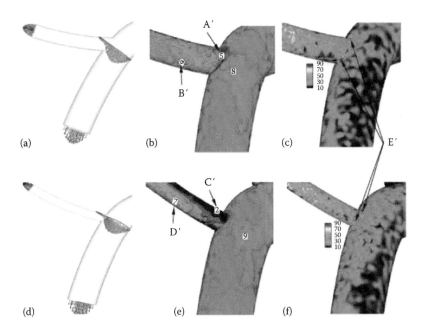

FIGURE 15.3
Time-averaged velocity vector profile (grid units/magnitude of velocity = 0.008), WSS (dyn/cm^2), and time-averaged WSSG (dyn/cm^3) at arterial bifurcations with diameter ratio = 0.5 (a–c) and diameter ratio = 0.3 (d–f). (From Huo, Y. et al., *J. Biomech.*, 42, 594, 2009.) Locations A′ and C′ are opposite to the flow divider, locations B′ and D′ are in the branch, and location E′ is at the orifice. As indicated in Table 15.1, the sites of predilection to atherosclerosis, due to presence of low WSS, are at the flow divider locations A′ and C′; the branch sites B′ and D′, of high values of WSSG, are susceptible to increased permeability of LDL.

show the transient changes of WSS and WSSG at locations A′ (opposite to the flow divider) and B′ (flow divider) in Figure 15.3b, respectively. Figure 15.3d through f shows the time-averaged velocity vector profile, WSS, and WSSG for diameter ratio of 0.3. Correspondingly, Figures 15.4c and d and 15.5c and d show the transient changes of WSS and WSSG, respectively, for diameter ratio of 0.3 at locations C′ and D′. Table 15.1 shows the time-averaged WSS and WSSG at locations A′–D′ in Figure 15.3.

It is found that WSS opposite to the flow divider (at locations A′ and C′) decreases with the diameter ratio. The WSSG in the flow divider (at locations B′ and D′) increases as the diameter ratio decreases. In particular, there is a strong WSSG around the orifice, as shown at locations E′ in Figure 15.3. The vessel compliance reduces the time-averaged WSSG by approximately 10% at the flow divider, as compared with the rigid wall model with no vessel wall movement [7]. The permeability of LDL is determined mainly by the flow parameters, that is, low WSS [45] and high WSSG [14]. The elasticity-induced decrease of time-averaged WSSG at the flow divider implies that the elasticity may reduce the permeability of LDL at bifurcations.

We have developed a FE model, based on CT scans and physiological measurements in the normal epicardial RCA tree, to predict the role of vessel compliance. Based on Table 15.1, the HPs indicate the sites A′ and C′ (at the flow divider) that are prone to atherosclerosis due to the presence of low WSS. The branch sites B′ and D′, of high values of WSSG, are susceptible to increased permeability of LDL [14–16]. In future, the model can be made patient-specific, through medical imaging to guide diagnosis, intervention, and therapy.

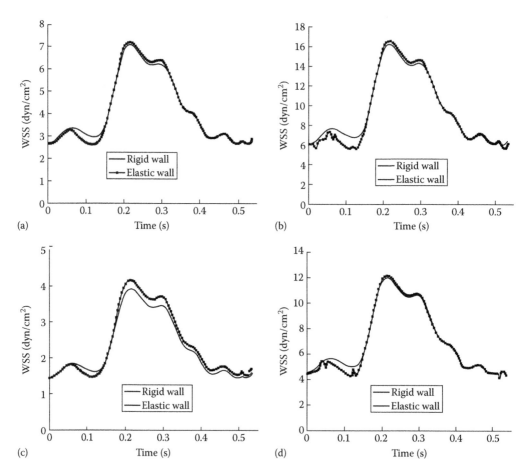

FIGURE 15.4
Transient WSS (dyn/cm²) in a cardiac cycle, where panels (a-d) show the changes of WSS at locations A′ to D′ in Figure 15.3. (From Huo, Y. et al., *J. Biomech.*, 42, 594, 2009.)

15.2.2 A Steady-State Flow Model in the Entire Coronary Arterial Tree of Porcine Model

We have earlier generated the spatial branching pattern and vascular geometry of the full 3D coronary arterial trees down to the first capillary vessels [46], using which a steady-state flow analysis was performed [3,35,36]. If we assume that the flow through a blood vessel is laminar, steady, and free from end effects, then the volumetric flow Q_{ij} in a vessel between any two nodes, represented by i and j, is given in terms of the pressure differential ΔP_{ij} and vessel conductance G_{ij} by

$$Q_{ij} = \frac{\pi}{128} \Delta P_{ij} G_{ij} \quad \text{with } \Delta P_{ij} = P_i - P_j \text{ and } G_{ij} = \frac{D_{ij}^4}{\mu_{ij} L_{ij}} \tag{15.17}$$

where
    D_{ij}, L_{ij}, and μ_{ij} are the diameter, length, and viscosity, respectively, between nodes i and j
    m_j is the number of vessels converging at the jth node

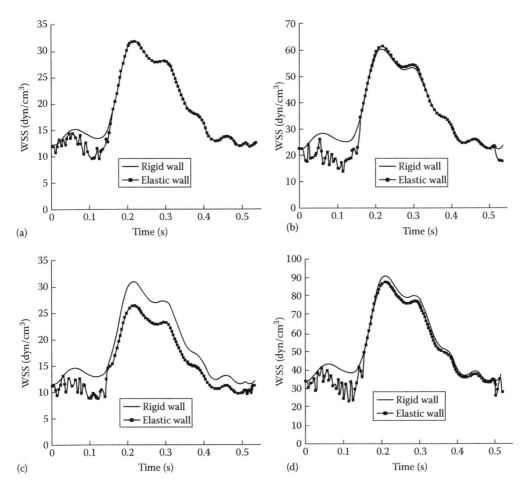

FIGURE 15.5
Transient WSSG (dyn/cm³) in a cardiac cycle, where panels (a-d) show the changes of WSSG at location A′ to D′ in Figure 15.3. (From Huo, Y. et al., *J. Biomech.*, 42, 594, 2009.)

TABLE 15.1

Time-Averaged WSS and WSSG at Bifurcations of RCA with Different Diameter Ratios, Where A′–D′ Correspond to Positions A′–D′ in Figure 15.3

	WSS (dyn/cm²)		WSSG (dyn/cm³)	
Positions	**Rigid wall**	**Elastic wall**	**Rigid wall**	**Elastic wall**
Low WSS position (opposite to flow divider)				
A′	4.18	4.18	18.9	18.4
C′	2.33	2.42	18.6	15.7
High WSS position (at flow divider)				
B′	9.61	9.53	35.9	34.1
D′	7.08	7.02	54.2	50.3

There are two or more vessels that emanate from the jth node anywhere in the tree, with the number of vessels converging at the jth node being m_j. By invoking conservation of mass, we have

$$\sum_{i=1}^{m_j} Q_{ij} = 0 \tag{15.18}$$

where the volumetric flow into a node is considered positive and the flow out of a node is negative for any branch. From Equations 15.17 and 15.18, we obtain a set of linear algebraic equations in pressure, for the M nodes in the network, namely,

$$\sum_{i=1}^{m_j} \left| P_i - P_j \right| G_{ij} = 0 \tag{15.19}$$

The set of equations represented by Equation 15.19 reduce to a set of simultaneous linear algebraic terms for the nodal pressures, once the conductances are evaluated from the geometry and suitable boundary conditions are specified. In matrix form, this set of equations is given by

$$GP = G_B P_B \tag{15.20}$$

where

    G is the matrix of conductance
    P is the column vector of the unknown nodal pressures
    $G_B P_B$ is the column vector of the conductance times the boundary pressure of their attached vessels

The pressures at the inlet and outlet (i.e., the first capillaries) of coronary arterial trees were set as 100 and 26 mmHg, respectively. The viscosity (μ_{ij}) was taken to be the viscosity of water at 37°C, because the experimental cardioplegic solution has similar hemodynamic properties to water.

Figure 15.6 illustrates the pressure distribution in two views (lateral left and posterolateral oblique left) of the entire coronary arterial tree model down to the first capillary segments [3]. It is clear that the pressure distribution is fairly uniform in larger vessels and changes significantly in smaller vessels (<100 μm), which is in agreement with experimental measurements [47,48]. This shows that the myocardial resistance mainly resides in the arteriolar bed. Moreover, the 3D coronary arterial model presented here provides a platform to analyze the flow distribution and heterogeneity in small neighboring regions of the myocardium.

15.2.3 A Hybrid Womersley-Type 1D Wave Propagation Model in the Entire Coronary Arterial Tree of a Porcine Model

The 1D wave propagation model has been used to study the pressure and flow wave propagation in the arterial tree under physiological and pathological conditions [49–54]. The 1D model of Hughes and Lubliner [55] is used to solve the blood flow in the entire epicardial coronary arterial tree of a vasodilated, arrested porcine heart by the finite difference (FD) method [41]. The governing equations are formulated for a Newtonian, incompressible fluid in an elastic tree. As shown in Figure 15.8, the 1D wave propagation analysis is carried out for large coronary arteries, every vessel of which is assumed to be cylindrical with impermeable wall. Hence, the fluid flow in every vessel segment is

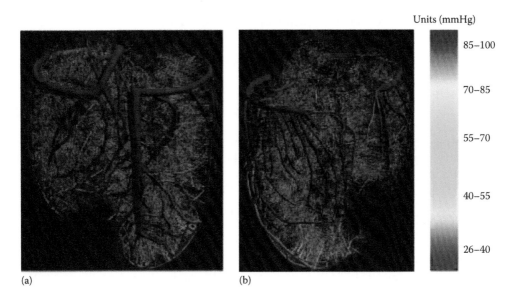

FIGURE 15.6
Pressure distribution in two views (lateral left and posterolateral oblique left) in the 3D entire coronary arterial trees consisting of the epicardial, transmural, and perfusion subnetworks: (a) lateral-left-view pressure and (b) posterolateral-oblique-left-view pressure. The 3D coronary arterial model presented here provides a platform to analyze the flow distribution and heterogeneity in small neighboring regions of the myocardium.

axisymmetric and laminar with no-slip boundary condition (i.e., the velocity of fluid at the wall equals the velocity of the wall).

The various geometrical parameters in a typical vessel can be represented as length L, radius R, cross-sectional area A, surface S, volume V, and wall thickness h, that can vary with time and space. Furthermore, the fluid mechanics parameters are represented as the velocities of fluid flow $[u_r(r, z, t), u_x(r, z, t)]$. The volumetric flow rate and the pressure in the vessel are $q(z, t)$ and $p(z, t) - p_0$ (intravascular pressure minus external pressure, which is assumed to be zero in diastole), respectively. A cylindrical coordinate system is used with radial (r) and axial (z) directions; the hemodynamic quantities $u_r(r, z, t)$, $u_z(r, z, t)$, $q(z, t)$, and $p(z, t)$ can be represented as u_r, u_z, q, and p.

In order to carry out the wave propagation analysis, the continuity (mass conversation) and momentum equations for tube flow can be simplified to

$$\frac{\partial u_z}{\partial x} + \frac{1}{r}\frac{\partial (r u_r)}{\partial r} = 0 \tag{15.21}$$

$$\frac{\partial u_z}{\partial t} + u_z \frac{\partial u_z}{\partial z} + u_r \frac{\partial u_z}{\partial r} + \frac{1}{\rho}\frac{\partial p}{\partial z} = \frac{\nu}{r}\frac{\partial}{\partial r}\left(r\frac{\partial u_z}{\partial r}\right) + \nu\frac{\partial^2 u_z}{\partial z^2} \tag{15.22}$$

where $\nu = \mu/\rho$ is the kinematic viscosity. For the no-slip boundary condition and the deformation of the elastic wall of the vessel, we put down the following boundary equations:

$$(u_z)_{r=\pm R} = 0 \quad \text{and} \quad (u_r)_{r=R} = \frac{\partial R}{\partial t} \tag{15.23}$$

The volumetric flow rate and cross-sectional area are given by

$$q = 2\pi \int_0^R u_z r\, dr \qquad (15.24)$$

$$A = \pi \cdot r^2 \qquad (15.25)$$

By integrating Equations 15.21 and 15.22 over the cross-sectional area of the vessel with the boundary conditions (Equation 15.23), with the assumption that ρ is constant over the area, we obtain

$$\frac{\partial A}{\partial t} + \frac{\partial q}{\partial z} = 0 \qquad (15.26)$$

$$\frac{\partial q}{\partial t} + \frac{\partial}{\partial z}\left(2\pi \int_0^R u_z^2 r\, dr\right) + \frac{A}{\rho}\frac{\partial p}{\partial z} = 2\pi v\left(r\frac{\partial u_z}{\partial r}\right)_{r=R} + v\frac{\partial^2 q}{\partial z^2} \qquad (15.27)$$

In the larger epicardial arteries, the velocity profile is assumed to be fully developed Poiseuille flow. We assume the parabolic velocity profile, as given by

$$u_z = C_1 r^2 + C_2 r + C_3 \qquad (15.28)$$

where C_1, C_2, and C_3 are integration constants. When the boundary conditions (Equation 15.23) are considered, we solve Equation 15.28 to obtain

$$u_z = C_1(R^2 - r^2) \qquad (15.29)$$

Using Equations 15.29 and 15.24, we find that

$$q = \frac{C_1 A R^2}{2} \qquad (15.30)$$

The second term of Equation 15.27 may be written as

$$\frac{\partial}{\partial z}\left(2\pi \int_0^R u_z^2 r\, dr\right) = \frac{\partial}{\partial z}\left(\frac{4}{3}\frac{q^2}{A}\right) \qquad (15.31)$$

and the viscous drag force (on the right side of Equation 15.27) can be expressed as

$$2\pi v\left(r\frac{\partial u_z}{\partial r}\right)_{r=R} = -8\pi v\frac{q}{A} \qquad (15.32)$$

Inserting Equations 15.30 and 15.31 into Equation 15.27, we obtain

$$\frac{\partial q}{\partial t} + \frac{\partial}{\partial z}\left(\frac{4}{3}\frac{q^2}{A}\right) + \frac{A}{\rho}\frac{\partial p}{\partial z} = -8\pi v\frac{q}{A} + v\frac{\partial^2 q}{\partial z^2} \qquad (15.33)$$

Also, the constitutive equation based on a pressure cross-sectional area relationship for every vessel can be obtained, by utilizing Laplace's law:

$$\tau_\theta = \frac{(p - p_0)R_0}{h_0} \tag{15.34}$$

where τ_θ is the mean circumferential stress that relates the transmural pressure $(p - p_0)$ (intravascular pressure minus external pressure, which is assumed to be zero in diastole), the original vessel radius $R_0 = D_0/2$, and the original wall thickness h_0. If we assume that the wall stress–strain relationship is linear, we can write

$$\tau_\theta = E_{stat} \frac{R^2 - R_0^2}{R_0^2} \tag{15.35}$$

where
  E_{stat} is the static Young's modulus obtained from measurements [41]
  $(R^2 - R_0^2)/R_0^2$ is the circumferential strain

If we combine Equations 15.34 and 15.35, we obtain the following constitutive equation for the wall:

$$p - p_0 = \frac{E_{stat}h_0}{R_0} \left(\frac{A}{A_0} - 1 \right) \tag{15.36}$$

where the radius is expressed in terms of cross-sectional area. Upon inserting Equation 15.36 into Equation 15.33, we obtain

$$\frac{\partial q}{\partial t} + \frac{\partial}{\partial z} \left(\frac{4}{3} \frac{q^2}{A} \right) + \frac{A}{\rho} \frac{E_{stat}h_0}{R_0 A_0} \frac{\partial A}{\partial z} = -8\pi\nu \frac{q}{A} + \nu \frac{\partial^2 q}{\partial z^2} \tag{15.37}$$

The governing Equations 15.21 and 15.22 can now be outlined as

$$\frac{\partial A}{\partial t} + \frac{\partial q}{\partial z} = 0 \tag{15.38}$$

$$\frac{\partial q}{\partial t} + \frac{\partial}{\partial z} \left(\frac{4}{3} \frac{q^2}{A} \right) + \frac{A}{\rho} \frac{E_{stat}h_0}{R_0 A_0} \frac{\partial A}{\partial z} = -8\pi\nu \frac{q}{A} + \nu \frac{\partial^2 q}{\partial z^2} \tag{15.39}$$

Equations 15.38 and 15.39 are the basic equations, which can be simplified to

$$\frac{\partial A}{\partial t} + \frac{\partial q}{\partial z} = 0$$

$$\frac{\partial q}{\partial t} + a \frac{\partial q}{\partial z} + b \frac{\partial A}{\partial z} = c + d \frac{\partial^2 q}{\partial z^2} \tag{15.40}$$

where

$$a = \frac{8}{3} \frac{q}{A}, \quad b = -\frac{4}{3} \left(\frac{q}{A} \right)^2 + \frac{A}{\rho} \frac{E_{stat}h_0}{R_0 A_0}, \quad c = -8\pi\nu \frac{q}{A}, \quad d = \nu$$

For large vessels, Equations 15.40 can be solved by the time-centered implicit (Trapezoidal) FD method. The detailed description of the FD solution can be found in Huo and Kassab [41]. The inlet pressure boundary condition is obtained from experimental measurements, as shown in Figure 15.7.

The Womersley-type model [40] is applied to the morphometric trees to represent the distal vascular beds for each of the outlets of the numerical domain (see Figure 15.8). The impedance/admittance [$Z(x, \omega)/Y(x, \omega)$] is calculated at each outlet of the numerical domain.

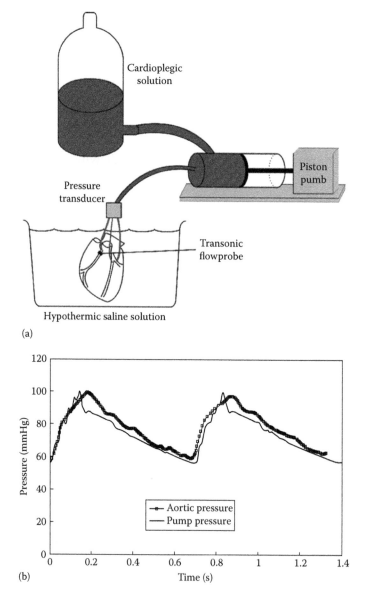

FIGURE 15.7

(a) Schematic diagram of apparatus of pulsatile flow preparation and (b) comparison of the profile of pressure produced by the piston pump with the measured in vivo aortic pressure. (From Huo, Y. and Kassab, G.S., *Am. J. Physiol. Heart Circ. Physiol.*, 291, H1074, 2006.)

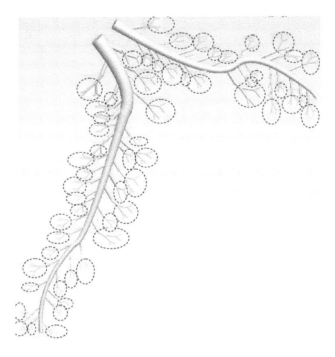

FIGURE 15.8
Schematic representation of the computational domains (the main trunk and primary branches) in the LMCA tree that consists of the LAD and LCx arterial trees. (From Huo, Y. and Kassab, G.S., *Am. J. Physiol. Heart Circ. Physiol.*, 292, H2623, 2007.)

By inverse Fourier transformation, $z(x, t)/y(x, t)$ can be obtained from $Z(x, \omega)/Y(x, \omega)$ [41]. Using the convolution theorem, the new resulting outflow boundary conditions can be obtained as follows:

$$p(x, t) = \int_{t-T}^{t} q(x, \tau) z(x, t-\tau) d\tau \quad \text{or} \quad q(x, t) = \int_{t-T}^{t} p(x, \tau) y(x, t-\tau) d\tau \qquad (15.41)$$

In the solution, the viscosity (μ) and density (ρ) are taken to be 1.1 cP and 1 g/cm³, respectively, to mimic our experimental studies using cardioplegic solution in the isolated arrested heart preparation [40]. The static Young's modulus is estimated to be 7×10^6 (dyn/cm²) [40]. Since the time-centered implicit FD method is stable and second order in both time and space, the mesh size (Δx) is selected as 0.05 cm and the time step (Δt) is set to 2×10^{-3} s.

Our 1D wave propagation model can accurately determine the transient blood flow at each discrete point of the main trunk and primary branches. Based on this model, Figure 15.9 shows the flow waves sequentially at different spatial positions along the main trunk starting from the inlet of LAD artery; Figure 15.10 shows the flow waves at the inlet of the various primary branches [41]. The decrease of flow amplitude along the main trunk is apparent, but the flow waveform remains relatively unchanged. This is because the primary branches shunt the flow away from the main trunk. Since the primary branches have different cross-sectional areas, the flow waves at the inlet of primary branches show different amplitudes. When the flow waves are normalized by

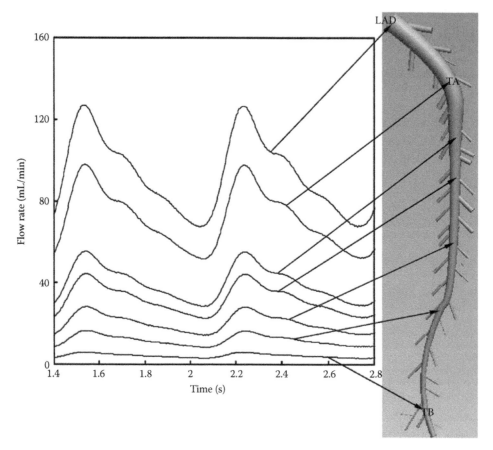

FIGURE 15.9
Flow waves sequentially along the main trunk, starting from the inlet of LAD artery. (From Huo, Y. and Kassab, G.S., *Am. J. Physiol. Heart Circ. Physiol.*, 292, H2623, 2007.)

the time-averaged flow rate, however, it is found that the flow waves tend to scale to a single curve, which reflects a structure–function relationship between the mean flow and vessel diameter [42,43].

The pulsatile pressure and flow waves have been widely studied from the aorta to the limb arteries in the classic book of *McDonald's Blood Flow in Arteries* [44]. In this study, the pressure and flow waves were calculated along the main trunk of LAD artery. The amplitude of the flow waves decreases gradually, and a small phase angle shift of the flow waves appears along the main trunk of LAD artery in the potassium-arrested heart. This is because the primary branches shunt the flow away from the main trunk. Since primary branches have different cross-sectional area, the flow waves at the inlet of primary branches show different amplitudes. When the flow waves are normalized by the time-averaged flow rate, however, it is found that the flow waves tend to scale to a single curve. This observation reflects an interesting scaling of flow to structure [42,43]. Specifically, we have found that Murray's exponential relation holds for the analysis but with an exponent of 2.4, 2.3, and 2.1 for RCA, LAD, and LCx arteries, respectively.

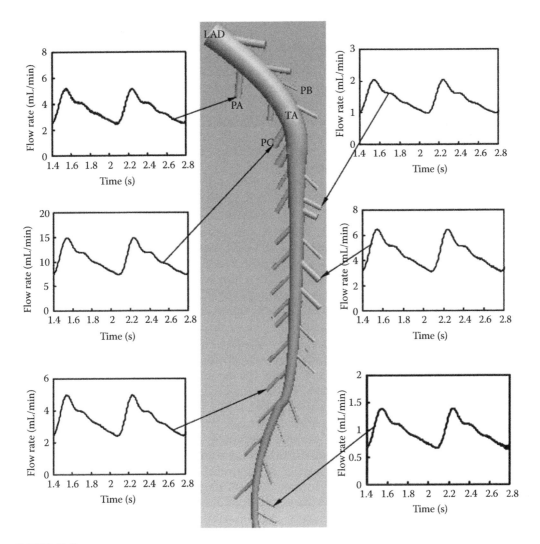

FIGURE 15.10
Flow waves of the primary branches of LAD arterial trunk. (From Huo, Y. and Kassab, G.S., *Am. J. Physiol. Heart Circ. Physiol.*, 292, H2623, 2007.)

This implies that we can predict the shape of the flow waves in the microcirculation that are not amenable to direct observations from knowledge of epicardial waveforms that can be measured.

Our present time-domain model is capable of predicting dynamic pulsatile flow based on detailed coronary morphometric data as demonstrated earlier. The 1D wave propagation model can be made patient-specific by interface with patient-specific anatomy of large epicardial vessels obtained from CT, MRI, or other imaging techniques. The smaller vessels that are beyond current clinical imaging resolution can be treated as a lumped model with less anatomical detail. When mass transport is coupled to the momentum equation mentioned earlier through the velocity components, the model can predict the distribution of cells and drugs to the ischemic myocardium.

15.3 Coronary Artery Bypass Graft Flow and Design for Enhanced Patency

Despite extensive research on cardiovascular disease (CVD) and in particular on the most prevalent serious disease of the heart, CAD, and its causative factors, CVD continues to be one of the leading causes of mortality in the world. According to American Heart Association (2012), an estimated 82,600,000 American adults (>1 in 3) have one or more types of CVD. Mortality data show that CVD, as the underlying cause of death, accounted for 1 of every 3 deaths and CAD caused 1 of every 6 deaths in the United States [56].

When the lumen of coronary artery is reduced, the cardiac muscle tissue perfused by the coronary artery beyond the point of the blockage is deprived of oxygen and nutrients. If a coronary obstruction persists for more than a few minutes, the affected cardiac muscle tissue will begin to die which is known as myocardial infarction or heart attack. Several alternative treatments exist for CAD, including medical therapy, rotablation, endarterectomy, percutaneous coronary intervention (PCI) or balloon angioplasty, stenting, and CABG. Depending on the severity, number and position of atherosclerotic lesions, and the clinical history of the patient, any of the aforementioned treatments may be chosen.

For high-risk patients, such as those with left main coronary artery (LMCA), severe three-vessel (LAD, LCx, and RCA), or diffuse disease not amendable to treat with a PCI, severe ventricular dysfunction (i.e., low ejection fraction), or diabetes mellitus, CABG is preferred [57]. Generally speaking, the greater the extent of coronary atherosclerosis and its diffuseness, the more compelling the choice of CABG, particularly if left ventricle function is depressed [58].

CABG is a surgical procedure performed to graft arteries or veins from the patient's body or synthetic conduits to the occluded coronary arteries, in order to bypass the atherosclerotic narrowing and improve the blood supply to the coronary circulation, for nourishing the myocardium. Figure 15.11 illustrates both arterial and venous grafts, each bypassing a coronary stenosis formed by cholesterol build-ups.

Although CABG is extremely effective for symptomatic relief and prognostic improvement in CAD and is the preferred remedy for high-risk patients, it is not devoid of complications and the long-term benefits are directly related to continuing conduit patency. Approximately 10%–15% of vein grafts occlude during the first year after operation [59]. About half of the vein grafts are only effective for a period of 5–10 years [60,61]. By 10 years after surgery, about 60% of vein grafts are patent, only 50% of which remain free of significant stenosis [62].

Early graft failure (within 30 days) of bypass grafts is attributable to surgical technical errors and thrombosis, while late graft failures are mainly caused by progression of atherosclerosis and intimal hyperplasia (IH) [63]. Various studies have found IH to be the major cause of graft stenosis [64]. IH is the abnormal, continued proliferation and overgrowth of smooth muscle cells (SMCs) in response to endothelial injury or dysfunction. Although the exact mechanism and pathophysiology of IH remains an enigma, there are indications that both *biological and biomechanical factors* are involved, which include endothelial injury [65], platelet activation [66], disturbed local hemodynamics [67,68], compliance mismatch between the graft and host vessel [69], and interactions between blood and graft material [70].

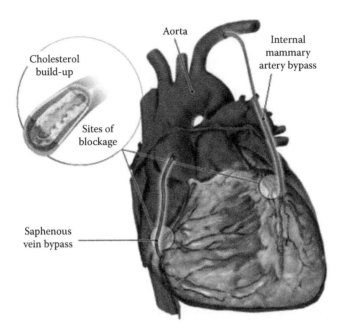

FIGURE 15.11

Illustration of coronary arterial bypass grafting: a saphenous vein graft is anastomosed proximally to aorta and distally to downstream of the stenosis of the right coronary artery (RCA). The internal mammary artery (IMA) that branches from aorta is anastomosed to the left anterior descending (LAD) coronary artery.

Among the aforementioned factors, *HPs* are believed to be highly important [71,72] in the genesis and development of IH. It has been shown that in end-to-side (ETS) graft–artery configurations, IH develops predominantly at the toe and heel of the anastomosis and on the artery bed across the junction where disturbed flow patterns and HPs are observed [71,73]. On the basis of this focal distribution of intimal thickening (IT), disturbed flow patterns and the associated HPs have been correlated with the onset and progression of atherosclerosis and distal anastomotic intimal hyperplasia (DAIH) [73,74]. Among the most *important HPs* are WSS, spatial and temporal gradients of WSS, and OSI.

Accordingly, several investigations have been conducted and different anastomotic geometries and devices have been designed to improve the flow fields and HPs' distribution at ETS anastomosis, in order to enhance the graft patency [75]. These investigations include studies on the effects of geometrical factors, such as anastomotic angle [76–82], modified configuration of distal anastomosis [83–86], graft-to-host artery diameter ratio [87–89], and out-of-plane graft [90–92], and effects of stenosis severity and proximal artery flow [93,94], irregularities of venous graft wall (due to venous valve sinus) [95], and distance of grafting (i.e., the distance of anastomosis from the occluded site) [96]. Considerable efforts toward attaining an optimal patency-enhancing CABG anastomotic configuration have been made, and continue to be made by investigators. This is because enhancement of the longevity and patency rate of CABGs (by means of an optimal anastomotic configuration) can result in considerable improvement in the left ventricular contractility index and ejection fraction of patients with CAD [97,98], elimination of the need for re-operation, reduced medical costs for patients suffering from coronary stenosis, and significantly lower morbidity.

Accordingly, this section reviews (1) the role of graft anastomotic configurations causing disturbed hemodynamic patterns and parameters associated with graft failure, followed by (2) various attempts to design an optimal anastomotic configuration for the distal CABG anastomosis. This section illuminates the impact of CABG layout designs toward obtaining higher long-term graft patency rates and the benefit of superior anastomotic designs for the improvement of global ejection fraction of patients with CAD.

The first subsection reviews the studies correlating different hemodynamic factors (and associated parameters) to the initiation and progression of atherosclerosis and IH. These studies include computational simulations of blood flow (and determination the HPs) in numerous in vitro and in vivo investigations, which have provided strong evidence on the influence of hemodynamic factors on the initiation and onset of IH.

The second subsection elaborates on the various attempts to design optimal anastomotic configurations for CABG. These attempts include adjustments of anastomotic angle and graft-to-host artery ratio, design of different cuffed and patched anastomotic configurations, and design and development of other novel configurations (such as the coupled sequential anastomoses [SQA]) and synthetic devices.

15.3.1 Graft Anastomosis Structural Configurations and Factors, Causing Disturbed Hemodynamics Patterns and Parameters Associated with Atherosclerosis and Intimal Hyperplasia, Responsible for Low Patency of Bypass Grafting

In vivo observations indicate that in an ETS graft–artery anastomotic configuration, IH occurs preferentially around the suture-line (especially at the toe and heel of the anastomosis), and also develops on the bed of the host artery across the junction [71,73,81,99–101] (Figure 15.12).

Arterial floor IT is attributable to altered flow conditions [71]. Although it has been suggested that suture-line IT might be related to vascular healing, an in vivo study by Sottiurai [101] has shown opposing results. He investigated the role of anastomotic configuration, using autogenous femoro-femoral bypass with ETS configuration and end-to-end (ETE) interposition graft in canine models. Since compliance mismatch is not an

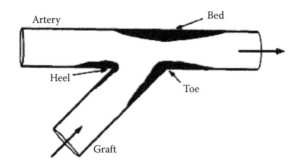

FIGURE 15.12
Outline of the spatial distribution of IH in an ETS distal anastomosis: IH occurs preferentially around the suture-line (especially at the toe and heel of the anastomosis) and on the bed of the host artery. (From Ojha, M., *J. Biomech.*, 26, 1377, 1993. With permission.)

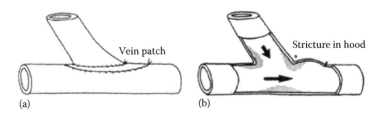

FIGURE 15.13
In vivo evidence that geometry of ETS anastomosis causes IH: (a) ETS distal anastomosis with a vein patch, (b) a section of distal ETS anastomosis; creation of an arbitrary stricture at the hood to simulate the toe (*) results in transferring the IH from the suture-line at the anastomotic toe to the stricture at the hood (physiologic toe); arrows indicate direction of blood flow. (From Sottiurai, V.S., *Int. J. Angiol.*, 8, 1, 1999. With permission.)

issue in the autogenous femoro-femoral bypass, for DAIH that exclusively occurs in the ETS (and not in the ETE) distal anastomoses, the geometry of the distal anastomosis has been concluded to be the logical causal factor.

Moreover, the creation of an arbitrary stricture on an extended hood of the arterial graft, to function as the "physiologic toe," has resulted in transferring DAIH to the site of the graft stricture (Figure 15.13). This attests to the fact that it is the ETS anastomotic configuration and its unnatural flow conditions, and not the trauma along the suture-line, which contributes to DAIH formation (more details are given in Section 15.3.1.4).

Several investigations have been conducted to better understand the relationship between blood flow-based stresses acting on the walls and IT in bypass grafts [67,71,73,103–106]. Subsequently, multiple HPs have been associated with occlusive formations in arterial bypass grafts and other branching blood vessel configurations, namely, (1) the bandwidth of WSS, (2) the magnitude of high-oscillatory WSS, (3) spatial and temporal gradients of WSS, and (4) vortex formation, flow separation and recirculation zones in the distal ETS anastomosis region based on its configuration.

15.3.1.1 Safe Bandwidth of WSS

Endothelial cells are constantly exposed to shear stress, induced by blood flow. Endothelial shear stress (i.e., WSS or τ_w) is the product of dynamic viscosity (μ) and shear rate ($\dot{\gamma} = \partial U/\partial r$) of blood at the vessel wall:

$$\tau_w = -\mu \frac{\partial U_{z\theta}}{\partial r}\bigg|_{r=R} \tag{15.42}$$

where
$U_{z\theta}$ is the velocity component parallel to the vessel wall
r is the radial axis
R is the radius of the blood vessel

The existence of a safe bandwidth of WSS has been suggested by Kleinstreuer et al. [107] to explain the localization of atherosclerotic plaques and IH, based on two contradictory hypotheses: (1) high shear stress theory and (2) low shear stress theory.

By experimental exposure of endothelium to high shear stresses, Fry [108,109] showed that a sufficiently high shear stress level would induce endothelial injury and promote the development of lesions, which were postulated to increase the permeability of endothelium and to alter the transport of molecular species across the endothelial barrier into the arterial wall, resulting in plaque formation.

On the other hand, Caro et al. [110] observed that atherosclerotic lesions occur along the inner wall of arterial curvature, where low shear stress exists. Hence, they proposed that (1) due to low WSS and enhanced particle residence time in flow separation and flow recirculation zones, excess cholesterol is deposited on the surface of the lumen, initiating atheroma growth, while (2) in the regions of moderately high WSS, more cholesterol is washed away by the blood flow.

Hence, combining the aforementioned opposing theories, it is suggested that there exists a safe bandwidth of WSS, and the wall shear that falls outside of this range will result in plaque formation. This hypothesis has successfully determined the sites and growth patterns of atherosclerotic lesions and IH in several arterial bifurcations and bypass graft configurations, respectively [111,112]. Moreover, study of numerical results of simulation of blood flow in the human aortic arch has suggested preferential development of early atherosclerotic lesions in regions of extreme (either maxima or minima) WSS and pressure [113]. In addition, it has been reported that the ECs in both low and high shear regions experience structural and functional abnormalities [114], thereby supporting the hypothesis of "safe bandwidth of WSS."

15.3.1.2 Low-Magnitude High-Oscillatory WSS

Based on the theory of Caro et al. [110], it is the "shear-dependent mass transfer," which is responsible for atheroma development and IT. Low shear stress acting on the vessel wall has been introduced as the key hemodynamic factor involved in the localization of IT, due to significant correlations found between the preferred sites of IT and the regions of slow recirculation flow (i.e., long particle residence time) with low WSS [68,106,115,116].

Morinaga et al. [117] investigated IT occurrence in autogenous vein grafts in dogs, by comparing the conditions of high flow rate and low WSS with low flow rate and high WSS. A comparatively significant intimal thickness was observed in high flow rate and low WSS condition, revealing that WSS, and not the rate of flow, is the essential hemodynamic factor related to IH.

Ku et al. [11] found a positive correlation between plaque location and low, oscillating shear stress, indicating that marked oscillations in the direction of wall shear may enhance atherogenesis. Consequently, they put forward the concept of "oscillatory shear index" to quantify the oscillatory nature of WSS. Based on its modified definition (Equation 15.43) [13], the OSI value varies between 0 and 0.5, where 0 corresponds to the regions experiencing no reverse flow, and 0.5 is for the case of fully oscillatory flow without net forward flow.

$$\text{OSI} = \frac{1}{2}\left(1 - \frac{\left|\int_0^T \vec{\tau}_w dt\right|}{\int_0^T \left|\vec{\tau}_w\right| dt}\right) \tag{15.43}$$

where
  T is the time period of a cardiac cycle
  $\vec{\tau}_w$ is the WSS vector

Li and Rittgers [118] compared the mechanical factors, obtained from in vitro study of pulsatile flow in a model of the distal ETS anastomosis of an arterial bypass graft, with histological findings of IH formation from earlier canine studies. Their results suggest that regions exposed to a combination of low-mean WSS and high-OSI may be most prone to IH formation. The same conclusion was obtained using in vitro preconditioned human umbilical vein ECs [119]. Besides, similar correlations of the HPs and sites of IT formation were observed by Zhang et al. [120] in a computational investigation of blood flow in a complete coronary artery bypass model.

Both low-mean shear and oscillatory shear stress contribute to an increased near-wall particle residence time, which may alter the mass transport of atherogenic substances to the vessel wall and increase the probability of deposition of platelets and macrophages, resulting in IT.

15.3.1.3 High Gradients of WSS

In an ETS graft–artery anastomosis, the floor typically experiences low oscillating WSS, due to the presence of a moving stagnation point during the cardiac cycle, as shown in Figure 15.14. However, this low-WSS–high-OSI hypothesis does not explain IH formation at the toe of the anastomosis (as the WSS is neither low nor oscillating at this location). Consequently, it has been postulated that the large spatial WSS gradient (WSSG), which is mainly observed at the toe of the anastomosis, induces morphological and functional changes in the endothelium that contribute to elevated wall permeability and hence possible atherosclerotic lesions [14]. The spatial gradient of WSS represents the nonuniformity of force distribution on the endothelium and implies a stretching force applied on the ECs, which can create local deformation of ECs and increase the wall permeability, leading to IH [83,102].

Moreover, the local WSSG is suggested as the single best indicator of nonuniform flow fields leading to atherogenesis [122]. Based on the biological evidence that non-uniform hemodynamic factors trigger an increase in wall permeability, Lei et al. [123] introduced an equation for wall permeability as a function of local WSSG magnitude. By employing the aorto-celiac junction of rabbits as a representative atherosclerotic model, their experimentally validated computer simulation model for enhanced LDL transport into the arterial wall showed that the WSSG is a reliable predictor of critical

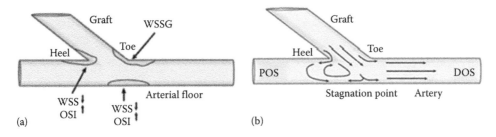

FIGURE 15.14
Typical flow patterns and HPs distribution in a distal ETS anastomosis: (a) outline of the typical spatial distribution of HPs and IT, and (b) flow patterns in the distal ETS anastomosis of arterial bypass grafts. A stagnation point forms on the arterial bed due to the bifurcation of the graft flow into the proximal and distal outlet segments (POS and DOS) of the coronary artery after impinging on the arterial bed. (Adapted from Haruguchi, H, and Teraoka, S., *J. Artif. Organs*, 6, 227, 2003. With permission.)

atherogenic sites in branching arteries [123]. Besides, it has been observed that IH tends to develop at sites having high spatial and temporal gradients in WSS [102].

15.3.1.4 Disturbed Flow Patterns Associated with Distal ETS Anastomosis

The configuration of distal ETS anastomosis is not naturally present in the arterial system (except for the patent ductus arteriosus). Although an ETS anastomosis is basically a bifurcation, it is different from naturally occurring blood vessel bifurcations. The angle between the daughter vessels is effectively obtuse and the flow division between the daughter branches in anastomoses can vary widely, which has a significant impact on the hemodynamics [124]. A distal ETS anastomosis is characterized by abnormal flow conditions, including flow oscillation at the heel, impingement on the artery floor, and flow separation at the toe.

Typically, there is a low-WSS region at the heel, where a vortex forms due to the interaction of the flow from the graft with the relatively slow flow in the occluded proximal artery, whose size changes with the flow phase (see Figure 15.14b). The presence of a slow recirculation flow (i.e., a vortex) increases the near-wall residence time and results in platelet activation [125] and fibrin thrombus formation [126,127], which leads to IH development [68,71,101,106,115,116].

Along with this vortex, there is a stagnation point on the artery bed, where the graft flow impinges the floor (Figure 15.14b) whose location oscillates (with the size of the vortex) during the cardiac cycle. This moving stagnation point provides a low-magnitude high-oscillatory WSS condition on the artery bed which is prone to enhancement of atherogenesis [11] and IH formation [118,128]. In addition, the flow impingement on the artery floor is known to be injurious to the endothelium and is believed to be a contributing factor to the graft failure, as there is evidence of change in the flow character once it impacts against the junction floor [129].

In a conventional ETS configuration, there are high flow shear rates at the toe of the anastomosis (causing high WSS at the toe), usually with a flow separation region just distal to the toe at the inner wall of the coronary artery (causing flow recirculation and low WSS at this area), as shown in Figure 15.15a. This results in a high spatial gradient of WSS at the toe of the anastomosis, which induces morphological and functional changes in the endothelium that contribute to elevated wall permeability and consequent atherosclerotic lesions [14,122,123] and IH development [102]. Moreover, in flow separation and

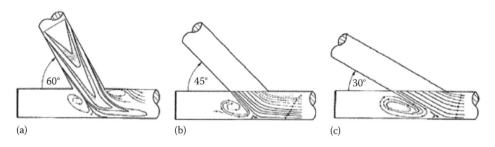

(a)   (b)   (c)

FIGURE 15.15

Effect of anastomotic angle on the flow regime: flow streamlines in the symmetry plane of distal ETS anastomoses with different anastomotic angles (a) 60°, (b) 45°, and (c) 30°. Flow separation at the toe and size of the reversed-flow region downstream of the anastomosis increases with anastomotic angle. (From Ghista, D.N. and Kabinejadian, F., *Biomed. Eng. Online*, 12, 129, 2013.)

flow recirculation zones, due to low WSS and enhanced particle residence time, excess cholesterol is deposited on the surface of the lumen, initiating atheroma growth [110] and IH [78,125].

Although an ETS anastomosis is essentially a bifurcation, being manmade, surgically created anastomoses can be modified (in contrast to arterial bifurcations) to yield a flow environment that improves graft longevity [124]. As reviewed earlier, investigations of blood flow and HPs and their comparison with focal locations of IT and IH formation in CABGs have resulted in correlation of some HPs with initiation and progression of IH. Consequently, HPs can, in turn, be utilized as indicators to show susceptible sites of IT and favorable conditions for thrombi and IH formation. Accordingly, using these indicators (i.e., by modification of HPs), extensive efforts have been put to obtain an optimal graft design, which is an end point for the study of correlations between hemodynamics and graft failure.

15.3.2 Attempts to Design an Optimal Anastomotic Configuration

The first efforts toward attaining an optimal anastomosis have been made by *changing the anastomotic angle*. It has been shown that tissue remodeling at ETS arterial anastomoses is highly sensitive to graft angle [79], and graft patency rates vary according to anastomotic angle. The anastomotic angle affects the flow regime and shear stress [76,80]. A smaller anastomotic angle reduces (1) the peaks and gradients of WSS [76], (2) the flow separation and disturbances at the toe [77,78,81,82], (3) secondary flow components [78], and (4) size of recirculation area (i.e., reversed flow) downstream of the anastomosis [80–82], as shown in Figure 15.15. Hence, a smaller distal ETS anastomotic angle (≤30°) seems to bring about a less disturbed and more uniform, smooth flow from the graft into the coronary artery.

The effect of graft caliber (i.e., graft-to-host diameter ratio) on the hemodynamics of CABGs has also been examined by investigators. It is observed that larger graft-to-host diameter ratios (5:3) have better hemodynamic performance than smaller ones (1:1) [87], as they can bring about relatively large positive longitudinal velocity, uniform and large WSS [88], and small WSSG [76,88]. Likewise, results of a computational study, using mesh-less CFD and genetic algorithms optimization, indicate that the graft caliber should always be maximized, in order to minimize the spatial and temporal gradients of WSS [89].

Besides, smaller grafts typically present an increased risk of early graft failure due to thrombosis [130]. Several clinical studies have demonstrated that small caliber (<3.5 mm) of vein grafts is the only independent risk factor for vein graft stenosis [131,132]. Idu et al. [131] suggested that a small caliber is a greater risk factor for graft failure than the use of arm or composite vein grafts, and that these alternative veins should be preferred if the saphenous vein graft is less than 3.5 mm in diameter.

It has been observed that a small-diameter (<3 mm) saphenous vein graft is associated with a 2.1-fold increased risk of early failure [133], and such conduits have a higher rate of occlusion in the perioperative (0–30 days) interval [134]. Moreover, observations from a large multicenter trial suggest that small size of vein graft is the dominant technical determinant of early graft failure [133].

In addition, a smaller graft diameter increases the graft resistance against the flow, which can elevate the flow portion through the native (partially stenosed) coronary and escalate the competitive flow problem [135], that eventually results in graft thrombosis and failure.

The effect of competitive flow (i.e., flow through a bypassed native coronary artery with low degree of stenosis) on the graft patency has been extensively investigated, but still is somewhat controversial. Many studies have demonstrated that the patency of bypass grafts on functionally significant lesions is considerably higher than the patency of bypass grafts on nonsignificant lesions [136–143]. They have confirmed the existence of a critical value for stenosis severity, below which the graft failure is expected, and above that, the recipient artery will be progressively occluded [135,144].

Although competitive flow (from patent native coronary vessels) is implicated in the failure of internal mammary artery (IMA) grafts, it is not thought to affect the patency of saphenous vein grafts (SVGs) [136,140,145]. This is because nonmuscular SVGs cannot adjust their lumens in response to metabolic requirements as much as arterial grafts. Thus, the response of vein grafts to low flow is limited [139].

On the other hand, some studies have demonstrated that despite significant correlation between (low) degree of proximal stenosis of the recipient coronary artery (i.e., presence of competitive flow) and occurrence of a string sign (where the graft conduit is patent but with only a thread of antegrade flow, due to narrowing of the graft), chronic native competitive flow does not significantly affect midterm graft status [146] and that the flow rates of the IMA grafts are comparable with and without stenosis or string phenomenon [147]. Also, limited studies have reported that competitive flow from a moderately stenotic coronary artery has not predisposed patients toward the string sign of the IMA graft in the presence of substantial diastolic IMA flow [148].

The effects of stenosis severity and distance of grafting on the hemodynamics of distal anastomosis have also been investigated. Computational simulations have shown that in the case of bypass grafting of partially stenosed coronary artery, the flow through partially occluded host artery interacts with the bypass graft flow at the anastomotic junction and that this combined flow can cause adverse hemodynamic effects, particularly when the distance of grafting is short [94,149–151]. The jet flow from a partially stenosed artery can increase the peak value of the axial velocity, if the stenosis is close to the anastomosis [150]. Also, interaction between the flows from the graft and the partially occluded artery results in steep variations of WSS near the heel and toe of the anastomosis, which can facilitate intimal proliferation and thrombogenesis around the suture-line when combined with flow recirculation in these regions [150]. Thus, it has been recommended that anastomosis be sutured with a sufficient distance of grafting, to enable the velocity profile to fully reattach before the heel so as to minimize the risks of IH at the anastomosis [149].

The influence of out-of-plane graft curvature has been studied by several investigators [91]. These investigations have revealed reductions in magnitudes of the peak time-averaged WSS [92] and mean oscillatory shear [90] in the nonplanar models as compared to the planar configurations, which imply a corresponding reduction in the spatial extent of wall regions exposed to physiologically unfavorable flow conditions [90]. Accordingly, in order to induce nonplanar flow effects, the use of grafts with intrinsic helical axis was suggested [152]. In vitro flow visualizations have shown significantly increased cross-plane mixing for the helical grafts (Figure 15.16a and b), and preliminary in vivo studies in arteriovenous bypass grafts have indicated that helical grafts offer the potential for improved patency (Figure 15.16c) [152,153]. This can be attributed to the swirling flow effects induced by helical grafts, which increase the magnitudes of velocity and WSS by adding a secondary (circumferential) velocity component to the axial velocity. This can enhance fluid-wall mass transport and render the spatial distribution of WSS relatively uniform in curved conduits, and potentially at anastomoses [152].

Nevertheless, the graft nonplanarity is often constrained by surgical considerations beyond hemodynamics (e.g., the stenosed artery, location of stenosis, etc.) [104].

Further efforts have been put to obtain a more favorable anastomosis by *design of cuffed and patched anastomotic configurations.* Miller et al. [154] introduced a vein cuff design that

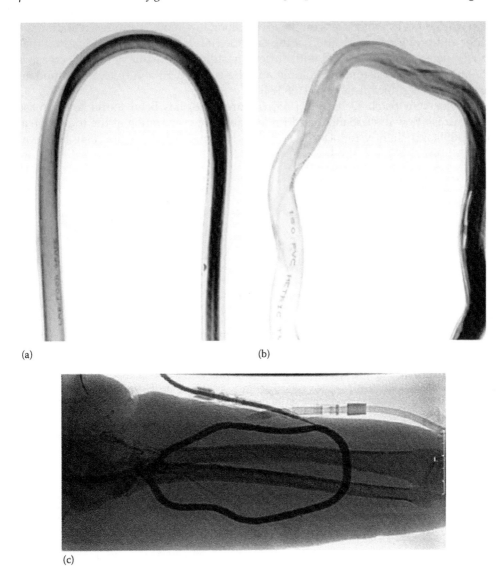

(a)   (b)

(c)

FIGURE 15.16
Helical graft. Flow mixing visualization by bolus injection into water flow (Re = 550) in U-tubes with (a) a conventional tube and (b) a helical tube. Significantly greater mixing can be observed in the helical tube, which can enhance fluid-wall mass transport and render the spatial distribution of WSS relatively uniform in curved conduits. (c) Angiogram of an arteriovenous access PTFE helical graft. Angiographic examinations have suggested that there exists reduction of helical geometry at or after implantation, which might be attributable to graft elongation under arterial pressure. (From Caro, C.G. et al., *J. Roy. Soc. Interf.*, 2, 261, 2005; Huijbregts, H.J.T.A.M. et al., *Eur. J. Vasc. Endovasc. Surg.*, 33, 472, 2007. With permission.)

produced good patency in femoral-distal grafts (Figure 15.17). However, the utility of this technique is somewhat controversial. While some studies found that grafts implanted with vein cuffs resulted in decreased developments of IH [155,156] and had better patency than those with a noncuffed anastomosis [157], other investigations showed that (1) the use of a Miller cuff caused no difference in IH thickness [158], (2) the improved patency was only in below-knee grafts (and not in above-knee popliteal bypasses) [154,159,160], and (3) the use of a cuff has adverse effects on hemodynamic factors around the anastomosis, such as large variations in shear stress on the artery floor, low-momentum recirculation within the cuff, and prominent separation at the cuff toe [161–163]. It is hence suggested that the improved patency rates achieved with cuffed anastomoses are due not to a decrease in IH but to an increased anastomotic volume and the consequent ability to accommodate IH, before it causes significant stenosis [158,164].

The Taylor vein patch technique [165] (Figure 15.18) has been found to decrease IH [166], diminish flow disturbances and undesirable flow separation at the toe of the anastomosis [83], and slightly reduce the WSSG in the anastomotic region [84]. However, its

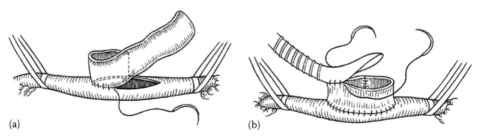

(a)   (b)

FIGURE 15.17
Miller cuff construction. (a) Vein cuff is sewn longitudinally around arteriotomy, (b) graft is then sutured end-to-cuff. Using a cuff has adverse effects on hemodynamic factors around the anastomosis (e.g., large variations in shear stress on the artery floor, low-momentum recirculation within the cuff, and prominent separation at the cuff toe), and any improved patency rates achieved with cuffed anastomoses have been attributed to increased anastomotic volume and the consequent ability to accommodate IH, before it causes significant stenosis, rather than any decrease in IH. (From Stonebridge, P.A. et al., *J. Vasc. Surg.*, 26, 543, 1997. With permission.)

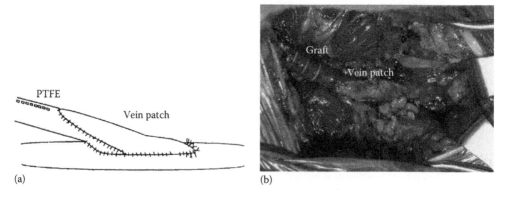

(a)   (b)

FIGURE 15.18
Taylor vein patch. (a) Schematic drawing of Taylor-patched anastomosis (b) Intraoperative photograph of distal Taylor vein patch (6 mm PTFE graft bypass to below knee popliteal artery). Patched grafts have not shown significant improvement in primary patency rates as compared to nonpatched grafts. (From Gentile, A.T. et al., *Am. J. Surg.*, 176, 601, 1998; Yeung, K.K. et al., *Am. J. Surg.*, 182, 578, 2001. With permission.)

improvement in hemodynamic factors is minor. Besides, patched and nonpatched grafts have shown similar primary patency rates [166].

Linton patch was introduced as a technique in which the conduit is patched with a venous segment of about 40–50 mm long [168], as shown in Figure 15.19, and it was frequently used in femoral artery to facilitate construction of the proximal anastomosis of femoropopliteal bypasses. Linton patch technique could considerably increase the compliance at the junction. However, its flow patterns have been shown to be similar to those of conventional ETS anastomosis. The clinical patency of this technique has been reported to be 65%–74% at 12–48 months post-operative [169].

Lei et al. [84], utilizing an iterative optimization procedure coupled with CFD simulations, further improved the geometric design of the Taylor patch to obtain smaller WSSGs. This improved design, whose anastomotic surface area was smaller than that of the Taylor patch, yielded a significant reduction in local time-averaged WSSG (ranging from two- to six-fold decrease, compared with standard and Taylor hooded configurations for a variety of flow splits between POS and DOS) both at the toe and on the floor. This reduction was due to the gradual S-shaped transition in wall curvature and cross-sectional area at the toe region, as shown in Figure 15.20.

The Tyrrell collar has been developed in attempts to incorporate the advantages of the Miller and Taylor anastomotic designs, by avoiding direct suturing of the graft and artery

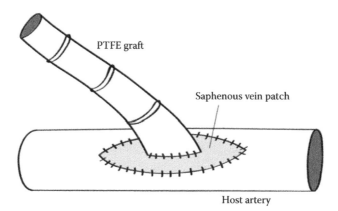

FIGURE 15.19
Linton patch. Schematic drawing of a Linton-patched anastomosis. The flow patterns of patched grafts are similar to those of conventional ETS anastomosis. The clinical patency of this technique has been reported to be 65%–74% at 12–48 months post-operative.

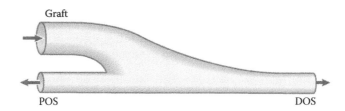

FIGURE 15.20
Lei's improved anastomotic geometry. Improved anastomotic geometry with S-shaped gradual transition in wall curvature and cross-sectional area at the toe region results in significant reduction of WSSG at the toe and on the floor as compared with standard ETS and Taylor patched configurations. (Adapted from Lei, M. et al., *J. Vasc. Surg.*, 25, 637, 1997. With permission.)

(which can cause high compliance mismatch in case a synthetic graft is used), and providing a more streamlined shape at the toe [170] (Figure 15.21). However, trials of Tyrrell collar venous anastomosis in arteriovenous grafts (AVGs) not only showed no improvements in graft patency [171], but also indicated that the use of the collar at the venous anastomosis of forearm loop AVGs resulted in early graft failure [172].

Longest and Kleinstreuer [86] numerically simulated the hemodynamics for a conventional ETS anastomosis (as the base case), the Venaflo™ graft, and an improved cuffed graft-end configuration for AVGs (Figure 15.22). The Venaflo graft demonstrated considerable improvements over the base case by enlarging the junction area and reducing the severity of disturbed flow patterns in predictive computer simulations. Considering the critical toe region, further improvements were achieved in the modified graft-end design by smoother wall curvatures and elimination of the graft bulges, which further reduced the maximum normalized WSSG to 6.4 from 18.1 for the Venaflo graft. However, results of clinical trials of

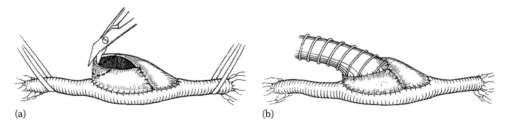

(a)   (b)

FIGURE 15.21
Tyrell vein collar. Diagram of a Tyrell vein collar (a) without and (b) with a PTFE graft. Trials of Tyrrell collar venous anastomosis in AVGs have not shown any improvement in graft patency. (From Tyrrell, M.R. and Wolfe, J.H.N., *Br. J. Surg.*, 78, 1016, 1991. With permission.)

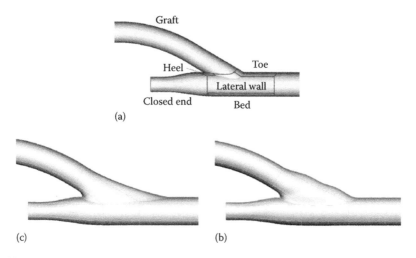

FIGURE 15.22
Numerical studies of three ETS anastomotic configurations. Geometric models of a conventional ETS anastomosis (a), Venaflo™ graft (b), and modified graft-end design (c). Venaflo graft provides larger junction area and less disturbed flow patterns than the conventional ETS anastomosis, and the modified graft-end design further reduces the WSSG by elimination of the graft bulges. Results of clinical trials of the Venaflo graft are controversial; some studies showed promising graft patency rates in the Venaflo grafts (58% versus 21% in the conventional standard grafts at 24 months), while other investigations demonstrated inferior 1-year patency rates of the Venaflo grafts (43% versus 47% for noncuffed ePTFE grafts). (Adapted from Longest, P.W. and Kleinstreuer, C., *J. Med. Eng. Technol.*, 24, 102, 2000.)

the Venaflo graft have been controversial. Some studies have shown promising graft patency rates in the Venaflo grafts (58% versus 21% in the conventional standard grafts at 24 months) [173], while other investigations have demonstrated the 1-year patency rates of the Venaflo grafts to be inferior to those of noncuffed ePTFE grafts (43% versus 47%) [174].

A streamlined anastomotic configuration in which the distal outlet segment (DOS) is aligned with the graft has been developed by Longest et al. [175]. This configuration, shown in Figure 15.23, resulted in an advantageous reduction of the peak normalized WSSG values in the vicinity of the toe (to 1.7 from 11.8 in a conventional ETS model). However, particle–wall interactions remained significant throughout the anastomosis, which can result in platelet activation and may lead to IH.

O'Brien et al. [176] have designed a configuration to replace the anastomosis with a synthetic bifurcation connected in an ETE fashion with the proximal outlet segment (POS) and DOS (Figure 15.24). Their numerical simulations indicated that the smoothly curving bifurcation improves the WSS environment by reducing flow separation and stagnation. Although this prosthetic graft configuration has primarily been designed for

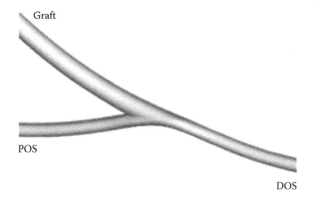

FIGURE 15.23
Streamlined anastomotic configuration. Streamlined arterial bypass graft configuration: although this geometric design can reduce the peak WSSG at the toe of the anastomosis, particle–wall interaction remains significant, which can result in platelet activation and may lead to IH. (Adapted from Longest, P.W. et al., *Ann. Biomed. Eng.*, 33, 1752, 2005.)

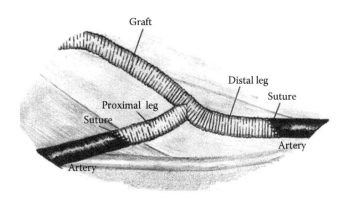

FIGURE 15.24
Prosthetic bifurcating graft-end configuration. Schematic drawing of the prosthetic graft-end configuration designed to reduce flow stagnation and flow separation zones. This prosthetic graft can be connected in an ETE fashion with the POS and DOS. (Adapted from O'Brien, T.P. et al., *J. Vasc. Surg.*, 42, 1169, 2005. With permission.)

femoral–popliteal bypasses, the concept may be relevant in other aspects of cardiovascular surgery. This prosthetic graft can be manufactured from clinically proven synthetic materials, does not require any additional training in its use, and combines attributes of ETS anastomoses with those of ETE anastomoses.

Chua et al. [177] designed a cuff-like sleeve for implantation at the distal anastomosis of CABGs as a connector between the graft and the host artery (Figure 15.25). Their computational simulation results suggested that the sleeve models with higher necks were preferred in terms of hemodynamics at the distal anastomosis.

In an attempt to alter the disturbed hemodynamic on the artery bed in the ETS anastomosis, O'Brien et al. [178] designed a flow-splitter to be placed into the junction of distal ETS anastomosis, as shown in Figure 15.26. This flow-splitter splits the flow profile entering the anastomosis into two channels and diverts the flow from artery bed toward the arterial side-walls. Although this flow-splitter could reduce the peaks of WSS and WSSG on the bed (by 36% and 49%, respectively) at particular phases (during deceleration) and also mitigate the flow separation at the toe, it caused large increases in WSS on both sides of the artery bed centerline, which can result in high values of time-averaged WSSG over the cardiac cycle near the centerline on the arterial bed. Besides, implantation of this flow-splitter may be practical only if integrated in a synthetic graft suite, and not along with autologous grafts.

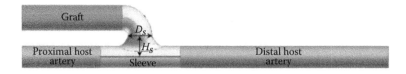

FIGURE 15.25
Cuff-like sleeve. Schematic view of a distal ETS anastomosis with an incorporated sleeve. Sleeve models with higher necks were deemed preferred in terms of hemodynamics at the distal anastomosis. (From Chua, L.P. et al., *Int. Commun. Heat Mass Transfer*, 32, 707, 2005. With permission.)

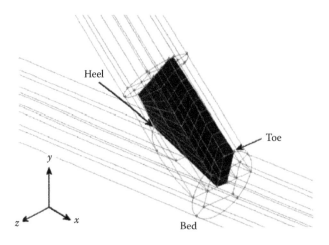

FIGURE 15.26
Flow-splitter. Schematic wire-frame view of a graft–artery junction and implanted flow-splitter. This flow-splitter can divert the flow from the arterial bed to avoid flow impingement on the bed, mitigate the flow separation at the toe, and reduce the size of flow recirculation areas. However, it causes flow impingements on the arterial side-walls and increases the WSS on both sides of the artery bed centerline, which can result in high values of time-averaged WSSG. (From O'Brien, T. et al., *Med. Eng. Phys.*, 28, 727, 2006. With permission.)

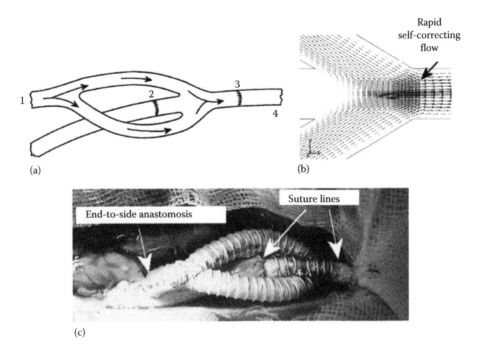

FIGURE 15.27
Prosthetic bifurcating vascular grafting device. (a) 1—Flow from the proximal anastomosis, 2,3—suture-lines of the end-to-end anastomoses of the distal section, 4—the host artery. (b) The bifurcated flows impinge upon each other at the central lumen of the distal anastomosis and avoid arterial bed impingement to reduce the possibility of IH formation. Also, flow separation at the toe is eliminated and the opposing self-correcting flows rapidly return to normal hemodynamic behavior. (c) Intraoperative photograph of the graft implanted into a porcine aorta. (Adapted from Walsh, M.T. et al., A vascular graft, US patent, University of Limerick, Ireland, 2010; O'Brien, T.P. et al., *Ann. Vasc. Surg.*, 21, 611, 2007. With permission.)

Walsh et al. [179] have designed a novel vascular grafting device with a bifurcating configuration (Figure 15.27a), in order to eliminate the flow impingement on the interior wall of the artery at the distal anastomosis. In this vascular device, the flow from the proximal anastomosis is bifurcated into two branches and these branch flows impinge upon each other at a central region of the lumen at the distal anastomosis. By avoiding arterial bed impingement, the possibility of disease formation is reduced. Besides, the opposing branch flows rapidly regain the normal hemodynamic behavior in the distal artery (Figure 15.27b). Another positive feature of this design is the mitigation of flow separation at the toe. This prosthetic vascular graft can be incorporated into the host artery by means of two ETE anastomoses (as shown by suture-lines 2 and 3 in Figure 15.27a) at the distal section and a side-to-end anastomosis at the proximal section (not shown here). Surgical feasibility of this design for treatment of peripheral arterial disease has been verified in vivo, by implantation of a PTFE graft into the aorta of a pig model (Figure 15.27c) [180]. However, a major limitation of this graft is its geometrical complexity.

15.3.2.1 Coupled Sequential Anastomoses Design

Based on the advantageous flow characteristics observed within the side-to-side (STS) anastomosis of typical sequential bypass grafts (i.e., a smoother flow with smaller spatial gradients of WSS than those in an ETS anastomosis [181]) and higher patency rates

Inlet axial velocity profile

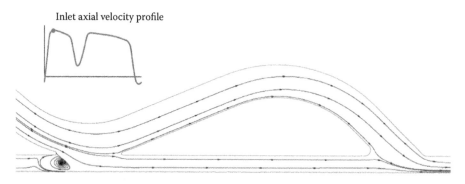

FIGURE 15.28
Coupled STS–ETS sequential anastomoses bypass graft design. Flow streamlines through the coupled STS–ETS sequential anastomoses bypass graft design. Part of the graft flow, which is diverted into the coronary artery at the STS anastomosis, lifts up the flow coming from the graft at the ETS anastomosis and directs it smoothly into the coronary artery; this prevents arterial bed impingement and eliminates the stagnation point and flow recirculation at the ETS anastomosis. This design provides a spare route for the blood flow to the coronary artery to avoid re-operation in case of restenosis in either of the anastomoses. (Adapted from Kabinejadian, F. et al., *Ann. Biomed. Eng.*, 38, 3135, 2010.)

in STS anastomoses than in ETS anastomoses [182], Kabinejadian et al. [183–185] developed a novel coupled STS–ETS sequential anastomoses bypass graft design, as shown in Figure 15.28. In this design, part of the graft flow is diverted into the coronary artery at the STS anastomosis, and when this flow in the coronary artery reaches the ETS anastomosis, it lifts up the flow coming from the graft and directs the graft flow smoothly into the coronary artery, which prevents impingement of blood flow on the arterial bed and eliminates the stagnation point and flow recirculation at the ETS anastomosis.

Computational simulations of blood flow through this novel design have shown improvements of HPs, especially at the heel and on the arterial bed of the ETS anastomosis. These improvements in distribution of HPs include an increase in the time-averaged WSS on the artery bed of the ETS anastomosis of the SQA (as compared to the conventional ETS anastomosis), reduction of the time-averaged WSSG at the heel and bed of the ETS component as well as at the toe and suture line of the STS component of the novel SQA (as compared to the conventional ETS and typical parallel STS anastomoses, respectively), and reduction of the OSI at the ETS anastomosis of the SQA at the heel region and on the artery wall and bed opposite to the heel (in comparison with the conventional ETS anastomosis). Besides, this design provides a spare route for the blood flow to the coronary artery in order to avoid re-operation in case of restenosis in either of the anastomoses. This design can be employed using autologous grafts without the need for any additional training.

15.4 Summary

In this chapter, we have first presented coronary blood flow analysis by employing computational methodologies and approaches, including lumped parameter, Womersley-type wave propagation, and 3D numerical methods. For the epicardial coronary tree pulsatile flow analysis, we have developed an FE model for pulsatile flow analysis, based on CT scans and physiological measurements in porcine models.

The HPs indicate that the sites at the flow divider are prone to atherosclerosis due to the presence of low WSS; the branch sites with high values of WSSG are susceptible to increased permeability of LDL. In future, the model can be made patient-specific through medical imaging to guide diagnosis, intervention, and therapy. For the steady-state laminar flow model in the entire coronary arterial tree of porcine model, we have determined the pressure distribution in the entire coronary arterial tree model down to the first capillary segments. It is seen that the pressure distribution is fairly uniform in larger vessels and changes significantly in smaller vessels (<100 μm), which shows that the myocardial resistance mainly resides in the arteriolar bed. Finally, we have carried out a hybrid Womersley-type 1D wave propagation model in the entire coronary arterial tree of a porcine model, using the inlet pulsatile pressure boundary condition obtained from experimental measurements. Our 1D wave propagation model can determine the transient blood flow waves sequentially at different spatial positions along the main trunk starting from the inlet of LAD artery into the various primary branches. There is decrease of flow amplitude along the main trunk, and the flow waves at the inlet of primary branches show different amplitudes. This wave propagation model can be made patient-specific by interface with patient-specific anatomy of large epicardial vessels obtained from CT, MRI, or other imaging techniques.

We have then provided an overview and analysis of CABG, the preferred treatment for high-risk CAD patients. The importance and role of HPs in restenosis of CABG is analyzed. We have presented various attempts to design an optimal distal anastomotic configuration, in terms of the anastomotic angle, graft caliber (i.e., graft-to-host diameter ratio), and influence of out-of-plane graft curvature. A smaller distal ETS anastomotic angle (≤30°) seems to bring about a less disturbed and more uniform, smooth flow from the graft into the coronary artery. Smaller grafts typically present an increased risk of early graft failure due to thrombosis; further results of computational studies indicate that the graft caliber should always be maximized, in order to minimize the spatial and temporal gradients of WSS. As regards the influence of out-of-plane graft curvature, investigations have revealed reductions in magnitudes of the peak time-averaged WSS and mean oscillatory shear in the nonplanar models as compared to the planar configurations, which imply a corresponding reduction in the spatial extent of wall regions exposed to physiologically unfavorable flow conditions.

This chapter provides the knowledge base on how coronary circulation and obstruction (stenosis) occurs, and how CABG can address the stenosis problem.

References

1. Fung YC. *Biomechanics: Circulation*. 2nd ed. New York: Springer; 1997.
2. Kaimovitz B, Huo Y, Lanir Y, Kassab GS. Diameter asymmetry of porcine coronary arterial trees: Structural and functional implications. *American Journal of Physiology: Heart and Circulatory Physiology*. 2008;294:H714–H723.
3. Huo Y, Kaimovitz B, Lanir Y, Wischgoll T, Hoffman JI, Kassab GS. Biophysical model of the spatial heterogeneity of myocardial flow. *Biophysical Journal*. 2009;96:4035–4043.
4. Thubrikar MJ, Robicsek F. Pressure-induced arterial-wall stress and atherosclerosis. *Annals of Thoracic Surgery*. 1995;59:1594–1603.

5. Asakura T, Karino T. Flow patterns and spatial distribution of atherosclerotic lesions in human coronary arteries. *Circulation Research*. 1990;66:1045–1066.

6. Huo Y, Wischgoll T, Kassab GS. Flow patterns in three-dimensional porcine epicardial coronary arterial tree. *American Journal of Physiology: Heart and Circulatory Physiology*. 2007;293: H2959–H2970.

7. Huo Y, Choy JS, Svendsen M, Sinha AK, Kassab GS. Effects of vessel compliance on flow pattern in porcine epicardial right coronary arterial tree. *Journal of Biomechanics*. 2009;42:594–602.

8. Chiu JJ, Chien S. Effects of disturbed flow on vascular endothelium: Pathophysiological basis and clinical perspectives. *Physiological Reviews*. 2011;91:327–387.

9. Davies PF. Hemodynamic shear stress and the endothelium in cardiovascular pathophysiology. *Nature Clinical Practice Cardiovascular Medicine*. 2009;6:16–26.

10. Caro CG, Fitzgera JM, Schroter RC. Proposal of a shear dependent mass transfer mechanism for atherogenesis. *Clinical Science*. 1971;40:P5.

11. Ku DN, Giddens DP, Zarins CK, Glagov S. Pulsatile flow and atherosclerosis in the human carotid bifurcation. Positive correlation between plaque location and low and oscillating shear stress. *Arteriosclerosis*. 1985;5:293–302.

12. Moore JE, Xu CP, Glagov S, Zarins CK, Ku DN. Fluid wall shear-stress measurements in a model of the human abdominal-aorta—Oscillatory behavior and relationship to atherosclerosis. *Atherosclerosis*. 1994;110:225–240.

13. He XJ, Ku DN. Pulsatile flow in the human left coronary artery bifurcation: Average conditions. *Journal of Biomechanical Engineering—Transactions of the ASME*. 1996;118:74–82.

14. Depaola N, Gimbrone MA, Davies PF, Dewey CF. Vascular endothelium responds to fluid shear-stress gradients. *Arteriosclerosis and Thrombosis*. 1992;12:1254–1257.

15. Herrmann RA, Malinauskas RA, Truskey GA. Characterization of sites with elevated LDL permeability at intercostal, celiac, and iliac branches of the normal rabbit aorta. *Arteriosclerosis and Thrombosis*. 1994;14:313–323.

16. Buchanan JR, Kleinstreuer C, Truskey GA, Lei M. Relation between non-uniform hemodynamics and sites of altered permeability and lesion growth at the rabbit aorto-celiac junction. *Atherosclerosis*. 1999;143:27–40.

17. Perktold K, Resch M, Florian H. Pulsatile non-Newtonian flow characteristics in a three-dimensional human carotid bifurcation model. *Journal of Biomechanical Engineering*. 1991;113:464–475.

18. Perktold K, Resch M, Peter RO. Three-dimensional numerical analysis of pulsatile flow and wall shear stress in the carotid artery bifurcation. *Journal of Biomechanics*. 1991;24:409–420.

19. Taylor CA, Hughes TJ, Zarins CK. Finite element modeling of three-dimensional pulsatile flow in the abdominal aorta: Relevance to atherosclerosis. *Annals of Biomedical Engineering*. 1998;26:975–987.

20. Santamarina A, Weydahl E, Siegel JM, Moore JE. Computational analysis of flow in a curved tube model of the coronary arteries: Effects of time-varying curvature. *Annals of Biomedical Engineering*. 1998;26:944–954.

21. WEYDAHL ES, MOORE JE. Dynamic curvature strongly affects wall shear rates in a coronary artery bifurcation model. *Journal of Biomechanics*. 2001;34:1189–1196.

22. Huo Y, Finet G, Lefevre T, Louvard Y, Moussa I, Kassab GS. Which diameter and angle rule provides optimal flow patterns in a coronary bifurcation? *Journal of Biomechanics*. 2012;45:1273–1279.

23. Peladeau-Pigeon M, Coolens C. Computational fluid dynamics modelling of perfusion measurements in dynamic contrast-enhanced computed tomography: Development, validation and clinical applications. *Physics in Medicine and Biology*. 2013;58:6111–6131.

24. Sun ZH, Xu L. Computational fluid dynamics in coronary artery disease. *Computerized Medical Imaging and Graphics*. 2014;38:651–663.

25. Hoffman JIE. Transmural myocardial perfusion. *Progress in Cardiovascular Diseases*. 1987;29:429–464.

26. Hoffman JIE, Baer RW, Hanley FL, Messina LM. Regulation of transmural myocardial blood-flow. *Journal of Biomechanical Engineering—Transactions of the ASME*. 1985;107:2–9.

27. Buckberg GD, Archie JP, Fixler DE, Hoffman JIE. Experimental subendocardial ischemia in dogs with normal coronary-arteries. *Circulation Research*. 1972;30:67–81.

28. Downey JM, Kirk ES. Inhibition of coronary blood-flow by a vascular waterfall mechanism. *Circulation Research.* 1975;36:753–760.
29. Flynn AE, Coggins DL, Goto M, Aldea GS, Austin RE, Doucette JW et al. Does systolic subepicardial perfusion come from retrograde subendocardial flow. *American Journal of Physiology.* 1992;262:H1759–H1769.
30. Bache RJ, Schwartz JS. Effect of perfusion-pressure distal to a coronary stenosis on transmural myocardial blood-flow. *Circulation.* 1982;65:928–935.
31. Spaan JAE, Breuls NPW, Laird JD. Diastolic-systolic coronary flow differences are caused by intramyocardial pump action in the anesthetized dog. *Circulation Research.* 1981;49:584–593.
32. Lee J, Chambers DE, Akizuki S, Downey JM. The role of vascular capacitance in the coronary arteries. *Circulation Research.* 1984;55:751–762.
33. Mates RE. The coronary circulation. *Journal of Biomechanical Engineering.* 1993;115:558–561.
34. Hoffman JI, Spaan JA. Pressure-flow relations in coronary circulation. *Physiological Reviews.* 1990;70:331–390.
35. Huo Y, Kassab GS. Effect of compliance and hematocrit on wall shear stress in a model of the entire coronary arterial tree. *Journal of Applied Physiology.* 2009;107:500–505.
36. Mittal N, Zhou Y, Linares C, Ung S, Kaimovitz B, Molloi S et al. Analysis of blood flow in the entire coronary arterial tree. *American Journal of Physiology: Heart and Circulatory Physiology.* 2005;289:H439–H446.
37. Algranati D, Kassab GS, Lanir Y. Mechanisms of myocardium-coronary vessel interaction. *American Journal of Physiology: Heart and Circulatory Physiology.* 2010;298:H861–H873.
38. Algranati D, Kassab GS, Lanir Y. Why is the subendocardium more vulnerable to ischemia? A new paradigm. *American Journal of Physiology: Heart and Circulatory Physiology.* 2011;300:H1090–H1100.
39. Kassab GS, Algranati D, Lanir Y. Myocardial-vessel interaction: Role of LV pressure and myocardial contractility. *Medical and Biological Engineering and Computing.* 2013;51:729–739.
40. Huo Y, Kassab GS. Pulsatile blood flow in the entire coronary arterial tree: Theory and experiment. *American Journal of Physiology: Heart and Circulatory Physiology.* 2006;291:H1074–H1087.
41. Huo Y, Kassab GS. A hybrid one-dimensional/Womersley model of pulsatile blood flow in the entire coronary arterial tree. *American Journal of Physiology: Heart and Circulatory Physiology.* 2007;292:H2623–H2633.
42. Huo Y, Kassab GS. A scaling law of vascular volume. *Biophysical Journal.* 2009;96:347–353.
43. Huo Y, Kassab GS. Intraspecific scaling laws of vascular trees. *Journal of the Royal Society Interface.* 2012;9:190–200.
44. Nichols WW, McDonald DA. *McDonald's Blood Flow in Arteries: Theoretic, Experimental, and Clinical Principles,* 6th ed. London, UK: Hodder Arnold; 2011.
45. Zeindler CM, Kratky RG, Roach MR. Quantitative measurements of early atherosclerotic lesions on rabbit aortae from vascular casts. *Atherosclerosis.* 1989;76:245–255.
46. Kaimovitz B, Lanir Y, Kassab GS. Large-scale 3-D geometric reconstruction of the porcine coronary arterial vasculature based on detailed anatomical data. *Annals of Biomedical Engineering.* 2005;33:1517–1535.
47. Chilian WM. Microvascular pressures and resistances in the left ventricular subepicardium and subendocardium. *Circulation Research.* 1991;69:561–570.
48. Kanatsuka H, Lamping KG, Eastham CL, Marcus ML, Dellsperger KC. Coronary microvascular resistance in hypertensive cats. *Circulation Research.* 1991;68:726–733.
49. Stergiopulos N, Young DF, Rogge TR. Computer simulation of arterial flow with applications to arterial and aortic stenoses. *Journal of Biomechanics.* 1992;25:1477–1488.
50. Avolio AP. Multi-branched model of the human arterial system. *Medical and Biological Engineering and Computing.* 1980;18:709–718.
51. Reymond P, Merenda F, Perren F, Rufenacht D, Stergiopulos N. Validation of a one-dimensional model of the systemic arterial tree. *American Journal of Physiology: Heart and Circulatory Physiology.* 2009;297:H208–H222.

52. Reymond P, Bohraus Y, Perren F, Lazeyras F, Stergiopulos N. Validation of a patient-specific one-dimensional model of the systemic arterial tree. *American Journal of Physiology: Heart and Circulatory Physiology.* 2011;301:H1173–H1182.

53. Olufsen MS, Peskin CS, Kim WY, Pedersen EM, Nadim A, Larsen J. Numerical simulation and experimental validation of blood flow in arteries with structured-tree outflow conditions. *Annals of Biomedical Engineering.* 2000;28:1281–1299.

54. Olufsen MS. Structured tree outflow condition for blood flow in larger systemic arteries. *American Journal of Physiology.* 1999;276:H257–H268.

55. Hughes TJR, Lubliner J. On the one-dimensional theory of blood flow in the larger vessels. *Mathematical Biosciences.* 1973;18:161–170.

56. Roger VL, Go AS, Lloyd-Jones DM, Benjamin EJ, Berry JD, Borden WB et al. Heart disease and stroke statistics—2012 update: A report from the American Heart Association. *Circulation.* 2012;125:e2–e220.

57. Rihal CS, Raco DL, Gersh BJ, Yusuf S. Indications for coronary artery bypass surgery and percutaneous coronary intervention in chronic stable angina: Review of the evidence and methodological considerations. *Circulation.* 2003;108:2439–2445.

58. Smith Jr SC, Dove JT, Jacobs AK, Kennedy JW, Kereiakes D, Kern MJ et al. ACC/AHA guidelines for percutaneous coronary intervention (revision of the 1993 PTCA guidelines)—Executive summary: A report of the American College of Cardiology/American Heart Association Task Force on Practice Guidelines (Committee to Revise the 1993 Guidelines for Percutaneous Transluminal Coronary Angioplasty) endorsed by the society for cardiac angiography and interventions. *Circulation.* 2001;103:3019–3041.

59. Braunwald H. *Heart Disease: A Textbook of Cardiovascular Medicine.* 5th ed. Philadelphia, PA: Saunders; 1997.

60. Davies MG, Hagen PO. Pathobiology of intimal hyperplasia. *British Journal of Surgery.* 1994;81:1254–1269.

61. Canver CC. Conduit options in coronary artery bypass surgery. *Chest.* 1995;108:1150–1155.

62. FitzGibbon GM, Kafka HP, Leach AJ, Keon WJ, Hooper GD, Burton JR. Coronary bypass graft fate and patient outcome: Angiographic follow-up of 5,065 grafts related to survival and reoperation in 1,388 patients during 25 years. *Journal of the American College of Cardiology.* 1996;28:616–626.

63. Whittemore AD, Clowes AW, Couch NP, Mannick JA. Secondary femoro-popliteal reconstruction. *Annals of Surgery.* 1981;193:35–42.

64. Butany JW, David TE, Ojha M. Histological and morphometric analyses of early and late aorto-coronary vein grafts and distal anastomoses. *Canadian Journal of Cardiology.* 1998;14:671–677.

65. Clowes AW, Reidy MA, Clowes MM. Kinetics of cellular proliferation after arterial injury. I. Smooth muscle growth in the absence of endothelium. *Laboratory Investigation.* 1983;49:327–333.

66. Liu MW, Roubin GS, King III SB. Restenosis after coronary angioplasty: Potential biologic determinants and role of intimal hyperplasia. *Circulation.* 1989;79:1374–1387.

67. Keynton RS, Evancho MM, Sims RL, Rodway NV, Gobin A, Rittgers SE. Intimal hyperplasia and wall shear in arterial bypass graft distal anastomoses: An in vivo model study. *Journal of Biomechanical Engineering.* 2001;123:464–473.

68. White SS, Zarins CK, Giddens DP, Bassiouny H, Loth F, Jones SA et al. Hemodynamic patterns in two models of end-to-side vascular graft anastomoses: Effects of pulsatility, flow division, Reynolds number, and hood length. *Journal of Biomechanical Engineering.* 1993;115:104–111.

69. Ballyk PD, Walsh C, Butany J, Ojha M. Compliance mismatch may promote graft-artery intimal hyperplasia by altering suture-line stresses. *Journal of Biomechanics.* 1997;31:229–237.

70. Clowes AW, Kirkman TR, Clowes MM. Mechanisms of arterial graft failure. II. Chronic endothelial and smooth muscle cell proliferation in healing polytetrafluoroethylene prostheses. *Journal of Vascular Surgery.* 1986;3:877–884.

71. Bassiouny HS, White S, Glagov S, Choi E, Giddens DP, Zarins CK. Anastomotic intimal hyperplasia: Mechanical injury or flow induced. *Journal of Vascular Surgery.* 1992;15:708–717.

72. Hofer M, Rappitsch G, Perktold K, Trubel W, Schima H. Numerical study of wall mechanics and fluid dynamics in end-to-side anastomoses and correlation to intimal hyperplasia. *Journal of Biomechanics*. 1996;29:1297–1308.

73. Sottiurai VS, Yao JST, Batson RC, Sue SL, Jones R, Nakamura YA. Distal anastomotic intimal hyperplasia: Histopathologic character and biogenesis. *Annals of Vascular Surgery*. 1989;3:26–33.

74. Ojha M, Cobbold RSC, Johnston KW. Influence of angle on wall shear stress distribution for an end-to-side anastomosis. *Journal of Vascular Surgery*. 1994;19:1067–1073.

75. Ghista DN, Kabinejadian F. Coronary artery bypass grafting hemodynamics and anastomosis design: A biomedical engineering review. *BioMedical Engineering Online*. 2013;12:129.

76. Brien TO, Walsh M, McGloughlin T. On reducing abnormal hemodynamics in the femoral end-to-side anastomosis: The influence of mechanical factors. *Annals of Biomedical Engineering*. 2005;33:310–322.

77. Fei DY, Thomas JD, Rittgers SE. The effect of angle and flow rate upon hemodynamics in distal vascular graft anastomoses: A numerical model study. *Journal of Biomechanical Engineering*. 1994;116:331–336.

78. Hughes PE, How TV. Effects of geometry and flow division on flow structures in models of the distal end-to-side anastomosis. *Journal of Biomechanics*. 1996;29:855–872.

79. Jackson ZS, Ishibashi H, Gotlieb AI, Lowell Langille B. Effects of anastomotic angle on vascular tissue responses at end-to-side arterial grafts. *Journal of Vascular Surgery*. 2001;34:300–307.

80. Pietrabissa R, Inzoli F, Fumero R. Simulation study of the fluid dynamics of aorto-coronary bypass. *Journal of Biomedical Engineering*. 1990;12:419–424.

81. Staalsen NH. The anastomosis angle does change the flow fields at vascular end-to-side anastomoses in vivo. *Journal of Vascular Surgery*. 1995;21:460–471.

82. Keynton RS, Rittgers SE, Shu MCS. The effect of angle and flow rate upon hemodynamics in distal vascular graft anastomoses: An in vitro model study. *Journal of Biomechanical Engineering*. 1991;113:458–463.

83. Cole JS, Watterson JK, O'Reilly MJG. Numerical investigation of the haemodynamics at a patched arterial bypass anastomosis. *Medical Engineering and Physics*. 2002;24:393–401.

84. Lei M, Archie JP, Kleinstreuer C. Computational design of a bypass graft that minimizes wall shear stress gradients in the region of the distal anastomosis. *Journal of Vascular Surgery*. 1997;25:637–646.

85. Leuprecht A, Perktold K, Prosi M, Berk T, Trubel W, Schima H. Numerical study of hemodynamics and wall mechanics in distal end-to-side anastomoses of bypass grafts. *Journal of Biomechanics*. 2002;35:225–236.

86. Longest PW, Kleinstreuer C. Computational haemodynamics analysis and comparison study of arterio-venous grafts. *Journal of Medical Engineering and Technology*. 2000;24:102–110.

87. Bonert M, Myers JG, Fremes S, Williams J, Ethier CR. A numerical study of blood flow in coronary artery bypass graft side-to-side anastomoses. *Annals of Biomedical Engineering*. 2002;30:599–611.

88. Qiao A, Liu Y. Influence of graft-host diameter ratio on the hemodynamics of CABG. *Bio-Medical Materials and Engineering*. 2006;16:189–201.

89. Zahab ZE, Divo E, Kassab A. Minimisation of the wall shear stress gradients in bypass grafts anastomoses using meshless CFD and genetic algorithms optimisation. *Computer Methods in Biomechanics and Biomedical Engineering*. 2010;13:35–47.

90. Papaharilaou Y, Doorly DJ, Sherwin SJ. The influence of out-of-plane geometry on pulsatile flow within a distal end-to-side anastomosis. *Journal of Biomechanics*. 2002;35:1225–1239.

91. Sankaranarayanan M, Ghista DN, Chua LP, Tan YS, Kassab GS. Analysis of blood flow in an out-of-plane CABG model. *American Journal of Physiology: Heart and Circulatory Physiology*. 2006;291:H283–H295.

92. Sherwin SJ, Shah O, Doorly DJ, Peiró J, Papaharilaou Y, Watkins N et al. The influence of out-of-plane geometry on the flow within a distal end-to-side anastomosis. *Journal of Biomechanical Engineering*. 2000;122:86–95.

93. Deplano V, Bertolotti C, Boiron O. Numerical simulations of unsteady flows in a stenosed coronary bypass graft. *Medical and Biological Engineering and Computing.* 2001;39:488–499.

94. Kute SM, Vorp DA. The effect of proximal artery flow on the hemodynamics at the distal anastomosis of a vascular bypass graft: Computational study. *Journal of Biomechanical Engineering.* 2001;123:277–283.

95. Kabinejadian F, Chua LP, Ghista DN, Tan YS. CABG models flow simulation study on the effects of valve remnants in the venous graft. *Journal of Mechanics in Medicine and Biology.* 2010;10:593–609.

96. Bertolotti C, Deplano V, Fuseri J, Dupouy P. Numerical and experimental models of postoperative realistic flows in stenosed coronary bypasses. *Journal of Biomechanics.* 2001;34:1049–1064.

97. Hida S, Chikamori T, Hirayama T, Usui Y, Yanagisawa H, Morishima T et al. Beneficial effect of coronary artery bypass grafting as assessed by quantitative gated single-photon emission computed tomography. *Circulation Journal.* 2003;67:499–504.

98. Zhong L, Tan RS, Ghista DN, Ng EYK, Chua LP, Kassab GS. Validation of a novel noninvasive cardiac index of left ventricular contractility in patients. *American Journal of Physiology: Heart and Circulatory Physiology.* 2007;292:H2764–H2772.

99. Sottiurai VS, Lim Sue S, Feinberg Ii EL, Bringaze WL, Tran AT, Batson RC. Distal anastomotic intimal hyperplasia: Biogenesis and etiology. *European Journal of Vascular Surgery.* 1988;2:245–256.

100. Trubel W, Moritz A, Schima H, Raderer F, Scherer R, Ullrich R et al. Compliance and formation of distal anastomotic intimal hyperplasia in Dacron mesh tube constricted veins used as arterial bypass grafts. *ASAIO Journal.* 1994;40:M273–M278.

101. Sottiurai VS. Distal anastomotic intimal hyperplasia: Histocytomorphology, pathophysiology, etiology, and prevention. *International Journal of Angiology.* 1999;8:1–10.

102. Ojha M. Spatial and temporal variations of wall shear stress within an end-to-side arterial anastomosis model. *Journal of Biomechanics.* 1993;26:1377–1388.

103. Fillinger MF, Reinitz ER, Schwartz RA, Resetarits DE, Paskanik AM, Bruch D et al. Graft geometry and venous intimal-medial hyperplasia in arteriovenous loop grafts. *Journal of Vascular Surgery.* 1990;11:556–566.

104. Giordana S, Sherwin SJ, Peiro J, Doorly DJ, Crane JS, Lee KE et al. Local and global geometric influence on steady flow in distal anastomoses of peripheral bypass grafts. *Journal of Biomechanical Engineering.* 2005;127:1087–1098.

105. Loth F, Jones SA, Zarins CK, Giddens DP, Nassar RF, Glagov S et al. Relative contribution of wall shear stress and injury in experimental intimal thickening at PTFE end-to-side arterial anastomoses. *Journal of Biomechanical Engineering.* 2002;124:44–51.

106. Rittgers SE, Karayannacos PE, Guy JF. Velocity distribution and intimal proliferation in autologous vein grafts in dogs. *Circulation Research.* 1978;42:792–801.

107. Kleinstreuer C, Nazemi M, Archie JP. Hemodynamics analysis of a stenosed carotid bifurcation and its plaque-mitigating design. *Journal of Biomechanical Engineering.* 1991;113:330–335.

108. Fry DL. Acute vascular endothelial changes associated with increased blood velocity gradients. *Circulation Research.* 1968;22:165–197.

109. Fry DL. Certain histological and chemical responses of the vascular interface to acutely induced mechanical stress in the aorta of the dog. *Circulation Research.* 1969;24:93–108.

110. Caro CG, Fitz-Gerald JM, Schroter RC. Atheroma and arterial wall shear. Observation, correlation and proposal of a shear dependent mass transfer mechanism for atherogenesis. *Proceedings of the Royal Society of London Series B: Biological Sciences.* 1971;177:109–159.

111. Nazemi M, Kleinstreuer C, Archie JP, Sorrell FY. Fluid flow and plaque formation in an aortic bifurcation. *Journal of Biomechanical Engineering—Transactions of the ASME.* 1989;111:316–324.

112. Nazemi M, Kleinstreuer C, Archie Jr JP. Pulsatile two-dimensional flow and plaque formation in a carotid artery bifurcation. *Journal of Biomechanics.* 1990;23:1031–1037.

113. Shahcheraghi N, Dwyer HA, Cheer AY, Barakat AI, Rutaganira T. Unsteady and three-dimensional simulation of blood flow in the human aortic arch. *Journal of Biomechanical Engineering—Transactions of the ASME.* 2002;124:378–387.

114. Nerem RM. Vascular fluid mechanics, the arterial wall, and atherosclerosis. *Journal of Biomechanical Engineering.* 1992;114:274–282.

115. Ishibashi H, Sunamura M, Karino T. Flow patterns and preferred sites of intimal thickening in end-to-end anastomosed vessels. *Surgery.* 1995;117:409–420.

116. Sunamura M, Ishibashi H, Karino T. Flow patterns and preferred sites of intimal thickening in diameter-mismatched vein graft interpositions. *Surgery.* 2007;141:764–776.

117. Morinaga K, Okadome K, Kuroki M. Effect of wall shear stress on intimal thickening of arterially transplanted autogenous veins in dogs. *Journal of Vascular Surgery.* 1985;2:430–433.

118. Li XM, Rittgers SE. Hemodynamic factors at the distal end-to-side anastomosis of a bypass graft with different POS:DOS flow ratios. *Journal of Biomechanical Engineering.* 2001;123:270–276.

119. Passerini AG, Milsted A, Rittgers SE. Shear stress magnitude and directionality modulate growth factor gene expression in preconditioned vascular endothelial cells. *Journal of Vascular Surgery.* 2003;37:182–190.

120. Zhang JM, Chua LP, Ghista DN, Yu SCM, Tan YS. Numerical investigation and identification of susceptible sites of atherosclerotic lesion formation in a complete coronary artery bypass model. *Medical and Biological Engineering and Computing.* 2008;46:689–699.

121. Haruguchi H, Teraoka S. Intimal hyperplasia and hemodynamic factors in arterial bypass and arteriovenous grafts: A review. *Journal of Artificial Organs.* 2003;6:227–235.

122. Lei M, Kleinstreuer C, Truskey GA. Numerical investigation and prediction of atherogenic sites in branching arteries. *Journal of Biomechanical Engineering.* 1995;117:350–357.

123. Lei M, Kleinstreuer C, Truskey GA. A focal stress gradient-dependent mass transfer mechanism for atherogenesis in branching arteries. *Medical Engineering and Physics.* 1996;18:326–332.

124. Loth F, Fischer PF, Bassiouny HS. Blood flow in end-to-side anastomoses. *Annual Review of Fluid Mechanics.* 2008;40:367–393.

125. Hughes PE, How TV. Flow structures at the proximal side-to-end anastomosis. Influence of geometry and flow division. *Journal of Biomechanical Engineering.* 1995;117:224–236.

126. Friedrich P, Reininger AJ. Occlusive thrombus formation on indwelling catheters: In vitro investigation and computational analysis. *Thrombosis and Haemostasis.* 1995;73:66–72.

127. Reininger AJ, Heinzmann U, Reininger CB, Friedrich P, Wurzinger LJ. Flow mediated fibrin thrombus formation in an endothelium-lined model of arterial branching. *Thrombosis Research.* 1994;74:629–641.

128. Li XM, Rittgers SE. Hemodynamic factors at the distal end-to-side anastomosis of a bypass graft with different POS:DOS ratios. *American Society of Mechanical Engineers, Bioengineering Division (Publication) BED.* 1999;42:225–226.

129. Bates CJ, O'Doherty DM, Williams D. Flow instabilities in a graft anastomosis: A study of the instantaneous velocity fields. *Proceedings of the Institution of Mechanical Engineers, Part H: Journal of Engineering in Medicine.* 2001;215:579–587.

130. Binns RL, Ku DN, Stewart MT, Ansley JP, Coyle KA. Optimal graft diameter: Effect of wall shear stress on vascular healing. *Journal of Vascular Surgery.* 1989;10:326–337.

131. Idu MM, Buth J, Hop WCJ, Cuypers P, Van De Pavoordt EDWM, Tordoir JMH. Factors influencing the development of vein-graft stenosis and their significance for clinical management. *European Journal of Vascular and Endovascular Surgery.* 1999;17:15–21.

132. Varty K, London NJM, Brennan JA, Ratliff DA, Bell PRF. Infragenicular in situ vein bypass graft occlusion: A multivariate risk factor analysis. *European Journal of Vascular Surgery.* 1993;7:567–571.

133. Schanzer A, Hevelone N, Owens CD, Belkin M, Bandyk DF, Clowes AW et al. Technical factors affecting autogenous vein graft failure: Observations from a large multicenter trial. *Journal of Vascular Surgery.* 2007;46:1180–1190; discussion 90.

134. Towne JB, Schmitt DD, Seabrook GR, Bandyk DF. The effect of vein diameter on patency of in situ grafts. *Journal of Cardiovascular Surgery.* 1991;32:192–196.

135. Yasuura K, Takagi Y, Ohara Y, Takami Y, Matsuura A, Okamoto H. Theoretical analysis of right gastroepiploic artery grafting to right coronary artery. *Annals of Thoracic Surgery.* 2000;69:728–731.

136. Bezon E, Choplain JN, Maguid YA, Aziz AA, Barra JA. Failure of internal thoracic artery grafts: Conclusions from coronary angiography mid-term follow-up. *Annals of Thoracic Surgery.* 2003;76:754–759.

137. Botman CJ, Schonberger J, Koolen S, Penn O, Botman H, Dib N et al. Does stenosis severity of native vessels influence bypass graft patency? A prospective fractional flow reserve-guided study. *Annals of Thoracic Surgery.* 2007;83:2093–2097.

138. Nakajima H, Kobayashi J, Toda K, Fujita T, Shimahara Y, Kasahara Y et al. A 10-year angiographic follow-up of competitive flow in sequential and composite arterial grafts. *European Journal of Cardio-Thoracic Surgery.* 2011;40:399–404.

139. Nordgaard H, Nordhaug D, Kirkeby-Garstad I, Løvstakken L, Vitale N, Haaverstad R. Different graft flow patterns due to competitive flow or stenosis in the coronary anastomosis assessed by transit-time flowmetry in a porcine model. *European Journal of Cardio-Thoracic Surgery.* 2009;36:137–142.

140. Pagni S, Storey J, Ballen J, Montgomery W, Chiang BY, Etoch S et al. ITA versus SVG: A comparison of instantaneous pressure and flow dynamics during competitive flow. *European Journal of Cardio-Thoracic Surgery.* 1997;11:1086–1092.

141. Sabik III JF, Lytle BW, Blackstone EH, Khan M, Houghtaling PL, Cosgrove DM et al. Does competitive flow reduce internal thoracic artery graft patency? *Annals of Thoracic Surgery.* 2003;76:1490–1497.

142. Speziale G. *Competitive Flow and Steal Phenomenon in Coronary Surgery. Intraoperative Graft Patency Verification in Cardiac and Vascular Surgery.* New York: Futura Publishing; 2001.

143. Villareal RP, Mathur VS. The string phenomenon: An important cause of internal mammary artery graft failure. *Texas Heart Institute Journal.* 2000;27:346–349.

144. Wiesner TF, Levesque MJ, Rooz E, Nerem RM. Epicardial coronary blood flow including the presence of stenoses and aorto-coronary bypasses II: Experimental comparison and parametric investigations. *Journal of Biomechanical Engineering.* 1988;110:144–149.

145. Sabik III JF, Lytle BW, Blackstone EH, Houghtaling PL, Cosgrove DM. Comparison of saphenous vein and internal thoracic artery graft patency by coronary system. *Annals of Thoracic Surgery.* 2005;79:544–551.

146. Gaudino M, Alessandrini F, Nasso G, Bruno P, Manzoli A, Possati G. Severity of coronary artery stenosis at preoperative angiography and midterm mammary graft status. *Annals of Thoracic Surgery.* 2002;74:119–121.

147. Hirotani T, Kameda T, Shirota S, Nakao Y. An evaluation of the intraoperative transit time measurements of coronary bypass flow. *European Journal of Cardio-Thoracic Surgery.* 2001;19:848–852.

148. Kawasuji M, Sakakibara N, Takemura H, Tedoriya T, Ushijima T, Watanabe Y. Is internal thoracic artery grafting suitable for a moderately stenotic coronary artery? *Journal of Thoracic and Cardiovascular Surgery.* 1996;112:253–259.

149. Bertolotti C, Deplano V. Three-dimensional numerical simulations of flow through a stenosed coronary bypass. *Journal of Biomechanics.* 2000;33:1011–1022.

150. Chen J, Lu XY, Wang W. Non-Newtonian effects of blood flow on hemodynamics in distal vascular graft anastomoses. *Journal of Biomechanics.* 2006;39:1983–1995.

151. Su CM, Lee D, Tran-Son-Tay R, Shyy W. Fluid flow structure in arterial bypass anastomosis. *Journal of Biomechanical Engineering.* 2005;127:611–618.

152. Caro CG, Cheshire NJ, Watkins N. Preliminary comparative study of small amplitude helical and conventional ePTFE arteriovenous shunts in pigs. *Journal of the Royal Society Interface.* 2005;2:261–266.

153. Huijbregts HJTAM, Blankestijn PJ, Caro CG, Cheshire NJW, Hoedt MTC, Tutein Nolthenius RP et al. A helical PTFE arteriovenous access graft to swirl flow across the distal anastomosis: Results of a preliminary clinical study. *European Journal of Vascular and Endovascular Surgery.* 2007;33:472–475.

154. Miller JH, Foreman RK, Ferguson L, Faris I. Interposition vein cuff for anastomosis of prosthesis to small artery. *Australian and New Zealand Journal of Surgery.* 1984;54:283–285.

155. Kissin M, Kansal N, Pappas PJ, DeFouw DO, Durán WN, Hobson Ii RW. Vein interposition cuffs decrease the intimal hyperplastic response of polytetrafluoroethylene bypass grafts. *Journal of Vascular Surgery.* 2000;31:69–83.

156. Suggs WD, Hendriques HF, DePalma RG. Vein cuff interposition prevents juxta-anastomotic neointimal hyperplasia. *Annals of Surgery.* 1988;207:717–723.

157. Brumby SA, Petrucco MF, Walsh JA, Bond MJ. A retrospective analysis of infra-inguinal arterial reconstruction: Three year patency rates. *Australian and New Zealand Journal of Surgery.* 1992;62:256–260.

158. Norberto JJ, Sidawy AN, Trad KS, Jones BA, Neville RF, Najjar SF et al. The protective effect of vein cuffed anastomoses is not mechanical in origin. *Journal of Vascular Surgery.* 1995;21:558–566.

159. Raptis S, Miller JH. Influence of a vein cuff on polytetrafluoroethylene grafts for primary femoropopliteal bypass. *British Journal of Surgery.* 1995;82:487–491.

160. Stonebridge PA, Prescott RJ, Ruckley CV. Randomized trial comparing infrainguinal polytetrafluoroethylene bypass grafting with and without vein interposition cuff at the distal anastomosis. *Journal of Vascular Surgery.* 1997;26:543–550.

161. Cole JS, Wijesinghe LD, Watterson JK, Scott DJA. Computational and experimental simulations of the haemodynamics at cuffed arterial bypass graft anastomoses. *Proceedings of the Institution of Mechanical Engineers, Part H: Journal of Engineering in Medicine.* 2002;216:135–143.

162. Henry FS, Küpper C, Lewington NP. Simulation of flow through a Miller cuff bypass graft. *Computer Methods in Biomechanics and Biomedical Engineering.* 2002;5:207–217.

163. Longest PW, Kleinstreuer C, Archie Jr JP. Particle hemodynamics analysis of Miller cuff arterial anastomosis. *Journal of Vascular Surgery.* 2003;38:1353–1362.

164. Wijesinghe LD, Mahmood T, Scott DJA. Axial flow fields in cuffed end-to-side anastomoses: Effect of angle and disease progression. *European Journal of Vascular and Endovascular Surgery.* 1999;18:240–244.

165. Taylor RS, Loh A, McFarland RJ, Cox M, Chester JF. Improved technique for polytetrafluoroethylene bypass grafting: Long-term results using anastomotic vein patches. *British Journal of Surgery.* 1992;79:348–354.

166. Gentile AT, Mills JL, Gooden MA, Hagerty RD, Berman SS, Hughes JD et al. Vein patching reduces neointimal thickening associated with prosthetic graft implantation. *American Journal of Surgery.* 1998;176:601–607.

167. Yeung KK, Mills Sr JL, Hughes JD, Berman SS, Gentile AT, Westerband A. Improved patency of infrainguinal polytetrafluoroethylene bypass grafts using a distal Taylor vein patch. *American Journal of Surgery.* 2001;182:578–583.

168. Linton RR, Darling RC. Autogenous saphenous vein bypass grafts in femoropopliteal obliterative arterial disease. *Surgery.* 1962;51:62–73.

169. Batson RC, Sottiurai VS, Craighead CC. Linton patch angioplasty. An adjunct to distal bypass with polytetrafluoroethylene grafts. *Annals of Surgery.* 1984;199:684–693.

170. Tyrrell MR, Wolfe JHN. New prosthetic venous collar anastomotic technique: Combining the best of other procedures. *British Journal of Surgery.* 1991;78:1016–1017.

171. Lemson MS, Tordoir JHM, Van Det RJ, Welten RJTJ, Burger H, Estourgie RJA et al. Effects of a venous cuff at the venous anastomosis of polytetrafluoroethylene grafts for hemodialysis vascular access. *Journal of Vascular Surgery.* 2000;32:1155–1163.

172. Gagne PJ, Martinez J, DeMassi R, Gregory R, Parent FN, Gayle R et al. The effect of a venous anastomosis Tyrell vein collar on the primary patency of arteriovenous grafts in patients undergoing hemodialysis. *Journal of Vascular Surgery.* 2000;32:1149–1154.

173. Sorom AJ, Hughes CB, McCarthy JT, Jenson BM, Prieto M, Panneton JM et al. Prospective, randomized evaluation of a cuffed expanded polytetrafluoroethylene graft for hemodialysis vascular access. *Surgery.* 2002;132:135–140.

174. Lumsden AB, Weaver FA, Hood DB. Prospective multi-center evaluation of VENAFLO ePTFE as compared to Impra ePTFE vascular graft in hemodialysis applications. In: Henry ML, ed. *Vascular Access for Hemodialysis,* 4th ed. Chicago, IL: Precept Press; 1997. pp. 242–249.

175. Longest PW, Kleinstreuer C, Deanda A. Numerical simulation of wall shear stress and particle-based hemodynamic parameters in pre-cuffed and streamlined end-to-side anastomoses. *Annals of Biomedical Engineering*. 2005;33:1752–1766.

176. O'Brien TP, Grace P, Walsh M, Burke P, McGloughlin T. Computational investigations of a new prosthetic femoral-popliteal bypass graft design. *Journal of Vascular Surgery*. 2005;42:1169–1175.

177. Chua LP, Tong JH, Zhou T. Numerical simulation of steady flows in designed sleeve models at distal anastomoses. *International Communications in Heat and Mass Transfer*. 2005;32:707–714.

178. O'Brien T, Walsh M, McGloughlin T. Altering end-to-side anastomosis junction hemodynamics: The effects of flow-splitting. *Medical Engineering and Physics*. 2006;28:727–733.

179. Walsh MT, McGloughlin TM, Grace P. A vascular graft. US patent. University of Limerick, Limerick, Ireland; 2010.

180. O'Brien TP, Walsh MT, Kavanagh EG, Finn SP, Grace PA, McGloughlin TM. Surgical feasibility study of a novel polytetrafluoroethylene graft design for the treatment of peripheral arterial disease. *Annals of Vascular Surgery*. 2007;21:611–617.

181. Sankaranarayanan M, Ghista DN, Chua LP, Tan YS, Sundaravadivelu K, Kassab GS. Blood flow in an out-of-plane aorto-left coronary sequential bypass graft. In: Guccione JM, Kassab GS, Ratcliffe M, eds. *Computational Cardiovascular Mechanics: Modeling and Applications in Heart Failure*. New York: Springer; 2010. pp. 277–295.

182. Vural KM, Sener E, Tasdemir O. Long-term patency of sequential and individual saphenous vein coronary bypass grafts. *European Journal of Cardio-Thoracic Surgery*. 2001;19:140–144.

183. Kabinejadian F, Chua LP, Ghista DN, Sankaranarayanan M, Tan YS. A novel coronary artery bypass graft design of sequential anastomoses. *Annals of Biomedical Engineering*. 2010;38:3135–3150.

184. Kabinejadian F, Ghista DN. Compliant model of a coupled sequential coronary arterial bypass graft: Effects of vessel wall elasticity and non-Newtonian rheology on blood flow regime and hemodynamic parameters distribution. *Medical Engineering and Physics*. 2012;34:860–872.

185. Kabinejadian F, Ghista DN, Su B, Kaabi Nezhadian M, Chua LP, Yeo JH et al. In vitro measurements of velocity and wall shear stress in a novel sequential anastomotic graft design model under pulsatile flow conditions. *Medical Engineering and Physics*. 2014;36:1233–1245.

16

Coupled Sequential Anastomotic Bypass Graft Design

Foad Kabinejadian, Dhanjoo N. Ghista, and Leok Poh Chua

CONTENTS

Acronyms

CABG	Coronary arterial bypass grafting
CCD	Charge coupled device
CFD	Computational fluid dynamic
CSABG	Coupled sequential anastomoses bypass graft
DV	Diameter variation
ETS	End-to-side
FFT	Fast Fourier transform
FSI	Fluid–structure interaction
HP	Hemodynamic parameter
IH	Intimal hyperplasia
IT	Intimal thickening
LAD	Left anterior descending coronary artery
LCA	Left coronary artery
LCx	Left circumflex coronary artery
LIMA	Left internal mammary artery
OSI	Oscillatory shear index
PDMS	Polydimethylsiloxane
PIV	Particle image velocimetry

RCA Right coronary artery
SMC Smooth muscle cell
SQA Sequential anastomoses
STS Side-to-side
SV Saphenous vein
TAWSS Time-averaged wall shear stress
TAWSSG Time-averaged wall shear stress gradient
TTL Transistor-transistor-logic
WSS Wall shear stress
WSSG Wall shear stress gradient

16.1 The Origin and Impetus of Our Modified Coupled Sequential Anastomotic Bypass Graft Design

The sequential bypass grafting technique, first described by Flemma et al. [1] and Bartley et al. [2], is a technique in which two or more coronary artery anastomoses are made with a single graft, usually the saphenous vein (SV). Intraoperative studies demonstrate a higher blood flow [3] and a higher velocity [4] in the proximal (pre-anastomotic) segment of a sequential graft than in a single coronary graft with an end-to-side (ETS) anastomosis. Higher patency rates have also been observed through post-angiograms in side-to-side (STS) anastomoses than in ETS anastomoses [5]. Moreover, according to results obtained by our group [6], STS anastomosis has a smoother flow with smaller spatial gradients of WSS as compared to ETS anastomosis, which may motivate the use of sequential bypass grafting over multiple bypass grafting.

It is well established that in the conventional ETS anastomotic region, impingement of blood flow on the artery floor and the flow recirculation at the heel play a critical role in the re-stenosis of the coronary artery bypass graft (CABG) distal anastomosis. Although many designs are suggested to improve the flow field at the distal anastomosis of the CABG, they do not exhibit large deviation from the general flow characteristics, such as the vortex formed at the heel or the impact of blood on the artery bed [7].

Our group has conducted numerous studies, both numerically and experimentally, in order to investigate the effects of geometrical parameters, including anastomotic angle [8], out-of-plane graft [9], and complete CABG modeling [10,11]. Optimization of these parameters in a conventional ETS anastomosis can improve the flow field and distributions of hemodynamic parameters (HPs) to some extent. However, in order to further improve the hemodynamics and alleviate the drawbacks of the available CABG anastomosis designs, a novel coupled sequential anastomosis (SQA) configuration design is developed, based on the beneficial results of sequential bypass grafts.

Investigation of the flow field in this SQA design (by means of numerical simulation and experimental measurements of pulsatile blood flow) and its comparison with a conventional CABG ETS anastomosis is presented here. After showing the advantages of the novel design, the effects of two design parameters, namely, the anastomotic angle and distance between the two anastomoses, on the distribution of HPs are studied. Also, the performance of the novel coupled SQA design is examined for an out-of-plane CABG model as well as for the case of a partial flow present through the proximal host artery.

Accordingly, this chapter presents (1) computational methodology and results of blood flow analysis in this novel SQA design (by means of numerical simulation of pulsatile Newtonian blood flow) and its comparison with conventional CABG ETS and parallel STS anastomoses, (2) in vitro measurements of velocity and wall shear stress in conventional and our coupled sequential anastomotic bypass graft (CSABG) design model under pulsatile flow conditions, and (3) effects of wall elasticity and non-Newtonian rheology on the blood flow regime and HPs in the compliant models of conventional and our CSABG designs.*

16.2 Coupled Sequential Anastomotic Bypass Graft Design: CFD Modeling of Blood Flow Pattern and Hemodynamic Parameters of CSABG Design in Comparison with Conventional ETS Anastomosis and Parallel STS Anastomosis Designs

16.2.1 CFD Geometric Models: Novel Coupled STS–ETS Model Design, Conventional ETS Anastomosis, and Parallel STS Anastomosis Designs

Based on the beneficial results of sequential bypass grafting, a novel configuration for the CABG is designed, to improve the flow field and HP distributions of the conventional ETS anastomoses. In this distal SQA design, shown in Figure 16.1a, there is initially an STS anastomosis distal to the stenosis, and then the graft end is anastomosed to the same coronary artery further downstream in an ETS fashion.

Three base models: In order to evaluate and compare the advantages and disadvantages of our suggested SQA design over a conventional ETS anastomosis configuration, three base CFD models are designed and evaluated: (1) the novel coupled anastomoses configuration, shown in Figure 16.1a, (2) a parallel STS anastomosis (Figure 16.1b), and (3) a conventional ETS anastomosis (Figure 16.1c). The latter two are the reference models to be compared, respectively, with the STS component of the new design (in order to study the possible effects of the ETS anastomosis of the new design on its STS component) and with its ETS component.

Models' dimensions: The dimensions of the three base models are listed in Table 16.1, where D_G, D_A, L_P, L_{STS}, L_{ETS}, L_D, and d stand, respectively, for the graft diameter, coronary artery diameter, length of the proximal section of the host artery, length of the STS anastomosis, length of the ETS anastomosis, length of the distal section of the host artery, and distance between the two anastomoses in the new SQA model, as shown in Figure 16.1.

The base models are considered to have an ETS anastomotic angle of 45° with the fully occluded proximal segment of the coronary artery. The models are designed to be planar, based on the study of Galjee et al. [13] who demonstrated that the typical location and course of SV in RCA bypass graft can be assumed to be approximately planar.

---

* This chapter is based *Coronary Artery Bypass Grafting Design Simulations: Emphasizing a Novel CABG Design of Sequential Anastomoses*, F. Kabinejadian and D.N. Ghista, Lambert Academic Publishing, Saarbrücken, Germany, 2012.

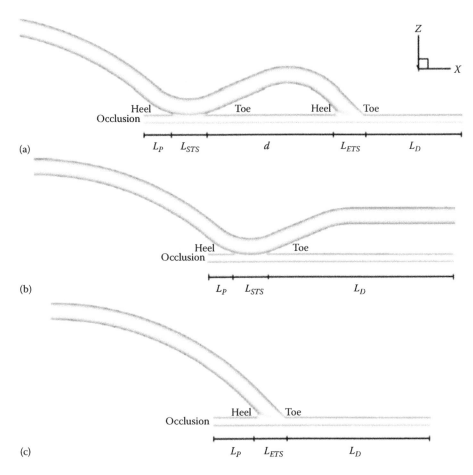

FIGURE 16.1
Various anastomotic models: (a) the new proposed coupled STS–ETS model design, (b) parallel STS anastomosis, (c) conventional ETS anastomosis model with an anastomotic angle of 45°. A fully developed pulsatile flow is applied at the graft inlet and outlets; in case of the parallel STS model (b), 85% of the blood flow is set to exit through the graft outlet. (From Kabinejadian, F. et al., *Ann. Biomed. Eng.*, 38, 3135, 2010.)

TABLE 16.1

Dimensions of the Base Models' Geometry (mm)

Model	D_G	D_A	L_P	L_{STS}	L_{ETS}	L_D	d
SQA design	4	2	6.5	8	7	48	30
Conventional ETS	4	2	10	N.A.	7	48	N.A.
Parallel STS	4	2	6.5	8	N.A.	48	N.A.

16.2.2 Computational Modeling and Flow Conditions

Blood flow through the CABG is assumed to have the characteristics of 3D, time-dependent, incompressible, isothermal, Newtonian and laminar flow, whose governing equations are

$$\text{Continuity equation,} \quad \nabla \cdot u = 0 \tag{16.1}$$

$$\text{Navier–Stokes equation,} \quad \rho\frac{\partial u}{\partial t} + \rho(u \cdot \nabla)u = -\nabla p + \mu\nabla^2 u \tag{16.2}$$

where
  u is the velocity vector
  t is the time
  p is the pressure

The density (ρ) and dynamic viscosity (μ) of blood are assumed to be 1050 kg/m³ and 0.00408 Pa s, respectively [14]. The vessel walls are assumed to be rigid at this stage.

The proximal anastomosis of the graft to the aorta is not analyzed in this study, and the focus is only on the distal anastomosis. Hence, a fully developed pulsatile flow is applied at the graft inlet; its flow waveform and the velocity profile are based on measurements by magnetic resonance phase velocity mapping within a CABG [15]. This waveform (with the time period of 0.9 s adapted for this study) is demonstrated in Figure 16.2. The Womersley solution [16] is assumed for the inlet axial velocity profile, which is derived as a fully developed pulsatile flow and implemented as the inlet boundary condition to calculate the velocity for the pulsatile flow (see Appendix 16A). The exit flow is assumed to be in a fully developed condition, due to the 48 mm long distal segment of the coronary artery models. Thereby, the FLUENT's outflow boundary condition is set to assume a zero normal gradient for all flow variables except pressure.

In the parallel STS model, 15% of the blood flow is set to pass through the STS anastomosis into the coronary artery, and the remaining 85% is assumed to pass through the graft to the (distally located) ETS anastomotic junction. The above percentage is adjusted to have the parallel STS model consistent with the novel coupled anastomoses configuration, since the flow is bifurcated with the same proportion through the coronary artery and the graft at the STS component (on average within each cycle), as observed in the results.

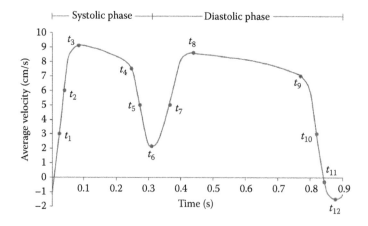

FIGURE 16.2
Average velocity values of the waveform used in the present study. Labels indicate times at which flow and HP are studied. (From Kabinejadian, F. et al., *Ann. Biomed. Eng.*, 38, 3135, 2010.)

16.2.3 CFD Results for CSABG Design in Comparison with Conventional ETS Anastomosis and Parallel STS Anastomosis Designs

16.2.3.1 Flow Behavior and Patterns

The flow field and HPs in all the three base models are studied at 12 instants of time, as shown on the waveform in Figure 16.2. At times t_3 of peak systole and t_{11} of late-diastole, samples of the computed streamlines of the flow field at the center plane of the three models are presented in Figures 16.3 and 16.4, respectively, wherein the novel SQA design, parallel STS, and conventional ETS models are labeled as (a), (b), and (c), respectively.

Acceleration phase: As the flow accelerates from t_1 to t_3 (the peak flow rate), in the conventional ETS anastomosis model, a vortex forms at the heel region, with a stagnation point on the artery floor due to the graft flow impacting the artery bed, as shown in Figure 16.3c for time t_3. However, in our novel SQA model (Figure 16.3a), the flow at the distal ETS anastomosis is very smooth without any vortex formation. There is no impingement on the artery floor. This is because the partial flow from the STS anastomosis along the coronary artery changes the velocity components of the ETS anastomosis flow toward the toe and the coronary artery axis rather than to the artery floor. This results in having no stagnation

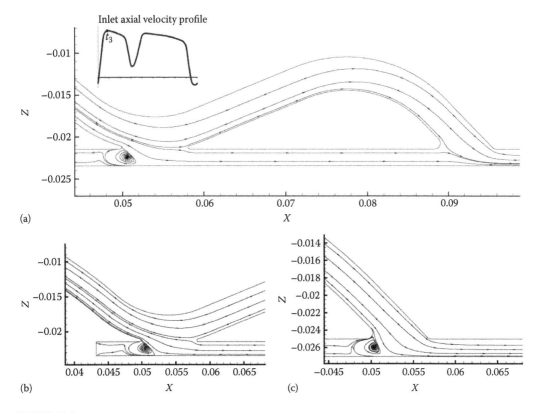

FIGURE 16.3
Streamlines at the symmetry plane at time t_3: (a) SQA design, (b) parallel STS model, (c) conventional ETS model. Strong impact of flow observed on the artery floor in the conventional ETS anastomosis compared to the flow at the STS anastomosis models. (From Kabinejadian, F. et al., *Ann. Biomed. Eng.*, 38, 3135, 2010.)

point formed on the bed. However, there would be some energy loss due to the collision of the two flows from the graft and coronary artery.

At the STS anastomosis of the novel SQA model (Figure 16.3a), a vortex forms at the heel region along with a stagnation point on the artery bed, due to the interaction of the flow from the graft with the relatively slow flow in the occluded end of the artery. This is consistent with our findings for the parallel STS anastomosis model (Figure 16.3b); Bonert et al. [17] have also shown similar results. At the peak flow rate (t_3) in the new design, 11% of the graft flow goes through the STS anastomosis, and 89% of that passes through the ETS anastomosis. The diversion of 11% of graft flow into the coronary artery at the STS anastomosis has the effect of smoothing the flow at the distal ETS anastomosis.

Deceleration and reversed flow phases: During the mid-deceleration, partial recirculation and back flow appear in the graft in all the models, particularly at the inner wall of the graft curvatures where the blood flow has low inertia, and exhibits oscillatory characteristics. At the ETS anastomosis of the new SQA model, the graft flow bifurcates into the distal and proximal segments of the coronary artery.

As the net flow rate just becomes negative (t_{11}), the blood flows back toward the aorta through the graft at near wall regions, while it still flows forward at the central regions near the graft axis, as shown in Figure 16.4. This is due to the high inertia of the fluid in the central region compared to the fluid near the wall having low inertia, as a result of the

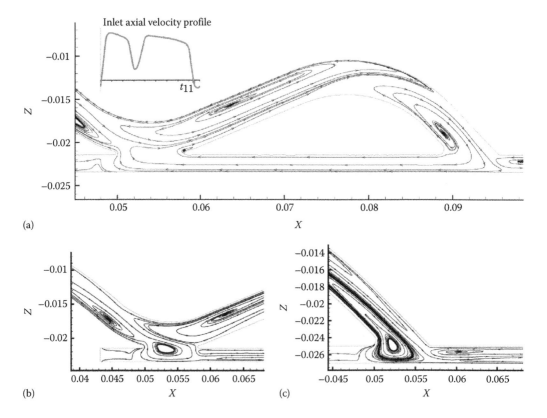

FIGURE 16.4
Streamlines at the symmetry plane at time t_{11}: (a) SQA design, (b) parallel STS model, (c) conventional ETS model. Larger vortices and recirculation areas are observed in models (b) and (c) compared to SQA design model (a). (From Kabinejadian, F. et al., *Ann. Biomed. Eng.*, 38, 3135, 2010.)

friction between the layers of the fluid within the boundary layer. At this time instant (t_{11}), there are large vortices and recirculation areas in all the models. At the ETS anastomosis of the new SQA model, there is a small vortex at the graft inner wall, upstream of the distal anastomosis, as shown in Figure 16.4a. However, in the conventional ETS anastomosis (Figure 16.4c), the vortex is much larger and occupies most of the anastomosis region and half of the graft near the inner wall. In the parallel STS anastomosis model (Figure 16.4b), a large vortex occupies the entire anastomosis region. On the other hand, in the STS anastomosis of the new SQA model, the size of the vortex is remarkably reduced and shifted over the toe of the anastomosis. This is due to the blood flow from the ETS component circulating within the vascular loop of the new SQA model, which eliminates the stagnation point on the artery bed as illustrated in Figure 16.4a.

16.2.3.2 Hemodynamic Parameters Distribution

It has been shown that (1) localized distribution of low-WSS and high-oscillatory shear index (OSI) strongly correlates with the focal locations of atheroma [18], (2) large spatial WSSG contributes to the elevated wall permeability and atherosclerotic lesions [19], and (3) prevailing development of these lesions and growth of plaque formation occur in regions of extreme (either maxima or minima) WSS [20,21]. Hence, in this study, the distributions of HPs, including time-averaged WSS (TAWSS), nondimensional TAWSSG [22], and OSI [18] are calculated according to their expressions in the following equations and compared in the three models.

$$WSS = \vec{\tau}_w = \mu \left(\frac{\partial \boldsymbol{u}}{\partial \boldsymbol{n}} \right) \Big|_{Wall} \tag{16.3}$$

$$TAWSS = \frac{1}{T} \int_0^T |\vec{\tau}_w| dt \tag{16.4}$$

$$TAWSSG = \frac{D_G}{\tau_0} \frac{1}{T} \int_0^T \sqrt{\left(\frac{\partial \tau_x}{\partial x} \right)^2 + \left(\frac{\partial \tau_y}{\partial y} \right)^2 + \left(\frac{\partial \tau_z}{\partial z} \right)^2} \, dt \tag{16.5}$$

$$OSI = \frac{1}{2} \left(1 - \frac{\left| \int_0^T \vec{\tau}_w dt \right|}{\int_0^T |\vec{\tau}_w| dt} \right) \tag{16.6}$$

where
   n is the inner unit vector normal to the wall
   $\vec{\tau}_w, \tau_x, \tau_y,$ and τ_z are the WSS vector (traction) and its components
   T is the time period of the flow cycle
   D_G is the graft diameter
   τ_0 is the WSS for Poiseuille flow at the mean flow Reynolds number, which is obtained
     as 0.48 Pa for the current study

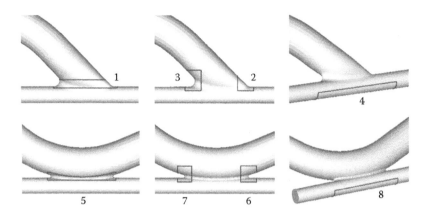

FIGURE 16.5
Critical regions of ETS and STS anastomoses, which are the susceptible sites of intimal hyperplasia and atherosclerotic lesion formation: 1,5—suture line, 2,6—toe, 3,7—heel, 4,8—bed. (From Kabinejadian, F. et al., *Ann. Biomed. Eng.*, 38, 3135, 2010.)

In order to compare the distribution of HPs quantitatively at the critical sites of the anastomosis such as toe, heel, bed, and the suture line (see Figure 16.5), the segmental averages of the HPs are calculated and listed in Table 16.2. In this table, the aforementioned calculated parameters are also presented for a few more studied models, which are introduced later in this section.

TAWSS: As shown in Table 16.2 for the base models (with anastomotic angle of 45° and $d = 30$ mm), TAWSS is increased on the artery bed of the ETS anastomosis of the new SQA model to 1.63 Pa, from 1.40 Pa in the conventional ETS model. Although this increase is marginal, Giddens et al. [23] have found a critical biological WSS value of 15 dyn/cm² (1.5 Pa) below which IT would develop; based thereon, the moderate improvement of TAWSS on the artery bed of the new SQA design can be deemed to be vital. The TAWSS in the STS anastomoses is generally low, with its peak located at the toe; the TAWSS is lower in the STS component of the new SQA model than in the parallel STS model. This depicts a more moderate distribution of WSS in the STS component of the new SQA model, which can reduce the probability of atherosclerotic lesion development.

TAWSSG: As shown in Table 16.2, TAWSSG at the heel and bed of the ETS component as well as at the toe and suture line of the STS component of the new SQA model is reduced, compared to the conventional ETS and parallel STS anastomoses, respectively. This manifests a more uniform distribution of WSS in the new SQA design at these critical locations, which can lessen the vessel wall permeability and atherosclerotic lesion development.

OSI: The OSI at the ETS anastomosis of the novel SQA model is lower at the heel region and the artery wall and bed opposite to the heel, than in the conventional ETS anastomosis model, as demonstrated in Figure 16.6. However, OSI is generally low at the ETS anastomoses, due to the flow having mostly a forward direction within the cycle. At the STS anastomosis region of the novel SQA model and in the parallel STS model, the OSI distribution is almost the same in the graft, at the heel, and the proximal part of the artery wall, as shown in Figure 16.6 and Table 16.2 for the base model. However, the OSI is increased on the artery bed and at the toe of

TABLE 16.2

Comparison of Segmental Average of <HP>s in Models with Fully Occluded Host Artery

		ETS anastomotic angle: 30°			45°			60°		
Model	Location	<OSI>	<TAWSS> (Pa)	<TAWSSG>	<OSI>	<TAWSS> (Pa)	<TAWSSG>	<OSI>	<TAWSS> (Pa)	<TAWSSG>
Conventional ETS model[a]	1—Suture line	0.03	2.59	20.1	0.02	3.08	44.8	0.02	3.49	64.4
	2—Toe	0.01	6.37	40.1	0.01	6.37	74.2	0.01	6.87	111.4
	3—Heel	0.07	0.54	7.0	0.05	0.59	9.0	0.05	0.63	10.7
	4—Bed	0.12	1.42	5.0	0.11	1.40	7.5	0.10	1.39	9.8
New design model with *d* = 30 mm	ETS component									
	1—Suture line	0.02	2.59	17.5	0.02	3.05	40.5	0.02	3.43	57.8
	2—Toe	0.01	6.40	40.7	0.01	6.43	78.6	0.01	6.91	109.4
	3—Heel	0.05	0.53	4.7	0.05	0.56	6.6	0.05	0.57	7.0
	4—Bed	0.05	1.60	4.1	0.05	1.63	6.2	0.05	1.66	7.6
	STS component									
	5—Suture line-STS	0.05	0.66	11.5	0.04	0.63	10.6	0.05	0.67	13.3
	6—Toe-STS	0.04	0.66	10.5	0.04	0.65	11.2	0.04	0.65	10.2
	7—Heel-STS	0.07	0.43	5.8	0.07	0.43	6.6	0.07	0.43	6.3
	8—Bed-STS	0.21	0.17	0.4	0.20	0.18	0.4	0.20	0.18	0.4
New design model with *d* = 20 mm	ETS component									
	1—Suture line	0.02	2.58	21.5	0.02	3.05	40.2	0.02	3.43	57.6
	2—Toe	0.01	6.40	55.9	0.01	6.44	79.0	0.01	6.21	87.3
	3—Heel	0.05	0.53	5.3	0.05	0.55	6.2	0.05	0.57	6.9
	4—Bed	0.05	1.62	4.3	0.05	1.65	6.4	0.05	1.68	7.6
	STS component									
	5—Suture line-STS	0.04	0.64	11.0	0.04	0.64	11.1	0.04	0.65	10.6
	6—Toe-STS	0.03	0.66	11.9	0.03	0.66	12.1	0.03	0.66	10.9
	7—Heel-STS	0.07	0.43	6.8	0.07	0.43	6.8	0.07	0.43	6.3
	8—Bed-STS	0.20	0.18	0.4	0.20	0.19	0.4	0.19	0.19	0.5
Non-planar new design model (with diamond STS component and *d* = 20 mm)	ETS component				Isolated STS models					
	1—Suture line	0.02	2.58	18.9						
	2—Toe	0.01	6.38	43.4						
	3—Heel	0.05	0.54	4.7						
	4—Bed	0.05	1.63	4.2	Diamond STS model[a]			Parallel STS model[a]		
	STS component									
	5—Suture line-STS	0.09	0.49	9.4	0.05	0.68	1.9	0.03	0.69	14.0
	6—Toe-STS	—	—	—	—	—	—	0.01	0.76	15.6
	7—Heel-STS	—	—	—	—	—	—	0.07	0.44	6.7
	8—Bed-STS	0.09	0.23	1.3	0.03	0.35	0.4	0.15	0.24	0.6

[a] Reference models.

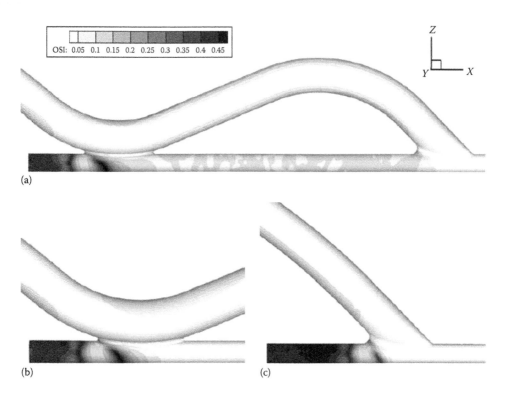

FIGURE 16.6
OSI distribution at the anastomotic regions of the three models: (a) new design, (b) parallel STS model, and (c) conventional ETS model. OSI is generally low in the graft and distal segment of the coronary artery, due to the waveform having mostly a forward flow. (From Kabinejadian, F. et al., *Ann. Biomed. Eng.*, 38, 3135, 2010.)

the STS component of the new design compared to those of the parallel STS model. As shown in Figure 16.6, the OSI is generally low within the graft; yet, there is a high-OSI area on the artery bed and wall just distal to the heel of the STS anastomosis, due to the vortex forming there and the moving stagnation point.

The OSI is also high at the occluded segment of the host artery, as illustrated in Figure 16.6; but, this is due to the very small mean WSS in this area rather than due to large changes in WSS over the cardiac cycle as reported by Bonert et al. [17]. The OSI distribution in the segment of the coronary artery between the two anastomoses of the new SQA model differs from that of the distal segment of the coronary artery in the parallel STS anastomosis model. In this segment as shown in Figure 16.6, the OSI value increases up to 0.15 in the new design, while it is below 0.05 in the parallel STS model. This increase in OSI can be due to the circulation of blood flow in the vascular loop of the novel SQA design.

16.2.3.3 Effects of the Design Parameters on the Hemodynamic Parameters Distribution

There are two types of parameters involved in the design of the suggested configuration. One group of parameters can be controlled by the surgeon such as the anastomotic angle at the ETS component, and the distance between the two anastomoses (*d*). The other group of parameters cannot be controlled as they are different from one patient to another, such as the diameter of the SV and coronary arteries, and the percentage and location of stenosis that can result in having parallel (where graft and host artery centerlines are approximately in plane) or diamond configuration (where the centerlines of the host artery and graft cross at approximately 90°) at the STS component.

Adjustable parameters: In order to obtain a better flow field and HP distributions, a number of models are simulated for a range of the adjustable parameters, involving anastomotic angle (of 30°, 45°, and 60°) at the ETS component and the distance (d = 20 and 30 mm) between the two STS and ETS components of the new design. Comprehensive information of the flow regime dependence on the design parameters (including the graft and coronary artery diameter) can enable tailoring an optimal design for a specific patient.

Non-planar model: In order to verify the advantage of the suggested design for the left coronary artery (LCA) bypasses (where the graft and coronary arteries cannot be assumed to be in the same plane), a non-planar model with a diamond configuration at the STS component is studied.

Variation in occlusion ratio: Anastomosis models with different percentages of coronary artery stenosis are simulated, in order to evaluate the performance of the new SQA graft design in the early post-operative stage. It is well known that during the first weeks following grafting (at least until 2 weeks [24]) a non-negligible residual flow remains through the stenosed host artery, which will progressively decrease until the stenosed vessel is completely occluded [25]. Hence, anastomosis models with two stenosis severity of 75% and 91% (equivalent to 50% and 70% diameter stenosis, respectively) are investigated in this study.

For this purpose, an axisymmetric stenosis with a Gaussian profile [26] is considered to be located 6 mm upstream from the heel in the models (with the ETS anastomotic angle of 30° and d = 30 mm). At the coronary artery inlet, Berne and Levy [27] flow waveform is imposed. According to Speziale [28] indicating that the flow rate in an internal thoracic artery graft increases with progressing stenosis of the native coronary artery, the distribution percentage of the flow rates issued from the graft and stenosed coronary artery are allocated to be 75 versus 25 and 91 versus 9 in the two studied cases, respectively, in order to simulate the progressive decrease of residual blood flow from a constricted host artery following the bypass surgery.

The segmental averages of the calculated HPs for the studied models with (1) fully occluded and (2) partially stenosed coronary arteries are, respectively, presented in Tables 16.2 and 16.3.

16.2.3.3.1 Inferences Drawn from the Results in Tables 16.2 and 16.3

The following features can be inferred from the results in Tables 16.2 and 16.3.

From Table 16.2, comparison of the conventional ETS models with different anastomotic angles indicates that the TAWSSG is considerably increased with the anastomotic angle, while the TAWSS is marginally increased (except on the artery bed where it is slightly decreased), and the OSI is almost remained constant. Therefore, a smaller anastomotic angle results in a more favorable HP distribution. This is in agreement with the results reported by Fei et al. [29] who studied the flow in distal ETS anastomoses with anastomotic angles of 20°, 30°, 40°, 45°, 50°, 60°, and 70°, and suggested that grafts should be placed with a minimal distal anastomotic angle.

Comparing the six planar SQA design models: As shown in Table 16.2, when the model anastomotic angle is changed from 30° to 60°, the TAWSSG is drastically increased mainly at the toe and suture line of the ETS component (by 169% and 230%, respectively), while

TABLE 16.3

Comparison of Segmental Average of <HP>s in Models with Partially Occluded Host Artery and ETS Anastomotic Angle of 30°

			75%				91%		
Occlusion ratio:									
Model		Location	<OSI>	<TAWSS> (Pa)	<TAWSSG>	<OSI>	<TAWSS> (Pa)	<TAWSSG>
Conventional ETS model[a]		1—Suture line	0.01	2.29	12.4	0.02	2.35	15.0
		2—Toe	0.004	5.59	28.8	0.01	5.78	29.8
		3—Heel	0.03	0.56	4.4	0.04	0.49	5.8
		4—Bed	0.003	1.55	3.5	0.02	1.32	4.0
New design model with $d = 30$ mm	ETS component	1—Suture line	0.01	2.25	12.9	0.02	2.34	13.6
		2—Toe	0.004	5.57	28.6	0.01	5.80	30.1
		3—Heel	0.04	0.47	4.0	0.05	0.49	4.4
		4—Bed	0.04	1.39	3.6	0.05	1.46	3.7
	STS component	5—Suture line-STS	0.02	0.64	7.2	0.04	0.60	8.0
		6—Toe-STS	0.03	0.52	5.4	0.04	0.59	7.4
		7—Heel-STS	0.02	0.52	4.4	0.03	0.41	4.1
		8—Bed-STS	0.03	0.38	0.4	0.11	0.18	0.3
Parallel STS model[a]		1—Suture line	0.01	0.93	16.5	0.02	0.67	10.5
		2—Toe	0.01	0.85	20.8	0.01	0.75	14.4
		3—Heel	0.02	0.52	4.9	0.03	0.41	4.7
		4—Bed	0.005	0.69	1.1	0.05	0.32	0.7

[a] Reference models.

generally the TAWSS is negligibly increased (8% and 32%, respectively) and OSI is not changed. This implies that the TAWSSG is the over-riding factor in the selection of the preferred anastomotic angle, which makes the case for the smaller anastomotic angle for the new design.

A change in the distance between the two components (*d*) has affected the TAWSSG mainly at the toe of the ETS component, with a different trend in each model depending on the anastomotic angle. A decrease in *d* (from 30 to 20 mm), has caused the TAWSSG (primarily at the toe) to (1) increase in the model with the anastomotic angle of 30°, (2) decrease in the model with the anastomotic angle of 60°, and (3) stay almost unchanged in the model with the anastomotic angle of 45°.

Neither the anastomotic angle nor the distance between the two components has any obvious effect on the HP distribution at the STS component of the new design.

The non-planar model with a diamond configuration at the STS component (with ETS anastomotic angle of 30° and d = 20 mm): This non-planar model (illustrated in Figure 16.7) depicts a lower TAWSSG distribution at the ETS component than the corresponding planar model, as shown in Table 16.2. On the artery bed of the STS component of this non-planar model, while the TAWSS and TAWSSG are slightly increased (to 0.23 and 1.3 from 0.18 and 0.4, respectively), the OSI is reduced to half (from 0.2 to 0.09) as compared to that of the corresponding planar model; this is beneficial to prevent the coincidence of low-WSS and high-OSI on the bed. However, on the suture line of the STS component of the non-planar

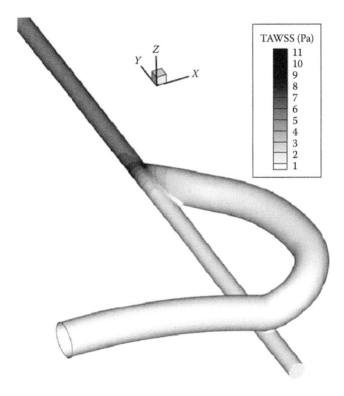

FIGURE 16.7
TAWSS distribution in the non-planar model. TAWSS is low in the graft and proximal segments of the coronary artery, and it is increased at the ETS component and downstream of the coronary artery, with its peak at the toe of the ETS anastomosis. (From Kabinejadian, F. et al., *Ann. Biomed. Eng.*, 38, 3135, 2010.)

model, the OSI becomes almost double (from 0.04 to 0.09), while TAWSS and TAWSSG are slightly decreased (from 0.64 and 11 to 0.49 and 9.4, respectively) compared to the corresponding planar model. In addition, the segmental average of TAWSSG on the graft wall across the STS anastomosis of the non-planar model is increased to 1.6 from 1 in the corresponding planar model (these latter values are not given in Table 16.2).

This is in agreement with the results reported by Bonert et al. [17], who demonstrated that the parallel configuration is more favorable than the diamond configuration for maintaining the graft patency at the STS anastomosis, while the diamond one is favorable for maintaining the host artery patency. Since graft patency is vital for the STS anastomosis of the new design, this design can be more beneficially applicable for the right CABG, wherein the graft and the coronary artery are approximately in the same plane. This fact is further proven by comparing the HP distributions in the STS component of the non-planar SQA model with the isolated diamond STS model, where all the HP distributions are more favorable both on the suture line and bed of the anastomosis, as shown in Table 16.2.

The models with partially stenosed coronary arteries: Comparison of the STS component of each new design model with the corresponding parallel STS model (in Table 16.3) indicates that the suggested SQA design configuration affects the distribution of HPs at the STS anastomosis of the partially occluded host artery models in exactly the same trend as in the fully occluded host artery models (shown in Table 16.2).

Comparison of the ETS component of each new design model with the corresponding conventional ETS model (in Table 16.3), indicates that in the case of 91% stenosed coronary artery, the change in the TAWSSG and TAWSS distributions due to the new design configuration has the same trend as in the fully stenosed host artery models (shown in Table 16.2). Yet, it does not hold for the OSI at the heel and bed of the coronary artery.

In the case of 75% stenosed coronary artery, the advantages of the new design concerning the distribution of HPs in its fully occluded and 91% stenosed models are not manifest. The TAWSSG on the bed and suture line, and the TAWSS and OSI on the heel and bed of the ETS component of the new design are inferior compared to those of the corresponding conventional ETS model.

This suggests that if the occlusion percentage of the stenosed artery is below a certain level, the overall advantages of the new configuration might be affected during the first few days following the bypass surgery, due to the competitive flows problem. This is in agreement with the results of the earlier studies [30–33], which have confirmed the existence of a critical value for stenosis severity, below which the graft failure is expected, and above that, the recipient artery will be progressively occluded.

In summary, the effects of the parameters above studied can be concluded as follows:

Comparison of each novel SQA model with the corresponding conventional ETS model depicts that in all the SQA design models (with different values of d and ETS anastomotic angle, illustrated in Figure 16.1 and Table 16.1) the HP distribution is improved on the bed, heel, and (in most of the models) suture line of the ETS component.

The variation of the design parameters of the new SQA graft design demonstrates that the combination of a smaller anastomotic angle at the ETS component and a longer distance (d) between the two components results in a better flow field and distribution of HPs. Yet, there are restrictions which inhibit surgeons from implementing a very acute anastomotic angle and adopting a long distance between the two components practically. Although some innovative suturing methods are proposed to obtain an acute anastomotic angle using prosthetic grafts [34], it is impractical in standard clinical practice to perform a very small anastomotic angle due to the large cross-sectional area of the graft section resulted in such an anastomosis.

Moreover, the lengths of coronary arteries are limited: the left anterior descending (LAD) coronary artery measures from 10 to 13 cm in length, whereas the LCx artery measures about 6 to 8 cm, and the dominant RCA is about 12 to 14 cm in length [35]. Therefore, taking into account the length of the coronary artery located proximal to the stenosis plus the distance of grafting (required distance between the stenosis and the STS anastomosis), in addition to the lengths of the two anastomoses of the new SQA design, there would be a restricted length of the coronary artery left to be adopted as the distance (d) between the two STS and ETS components of the new graft design practically.

Hence, in this study, the minimum anastomotic angle and maximum distance between the two components are adopted to be 30° and 30 mm, respectively, which result in a better flow field and distribution of HPs than the other models investigated.

The simulation results for the models with partially stenosed coronary arteries further confirm that there is a critical value for stenosis severity, below which graft failure is expected due to the competitive flow problem. Note that the effect of the partial flow through the coronary artery is only studied on the models with anastomotic angle of 30° and $d = 30$ mm, whose results are shown to be the most favorable among the investigated models.

16.3 In Vitro Pulsatile Flow Studies Measurements of Velocity and Wall Shear Stress in the CSABG Design in Comparison with Conventional ETS Anastomosis and Parallel STS Anastomosis Designs

In order to verify the hemodynamic advantages of the novel CSABG design (over the routine conventional ETS anastomoses), which were observed in the simulation results, the flow fields inside polydimethylsiloxane (PDMS) models of the three base CABG designs (i.e., the coupled SQA graft design, the conventional ETS anastomosis, and the parallel STS anastomosis) are investigated under pulsatile flow conditions, using a particle image velocimetry (PIV) technique. The velocity field and distributions of WSS in the three base models are studied and compared with each other, to complement the computational results.

16.3.1 Geometric Models

The silicone rubber (i.e., PDMS) models were fabricated, using the method introduced by Chong et al. [36], and are shown in Figure 16.8. The dimensions of the models are listed earlier in Table 16.1. The physical models were bilaterally symmetric with respect to the *XZ* plane, and the outlet of the proximal segment of the coronary artery was fully occluded during the experiments.

16.3.2 Working Fluid, Flow Conditions, and Flow Circuit

A mixture of 30% glycerin and 70% sodium chloride (NaCl) solution by volume was used as the working fluid in this study (the NaCl solution was made up of 1 part NaCl and 3 parts water by weight). This Newtonian mixture's density was 1156 kg/m³ and its dynamic viscosity at the working temperature of 25°C was quantified by a controlled shear

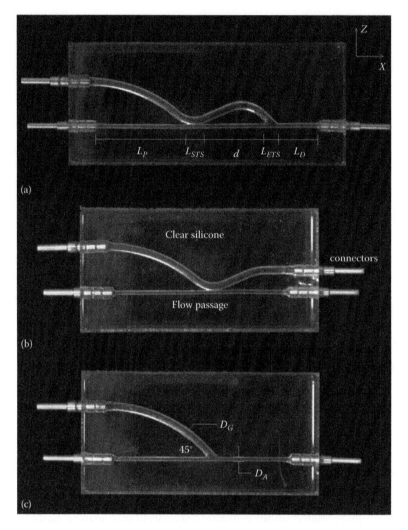

FIGURE 16.8
Fabricated silicone rubber (PDMS) models of (a) the novel coupled SQA graft design, (b) parallel STS, and (c) conventional ETS anastomosis. (From Kabinejadian, F. et al., *Med. Eng. Phys.*, 36, 1233, 2014.)

rate rheometer (Contraves low rate 40) to be 0.0054 Pa s (5.4 cP). The refractive index of the mixture was measured by a commercial refractometer (Atago 3T; High-Precision Model) to be 1.409, which matches that of the PDMS model.

Each PDMS model was incorporated into the flow circuit, as shown schematically in Figure 16.9, and a computer-controlled gear pump system (Micropump Inc., Vancouver, WA), including one varying flow pump (Model HG0024-N23 PF1SGB1) and one steady flow pump (Model HG0024-G050), was used to generate the physiological inlet flow waveform, demonstrated earlier in Figure 16.2 [12]. The flow rate was measured and monitored by means of an electromagnetic flow meter (Promag 53, Endress+Hauser, Germany) immediately upstream of the test section.

The peak flow rate during systole was $Q_{max} = 70$ mL/min. The maximum Reynolds and Womersley numbers at the peak systole were calculated to be $Re_{max} = 79$ and $\alpha_{max} = 2.45$, respectively, based on the graft diameter of 4 mm. This suggested that the flow was

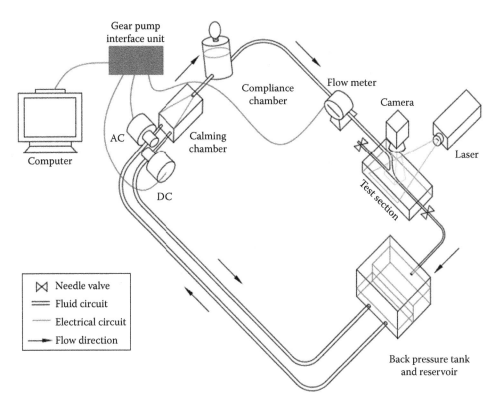

FIGURE 16.9
Schematic of the mock circulation loop and PIV system. (From Kabinejadian, F. et al., *Med. Eng. Phys.*, 36, 1233, 2014.)

laminar, which was further proven by PIV results, as no turbulence was observed in the flow field.

In the parallel STS model, 15% of the blood flow (on average within each cardiac cycle) was set to pass through the STS anastomosis into the coronary artery, and the remaining 85% was allowed to pass through the graft, by adjusting the resistance at the outlets of the graft and coronary artery of this model. The aforementioned flow division was adjusted to make the parallel STS model consistent with the novel coupled SQA configuration, since the flow was bifurcated in the same proportion through the coronary artery and the graft at the STS component of the SQA model.

In this experiment, hollow glass spheres with mean diameter of 10 μm, density of 1.1 g/cm³, and refractive index of 1.52 (HGS-10, Dantec Dynamics, Denmark) were used as tracer particles and seeded into the working fluid.

16.3.3 Particle Image Velocimetry System

The PIV is an optical measurement technique, allowing the instantaneous acquisition of an entire planar section of a flow field [38]. The PIV system used in this study, consisted of a 15 Hz Q-switched, double-cavity pulsed Nd:YAG laser (Minilase-III, New Wave Research, United States) with an energy of 150 mJ at a wavelength of 1064 nm, producing a light sheet, which was adjusted to illuminate the tracer particles in the symmetry plane of the models, as shown schematically in Figure 16.9.

The particles' motion was recorded by means of a synchronized charge coupled device (CCD) camera (FlowSense, Dantec Dynamics, Denmark), with a spatial resolution of 1600×1200 pixel^2, and a Nikon lens (AF Micro Nikkor, 60/2.8) positioned normal to the laser sheet. The image acquisition in this phase-resolved PIV measurement was triggered by a TTL signal (5 V), generated by the gear pump interface unit, in order to phase-lock the measurements. The flow data were acquired at different phase points during the cardiac cycle, and presented for six distinct points, namely, t_2, t_3, t_5, t_6, t_{11}, and t_{12}, as shown on the waveform in Figure 16.2. For statistical convergence, 100 measurements were found to be sufficient for each time instant, in order to generate a stable velocity vector map.

16.3.3.1 Post-Processing of the Data

16.3.3.1.1 Image Processing

After minimum background subtraction, Gaussian smoothing, intensity normalization, and masking [38], the recorded image pairs were analyzed by a two-frame FFT cross-correlation algorithm (DynamicStudio, Version 2.20.18, Dantec Dynamics, Denmark) with interrogation areas of 32×32 pixel^2, overlapped by 50% on each side, to yield the local displacement vector for each interrogation area [39]. This method provided a total of 7326 velocity vectors for an area of 13×9 mm^2. The validation of the PIV method in relation to the corresponding Womersley solution is provided in Appendix 16B.

16.3.3.1.2 Derivation of WSS

The velocity field obtained by PIV was used to estimate the rate-of-shear ($\dot{\gamma}$) along the wall from the near wall velocity gradient, and thereby the WSS, using Equation 16.7:

$$WSS = \mu \frac{du_\xi}{d\eta} \tag{16.7}$$

where
   μ is the dynamic viscosity of the blood analogue
   u_ξ is the component of the velocity vector tangential to the wall
   η is the direction normal to the wall

The ξ–η coordinate system was utilized for ease of calculation and presentation of the results. As shown in Figure 16.10, the origins of coordinates ξ_1–ξ_3 were chosen on the heel, toe, and artery bed of the anastomosis, respectively.

A computer code, developed in-house, was utilized to interpolate the near-wall velocities within the viscous boundary layer based on the finite element shape functions [40]. Briefly, the discrete pixel wall location for each data set was extracted (no wall movement was detected in this study); by marching on these wall points (Figure 16.10), the slope of each wall section, located between two neighboring wall points, was calculated. Then, on the perpendicular bisector of each wall section, two points with an increment of 0.13 mm (16 pixels) between the subsequent points were located within the flow boundary layer, and the tangential components of the velocity vectors (with respect to the corresponding wall section) were interpolated at these points based on the three nearest adjacent velocity vectors, using finite element shape functions. Subsequently, velocity gradients were calculated from a surface fit of the velocity by using generalized multiquadratic radial basis functions, optimized to minimize the surface roughness of the resultant fit [41], assuming

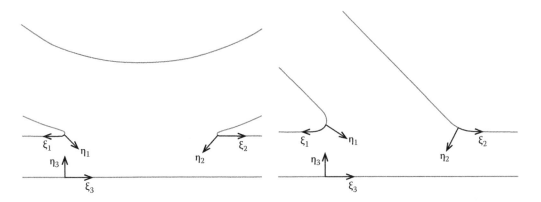

FIGURE 16.10
The origin and direction of ξ–η coordinate system at (1) heel, (2) toe, and (3) artery bed of the STS and ETS anastomoses. (From Kabinejadian, F. et al., *Med. Eng. Phys.*, 36, 1233, 2014.)

no-slip condition at the wall. Appendix 16C provides the validation of the WSS estimation method in relation to the corresponding analytically calculated WSS values obtained from the Womersley solution.

16.3.4 Comparison of the Velocity Profiles in the Anastomotic Region of the Models

The velocity field in the symmetry plane was measured at the anastomotic region of the models, as shown in Figures 16.11 through 16.16, correspondingly, for the six instants of time, t_2, t_3, t_5, t_6, t_{11}, and t_{12}. Therein, the STS and ETS components of the novel SQA design, parallel STS, and conventional ETS models are labeled as (a), (b), (c), and (d), respectively.

For the purpose of visualization, the velocity fields obtained by a lower resolution (interrogation area of 64×64 pixel^2) are shown in Figures 16.11 through 16.16. However, for calculation of WSS, the velocity fields of a higher resolution (interrogation area of 32×32 pixel^2) were used, in order to attain a higher accuracy.

16.3.4.1 Acceleration Phase

During the systolic mid-acceleration (t_2) and at the peak flow rate (t_3) in the conventional ETS anastomosis model, a vortex was formed at the heel region within the coronary artery, with a stagnation point on the artery floor at $\xi_3 = 0.5$ and $\xi_3 = 1.5$ mm, respectively, due to the graft flow impacting the artery bed, as shown in Figures 16.11d and 16.12d, correspondingly. However, in the novel SQA graft design model, the flow at the distal ETS anastomosis (Figures 16.11b and 16.12b) was very smooth without any vortex formation. There was no impingement on the artery floor, because the partial flow from the STS anastomosis along the coronary artery changed the velocity components of the ETS anastomosis flow toward the axis of the coronary artery rather than to the artery floor. This resulted in having no stagnation point formed on the bed, which is a positive feature of the SQA design, as a stagnation point is associated with low-magnitude high-oscillatory WSS condition on the artery bed which is prone to enhancement of atherogenesis [42] and IH formation [43].

At the STS anastomosis of the novel SQA model (Figures 16.11a and 16.12a), a vortex was formed at the heel region along with a stagnation point on the artery bed. This was consistent with the flow field in the parallel STS anastomosis model (Figures 16.11c and 16.12c).

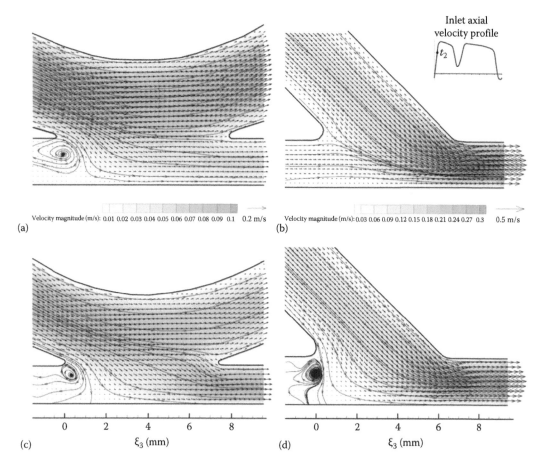

FIGURE 16.11
Measured flow field and velocity vectors in the anastomotic region of the models at systolic mid-acceleration (time t_2): (a) STS component of the SQA model, (b) ETS component of the SQA model, (c) parallel STS model, and (d) conventional ETS model. Note that there is a vortex in the heel region of the conventional ETS model. However, in the ETS component of the SQA model, the flow is smooth without any vortex formation. (From Kabinejadian, F. et al., *Med. Eng. Phys.*, 36, 1233, 2014.)

16.3.4.2 Deceleration and Reversed Flow Phases

During the systolic mid-deceleration phase (t_5), the vortex at the heel region of the parallel STS model was increased in size (relative to that at the peak flow rate) and was stretched toward the center of the anastomosis, as demonstrated in Figure 16.13c; however, there was only a mild vortex on the artery floor at the STS component of the SQA model, as shown in Figure 16.13a.

At time t_6, the fluid at the ETS anastomosis of the SQA model bifurcated into the distal part and into the proximal segment of the coronary artery toward the STS component (Figure 16.14b). This backflow (from the ETS component through the coronary artery) was so strong that not only did it prevent the fluid flow from the graft into the coronary artery at the STS anastomosis of the SQA model, but also some fluid flowed from the coronary artery back into the graft toward the ETS anastomosis, located downstream, as demonstrated in Figure 16.14a. In the parallel STS model, illustrated in Figure 16.14c,

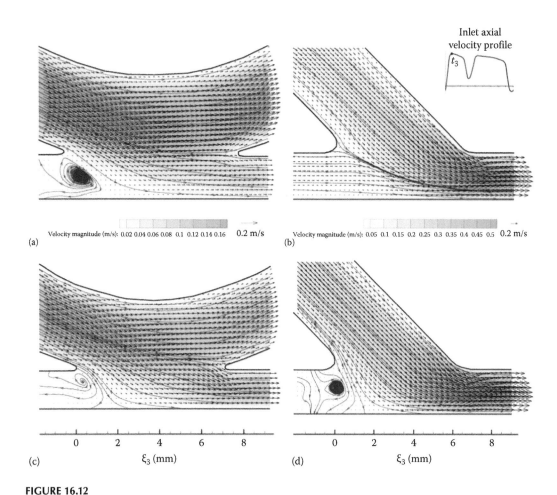

FIGURE 16.12
Measured flow field and velocity vectors in the anastomotic region of the models at the peak flow rate (time t_3): (a) STS component of the SQA model, (b) ETS component of the SQA model, (c) parallel STS model, and (d) conventional ETS model. Again, a vortex is present in the heel region of the conventional ETS model with the blood flow impacting the artery bed, whereas the flow at the ETS component of the SQA model is smooth and devoid of any vortex or impact on the artery floor. (From Kabinejadian, F. et al., *Med. Eng. Phys.*, 36, 1233, 2014.)

the vortex at the heel of the anastomosis further increased in size and covered about 70% of the anastomosis (along with a stagnation point on the arterial bed at $\xi_3 = 6$ mm), with the fluid flowing from the graft into the coronary artery. Comparison of the STS anastomosis of the novel SQA design (Figure 16.14a) with the parallel STS anastomosis (Figure 16.14c) demonstrated that in the novel SQA design the backflow from the ETS component into the coronary artery wiped out the vortex at the STS anastomosis, and thereby eliminated the stagnation point on the artery bed. This indicates a higher WSS on the artery bed and lower particle residence time in the SQA model than those in the parallel STS model. It is to be noted that enhanced particle residence time may alter the mass transport of atherogenic substances to the vessel wall and increase the probability of deposition of platelets and macrophages, resulting in intimal thickening.

The flow fields during the diastolic acceleration and deceleration phases were similar to those of corresponding systolic phases; hence, for brevity, they are not presented here.

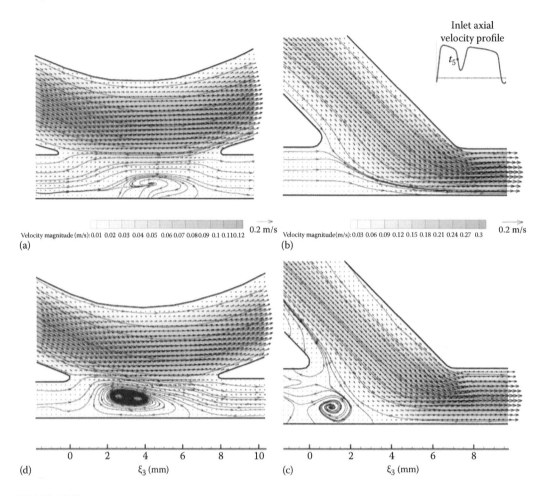

FIGURE 16.13
Measured flow field and velocity vectors in the anastomotic region of the models at systolic mid-deceleration (time t_5): (a) STS component of the SQA model, (b) ETS component of the SQA model, (c) parallel STS model, and (d) conventional ETS model. Note the weak vortex in the STS component of the SQA design model versus the large vortex in the parallel STS model. (From Kabinejadian, F. et al., *Med. Eng. Phys.*, 36, 1233, 2014.)

As the net flow rate just became negative at t_{11}, large vortices and recirculation areas appeared in all the models. At the ETS anastomosis of the SQA model, a vortex formed at the graft inner wall, upstream of the distal anastomosis, as shown in Figure 16.15b. However, in the conventional ETS anastomosis (Figure 16.15d), the vortex was much larger in size, and occupied most of the anastomotic region and two-thirds of the graft near the inner wall. In the parallel STS anastomosis model (Figure 16.15c), a large vortex occupied the entire anastomosis region. On the other hand, in the STS anastomosis of the SQA model, the vortex was almost negligent and was shifted over the toe of the anastomosis, as illustrated in Figure 16.15a. This was due to the fluid flow circulation within the vascular loop of the SQA model, which eliminated the stagnation point on the artery bed.

At the peak reversed flow (t_{12}), in the ETS anastomosis of the SQA design (unlike the conventional ETS model) at the heel there was no fluid trapped in the coronary artery.

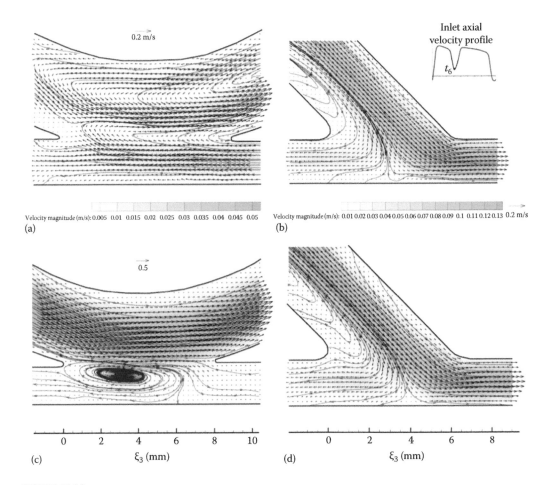

FIGURE 16.14
Measured flow field and velocity vectors in the anastomotic region of the models at time t_6: (a) STS component of the SQA model, (b) ETS component of the SQA model, (c) parallel STS model, and (d) conventional ETS model. There is a large vortex in the parallel STS model. However, in the SQA design model, the backflow into the coronary artery from the ETS component emerges into the STS component and eliminates the possibility of vortex formation. (From Kabinejadian, F. et al., *Med. Eng. Phys.*, 36, 1233, 2014.)

However, a stagnation point formed at the heel region ($\xi_1 = 0$ mm) where the backward flow bifurcated into the graft and the coronary artery, as shown in Figure 16.16b.

16.3.5 Comparison of the WSS Distribution in the Anastomotic Region of the Models

The local WSS was evaluated at the heel, toe, and coronary artery bed of the anastomosis in all the models at the six time instants, as shown in Figures 16.17 through 16.20, wherein the WSS distributions at the heel, toe, and artery bed of the anastomosis are shown, respectively, in panels (a)–(c).

16.3.5.1 WSS Distribution in the Heel Region of the ETS Anastomoses

Comparison of the WSS distribution in the heel region of the ETS component of the SQA design with that of the conventional ETS model (Figures 16.17a and 16.18a) indicated

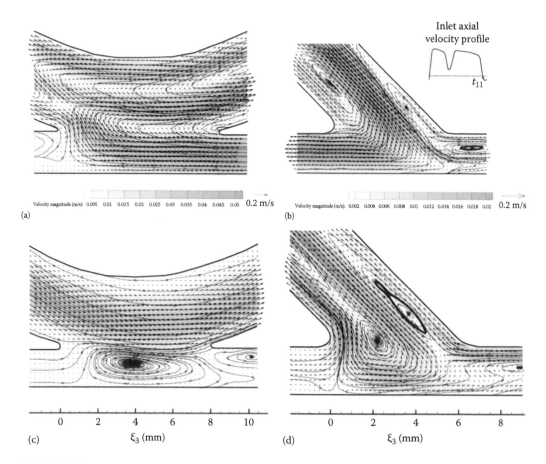

FIGURE 16.15
Measured flow field and velocity vectors in the anastomotic region of the models at time t_{11}, when the graft average velocity has just become negative: (a) STS component of the SQA model, (b) ETS component of the SQA model, (c) parallel STS model, and (d) conventional ETS model. There are remarkably larger vortices in the conventional ETS and parallel STS models, compared to those in the corresponding ETS and STS components of the SQA design model. (From Kabinejadian, F. et al., *Med. Eng. Phys.*, 36, 1233, 2014.).

that the peak value of WSS was slightly reduced on the graft inner wall ($\xi_1 < 0$ mm) of the SQA design as compared to the conventional ETS model (for instance from 3 to 2 Pa at t_3). This was due to the lower flow rate passing through the graft toward ETS anastomosis in the novel design compared to the conventional ETS model, since part of the flow was diverted into the coronary artery at the STS anastomosis of the SQA design. However, the WSS at the heel of the ETS anastomosis of the SQA model within the coronary artery ($\xi_1 > 0$ mm) was considerably increased in magnitude compared to the conventional ETS model. This was because in the conventional ETS model, the blood was almost stagnant in the proximal segment of the coronary artery, while in the novel SQA design model the partial flow from the STS component through the coronary artery increased the magnitude of WSS at this location (note that the change in the sign of the WSS is due to the definition of the coordinate system and the location of the origin at the heel region of the models with respect to the flow directions). It is to be noted that a number of studies have indicated a strong relationship between the

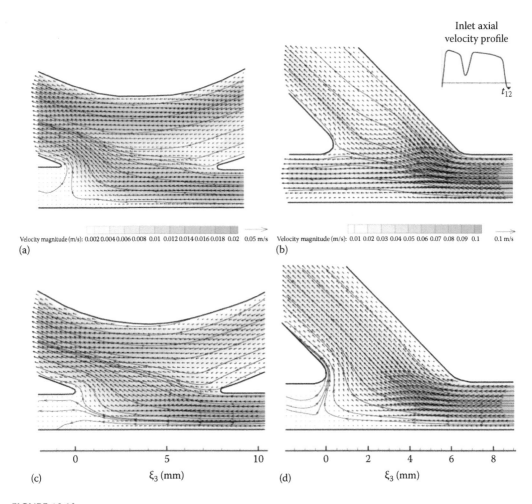

Inlet axial
velocity profile

t_{12}

Velocity magnitude (m/s): 0.002 0.004 0.006 0.008 0.01 0.012 0.014 0.016 0.018 0.02   0.05 m/s
(a)

Velocity magnitude (m/s): 0.01 0.02 0.03 0.04 0.05 0.06 0.07 0.08 0.09 0.1   0.1 m/s
(b)

0   5   10
(c) ξ_3 (mm)

0   2   4   6   8
(d) ξ_3 (mm)

FIGURE 16.16
Measured flow field and velocity vectors in the anastomotic region of the models at the peak reversed flow (time t_{12}): (a) STS component of the SQA model, (b) ETS component of the SQA model, (c) parallel STS model, and (d) conventional ETS model. There is a stagnation point at the heel of the ETS anastomosis of the SQA model where the backward flow bifurcates between the graft and the coronary artery. (From Kabinejadian, F. et al., *Med. Eng. Phys.*, 36, 1233, 2014.)

localized distribution of low-WSS and IT development; as a result, this increase of WSS magnitude at the heel of the ETS anastomosis is a positive feature of the SQA design.

16.3.5.2 WSS Distribution in the Toe Region of the ETS Anastomoses

At the toe of the ETS anastomosis of the SQA model and the conventional ETS model, the qualitative distribution of WSS was similar, as shown in Figures 16.17b and 16.18b. There was a sharp increase in the WSS magnitude to its peak at the toe, and then a rapid drop to form an apex, continued by a slow increase to an asymptotic value further downstream along the toe within the coronary artery mainly during the forward flow phases. The peak value of the WSS at the toe during the peak flow rate (t_3) was higher in the conventional ETS model (44 Pa) than that in the ETS component of the SQA model (34 Pa).

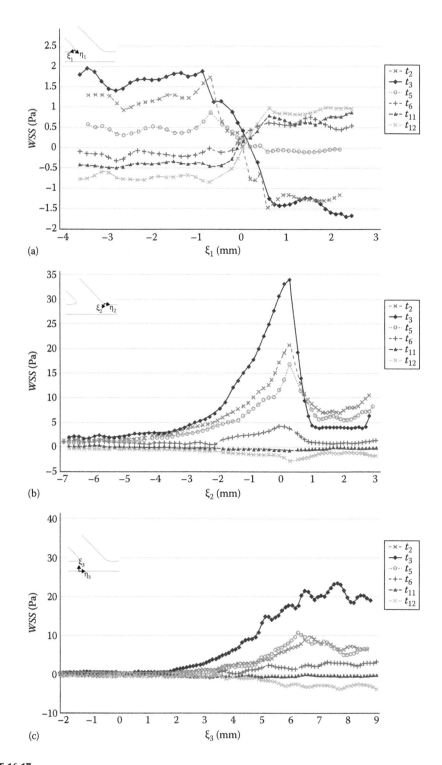

FIGURE 16.17
WSS distribution in the ETS component of the SQA model, along the (a) heel, (b) toe, and (c) artery bed. (From Kabinejadian, F. et al., *Med. Eng. Phys.*, 36, 1233, 2014.)

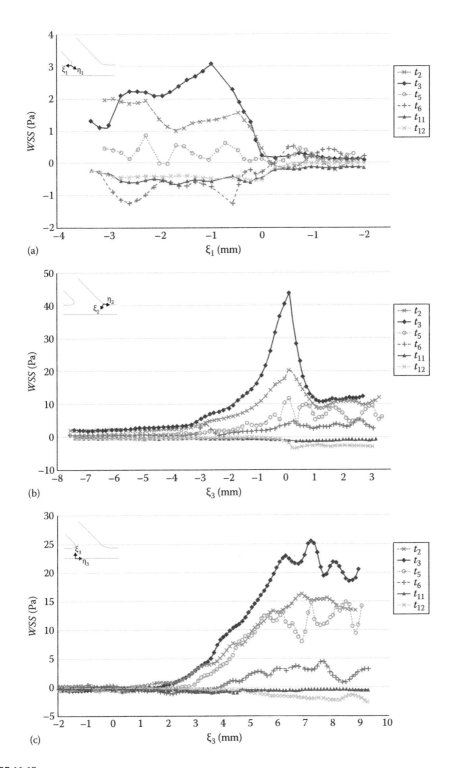

FIGURE 16.18
WSS distribution in the conventional ETS model, along the (a) heel, (b) toe, and (c) artery bed. (From Kabinejadian, F. et al., *Med. Eng. Phys.*, 36, 1233, 2014.)

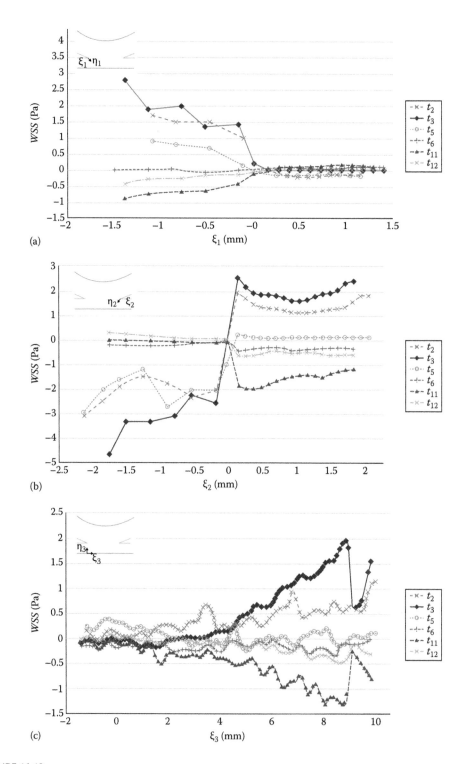

FIGURE 16.19
WSS distribution in the STS component of the SQA model, along the (a) heel, (b) toe, and (c) artery bed. (From Kabinejadian, F. et al., *Med. Eng. Phys.*, 36, 1233, 2014.)

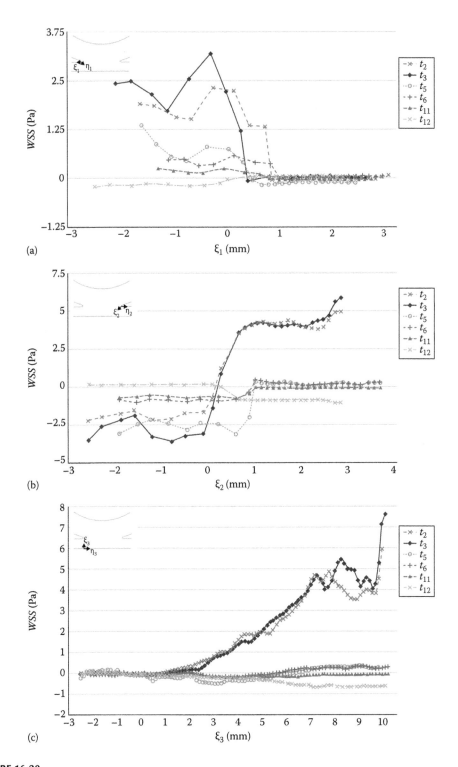

FIGURE 16.20
WSS distribution in the parallel STS model, along the (a) heel, (b) toe, and (c) artery bed. (From Kabinejadian, F. et al., *Med. Eng. Phys.*, 36, 1233, 2014.)

This represents a more moderate distribution of WSS (with lower spatial and temporal gradients) at the toe of the ETS component of the SQA model, which may reduce the probability of atherosclerotic lesion development, since it has been postulated that the progress of atherosclerotic lesions and growth of plaque formation occurs mainly in regions of extreme (either maxima or minima) WSS [20,21].

16.3.5.3 WSS Distribution on the Coronary Artery Bed of the ETS Anastomoses

On the coronary artery bed opposite to the heel of the ETS anastomosis ($-2 \leq \xi_3 \leq 3$ mm), the WSS was slightly higher in magnitude in the SQA model than that in the conventional ETS model, as shown in Figures 16.17c and 16.18c, respectively. This is due to the fluid flowing through the coronary artery segment between the two anastomoses of the novel SQA model (contrasted with the flow circulation in the conventional ETS model). This moderate increase in the WSS magnitude, conjugated by the absence of the stagnation point on the artery bed in the ETS anastomosis of the SQA model (as mentioned earlier) can reduce the risk of IT and atherosclerosis development at this critical location. On moving downstream along the artery bed, the WSS magnitude increased, reaching its peak value opposite to the toe of the ETS anastomosis as shown in Figures 16.17c and 16.18c, and then reduced to an asymptotic value in both models (not shown here). These values of WSS at the downstream of the artery bed in the ETS anastomosis of the conventional ETS model ($\xi_3 \geq 6.5$ mm) were higher than those along the toe of the anastomosis within the coronary artery ($\xi_2 \geq 1$ mm in Figures 16.17b and 16.18b) during the forward flow phases, indicating that the velocity profile was skewed toward the artery floor, inducing larger velocity gradients on the floor side. However, this phenomenon was less pronounced in the SQA model (Figure 16.17) than in the conventional ETS model (Figure 16.18), due to the partial flow from the coronary artery changing the direction of the graft flow toward the coronary artery axis and reducing the velocity profile skew toward the artery bed at the ETS component (as shown earlier in Figure 16.12).

16.3.5.4 WSS Distribution in the Heel Region of the STS Anastomoses

Upon comparing the distribution of WSS in the STS anastomosis of the SQA model and the parallel STS model, shown in Figures 16.19a and 16.20a, respectively, the qualitative distribution of the WSS was mostly similar in the heel region of the STS anastomosis of the two models. However, at time t_{11} the WSS in the graft over the heel region ($\xi_1 \leq 0$) was positive (with respect to ξ_1 coordinate at the heel, shown in Figure 16.10) in the parallel STS model, while it had negative values in the STS component of the SQA model. This was consistent with the opposing flow directions over the heel region in the two models at this time instant (as shown in Figure 16.15).

16.3.5.5 WSS Distribution in the Toe Region of the STS Anastomoses

At the toe of the STS anastomosis of the two models, the distribution of WSS was about the same. However, at times t_6 and t_{11}, the magnitude of WSS on the graft and the coronary artery walls had different distributions in the two models, as demonstrated in Figures 16.19b and 16.20b. In the STS component of the novel SQA model, due to the strong backflow through the coronary artery at these time instants, the WSS magnitude was higher on the coronary artery wall at the toe of the anastomosis ($\xi_2 \geq 0$) than on the graft wall at the toe ($\xi_2 \leq 0$), where a small recirculation zone resulted in a low WSS magnitude at time t_{11} (as shown in Figure 16.15). However, in the parallel STS model, owing to the large vortices within the coronary artery, the WSS magnitude was lower on the artery wall at the toe ($\xi_2 \geq 0$) than on the graft wall ($\xi_2 \leq 0$) on account of the higher flow rate in the graft (than in the coronary artery).

16.3.5.6 *WSS Distribution on the Coronary Artery Bed of the STS Anastomoses*

On the coronary artery bed, during the acceleration phase and the peak flow, the magnitude of WSS was higher in the parallel STS model than that in the STS anastomosis of the SQA model (e.g., 5 versus 2 Pa at $\xi_3 = 8.8$ mm at time t_3), as shown in Figures 16.20c and 16.19c, respectively. During the deceleration phase (t_5), in the parallel STS model (Figure 16.20c), the WSS magnitude was generally low, with a region of negative values at the middle of the bed opposite to the anastomosis junction ($-0.9 \leq \xi_3 \leq 6.2$ mm), indicating that the shear was directed proximally. This was due to the large vortex, formed in the coronary artery at this time instant (see Figure 16.13). The zero value of WSS at point $\xi_3 = 6.2$ mm corresponded to the stagnation point, created just distal to the vortex. However, in the STS anastomosis of the SQA model (Figure 16.19c) at this time (t_5), the results showed fluctuations in the WSS values on the artery bed. This could possibly be due to the inaccuracy inducted into the PIV results, caused by scattering of the laser light sheet due to the unevenness of the inner surfaces of this fabricated model at this particular region. Another possible reason for this inaccuracy can be the accumulation of some seeding particles in this low-velocity region, which would induce errors into the velocity measurement, and consequently, the WSS calculation. These oscillations also resulted in fluctuations in the sign of WSS, due to the very small (nearly zero) velocity magnitude at this time (t_5). Some fluctuations in the magnitude of WSS could also be observed in this model at other time instants. At time t_{11}, the WSS magnitude on the artery bed of the parallel STS model (Figure 16.20c) was much lower than that in the STS anastomosis of the novel SQA model (Figure 16.19c), due to the recirculation zones and low velocity regions created within the coronary artery in the parallel STS model (as shown in Figure 16.15c). However, during the backflow phase (t_{12}), both models showed similar WSS distributions.

The presented PIV measurements and calculated WSS distributions complement the computational modeling of the blood flow through this novel CSABG design, from which more complex HPs have been derived to quantify hemodynamics in the novel CSABG design models with a variety of the design parameters. In the following section, the effects of the vessel wall compliance and non-Newtonian rheology of blood on the distribution of HPs in the CSABG design are presented.

16.4 CSABG Design Model Incorporating Vessel Wall Elasticity and Non-Newtonian Rheology: Analysis for Blood Flow Regime and Hemodynamic Parameters Distribution

In the earlier described computational simulations of blood flow of the CSABG design, the graft and the artery were adopted to be rigid vessels and the blood was assumed to be a Newtonian fluid. However, the arterial wall is a viscoelastic deformable tissue, and

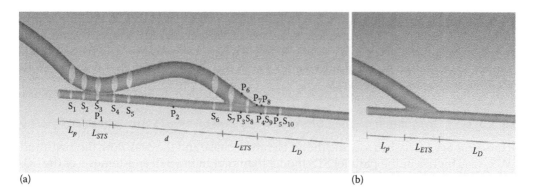

FIGURE 16.21
(a) Coupled STS–ETS sequential anastomoses model. S_1–S_{10} and P_1–P_7 indicate, respectively, the cross sections and the points at which velocity profiles and WSS variations are discussed and (b) conventional ETS anastomosis model. (From Kabinejadian, F. and Ghista, D.N., *Med. Eng. Phys.*, 34, 860, 2012.)

its deformation interacts with the pulsatile blood flow. As a result of this interaction, hemodynamic factors of the blood flow are influenced by the mechanical behavior of the wall, and the dynamic properties of the wall are affected by the transient behavior of the blood flow. Hence, in order to (1) investigate the effects of wall compliance and non-Newtonian rheology on the local flow field and HPs distribution, and (2) verify the advantages of the CSABG design over the conventional ETS configuration in a more realistic bio-mechanical condition, a two-way fluid–structure interaction (FSI) analysis has been carried out.

In this study, the superior CSABG model (with the anastomotic angle of 30° and 30 mm distance between the two [STS and ETS] anastomoses) and its corresponding conventional ETS model, shown in Figure 16.21, are utilized to verify the previously observed advantages of this novel CSABG design over the conventional ETS configuration in a more realistic bio-mechanical condition. For this purpose, the transient wall equations and the flow equations are solved in an implicitly coupled approach, using an iterative procedure.

16.4.1 Blood Flow Simulation by Fluid–Structure Interaction (FSI): Computational Models and Boundary Conditions

A two-way (bi-directional) FSI simulation of blood flow in compliant-wall CABG models is conducted using the commercial computational software ANSYS Workbench (ANSYS Inc.) for the coupling of the finite-element-based software, ANSYS, with the finite-volume-based software, ANSYS CFX. Therein, the calculated displacements of the solid (vessel) structure are transferred to the boundary walls of the fluid domain, and the computed forces in CFX are sent back to the solid domain during each stagger (coupling) iteration.

16.4.1.1 Vessel Wall Model

Blood vessels experience large strain in vivo, particularly near branches and graft artery junctions [45]. However, as the focus of this investigation is on the flow fields and HPs distribution rather than the intramural stress distributions, a small strain (large deformation) approximation of blood vessel mechanics is utilized, as commonly used in other earlier studies [46–48]. The transient structural equilibrium equation is

$$\{F_{(t)}\} = [M]\{\ddot{u}_{(t)}\} + [K]\{u_{(t)}\} \tag{16.8}$$

where
  $\{F\}$ is the load vector
  $[M]$ is the structural mass matrix
  $[K]$ is the structural stiffness matrix
  $\{u\}$ is the nodal displacement vector
  $\{\ddot{u}\}$ is the nodal acceleration vector

The equilibrium equations for the vessel wall structure are solved with stress boundary conditions (the calculated pressure and WSS values from the fluid domain) at the fluid–structure interface and constraint conditions (at the graft inlet and the coronary artery outlet to prevent rigid body motion), in order to estimate the vessel wall displacements.

The vessel walls are assumed to be isotropic, incompressible, and homogeneous with a density of 1060 kg/m³ [49], and modeled as a linearly elastic, geometrically nonlinear shell structure [50,51]. Poisson's ratio is regarded as $v \approx 0.5$ to express the incompressibility of the isotropic vessel wall material.

The stiffness of venous walls is highly nonlinear, exhibiting an increasing elastic modulus for higher strains. At low (venous) pressures, veins have a lower stiffness than arteries; however, at arterial pressures, the stiffness of arterialized vein grafts increases to a level even higher than that of arteries. Wesly et al. [52] have measured the incremental elastic moduli (Young's modulus) of human SV in both longitudinal and circumferential directions at different transmural pressures. As the vessels are strongly restricted in the axial direction under in vivo conditions [53], the value of circumferential elastic modulus at a mean physiologic transmural arterial wall pressure of 100 mmHg, is interpolated (to be $E_\theta = 2.2$ MPa) in this study, and used as Young's modulus for the isotropic graft wall material. Also, as the arterial wall stiffness is increased in atherosclerotic arteries and in this study we are not investigating the effects of compliance mismatch, the same value of elastic modulus is employed for the arterial wall too.

The wall thickness of human LAD coronary artery has been measured in atherosclerotic patients both by high-frequency, 2D transthoracic echocardiography (to be $t = 1.9 \pm 0.3$ mm) and by high-frequency epicardial echocardiography (to be $t = 1.8 \pm 0.2$ mm) [54]. Further, it has been demonstrated that autogenous veins undergo medial thickening when used as arterial bypass grafts [55]. Accordingly, the wall thickness of both the graft and artery is taken to be 2 mm in this investigation.

16.4.1.2 Blood Flow Model

Blood flow through the CABG is assumed to be a 3D, time-dependent, incompressible, isothermal, and laminar flow. In distensible models, the modified equations of motion for fluid mechanics computations (with corrected convective velocity due to moving boundaries [56]), which are obtained by applying the Leibnitz Rule on the integral conservation equations [57], are as follows.

$$\frac{d}{dt}\int_{V(t)} \rho dV + \int_S \rho(U_j - W_j)dn_j = 0 \tag{16.9}$$

$$\frac{d}{dt}\int_{V(t)} \rho U_i dV + \int_S \rho(U_j - W_j)U_i dn_j = -\int_S P dn_i + \int_S \eta\left(\frac{\partial U_i}{\partial x_j} + \frac{\partial U_j}{\partial x_i}\right)dn_j \tag{16.10}$$

where
  U_j and W_j are the components of the flow velocity and the velocity of the control volume
    boundary (mesh velocity), respectively
  ρ is density (assumed to be 1050 kg/m³ for blood in this study)
  P is pressure
  η is the dynamic viscosity of the fluid
  V and S denote volume and surface regions of integration, respectively
  dn_j are the differential Cartesian components of the outward normal surface vector

The mesh velocity at an inner point of the flow domain is calculated from the wall movement by a "Displacement Diffusion" mesh motion model, in which the displacements applied on the boundaries are diffused to other mesh points in a way that the relative mesh distribution of the initial mesh is preserved. For instance, as the initial mesh is relatively fine in boundary layers, it remains comparatively fine after the mesh motion model is applied.

To model the shear thinning behavior of blood, the Carreau–Yasuda model [58] is employed as

$$\eta = \eta_\infty + (\eta_0 - \eta_\infty)[1 + (\lambda\dot{\gamma})^a]^{((n-1)/a)} \tag{16.11}$$

where $\dot{\gamma}$ represents a scalar measure of the rate of deformation tensor ($D = [\nabla U + (\nabla U)^T]/2$), defined as

$$\dot{\gamma} = \sqrt{2\mathrm{tr}(D^2)} \tag{16.12}$$

and the other parameters are obtained from the experimental data of a blood analogue by Gijsen et al. [59] to be: $\eta_0 = 22 \times 10^{-3}$ Pa s, $\eta_\infty = 2.2 \times 10^{-3}$ Pa s, $\lambda = 0.11$ s, $a = 0.644$, and $n = 0.392$. In the case of Newtonian flow, the dynamic viscosity of blood is taken to be $\eta = 0.00408$ Pa s.

A fully developed pulsatile flow is applied at the graft inlet with the same flow waveform shown earlier in Figure 16.2. The Womersley solution [16] is assumed for the inlet axial velocity profile, which is derived as a fully developed pulsatile flow and implemented as the inlet boundary condition. At the coronary artery outlet, the traction-free outflow boundary condition is applied. Also, the no-slip boundary condition is applied to all the walls.

The governing equations are solved numerically by a finite volume method and the computational fluid dynamic (CFD) software, ANSYS CFX, using a fully implicit second-order backward Euler differencing scheme.

The convergence criterion (a normalized residual, obtained based on the imbalance in the linearized system of discrete equations) is set to 10^{-5} in this study.

The mesh sensitivity is tested on the velocity and WSS, by varying the number of grid cells. The computational domain is considered to be sufficient for this study, when further mesh refinement can only result in less than 2% change in velocity and 1% change in WSS at some examined sections.

The time-step size is taken to be 0.01 s, and the results are recorded at the end of each time-step. In order to eliminate the start-up effects of transient flow, the computation is carried out for five periods, and the fifth period results are presented. Validation of this FSI methodology is presented in Appendix 16D.

16.4.2 FSI Results

16.4.2.1 Wall Deformation

The mesh displacement contour in the SQA model at the peak internal pressure during diastole ($t/T = 0.43$) is shown in Figure 16.22. The wall deformation pattern remains

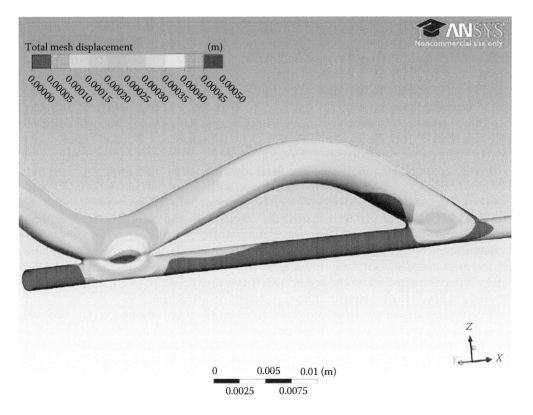

FIGURE 16.22
Mesh displacement contour in the SQA model at the peak pressure ($t/T = 0.43$), with the maximum value occurring at the side walls of the STS anastomosis. The wall deformation pattern remains qualitatively unchanged during the cardiac cycle. (From Kabinejadian, F. and Ghista, D.N., *Med. Eng. Phys.*, 34, 860, 2012.)

qualitatively unchanged during the cardiac cycle. The maximum mesh displacement is about 0.5 mm, occurring at the side walls of the STS anastomosis of the SQA model in the middle of the suture line, where the normal pressure causes the maximum moment (about axes X and Z) on the artery and the graft wall structure, due to the high pressure and long scissor ($L_{STS} = 9$ mm) on the blood vessels at this location. Likewise, at the ETS component of the SQA model and in the conventional ETS model, the maximum displacement occurs on the side walls of the anastomosis, nearer to the heel rather than to the toe.

At the peak internal pressure, the increase in the diameter of the graft and of the coronary artery at locations immediately proximal and distal to the anastomosis of the conventional ETS model is about 0.16, 0.06, and 0.04 mm (equivalent to 4%, 3%, and 2% diameter variation [DV] ratio), respectively. This value increases up to 5% in the coronary artery of the SQA model proximal to the STS anastomosis. Schaar et al. [60] reported up to 2% circumferential strain (equivalent to 2% DV) in human coronary arteries using 3D ultrasound-based intravascular palpography. Zeng et al. [61] measured 15% of maximum temporal cross-sectional area variation averaged along the RCA (which corresponds to about 8% DV) using multi-slice CT. Also, canine elastic arteries have been reported to experience 6%–10% DV over a cardiac cycle driven by the pressure pulse [62,63]. Hence, the calculated diameter variations in the present FSI simulation are comparable to experimental findings.

16.4.2.2 Flow Patterns

The flow patterns in the rigid-wall model have been discussed in detail earlier in this chapter. However, there are substantial differences between certain flow characteristics of the rigid-wall–Newtonian-fluid and compliant-wall–non-Newtonian-fluid models, which are manifested in this section.

Less flow separation is observed in the compliant models. This is consistent with the results of earlier studies; Perktold and Rappitsch [51,64] reported reduction of flow separation at the outer wall of a distensible carotid artery bifurcation model in comparison with the corresponding rigid-wall model. The very advantages that had been observed in the flow fields of the SQA configuration in comparison with that of the conventional ETS anastomosis in the case of rigid-wall model with Newtonian fluid [12] are present in the compliant model as well. For instance, during the acceleration and early deceleration phases, part of the graft flow is diverted into the coronary artery at the STS anastomosis; when this flow in the coronary artery reaches the ETS anastomosis, it lifts up the flow coming from the graft and directs it smoothly into the coronary artery, as shown in Figure 16.23. Thereby, there is no impact on the artery bed; this is an important point, as the impact on the floor is believed to be a contributing factor to the graft failure.

In order to investigate the effect of non-Newtonian rheology of blood on the flow field, the axial velocity profiles at various sections in the symmetry plane of the SQA model at the end of systole (t_6) are demonstrated in Figure 16.24 for both the Newtonian and non-Newtonian fluid models. The axial velocity profile of the non-Newtonian fluid is somewhat flattened due to its shear thinning behavior, and is less skewed toward the outer wall of the graft curvature, as compared to that of the Newtonian fluid, especially at sections S_3, S_4, and S_5 at the STS component (Figure 16.24a) and at section S_6 at the ETS component (Figure 16.24b) of the SQA model.

To exemplify the effect of wall compliance and non-Newtonian rheology of blood on the reversed flow, the axial velocity profile at section S_{10}, located distal to the ETS anastomosis

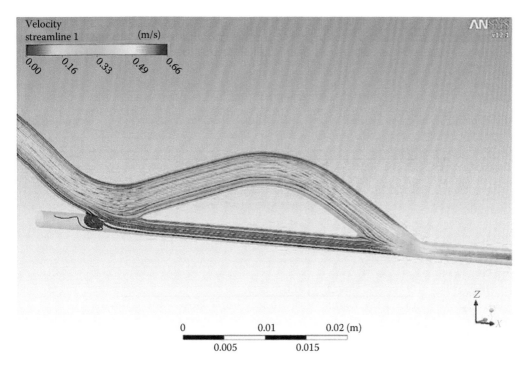

FIGURE 16.23
Flow streamlines in the SQA model at the peak flow rate (t_3). No impact of the flow observed on the artery floor at the ETS anastomosis, as the partial flow from the coronary artery segment located between the two anastomoses changes the velocity components of the graft flow and smoothly directs it into the coronary artery. (From Kabinejadian, F. and Ghista, D.N., *Med. Eng. Phys.*, 34, 860, 2012.)

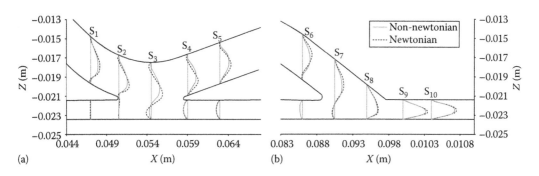

FIGURE 16.24
Axial velocity profiles at various sections in the symmetry plane of the SQA model at the end of systole (t_6) for the non-Newtonian (continuous line) and Newtonian (dashed line) fluid models. (a) STS anastomosis of the SQA model and (b) ETS anastomosis of the SQA model. (From Kabinejadian, F. and Ghista, D.N., *Med. Eng. Phys.*, 34, 860, 2012.)

of the SQA model, at time t_{11}, when the graft net flow rate just becomes negative, is shown in Figure 16.25. Comparison between the Newtonian and non-Newtonian fluid models (in both the rigid and compliant models) demonstrates that the velocity profile of the non-Newtonian fluid is somewhat flattened, due to its shear-thinning behavior. Comparison between the rigid and compliant models (for both the Newtonian and non-Newtonian

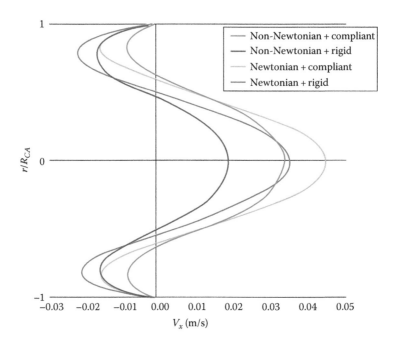

FIGURE 16.25

Axial velocity profiles in different models at section S_{10}, located distal to the ETS anastomosis of the SQA model at time t_{11}, when the graft net flow rate has just become negative. A considerable decrease of the reversed flow is obvious in the distensible model compared to that in the rigid-wall model. (From Kabinejadian, F. and Ghista, D.N., *Med. Eng. Phys.*, 34, 860, 2012.)

fluid models) illustrates a considerable reduction of reversed flow in the distensible model. This is because when the graft flow rate decreases during the deceleration phase, in order to satisfy the fluid's mass conservation in the rigid-wall model, this decrease can be compensated for only by means of reducing the flow velocity. However, in the compliant model, the vessel's contraction partially compensates the flow rate drop by reducing the cross-sectional area; consequently, less flow rate would be left to be compensated for by reducing the velocity. As a result, less reversed flow is present in the distensible-wall models. These results are consistent with those of earlier studies [50,65].

Figure 16.26 shows the secondary flows at two cross sections (S_3 and S_9) in the SQA model for both the Newtonian and non-Newtonian fluid models at the peak flow rate (t_3). At both sections, counter-rotating vortices (Dean vortices) are evident, with nearly symmetric streamlines due to the planarity of the models. At section S_3, the secondary flows are weakened in the case of non-Newtonian fluid as compared to those of Newtonian fluid, which is consistent with the results of earlier studies [65]. However, as the cross-sectional area is reduced at section S_9, the velocity, and consequently, the near-wall shear rates are increased at this section where the flows from the coronary artery and the graft are merged.

Hence, the shear-thinning property of the non-Newtonian fluid reveals an opposing effect on the secondary flows at different locations of this section: the secondary velocity is increased at locations near to the wall; but, it is slightly decreased in the central region as compared to the case of Newtonian fluid model. This is because in the near-wall region of this section at this time instant, the fluid shear rate is higher than the threshold value (calculated to be = 382 s^{-1} in this study), above which the viscosity of the non-Newtonian

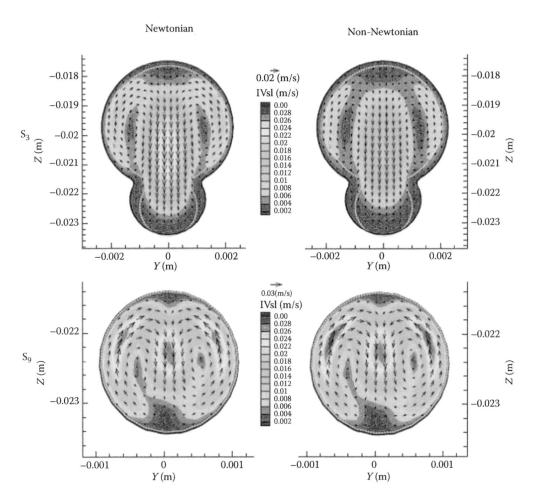

FIGURE 16.26
Secondary flows at two cross sections in the SQA model (S_3 at the middle of the STS anastomosis [upper panel] and S_9 located distal to the ETS anastomosis [lower panel]) for the Newtonian (on the left) and non-Newtonian (on the right) fluid models at the peak flow rate (t_3). The shape of the rigid wall model is shown by dashed lines to illustrate the deformation of the vessel walls. The contours demonstrate the magnitude of the secondary flow, and they have the same scale for both the sections to facilitate the comparison. (From Kabinejadian, F. and Ghista, D.N., *Med. Eng. Phys.*, 34, 860, 2012.)

fluid falls below the constant viscosity of the Newtonian fluid; however, in the central region, the shear rate is below the threshold. In all cases, the secondary flows are weakened along the coronary artery (distal to the ETS anastomosis) owing to the effect of the fluid viscosity.

16.4.2.3 Temporal and Spatial Variations of WSS

The temporal variations of WSS are investigated at some particular points on the vessel wall (P_1–P_8 whose locations are shown in Figure 16.21) throughout the cardiac cycle, and are compared for the non-Newtonian fluid between the rigid and compliant models, as demonstrated in Figure 16.27. Among all the points studied (including those whose graphs are not shown in Figure 16.27), P_7, located at the toe of the ETS anastomosis,

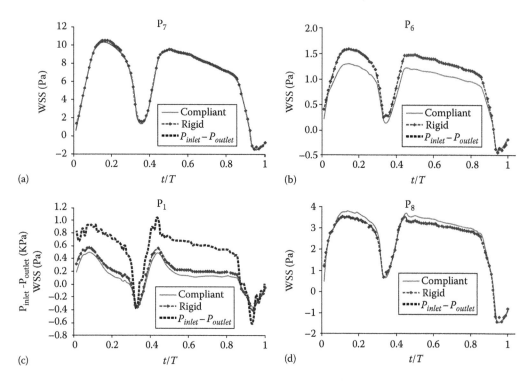

FIGURE 16.27

Temporal variations of WSS throughout the cardiac cycle at various points on the wall. (a) At P_7, located at the toe of the ETS anastomosis, (b) at P_6, located on the graft outer wall proximal to the ETS anastomosis, (c) at P_1, located on the artery bed in the middle of the STS anastomosis, (d) at P_8, located on the ceiling wall of the coronary artery just distal to the toe of the ETS anastomosis. The calculated pressure waveform is shown by dashed line in panel c. (From Kabinejadian, F. and Ghista, D.N., *Med. Eng. Phys.*, 34, 860, 2012.)

shows the minimum disparity between the WSS time-history of the rigid and compliant models where the two graphs are almost identical (Figure 16.27a). On the other hand, P_6, located on the graft outer wall proximal to the ETS anastomosis, demonstrates the most discrepancy with up to 21% increase in the WSS magnitude in the rigid model compared to that of the distensible model (Figure 16.27b), which can be attributable to the higher DV in the graft than in the coronary artery.

The profile of the WSS curves at proximal locations such as P_1 is more analogous to the calculated pressure waveform (see Figure 16.27c), than those at distal locations. The overall shape of the WSS time-history curves is similar between the rigid and distensible models, with the WSS magnitude being generally higher in the rigid-wall model due to its smaller vessel diameter and the consequent higher velocity. However, at point P_8, located on the ceiling wall of the coronary artery just distal to the toe of the ETS anastomosis, the magnitude of the WSS in the compliant model is higher than that in the rigid model (Figure 16.27d), unlike the other points. This is due to the higher flow separation at this point in the rigid-wall model compared to the distensible model, which results in a significant reduction of WSS magnitude, and is in agreement with the aforementioned observations.

Figure 16.28 demonstrates instantaneous WSS distributions along the coronary artery bed of the SQA model for the four cases of the rigid and compliant wall with the Newtonian and non-Newtonian fluid models at four different time points. During the systolic acceleration phase (t_2) as shown in Figure 16.28a, on the artery bed before the middle of the

ETS anastomosis ($x \leq 0.0941$ m), the WSS is higher for the non-Newtonian fluid due to its shear thinning behavior and the low shear rate in this region (in both the rigid and compliant models). However, on the artery bed opposite to the ETS anastomosis and further distal, the shear thinning behavior causes the WSS for the non-Newtonian fluid to become smaller than that for the Newtonian fluid, owing to the high shear rate in this region caused by the flow from the graft merging with that from the coronary artery at the ETS anastomosis. The WSS is somewhat higher in the rigid-wall model than that in the distensible model for both the Newtonian and non-Newtonian fluid models. At this time instant, the shear rate in the segment of the coronary artery located between the two anastomoses, and at the location distal to the ETS anastomosis is, respectively, lower and higher than the aforementioned threshold (above which the viscosity of non-Newtonian

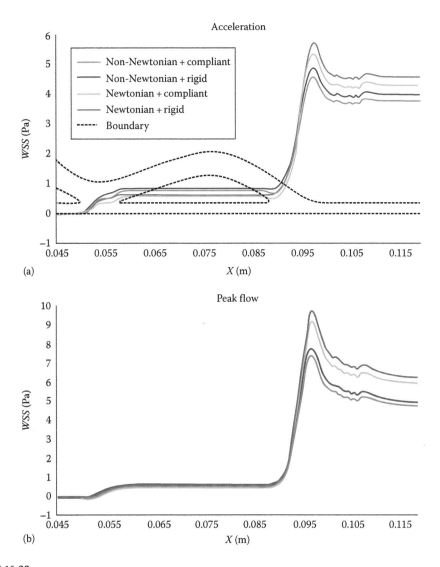

FIGURE 16.28
Instantaneous WSS distributions along the coronary artery bed of the SQA model at different time points. (a) During systolic acceleration phase (t_2), (b) at systolic peak flow (t_3). *(Continued)*

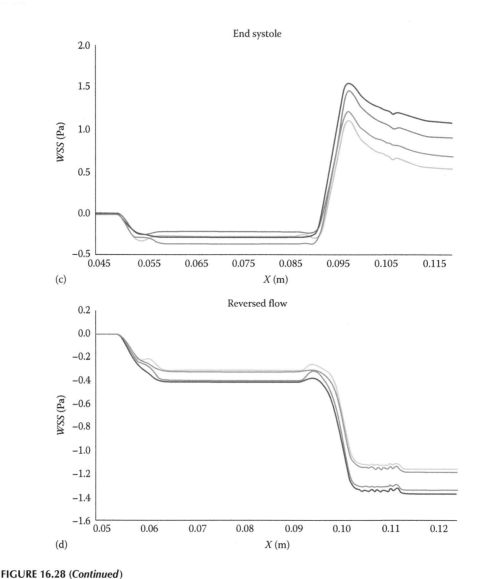

FIGURE 16.28 (*Continued*)
Instantaneous WSS distributions along the coronary artery bed of the SQA model at different time points.
(c) End of systole (t_6), (d) at peak reversed flow (t_{12}). The shape of the vessel walls is shown by dashed line in panel (a). (From Kabinejadian, F. and Ghista, D.N., *Med. Eng. Phys.*, 34, 860, 2012.)

fluid becomes lower than that of the Newtonian fluid). Therefore, as the flow rate increases to its peak value (t_3), the difference between the WSS magnitudes for the Newtonian and non-Newtonian fluids decreases in the coronary artery segment between the two anastomoses, while it increases in the coronary artery segment distal to the ETS anastomosis, as shown in Figure 16.28b. Nevertheless, the qualitative distribution of WSS on the artery bed at the peak flow rate is similar to that during the acceleration phase, with the peak value occurring opposite to the toe of the ETS anastomosis.

Figure 16.28c demonstrates the WSS distribution on the artery bed at the end of systole (t_6). The magnitude of the WSS for the non-Newtonian fluid is generally higher than that for the Newtonian fluid in both the compliant and rigid-wall models, as a result of the low shear rate at this time instant (negative values of WSS indicate reversed flow). At locations distal to the ETS anastomosis, the WSS magnitude in the rigid-wall model is higher than that in the compliant model for both Newtonian and non-Newtonian fluids. However, in the coronary artery segment located between the two anastomoses, the WSS magnitude in the distensible model is higher than that in the rigid model. This is because at this moment (late systolic deceleration), the low pressure results in the coronary artery contraction and reduction of the vessel diameter (to a value even smaller than that of the rigid model in this segment), and consequently, an increase in the WSS magnitude. The same phenomenon occurs in the late diastole too (not shown here). This is in agreement with the results of earlier FSI simulation studies of the blood flow in the right coronary artery reported by Zeng et al. [61] and Torii et al. [66]. Also, similar result can be observed in an ETS anastomosis FSI study by Hofer et al. [50], albeit this aspect (the opposing effect of wall distensibility on WSS distribution) has not been pointed out.

At the peak reversed flow (t_{12}), the WSS magnitude for the non-Newtonian fluid is considerably higher than that for the Newtonian fluid along the artery bed in both the rigid and distensible models, due to the low shear rate at this time instant, as shown in Figure 16.28d. Also, the WSS magnitude is slightly higher in the rigid-wall model than in the compliant model.

16.4.2.4 *Hemodynamic Parameters Distribution*

In order to investigate the effect of wall distensibility and non-Newtonian rheology on the distribution of HPs at the critical sites of the anastomosis, namely, toe, heel, bed, and the suture line (shown earlier in Figure 16.5), the segmental averages of the HPs, including TAWSS, nondimensional time-averaged WSS gradient (TAWSSG) [22], and oscillatory shear index (OSI), are calculated and presented in Table 16.4. The following features can be inferred from the tabulated results.

TAWSS: Comparison of the TAWSS between the rigid and compliant models (both for the Newtonian and non-Newtonian fluid models) demonstrates a decrease in the TAWSS at all critical locations in the compliant model, which ranges between 3% (on the suture line) and 32% (on the heel) in the conventional ETS model, and from 4% (at the toe of the STS anastomosis) to 27% (on the suture line of the STS anastomosis) in the SQA model. This is consistent with the results of earlier studies reporting that wall motion reduces the mean WSS in a straight elastic tube model [67], and in an elastic abdominal aortic bifurcation model [68].

Upon comparing the TAWSS between the Newtonian and non-Newtonian fluid models (in both compliant and rigid-wall models), it is seen that at the ETS anastomosis (of both the conventional and SQA models) in the case of non-Newtonian fluid, the TAWSS is decreased at the toe, suture line, and on the bed, while it is increased at the heel. On the other hand, at the STS anastomosis, the TAWSS is increased at all the critical locations. This reduction at the ETS anastomosis and increase at the STS anastomosis are due to the shear thinning behavior of the non-Newtonian fluid, as the shear rate is generally high at the ETS anastomosis (except at the heel) while it is low at the STS anastomosis.

TAWSSG: Comparison of the TAWSSG between the rigid and compliant models (both for the Newtonian and non-Newtonian fluid models) indicates that the TAWSSG is generally decreased in compliant models at the ETS anastomosis of both the

TABLE 16.4

Comparison of the Segmental Averages of <HP>s

Wall model:								Rigid[a]								Distensible[a]					
Fluid model:			Newtonian[b]			Non-Newtonian[b]				Newtonian[b]			Non-Newtonian[b]		
Anastomosis model		Location	<OSI>	<TAWSS> (Pa)	<TAWSSG>	<OSI>	<TAWSS> (Pa)	<TAWSSG>	<OSI>	<TAWSS> (Pa)	<TAWSSG>	<OSI>	<TAWSS> (Pa)	<TAWSSG>
Conventional ETS model		1—Toe	0.01	6.69	34.02	0.01	5.65	28.47	0.01	6.14	31.00	0.02	5.23	26.34
		2—Heel	0.09	0.56	8.29	0.07	0.71	9.57	0.11	0.38	6.10	0.09	0.52	7.97
		3—Bed	0.09	1.67	5.46	0.08	1.55	4.64	0.11	1.47	5.01	0.09	1.40	4.29
		4—Suture line	0.04	2.12	15.09	0.04	2.06	14.94	0.05	2.05	13.30	0.04	1.99	13.66
Coupled sequential anastomoses model	ETS component	1—Toe	0.01	6.33	36.95	0.02	5.36	31.23	0.01	5.85	29.71	0.02	5.01	25.24
		2—Heel	0.08	0.49	4.39	0.07	0.69	6.26	0.08	0.40	3.52	0.07	0.61	5.50
		3—Bed	0.05	1.86	4.93	0.05	1.76	4.05	0.06	1.76	5.02	0.06	1.59	3.88
		4—Suture line	0.03	2.51	15.12	0.03	2.39	15.00	0.03	2.10	11.44	0.04	2.05	11.61
	STS component	5—Toe-STS	0.04	0.70	6.03	0.05	0.80	6.00	0.04	0.67	7.32	0.05	0.77	7.44
		6—Heel-STS	0.08	0.41	4.42	0.08	0.54	5.38	0.09	0.32	3.44	0.07	0.45	4.89
		7—Bed-STS	0.22	0.17	0.40	0.18	0.25	0.50	0.24	0.15	0.45	0.18	0.22	0.55
		8—Suture line-STS	0.05	0.65	5.94	0.05	0.80	6.54	0.05	0.47	5.37	0.05	0.62	6.39

[a] Wall model.
[b] Fluid model.

conventional and SQA models (except on the artery bed of ETS anastomosis of SQA model in the case of Newtonian fluid). At the STS anastomosis of the SQA model, the TAWSSG is decreased at the heel and on the suture line, while it is increased at the toe and on the artery bed of the distensible models.

Comparison of the TAWSSG between the Newtonian and non-Newtonian fluid models (in both compliant and rigid-wall models) demonstrates that the TAWSSG at the ETS anastomosis (of both the conventional and SQA models) is reduced at the toe and on the artery bed, while it is increased at the heel, and is negligibly (<3%) changed on the suture line in the case of the non-Newtonian fluid model. At the STS anastomosis, the TAWSSG is increased on the artery bed, suture line, and at the heel, while it experienced less than 2% change at the toe in the case of non-Newtonian fluid.

OSI: As shown in Table 16.4, the wall compliance somewhat increases the OSI in all the models, albeit the OSI value is generally low due to the waveform having mostly a forward flow during the cardiac cycle. The non-Newtonian rheology has an opposing effect on the OSI, in accordance with the shear thinning behavior. At locations with high shear rate where the shear thinning effect reduces the fluid viscosity and facilitates the oscillation of the flow (such as at the toe of the anastomosis), the OSI is increased in the case of non-Newtonian fluid model. Conversely, at locations with low shear rate where the shear thinning effect increases the fluid viscosity and impedes the flow oscillation (for instance at the heel and on the artery bed), the non-Newtonian rheology reduces the OSI. This effect is mostly pronounced on the artery bed at the STS anastomosis of the SQA model, where the OSI is reduced from 0.24 to 0.18 in the distensible model and from 0.22 to 0.18 in the rigid-wall model.

The OSI is slightly lower at the heel and on the artery bed of the ETS anastomosis of the SQA model, than in the conventional ETS anastomosis. Moreover, the OSI on the artery bed at the STS anastomosis of the SQA configuration is lower in the case of compliant model with non-Newtonian fluid, than in the case of the rigid-wall model with Newtonian fluid.

16.4.3 Model Assumptions and Limitations

In this study, a two-way coupled FSI analysis of a novel CABG SQA is performed. The effects of vessel wall compliance and shear thinning property of blood are investigated on the flow field and HP distributions, and the performance of this coupled SQA configuration in comparison with the conventional ETS anastomosis is evaluated in a more realistic bio-mechanical condition.

As the focus of this investigation is on the flow fields and HPs distribution rather than on the intramural stress distributions, a small strain (large deformation) approximation of blood vessel mechanics is utilized. The vessel walls are assumed to be isotropic and homogeneous, and modeled as a linearly elastic, geometrically non linear shell structure [50,51], and the same value of elastic modulus is employed for both the graft and the arterial wall.

The cardiac motion is ignored in this investigation, as it is indicated that a static geometry can predict the mean wall shear rates with a reasonable accuracy and the dynamic behavior is not significant at the base cardiac frequency of 1 Hz [69], and the motion of the RCA has minor effect on TAWSS patterns [70].

16.4.4 Evaluation of Results

As described earlier in the FSI results, the velocity profiles of non-Newtonian flow are flattened (as illustrated in Figures 16.24 and 16.25) and the TAWSS is reduced at high shear rates due to shear thinning behavior of the blood (as shown in Table 16.4). In simple language, the blood has the property of losing its viscosity at high variations of velocity, which makes it less sticky and more fluent, and lets the fluid layers flow more easily over each other.

Since the change in the velocity is higher in the near wall region and lower in the core region, this characteristic facilitates the flow in the former region and impedes it in the latter one. Hence, the velocity profile is flattened as compared to the parabolic velocity profile of a Newtonian fluid.

Likewise, in the case of high velocity gradients at the wall, the less sticky layers of the fluid can easily flow over each other near to the wall and induce less shear forces onto the wall than in the case of low velocity gradients where the flow of the viscous fluid layers exerts higher shear forces onto the wall. When a non-Newtonian fluid is approximated by a Newtonian model, the constant viscosity of the Newtonian model represents the average viscosity of the non-Newtonian fluid within its working range of shear rates. Thus, comparison of the two fluids results in lower viscosity (and WSS values) at high shear rates and higher viscosity (and WSS values) at low shear rates for the non-Newtonian fluid as compared to the equivalent Newtonian fluid.

As observed and discussed in the FSI results, at some locations, the effects of wall compliance and non-Newtonian rheology on the HPs distribution are in synchrony, while at some other locations these effects are opposing. For instance, the wall compliance and non-Newtonian rheology both decrease the TAWSSG at the toe of the ETS anastomosis (from 36.95 to 29.71 and from 36.95 to 31.23, respectively, in the SQA model), which result in a further reduction (to 25.24) when comparing the "compliant wall with non-Newtonian fluid" model with the "rigid-wall with Newtonian fluid" model, due to the accumulation of these effects. However, at the heel of the ETS anastomosis, for example, the non-Newtonian rheology increases the TAWSS (from 0.56 to 0.71 Pa in the rigid model), while the wall compliance decreases this parameter (from 0.56 to 0.38 Pa in the case of Newtonian fluid); and the accumulation of these opposing effects results in a negligible overall change (from 0.56 to 0.52 Pa) when a comparison between the aforementioned models is made.

Nevertheless, the interesting point is that at some particular locations, the accumulation of the two effects does not result in an expected outcome as shown to have happened earlier. For instance, at the toe of the STS anastomosis of the SQA model, the non-Newtonian rheology slightly decreases the TAWSSG in the rigid model from 6.03 to 6, while the wall compliance increases this HP from 6.03 to 7.32. Nonetheless, the accumulation of the two effects does not result in a value between 6 and 7.32, but in a higher value of 7.44. This fact demonstrates that the effect of one parameter (either non-Newtonian rheology or wall compliance) is not independent from the other one. As in this example, the non-Newtonian rheology has slightly decreased the TAWSSG in the rigid-wall model (from 6.03 to 6), while it has increased this HP in the compliant model (from 7.32 to 7.44). Likewise, on the artery bed of the ETS anastomosis of the SQA model for instance, the wall compliance has slightly increased the TAWSSG (from 4.93 to 5.02) in the case of the Newtonian fluid model, while it has decreased this HP (from 4.05 to 3.88) in the case of the non-Newtonian fluid model.

This phenomenon might be attributable to the interaction of the shear thinning property of the blood with the sudden, local variations of shear rate due to expansions and contractions of the compliant vessel wall during the cardiac cycle. As the vessel wall moves, the shear rate may increase or decrease at different points, depending on the relative movement of the wall and the fluid. This results in some instantaneous local variations of WSS that results in some extreme (high or low) spatial WSSG that unexpectedly affects the value of TAWSSG over the cardiac cycle. This phenomenon suggests that it is essential to study and incorporate the effects of these parameters (wall compliance and non-Newtonian rheology) simultaneously, rather than discretely and individually, as they are not independent and cannot be superimposed.

The HPs distribution illustrates that the advantages of the SQA model over the conventional ETS anastomosis, which had been observed in the rigid-wall model with the Newtonian fluid previously and reported in our earlier study [12], are present in the compliant model with the non-Newtonian fluid too. The TAWSS is increased on the artery bed of the ETS anastomosis of the SQA model to 1.59 Pa, from 1.40 Pa in the conventional ETS model. Although this increase is marginal, a critical biological WSS value of 1.5 Pa has been reported [23,71] below which intimal thickening would develop. Based thereon, the moderate improvement of TAWSS on the artery bed of the SQA design is deemed to be vital. In addition, the TAWSS at the heel of the ETS anastomosis is slightly reduced in the conventional ETS anastomosis (from 0.56 to 0.52), while it is increased in the SQA configuration (from 0.49 to 0.61) in the compliant model with non-Newtonian fluid, as compared to those in the rigid-wall model with Newtonian fluid. This results in having the TAWSS at the heel of the ETS anastomosis, in the SQA model to be higher than that in the conventional ETS model, while it is opposite in the rigid-wall model with Newtonian fluid. This reveals another advantage of the SQA configuration over the conventional ETS anastomosis which had not been disclosed in our previous study.

As shown in Table 16.4, the TAWSSG is decreased at all the critical locations of the ETS anastomosis in the SQA configuration as compared to the conventional ETS anastomosis in the case of compliant model with non-Newtonian fluid, while this advantage can be observed only at the heel and on the artery bed in the case of the rigid-wall model with Newtonian fluid. This manifests a more uniform distribution of WSS at the ETS anastomosis of the SQA configuration, which can lessen the vessel wall permeability and atherosclerotic lesion development, and further unveils the advantages of the SQA design over the conventional ETS anastomosis.

16.4.5 Results Review

A two-way coupled FSI analysis of a novel CABG SQA is carried out in conjunction with the shear thinning property of blood, to investigate the performance of this coupled SQA configuration in comparison with the conventional ETS anastomosis in a more realistic bio-mechanical condition, with an emphasis on the effects of wall compliance and non-Newtonian rheology on the HPs distribution.

The simulation results indicate that the velocity patterns and qualitative distribution of WSS parameters do not change significantly in the compliant model, despite quite large side-wall deformations in the anastomotic regions. The WSS magnitude is generally reduced in the distensible model, as compared to that in the rigid-wall model, resulting in a lower TAWSS in the compliant model. The wall compliance has generally decreased the TAWSSG, while it has somewhat increased the oscillatory nature of the flow.

The effect of non-Newtonian rheology on the HPs is heterogeneous. The ETS anastomosis (of both the conventional and SQA models) experiences mostly a decrease in the TAWSS (except at the heel), while the STS anastomosis of the SQA model undergoes an increase in this HP. The flow oscillation is increased at the toe of the anastomosis, whereas it is decreased at the heel and on the artery bed, due to the shear thinning behavior of the blood.

It is observed that the effects of wall compliance and non-Newtonian rheology are not independent, and that they influence each other. Hence, it is essential to investigate the effects of these parameters simultaneously (and not individually) in each particular model.

Although vessel wall compliance and non-Newtonian rheology have shown modest influence on the HPs in each model, they have unveiled further advantages of the coupled SQA model over the conventional ETS anastomosis, which had not been revealed in our previous study with the rigid-wall and Newtonian fluid models [12]. Therefore, we conclude that the inclusion of wall compliance and non-Newtonian rheology in flow simulation of blood vessels can be essential in quantitative and comparative analyses. This investigation further verifies the hemodynamic benefits of the blood flow in the coupled SQA configuration in a more realistic biomechanical condition.

16.5 Conclusion

In this chapter, a novel coupled SQA configuration for the distal CABG anastomoses is presented, based on the advantageous flow characteristics observed within the STS anastomosis in sequential bypass grafts. The flow fields and HPs are studied within the model, and compared to those of the conventional ETS distal anastomosis and parallel STS anastomosis by means of CFD simulation. Also, sensitivity analysis for the suggested SQA design is conducted by computational simulations and comparison of several models within the physiological range of the parameters involved.

Subsequently, to complement and validate the flow-simulation results, experimental measurements are conducted in vitro, using the PIV technique. The measured velocity fields and the calculated WSS are studied and compared with those obtained from the preliminary computational simulations, in which the graft and the artery are adopted to be rigid vessels and the blood is assumed to be a Newtonian fluid.

Finally, a two-way coupled FSI analysis is carried out in conjunction with the shear thinning property of blood to investigate the performance of the coupled SQA configuration in a more realistic biomechanical condition, in the presence of wall compliance and non-Newtonian blood rheology.

Computational simulations of blood flow through this novel design have shown improvements of HPs, especially at the heel and on the arterial bed of the ETS anastomosis. These improvements in distribution of HPs include (1) an increase in the TAWSS on the artery bed of the ETS anastomosis of the SQA (as compared to the conventional ETS anastomosis), (2) reduction of the TAWSSG at the heel and bed of the ETS component as well as at the toe and suture line of the STS component of the novel SQA (as compared to the conventional ETS and typical parallel STS anastomoses, respectively), and (3) reduction of the OSI at the ETS anastomosis of the SQA at the heel region and on the artery wall and bed opposite to the heel (in comparison with the conventional ETS anastomosis). In addition, this design provides a spare route for the blood flow to the coronary artery, in order to avoid re-operation in case of re-stenosis in either of the anastomoses. This design can also be employed by using autologous grafts without the need for any additional training.

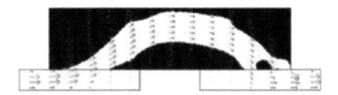

FIGURE 16.29
Optimized topological layout for bypass graft having two outlet channels, resembling the coupled sequential STS–ETS anastomotic design. (Adapted from Hyun, J. et al., *Comput. Math. Appl.*, 67, 1154, 2014. With permission).

A recent study on topology optimization with application to bypass graft geometries [72] has shown that among the different investigated geometric models, the optimized bypass graft has two outlet channels (shown in Figure 16.29), resembling our proposed CSABG design. This optimized model has shown the best performance among the studied models in terms of WSS, with a relatively uniform WSS distribution and the smallest maximum value of WSS. The study has referred to our proposed novel sequential anastomoses design and concluded that their topology optimization method leads to this sequential anastomotic design, further confirming the hemodynamic potential of this novel sequential anastomotic design.

16.5.1 Surgical Aspects of CSABG Design

The surgical procedure required to perform the coupled SQA configuration is the same as that of a typical sequential bypass grafting; the only difference is that both the anastomoses are sutured on the same coronary artery. Usually, surgeons start the suturing with the furthest anastomosis; for instance, in the case of left coronary arteries, the distal ETS anastomosis is performed first, and then the STS anastomosis is sutured.

The angle at which a surgeon cuts the graft end determines the angle of implantation (ETS anastomotic angle) which can be adjusted to an optimum value. The length of arteriotomy is about 5 mm, and most superficial coronary arteries have at least 2–3 cm of visible course on the surface of the heart. Hence, the proposed grafting configuration would be technically feasible in general.

This design does involve one additional anastomosis that results in a prolonged operation time. However, apart from the distinct advantages it brings about in the flow field and distribution of HPs, it provides a spare route for the blood flow to the coronary artery, to avoid re-operation in case of re-stenosis in either of the anastomoses.

16.5.2 Optimal CABG Design Criteria

The search for an ideal distal anastomotic configuration for coronary bypass grafting has led to numerous designs. An optimal anastomosis design must take into account practical issues such as surgical construction. An anastomotic design should be feasible to be implemented by surgeons in a reasonable time. In conclusion, the following aspects should be considered in the design of an optimal CABG:

1. *Compatibility of the graft with the arterial pressure and the supplied blood flow rate*, to ensure a physiologic range of intramural stresses and hemodynamic forces in the graft itself. Arterial grafts, such as left internal mammary artery (LIMA), have demonstrated considerably higher patency rates than the most commonly used SV

grafts [73]. However, due to lack of arterial conduits, veins are currently used most commonly as grafts. With technological advances, the time required for production of matured implantable tissue-engineered grafts, which could fulfill the ideal characteristics present in the arteries, will be shortened [74]; and they can replace the vein grafts in CABG.

2. *Arterial compliance of the graft*, to avoid compliance mismatch with the host artery at the anastomotic junction, to prevent escalation of intramural stresses in the artery and the graft, which can result in IH formation especially on the suture line. Compliance mismatch between the graft and the host artery results in an increase of intramural stresses, which in turn promotes IH. Use of arterial conduits can (to some extent) address this issue too. However, as mentioned earlier, tissue-engineered grafts might be the future solution to this problem.

3. *Hemodynamic performance driven design of anastomotic configuration of the distal anastomosis*, to regulate the HPs and wall shear stress indices, in order to avoid triggering of the pathogenic factors of IH and thrombosis (e.g., platelet activation, long near-wall residence time, etc.). As reviewed in this section, it is well established that HPs play an important role in the initiation and progression of atherosclerosis and IH. A hemodynamically optimized anastomotic configuration can provide moderate shear stress parameters and smooth blood flow without flow disturbances, to avoid triggering the associated atherogenic phenomena.

4. *Minimal vascular injury*, to minimize proliferation of smooth muscle cells (SMCs) as a wound healing response. Technological advances may further develop the suggested alternatives to sutures (e.g., biological glues, laser generated solders, etc.) to a practicable level for routine clinical use. Not only can such products minimize vascular injury, but also they can eliminate the para-anastomotic hyper-compliant zone and the associated elevating intramural stresses, which are caused by the stiff sutures.

5. *Patient-specific designs*, to tailor the design considerations to each particular patient's cardiovascular characteristics. Development of clinical imaging (e.g., magnetic resonance and computed tomography) enables a detailed patient-specific description of the actual hemodynamics and structural behavior of living tissues. Coupling of these data with engineering analyses is becoming a standard evaluation that is expected to become part of clinical practice in diagnosis and surgical planning in advanced medical centers [75]. This would optimize the design considerations and choice of graft for each particular patient, depending on the number, location, and severity of stenosis, etc.

16A Appendix: Derivation of Womersley Solution

Analytical solutions to the Navier–Stokes equations are possible in only a few selected cases with very special geometry and boundary conditions. These solutions are essential for making the assumption of the inlet velocity profile and the validation of numerical methods. Moreover, most of these analytical solutions require the assumption of steady flow conditions and are thus of no use in addressing time-dependent issues for transient problems such as blood flow. Fortunately, a canonical solution for pulsatile flow does exist, that is, the Womersley solution [16] for fully developed pulsatile flow in a straight circular tube.

Consider a long circular tube, which is subject to (1) a time-varying flow rate at inlet and (2) a constant but arbitrary pressure over the outflow boundary. With a sufficient distance from the inlet (which depends on the geometric and flow parameters), the radial and circumferential components of velocity vanish, the only non-zero component of the velocity vectors is in the axial direction and is denoted as u. Using cylindrical polar coordinates, and taking the problem to be axis-symmetric (i.e., $u = u(r, x, t)$, $p = p(r, x, t)$), the continuity equation reduces to

$$\frac{\partial u}{\partial x} = 0 \tag{16A.1}$$

The Navier–Stokes equations become

$$\rho \frac{\partial u}{\partial t} = -\frac{\partial p}{\partial x} + \frac{\mu}{r} \frac{\partial}{\partial r}\left(r \frac{\partial u}{\partial r} \right) \tag{16A.2}$$

$$0 = -\frac{\partial p}{\partial r} \tag{16A.3}$$

The above equations imply that

$$u = u(r, t), \quad p = p(x, t) \tag{16A.4}$$

Therefore, Equation 16A.2 can be rearranged into

$$\frac{\mu}{r} \frac{\partial}{\partial r}\left(r \frac{\partial u}{\partial r} \right) - \rho \frac{\partial u}{\partial t} = \frac{\partial p}{\partial x} \tag{16A.5}$$

It is observed that the left-hand side of Equation 16A.5 is a function of r and t while the right-hand side is the function of x and t. Hence, in order to maintain the equality of Equation 16A.5, both sides must be a function of t only.

Consider now a pulsatile sinusoidal flow with the pressure gradient and the axial velocity as

$$\frac{\partial p}{\partial x} = -Pe^{i\omega t} \tag{16A.6}$$

$$u(r, t) = U(r)e^{i\omega t} \tag{16A.7}$$

where
$\omega = 2\pi f$ is angular frequency in radian per second of the oscillatory motion, with f the frequency in Hz
P is a constant
$U(r)$ is the distribution of axial velocity across the tube of radius R

When the flow is fully developed, it is assumed to be identical at each section along the tube. Therefore, a traveling wave solution can be neglected. It is clear that when $\omega = 0$ (the steady case), the flow becomes the Poiseuille flow.

From Equations 16A.6 and 16A.7, it is clear that real part gives the velocity for pressure gradient $P(\cos \omega t)$ and the imaginary part gives the velocity for the pressure gradient $P(\sin \omega t)$. Upon substituting Equations 16A.6 and 16A.7 into Equation 16A.5, and after some arrangements, the following equation can be obtained.

$$\frac{d^2U}{dr^2} + \frac{1}{r}\frac{dU}{dr} - \frac{i\omega\rho}{\mu}U = -\frac{P}{\mu} \tag{16A.8}$$

The general solution of an ordinary differential equation in the form of

$$\frac{d^2y}{dx^2} + \frac{1}{x}\frac{dy}{dx} + y = 0 \tag{16A.9}$$

is

$$y = AJ_0(x) + BY_0(x) \tag{16A.10}$$

which involves the first kind and second kind of Bessel functions J_0 and Y_0, respectively, of complex argument. By assuming $x = iKX$, we have

$$\frac{dy}{dx} = \frac{1}{iK}\frac{dy}{dX}, \quad \frac{d^2y}{dx^2} = -\frac{1}{K^2}\frac{d^2y}{dX^2}$$

Equation 16A.9 can then be modified as Equation 16A.11:

$$\frac{d^2y}{dX^2} + \frac{1}{X}\frac{dy}{dX} - K^2y = 0 \tag{16A.11}$$

and the corresponding solution becomes

$$y = AJ_0(iKX) + BY_0(iKX) \tag{16A.12}$$

Thus, the solution of Equation 16A.8 is

$$U(r) = AJ_0\left(i\sqrt{\frac{i\omega\rho}{\mu}}r\right) + BY_0\left(i\sqrt{\frac{i\omega\rho}{\mu}}r\right) + \frac{P}{i\omega\rho} \tag{16A.13}$$

Note that X and K in Equation 16A.11 are equivalent to r and $\sqrt{i\omega\rho/\mu}$, respectively, in Equation 16A.8. As U must be finite on the axis (i.e., at $r = 0$) and since $Y_0(0)$ is not finite, then B has to be zero. Also because of the no-slip condition $U(r)|_{r=R} = 0$, so that the following result is obtained

$$AJ_0\left(i^{3/2}\sqrt{\frac{\omega\rho}{\mu}}R\right) + \frac{P}{i\omega\rho} = 0 \tag{16A.14}$$

To simplify this expression, a nondimensional parameter α, known as the Womersley number, is introduced

$$\alpha = R\sqrt{\frac{\omega\rho}{\mu}} \quad \text{or} \quad \alpha = R\sqrt{\frac{\omega}{\nu}} \tag{16A.15}$$

where $\nu = \mu/\rho$ is the kinematic viscosity. Then, from Equation 16A.14

$$A = -\frac{P}{i\omega\rho}\frac{1}{J_0(i^{3/2}\alpha)} \quad \text{or} \quad A = \frac{iP}{\omega\rho}\frac{1}{J_0(i^{3/2}\alpha)} \tag{16A.16}$$

and finally, from Equation 16A.13 the axial velocity can be expressed as

$$U(r) = -\frac{iP}{\omega\rho}\left(1 - \frac{J_0(i^{3/2}\alpha r/R)}{J_0(i^{3/2}\alpha)}\right) \tag{16A.17}$$

In the limit as α approaches zero, that is, $\omega \to 0$, the velocity profile becomes parabolic. As α tends to infinity, that is, viscosity becomes not important ($\mu \to 0$), it can be shown that

$$\frac{J_0(i^{3/2}\alpha r/R)}{J_0(i^{3/2}\alpha)} \to 0 \tag{16A.18}$$

which implies that

$$U(r) \to -\frac{iP}{\omega\rho} \tag{16A.19}$$

In fact, by introducing the idea that a Stokes boundary layer of thickness δ is proportional to $1/\alpha$, it can be concluded that in this case the boundary layer thickness at the cylindrical tube inner wall disappears.

It is interesting to note that the earlier given expression is independent of viscosity μ, and exactly 90° out of phase with P. Actually, this result corresponds to the Euler equation (which only holds for $\mu = 0$, i.e., inviscid fluids), namely,

$$\frac{\partial u}{\partial t} = -\frac{1}{\rho}\frac{\partial p}{\partial x} \tag{16A.20}$$

Substituting Equations 16A.6 and 16A.7 into Equation 16A.20, it can be easily shown that

$$U = \frac{P}{i\omega\rho} = -\frac{iP}{\omega\rho} \tag{16A.21}$$

which is the same as the result in Equation 16A.19.

Hence, the final result for the velocity of pulsatile flow in a cylindrical tube of radius R is

$$u(r, t) = -\frac{iP}{\omega\rho}\left(1 - \frac{J_0(i^{3/2}\alpha r/R)}{J_0(i^{3/2}\alpha)}\right)e^{i\omega t} \tag{16A.22}$$

To obtain the volume flow rate Q, it is necessary to integrate the velocity *across* the lumen of the tube. After the integration, Q can be expressed as Equation 16A.23 [49].

$$Q = \frac{\pi R^2 P}{i\omega\rho}\left(1 - \frac{2J_1(\alpha i^{3/2})}{\alpha i^{3/2} J_0(i^{3/2}\alpha)}\right)e^{i\omega t}$$ (16A.23)

where J_1 is the first kind Bessel function with order 1.

Dividing Equation 16A.22 by Equation 16A.23, and if the volume flow rate is known, the axial velocity can be expressed as

$$u(r,t) = \frac{Q}{\pi R^2}\left(\frac{1 - ((J_0(i^{3/2}\alpha r/R))/J_0(\alpha i^{3/2}))}{1 - ((2J_1(\alpha i^{3/2}))/(\alpha i^{3/2} J_0(\alpha i^{3/2})))}\right)e^{i\omega t}$$ (16A.24)

Similarly, if pressure gradient and the axial velocity are assumed to be cosinusoidal flow as follows:

$$\frac{\partial p}{\partial x} = -Pe^{i\omega t}$$ (16A.25)

$$u(r,t) = U(r)e^{i\omega t}$$ (16A.26)

the axial velocity can be expressed as

$$u(r,t) = \frac{Q}{\pi R^2}\left(\frac{1 - ((J_0(i^{5/2}\alpha r/R))/J_0(\alpha i^{5/2}))}{1 - ((2J_1(\alpha i^{5/2}))/(\alpha i^{5/2} J_0(\alpha i^{5/2})))}\right)e^{i\omega t}$$ (16A.27)

In the case where the flow rate or average velocity is known, Fourier transform can be used to extract the frequency content of volume flow waveform when the fundamental frequency ω is given. Thus, if $Q(t)$ is assumed as the Fourier series,

$$Q(t) \approx \sum_{n=-N}^{n=N} B_n e^{i\omega t}$$ (16A.28)

the Fourier coefficients, B_n can be determined. The axial velocity is then given as

$$u(r,t) = \frac{2B_0}{\pi R^2}\left[1 - \left(\frac{r}{R}\right)^2\right] + \sum_{n=-N}^{n=-1}\left\{\frac{B_n}{\pi R^2}\left(\frac{1 - ((J_0(i^{5/2}\alpha_n r/R))/J_0(i^{5/2}\alpha_n))}{1 - ((2J_1(i^{5/2}\alpha_n))/(i^{5/2}\alpha_n J_0(i^{5/2}\alpha_n)))}\right)\right\}e^{in\omega t}$$
$$+ \sum_{n=1}^{n=N}\left\{\frac{B_n}{\pi R^2}\left(\frac{1 - ((J_0(i^{3/2}\alpha_n r/R))/J_0(i^{3/2}\alpha_n))}{1 - ((2J_1(i^{3/2}\alpha_n))/(i^{3/2}\alpha_n J_0(i^{3/2}\alpha_n)))}\right)\right\}e^{in\omega t}$$ (16A.29)

where
R is the radius of cylinder
J_0 and J_1 are first kind Bessel functions of order 0 and 1, respectively
$\alpha_n = R\sqrt{(n\omega)/\nu}$

Equation 16A.30 shows the complex conjugate characters of the following parameters.

$$J_0\left(i^{5/2}\frac{\alpha_n r}{R}\right) = \overline{J_0\left(i^{3/2}\frac{\alpha_n r}{R}\right)} \quad J_1(i^{5/2}\alpha_n) = \overline{J_1(i^{3/2}\alpha_n)} \quad B_{-n} = \overline{B_n}$$
$$J_0(i^{5/2}\alpha_n) = \overline{J_0(i^{3/2}\alpha_n)} \quad i^{5/2} = \overline{i^{3/2}} \quad e^{-in\omega t} = \overline{e^{-in\omega t}}$$
(16A.30)

Thus, the axial velocity can be simplified to

$$u(r,t) = \frac{2B_0}{\pi R^2}\left[1-\left(\frac{r}{R}\right)^2\right] + 2*\text{Real}\left\{\sum_{n=1}^{n=N}\left\{\frac{B_n}{\pi R^2}\left(\frac{1-((J_0(i^{3/2}\alpha r/R))/(J_0(i^{3/2}\alpha)))}{1-((2J_1(i^{3/2}\alpha))/(i^{3/2}\alpha J_0(i^{3/2}\alpha)))}\right)\right\}e^{in\omega t}\right\}$$
(16A.31)

Here, Real{} means the real part of a complex value.

16B Appendix: Validation of PIV Method

In order to validate the accuracy and precision of the PIV measurements, a comparison was conducted between the PIV results for a fully developed sinusoidal flow ($Q = 140(1 + \sin(4.2t))$ mL/min) in a straight tube (with an inner diameter of 3 mm) and the corresponding Womersley solution [16].

As shown in Figure 16.30, a good qualitative match was observed between the experimentally obtained and analytical velocity profiles at different phases of the flow cycle. The quantitative comparison of the results revealed an average relative difference of 8.6% in the velocity magnitude between the two sets of data. This reasonable discrepancy confirmed that the accuracy of the PIV results was acceptable.

16C Appendix: Validation of the WSS Estimation Method

In order to validate the accuracy of the WSS estimation method, a comparison was conducted between the WSS values estimated from PIV results for the fully developed sinusoidal flow, mentioned earlier, in a straight tube (with an inner diameter of 3 mm) and the corresponding analytically calculated WSS values obtained from the Womersley solution at the very time instants for which the PIV results were validated (i.e., $t/T = 0.2, 0.75, 0.856,$ and 1, as shown in Figure 16.30).

The WSS calculation method was applied to data points obtained from the analytical solution (rather than the PIV data) at the aforementioned time points and compared with those obtained from the analytical solution and from the PIV data (Table 16.5). The WSS values obtained from the analytical data points do not include (and are not influenced by) the PIV measurement error; hence they can indicate the accuracy/error of the WSS calculation method. On the other hand, the WSS values obtained from the PIV results are highly influenced by the near-wall error of the PIV measurement results.

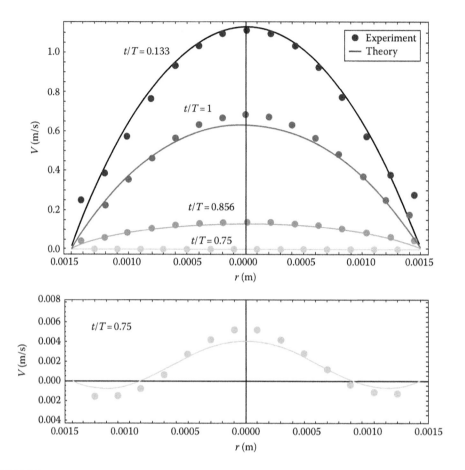

FIGURE 16.30

Comparison of the PIV measurement results with the analytical Womersley solution for a sinusoidal flow in a straight tube for different phases of the flow cycle. Lower panel shows the up-scaled graph at $t/T = 0.75$ for a better illustration of the velocity profile. (From Kabinejadian, F. et al., *Med. Eng. Phys.*, 36, 1233, 2014.)

TABLE 16.5

Comparison of the WSS Values Obtained by Different Methods

t/T	0.2	0.75	0.856	1
Theory	8.56	−0.03	1.25	5.15
Estimation (based on experimental PIV data)	12.73	−0.04	1.94	6.98
Estimation (based on theoretical data points)	7.79	−0.02	1.09	4.59

As shown in Table 16.5, the estimated WSS values based on the analytical data points showed a good agreement with the analytically calculated WSS values with an error of <13% (except for $t/T = 0.75$ with an error of <33%; this was mainly due to the small magnitude of the WSS at this time point, resulting in higher percentage of error even for small differences between the two sets of data). However, the WSS values estimated based on the PIV data (which include the near-wall PIV measurement errors) had relative errors of up to about 55% with respect to the analytically calculated WSS values. Nevertheless, the trend of the WSS variations was identical among the different sets of data, which made the comparison of the WSS variation among different geometric models valid in the present study.

16D Appendix: Validation of FSI Methodology

In order to validate the FSI simulations and the method used in this study, a simple sinusoidal flow in a straight compliant tube is modeled, and the numerical results are compared with the corresponding analytical solution due to Zamir [76].

The length and radius of the tube, and the thickness and elastic modulus of the wall are, respectively, 0.42, 0.005, 0.0005 m, and 20 MPa; and the fluid has the same properties as the Newtonian blood in the present study. The frequency of oscillation is set to be 1 Hz.

The applied boundary pressure waveforms are

$$P_{inlet} = 30 + 1000\sin(2\pi t) \text{ Pa} \tag{16D.1}$$

$$P_{outlet} = 1000\sin(2\pi t - 0.0139456) \text{ Pa} \tag{16D.2}$$

Figure 16.31 demonstrates the comparison of the calculated nondimensional velocity profiles at a cross section located at 0.4 m distance from the entrance of the tube. The velocity is normalized using $R^*\omega$ as the characteristic scale, where R^* is the radius of the tube plus half the thickness of the tube wall, and ω is the angular frequency of oscillation. There is an excellent agreement between the analytical solution and the obtained numerical solution with an average relative error of 5.1%.

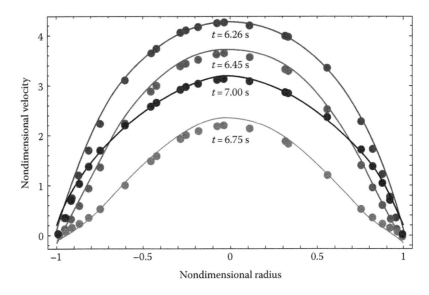

FIGURE 16.31
Comparison of analytical solution due to Zamir [76] and the current numerical solution at $t = 6.26$, 6.45, 6.75, and 7.00 s. The symbols are due to the current numerical solution and the solid lines are due to the analytical solution.

Based on these validation results, it is concluded that the FSI method used in the present study is accurate in predicting the fluid dynamics of the coronary arterial bypass graft models investigated.

References

1. Flemma RJ, Johnson WD, Lepley D. Triple aorto-coronary vein bypass as treatment for coronary insufficiency. *Archives of Surgery.* 1971;103:82–83.
2. Bartley TD, Bigelow JC, Page US. Aortocoronary bypass grafting with multiple sequential anastomoses to a single vein. *Archives of Surgery.* 1972;105:915–917.
3. Grondin CM, Limet R. Sequential anastomoses in coronary artery grafting: Technical aspects and early and late angiographic results. *Annals of Thoracic Surgery.* 1977;23:1–8.
4. O'Neill Jr MJ, Wolf PD, O'Neill TK, Montesano RM, Waldhausen JA. A rationale for the use of sequential coronary artery bypass grafts. *Journal of Thoracic and Cardiovascular Surgery.* 1981;81:686–690.
5. Vural KM, Sener E, Tasdemir O. Long-term patency of sequential and individual saphenous vein coronary bypass grafts. *European Journal of Cardio-Thoracic Surgery.* 2001;19:140–144.
6. Sankaranarayanan M, Ghista DN, Chua LP, Tan YS, Sundaravadivelu K, Kassab GS. Blood flow in an out-of-plane aorto-left coronary sequential bypass graft. In: Guccione JM, Kassab GS, Ratcliffe M, eds. *Computational Cardiovascular Mechanics: Modeling and Applications in Heart Failure.* New York: Springer; 2010. pp. 277–295.
7. Ghista DN, Kabinejadian F. Coronary artery bypass grafting hemodynamics and anastomosis design: A biomedical engineering review. *BioMedical Engineering Online.* 2013;12:129.
8. Chua LP, Zhang JM, Yu SCM, Ghista DN, Tan YS. Numerical study on the pulsatile flow characteristics of proximal anastomotic models. *Proceedings of the Institution of Mechanical Engineers, Part H: Journal of Engineering in Medicine.* 2005;219:361–379.
9. Sankaranarayanan M, Ghista DN, Chua LP, Tan YS, Kassab GS. Analysis of blood flow in an out-of-plane CABG model. *American Journal of Physiology: Heart and Circulatory Physiology.* 2006;291:H283–H295.
10. Zhang JM, Chua LP, Ghista DN, Yu SCM, Tan YS. Numerical investigation and identification of susceptible sites of atherosclerotic lesion formation in a complete coronary artery bypass model. *Medical and Biological Engineering and Computing.* 2008;46:689–699.
11. Sankaranarayanan M, Chua LP, Ghista DN, Tan YS. Computational model of blood flow in the aorto-coronary bypass graft. *BioMedical Engineering Online.* 2005;4:14.
12. Kabinejadian F, Chua LP, Ghista DN, Sankaranarayanan M, Tan YS. A novel coronary artery bypass graft design of sequential anastomoses. *Annals of Biomedical Engineering.* 2010;38:3135–3150.
13. Galjee MA, vanRossum AC, Doesburg T, vanEenige MJ, Visser CA. Value of magnetic resonance imaging in assessing patency and function of coronary artery bypass grafts—An angiographically controlled study. *Circulation.* 1996;93:660–666.
14. Kabinejadian F, Chua LP, Ghista DN, Tan YS. CABG models flow simulation study on the effects of valve remnants in the venous graft. *Journal of Mechanics in Medicine and Biology.* 2010;10:593–609.
15. Galjee MA, Van Rossum AC, Doesburg T, Hofman MBM, Falke THM, Visser CA. Quantification of coronary artery bypass graft flow by magnetic resonance phase velocity mapping. *Magnetic Resonance Imaging.* 1996;14:485–493.
16. Womersley JR. Method for the calculation of velocity, rate of flow and viscous drag in arteries when the pressure gradient is known. *Journal of Physiology.* 1955;127:553–563.

17. Bonert M, Myers JG, Fremes S, Williams J, Ethier CR. A numerical study of blood flow in coronary artery bypass graft side-to-side anastomoses. *Annals of Biomedical Engineering.* 2002;30:599–611.
18. He X, Ku DN. Pulsatile flow in the human left coronary artery bifurcation: Average conditions. *Journal of Biomechanical Engineering.* 1996;118:74–82.
19. DePaola N, Gimbrone Jr MA, Davies PF, Dewey Jr CF. Vascular endothelium responds to fluid shear stress gradients. *Arteriosclerosis and Thrombosis.* 1992;12:1254–1257.
20. Kleinstreuer C, Nazemi M, Archie JP. Hemodynamics analysis of a stenosed carotid bifurcation and its plaque-mitigating design. *Journal of Biomechanical Engineering.* 1991;113:330–335.
21. Shahcheraghi N, Dwyer HA, Cheer AY, Barakat AI, Rutaganira T. Unsteady and three-dimensional simulation of blood flow in the human aortic arch. *Journal of Biomechanical Engineering—Transactions of the ASME.* 2002;124:378–387.
22. Buchanan JR, Kleinstreuer C, Hyun S, Truskey GA. Hemodynamics simulation and identification of susceptible sites of atherosclerotic lesion formation in a model abdominal aorta. *Journal of Biomechanics.* 2003;36:1185–1196.
23. Giddens DP, Zarins CK, Glagov S. Response of arteries to near-wall fluid dynamics behavior. *Applied Mechanics Review.* 1990;43:S98–S102.
24. Bertolotti C, Deplano V. Three-dimensional numerical simulations of flow through a stenosed coronary bypass. *Journal of Biomechanics.* 2000;33:1011–1022.
25. Kakos GS, Sabiston DC, Hagen PO, Davis RW, Dixon SH, Oldham HN. Coronary artery hemodynamics after aorto-coronary artery vein bypass. An experimental evaluation. *Journal of Thoracic and Cardiovascular Surgery.* 1972;63:849–853.
26. Siouffi M, Deplano V, Pélissier R. Experimental analysis of unsteady flows through a stenosis. *Journal of Biomechanics.* 1998;31:11–19.
27. Berne RM, Levy MN. *Cardiovascular Physiology.* 8th ed. St. Louis, MO: Mosby; 2001.
28. Speziale G. *Competitive Flow and Steal Phenomenon in Coronary Surgery. Intraoperative Graft Patency Verification in Cardiac and Vascular Surgery.* New York: Futura Publishing; 2001.
29. Fei DY, Thomas JD, Rittgers SE. The effect of angle and flow rate upon hemodynamics in distal vascular graft anastomoses: A numerical model study. *Journal of Biomechanical Engineering.* 1994;116:331–336.
30. Einav S, Avidor J, Vidne B. Haemodynamics of coronary artery—Saphenous vein bypass. *Journal of Biomedical Engineering.* 1985;7:305–309.
31. Furuse A, Klopp EH, Brawley RK, Gott VL. Hemodynamics of aorta-to-coronary artery bypass: Experimental and analytical studies. *Annals of Thoracic Surgery.* 1972;14:282–293.
32. Wiesner TF, Levesque MJ, Rooz E, Nerem RM. Epicardial coronary blood flow including the presence of stenoses and aorto-coronary bypasses. II: Experimental comparison and parametric investigations. *Journal of Biomechanical Engineering.* 1988;110:144–149.
33. Yasuura K, Takagi Y, Ohara Y, Takami Y, Matsuura A, Okamoto H. Theoretical analysis of right gastroepiploic artery grafting to right coronary artery. *Annals of Thoracic Surgery.* 2000;69:728–731.
34. Hakaim AG, Nalbandian MN, Heller JK, Chowla AC, Oldenburg WA. Improved patency of prosthetic arteriovenous grafts with an acute anastomotic angle and flow diffuser. *Journal of Vascular Surgery.* 2003;37:1032–1035.
35. Waller B, Schlant R. *Anatomy of the Heart. Hurst's the Heart.* London, UK: McGraw-Hill; 1986.
36. Chong CK, Rowc CS, Sivancsan S, Rattray A, Black RA, Shortland AP et al. Computer aided design and fabrication of models for in vitro studies of vascular fluid dynamics. *Proceedings of the Institution of Mechanical Engineers, Part H: Journal of Engineering in Medicine.* 1999;213:1–4.
37. Kabinejadian F, Ghista DN, Su B, Kaabi Nezhadian M, Chua LP, Yeo JH et al. In vitro measurements of velocity and wall shear stress in a novel sequential anastomotic graft design model under pulsatile flow conditions. *Medical Engineering and Physics.* 2014;36:1233–1245.
38. Raffel M, Willert CE, Wereley ST, Kompenhans J. *Particle Image Velocimetry.* 2nd ed. Berlin, Germany: Springer-Verlag; 2007.

39. Kabinejadian F, Cui F, Zhang Z, Ho P, Leo HL. A novel carotid covered stent design: In vitro evaluation of performance and influence on the blood flow regime at the carotid artery bifurcation. *Annals of Biomedical Engineering.* 2013;41:1990–2002.

40. Ethier CR, Steinman DA, Zhang X, Karpik SR, Ojha M. Flow waveform effects on end-to-side anastomotic flow patterns. *Journal of Biomechanics.* 1998;31:609–617.

41. Karri S, Charonko J, Vlachos PP. Robust wall gradient estimation using radial basis functions and proper orthogonal decomposition (POD) for particle image velocimetry (PIV) measured fields. *Measurement Science and Technology.* 2009;20:045401.

42. Ku DN, Giddens DP, Zarins CK, Glagov S. Pulsatile flow and atherosclerosis in the human carotid bifurcation. Positive correlation between plaque location and low and oscillating shear stress. *Arteriosclerosis.* 1985;5:293–302.

43. Li XM, Rittgers SE. Hemodynamic factors at the distal end-to-side anastomosis of a bypass graft with different POS:DOS flow ratios. *Journal of Biomechanical Engineering.* 2001;123:270–276.

44. Kabinejadian F, Ghista DN. Compliant model of a coupled sequential coronary arterial bypass graft: Effects of vessel wall elasticity and non-Newtonian rheology on blood flow regime and hemodynamic parameters distribution. *Medical Engineering and Physics.* 2012;34:860–872.

45. Ballyk PD, Walsh C, Ojha M. *Effect of Intimal Thickening on the Stress Distribution at an End-to-Side Graft-Artery Junction.* San Francisco, CA: ASME; 1995.

46. Aoki T, Ku DN. Collapse of diseased arteries with eccentric cross section. *Journal of Biomechanics.* 1993;26:133–142.

47. Salzar RS, Thubrikar MJ, Eppink RT. Pressure-induced mechanical stress in the carotid artery bifurcation: A possible correlation to atherosclerosis. *Journal of Biomechanics.* 1995;28:1333–1340.

48. Vorp DA, Raghavan ML, Borovetz HS, Greisler HP, Webster MW. Modeling the transmural stress distribution during healing of bioresorbable vascular prostheses. *Annals of Biomedical Engineering.* 1995;23:178–188.

49. Nichols WW, O'Rourke MF. *McDonald's Blood Flow in Arteries. Theoretical, Experimental and Clinical Principles.* 3rd ed. London, UK: Edward Arnold; 1990.

50. Hofer M, Rappitsch G, Perktold K, Trubel W, Schima H. Numerical study of wall mechanics and fluid dynamics in end-to-side anastomoses and correlation to intimal hyperplasia. *Journal of Biomechanics.* 1996;29:1297–1308.

51. Perktold K, Rappitsch G. Computer simulation of local blood flow and vessel mechanics in a compliant carotid artery bifurcation model. *Journal of Biomechanics.* 1995;28:845–856.

52. Wesly RLR, Vaishnav RN, Fuchs JCA, Patel DJ, Greenfield Jr JC. Static linear and nonlinear elastic properties of normal and arterialized venous tissue in dog and man. *Circulation Research.* 1975;37:509–520.

53. Hasegawa H, Kanai H. Measurement of elastic moduli of the arterial wall at multiple frequencies by remote actuation for assessment of viscoelasticity. *Japanese Journal of Applied Physics, Part 1: Regular Papers and Short Notes and Review Papers.* 2004;43:3197–3203.

54. Gradus-Pizlo I, Bigelow B, Mahomed Y, Sawada SG, Rieger K, Feigenbaum H. Left anterior descending coronary artery wall thickness measured by high-frequency transthoracic and epicardial echocardiography includes adventitia. *American Journal of Cardiology.* 2003;91:27–32.

55. Dobrin PB, Littooy FN, Endean ED. Mechanical factors predisposing to intimal hyperplasia and medial thickening in autogenous vein grafts. *Surgery.* 1989;105:393–400.

56. Hughes TJR, Liu WK, Zimmermann TK. Lagrangian-Eulerian finite element formulation for incompressible viscous flows. *Computer Methods in Applied Mechanics and Engineering.* 1981;29:329–349.

57. Kabinejadian F, Cui F, Su B, Danpinid A, Ho P, Leo HL. Effects of a carotid covered stent with a novel membrane design on the blood flow regime and hemodynamic parameters distribution at the carotid artery bifurcation. *Medical and Biological Engineering and Computing.* 2015;53:165–177.

58. Bird RB, Armstrong RC, Hassager O. *Dynamics of Polymer Liquids.* 2nd ed. New York: Wiley; 1987.

59. Gijsen FJH, Van De Vosse FN, Janssen JD. The influence of the non-Newtonian properties of blood on the flow in large arteries: Steady flow in a carotid bifurcation model. *Journal of Biomechanics.* 1999;32:601–608.

60. Schaar JA, Regar E, Mastik F, McFadden EP, Saia F, Disco C et al. Incidence of high-strain patterns in human coronary arteries: Assessment with three-dimensional intravascular palpography and correlation with clinical presentation. *Circulation.* 2004;109:2716–2719.

61. Zeng D, Boutsianis E, Ammann M, Boomsma K, Wildermuth S, Poulikakos D. A study on the compliance of a right coronary artery and its impact on wall shear stress. *Journal of Biomechanical Engineering.* 2008;130:1–11.

62. Atabek HB, Ling SC, Patel DJ. Analysis of coronary flow fields in thoracotomized dogs. *Circulation Research.* 1975;37:752–761.

63. Patel DJ, Fry DL. In situ pressure-radius-length measurements in ascending aorta of anesthetized dogs. *Journal of Applied Physiology.* 1964;19:413–416.

64. Perktold K, Rappitsch G. Numerical analysis of arterial wall mechanics and local blood flow phenomena. In: Tarbell JM, ed. *Advances in Bioengineering.* New York: ASME; 1993. pp. 127–130.

65. Chen J, Lu XY, Wang W. Non-Newtonian effects of blood flow on hemodynamics in distal vascular graft anastomoses. *Journal of Biomechanics.* 2006;39:1983–1995.

66. Torii R, Wood NB, Hadjiloizou N, Dowsey AW, Wright AR, Hughes AD et al. Fluid-structure interaction analysis of a patient-specific right coronary artery with physiological velocity and pressure waveforms. *Communications in Numerical Methods in Engineering.* 2009;25:565–580.

67. Wang DM, Tarbell JM. Nonlinear analysis of oscillatory flow, with a nonzero mean, in an elastic tube (artery). *Journal of Biomechanical Engineering.* 1995;117:127–135.

68. Lee CS, Tarbell JM. Wall shear rate distribution in an abdominal aortic bifurcation model: Effects of vessel compliance and phase angle between pressure and flow waveforms. *Journal of Biomechanical Engineering.* 1997;119:333–342.

69. Santamarina A, Weydahl E, Siegel Jr JM, Moore Jr JE. Computational analysis of flow in a curved tube model of the coronary arteries: Effects of time-varying curvature. *Annals of Biomedical Engineering.* 1998;26:944–954.

70. Zeng D, Ding Z, Friedman MH, Ross Ethier C. Effects of cardiac motion on right coronary artery hemodynamics. *Annals of Biomedical Engineering.* 2003;31:420–429.

71. Lieber BB, Giddens DP. Post-stenotic core flow behavior in pulsatile flow and its effects on wall shear stress. *Journal of Biomechanics.* 1990;23:597–605.

72. Hyun J, Wang S, Yang S. Topology optimization of the shear thinning non-Newtonian fluidic systems for minimizing wall shear stress. *Computers and Mathematics with Applications.* 2014;67:1154–1170.

73. Goldman S, Zadina K, Moritz T, Ovitt T, Sethi G, Copeland JG et al. Long-term patency of saphenous vein and left internal mammary artery grafts after coronary artery bypass surgery: Results from a Department of Veterans Affairs Cooperative Study. *Journal of the American College of Cardiology.* 2004;44:2149–2156.

74. Sarkar S, Schmitz-Rixen T, Hamilton G, Seifalian AM. Achieving the ideal properties for vascular bypass grafts using a tissue engineered approach: A review. *Medical and Biological Engineering and Computing.* 2007;45:327–336.

75. Migliavacca F, Dubini G. Computational modeling of vascular anastomoses. *Biomechanics and Modeling in Mechanobiology.* 2005;3:235–250.

76. Zamir M. *The Physics of Pulsatile Flow.* New York: Springer-Verlag; 2000.

Index

Printed and bound by CPI Group (UK) Ltd, Croydon, CR0 4YY

01/11/2024

01782604-0013